Ricardo Ramina, Paulo Henrique Pires Aguiar, Marcos Tatagiba (Eds.)

Samii's Essentials in Neurosurgery

Ricardo Ramina, Paulo Henrique Pires Aguiar,
Marcos Tatagiba
Editors

# Samii's Essentials in Neurosurgery

With 550 Figures and 37 Tables

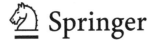 Springer

**Ricardo Ramina**
Chief of Department of Neurosurgery
Neurological Institute of Curitiba, Curitiba, Brazil
Pontifical Catholic University of Parana
Postgraduate Course in Surgery, Curitiba, Brazil
R. Jeremias Maciel Perretto 300
80210-310 Curitiba
Brazil
ramina@inc-neuro.com.br

**Marcos Tatagiba**
Direktor
Klinik für Neurochirurgie
Universitätsklinikum Tübingen
Hoppe-Seyler-Straße 3
D-72076 Tübingen
Germany
marcos.tatagiba@med.uni-tuebingen.de

**Paulo Henrique Aguiar**
Associated Professor of Division of Neurosurgery
of Hospital das Clínicas of São Paulo Medical School
Department of Neurology
University of São Paulo
Director of Division of Neurosurgery of Hospital Santa
Paula, São Paulo Brasil
Research and Clinic Fellowship Nordstadt
Krankenhaus, Hannover, Germany 1992–1993
R. David Ben Gurion, 1077 – apt 11
015634-001 São Paulo
Brazil
phpaneurocir@gmail.com

ISBN 978-3-642-08041-8          ISBN 978-3-540-49250-4 (eBook)

Springer is a part of Springer Science+Business Media
springer.com

Editor: Gabriele Schröder, Heidelberg, Germany
Desk Editor: Stephanie Benko, Heidelberg, Germany

Cover design: Frido Steinen-Broo, EStudio, Calamar, Spain

Printed on acid-free paper 24/3180/YL 5 4 3 2 1 0

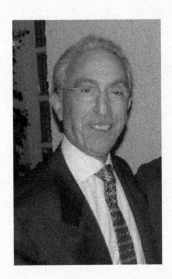

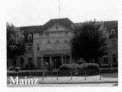
Mainz

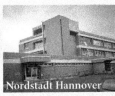
Nordstadt Hannover

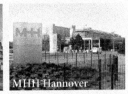
MHH Hannover

INI Hannover

# Foreword I

It is a privilege to write a foreword for the Festschrift of a dear friend, who also happens to be a living legend.

In 1969 in Japan, we were examining the usual international meeting papers, often geographically and politically selected, when suddenly we came across some excellent scientific papers by a group of young investigators from Mainz Germany, led by a young neurosurgeon named Madjid Samii. The papers dealt with peripheral nerve physiology. They described important basic research and the findings have stood the test of time. I felt intrigued and felt that I should get to know this man, who has since become one of my best friends, if not my best friend. I went to him, introduced myself and we started talking. We have been in conversation ever since.

Madjid Samii rapidly became a world-leading, world-class neurosurgeon. He has boundless energy, a will to succeed, and a talent for doing everything well. He went to the Nordstadt Hospital in Hannover as Chairman of Neurosurgery in 1977, and developed a superior neurosurgical training program, some of the fruits of which you will see in this volume. He and his wife, Mahschid, raised two fine children. They are now grandparents and are happy in this phase in their lives.

Professionally, Madjid was President of the German Society of Neurological Surgery for 2 years between 1996 and 1998. Also in 1996, he combined the Department of Neurosurgery at the Nordstadt Hospital and the Hannover School of Medicine. When he was nominated for President of the World Federation of Neurological Societies, I told him he should not do this because he was too busy and too much important work would otherwise not be done. However, his energy succeeded and he was able to show that he could stay busy and productive as a neurosurgeon, teacher, investigator, and lecturer while he did an extraordinary job as President of the World Federation.

On retirement from the neurosurgical department chair, he became President of the International Neuroscience Institute (INI) in July of 2000. He has continued to work productively in the INI and continues to do new work and to train excellent people.

Madjid Samii is one of the best technical neurosurgeons I have ever known, if not the best. Any neurosurgeon can learn from him. He has created a system of sharing information that puts many other professors to shame.

This is the professional side. How about the personal side of Madjid? He is a generous, giving man. He gives gifts to people, but more importantly, gives the gift of himself to friends and acquaintances. He has a talent for hospitality that is remarkable. He is fun to be around and although quiet and reserved, he is able to spin a wonderful story and to share with others his wisdom and his joy in life. He astoundingly, and despite his ego (which one needs to be a good neurosurgeon) also listens, and therefore, one can have a real conversation, a dialogue, with Samii. It has been my pleasure to have had many such dialogues, to have spent much time with him, to have learned from him, and to have tried to teach him as we have matured (I cannot say grow old) together. I treasure his friendship, I am amazed at his contributions, and I am impressed by his energy level.

If one is to be a leader, especially an innovative leader, and most especially in a surgical field, several factors are operant. That person must understand, but usually cannot fully comprehend what a serious effect he has on others. To put this another way, we do not know the importance of what we do when we do it. We may not understand this at any time or for some time. We often do not understand the proper use of new technology until it becomes old technology.

We must command the respect of others, and to do this demands an attitude of seriousness without self-absorption and ego. We must have the ability to have others work with us as much as for us. We must have organizational skills. Without these, we can accomplish nothing and all the best ideas and talent in the world will be wasted.

We must decisively do the right thing in any situation, despite the fact that this is often more difficult, and despite the consequences. This is most serious, most important, and most constructive in the long run. We must have the ability to walk in high places without fear and with the understanding of relationships. We must not be seduced by false technology and gimmickry. Speaking for neurosurgery, one can look at lasers gathering dust, capricious use of focal irradiation, and misinformed use of monocular endoscopy for neurosurgical procedures as examples.

As neurosurgeons, we must understand that operative technique is important. Simplicity and economy of movement are paramount to excellent understanding of three-dimensional anatomy and pathology and treatment thereof. We must be able to separate dogma from claptrap, as underlying dogma has frequently been lost in the development of surgery over the years. We must be paragons of virtue to our students, residents, and associates. We must be absolutely honest in all our approaches.

In all of the above, Dr. Madjid Samii stands as a towering figure, able to comprehend, organize, develop, and teach neurosurgery to others. Witness the superb group of people doing superb work in this volume. They are not necessarily a reflection of Dr. Samii's own work, but they are developments of thinking, of operative technique, and of management principles, which have, with Dr. Samii's blessing, gone beyond and beside his superb level of practice and teaching. This writer is proud to be a friend of Dr. Samii's, to be a comrade in the field of microneurosurgery, and to have written a foreword for this magnificent volume.

**Peter Janetta**

# Foreword II

The first time I was confronted with a brain tumor was when I was a medical student at the Pathological Institute of Nordstadt Krankenhaus in Hannover, Germany, while observing Professor Erdmann performing an autopsy of a patient who had been operated by Dr. Brunngraber, chief of the Neurosurgical Department of the Nordstadt Krankenhaus. At that time, in the early 1960s, I could not imagine how this event would influence my life or how this special place, Nordstadt Krankenhaus, would influence the world of neurosurgery. Guidelines for the treatment of neurosurgical pathologies and development of leadership would arise from that hospital.

This book reflects all of the teachings and the neurosurgical techniques initially introduced and developed by Madjid Samii. The chapters herein are presented by his earlier coworkers, co-operators, pupils, and friends, each one an expert and master in his or her own right; following the motto of the famous poet Hans Sachs from Nuremberg:

"Ehret Eure Meister, dann bannt Ihr böse Geister" (Honor your master and banish your bad spirits).

Standing on shoulders of their teachers, senior neurosurgeons are, over time, able to further develop and improve on their results.

Madjid Samii became involved with peripheral nerve surgery, including peripheral nerve regeneration by autologous transplantation, at the University of Mainz, Germany. For a short time I was also interested in this field, but following the orientation of my teacher, Frank Marguth, at the University of Munich, Germany, I changed to pituitary surgery and neuroendocrinology. Madjid Samii continued with peripheral nerve surgery. Frank Marguth was a good friend of Kurt Schürmann, Samii's teacher in Mainz.

Madjid Samii accepted with great enthusiasm a call to work in Hannover. From the beginning he was able to convince the local authorities that something special and extraordinary could be created here.

I discovered the skull base "from and around the sella turcica" following the advice of one of the pioneers of skull-base surgery, Patrick Derome, from Paris, France. Madjid expanded his interests in neurosurgery from the peripheral nerves to the cranial nerves. He was one of the founders of an interdisciplinary and international study group on skull-base surgery, and later of national and international societies. These organizations have become important structures of teaching worldwide.

It was the facial nerve that led Madjid Samii to worldwide success with acoustic neurinoma surgery. His unsurpassed (probably unsurpassable) series of more than 3500 operated acoustic neurinomas started in Nordstadt Krankenhaus, Hannover. In the beginning these surgeries were very time consuming, lasting from the morning until evening. Today, almost daily, Madjid Samii is resecting such tumors in about 1 hour. After experience with more than 4000 surgeries for pituitary adenomas, that is also the time I need to totally remove such a tumor. The techniques he has taught his pupils, the authors of this book, will also be passed on to their pupils.

My congratulations to Madjid on his more than 40 years in neurosurgical practice and on his 70th birthday. All my best wishes to a brilliant leader and friend, who with continuous enthusiasm and total dedication to neurosurgery fulfils his global responsibility to his medical field and even more to his patients. He has introduced to neurosurgery new ways, environments, and structures, both locally and internationally, and is the best of all at the International Neuroscience Institute in Hannover.

Ad multos annos! To Madjid and his teaching generation.

**Rudolf Fahlbusch**

The idea to write a book in honor of Professor Madjid Samii's 70th birthday evolved after talking to several of his former colleagues. This book shares with the readers his method of teaching surgical techniques as well as his management philosophy.

The last 40 years will be remembered among neurosurgeons for the remarkable development of new surgical techniques and technological advances. The introduction of the binocular dissection microscope for neurosurgery was a monumental advance; it opened up new horizons and possibilities for the safe treatment of most neurosurgical diseases. One of the pioneers of this "new era" of neurosurgery is Professor Madjid Samii. Very early in his career he started to use the operative microscope and developed new approaches for peripheral nerves, skull-base surgery, brain tumors, vascular pathologies of the brain and spinal cord, and spine diseases.

Writing about the professional career of one of the best surgeons in the history of neurosurgery is not difficult. Several hundred neurosurgeons had the opportunity to observe his skills as he operated on the most difficult cases in Germany and in many other countries. He is a great teacher. He has trained several surgeons who have since become outstanding neurosurgeons in Germany and the rest of the world. He is a master in the management of all neurosurgical pathologies and his scientific production is extraordinary. I have known him since 1979, initially as a resident, then as his associate ("Oberarzt") until 1986, and finally as a close friend. My first impression of his character as a person and a neurosurgeon goes back to 1979. I had been at the clinic (Nordstadt Krankenhaus) for only a few weeks, and after a "chief visit" he said to all of his staff: "The only real treasures a neurosurgeon can have in his life are his patients." Through the many years that I have known Madjid Samii, I can testify that he practiced what he preached, treating each patient, regardless of his/her status, with the same dedication, respect, and tenderness.

Madjid Samii is a very gentle and elegant person, but at the same time very exigent. He has never tolerated negligence and disrespect, especially with patients. He handles everyone in his clinic with honesty, justice, and a tender heart, and everybody in the clinic trusts him. He also has a special ability to motivate people to work together as a team. In addition to all of the medical colleagues he has worked with during his life, he has also been able to put together a "first-class team" of administrative support (e.g., Frau Plünecke and Frau Krümmel) and nurses (e.g., Schwester Hanna, Schwester Birgit, and especially Schwester Gisela).

Professor Samii feels "at home" and relaxed in the operating theater. For example, he is not concerned if during a very complicated surgery somebody asks him something about the procedure. He will pay attention and answer in a polite way. Some years ago, Professor Yasargil told me that he was surprised at the relaxed way Professor Samii went into the operating room to perform a difficult surgery: "It was like he was going to play golf!" He loves to show and teach his surgical technique and is very proud of his pupils, always giving them his undying support. I remember a situation that arose during a congress of the German Neurosurgical Society in Hannover. At that time, I had just finished my neurosurgical training and was on call. A patient with a difficult ruptured anterior communicating aneurysm came into our clinic and emergency surgery was indicated. Professor Samii had brought six neurosurgical professors from Germany and Austria to visit the clinic, when I started the aneurysm dissection, all of them came into the operating room to observe the surgery. Professor Samii told me I should continue on and clip the aneurysm. It was a difficult case but I succeeded in clipping it very nicely. After the clipping, all of the visitors left the room with the exception of an old professor from Vienna. He came to me and whispered in my ear, "My young man, I would not like to have been in your position today!" Yet I was very confident because I knew Professor Samii would have helped me if I had needed him.

Madjid Samii is a very optimistic person who believes in what he does. Patients love him; he is attentive to their needs and is always trying to do his best to help solve their problems. He is an honest man. In his scientific publications and conferences he has always presented true complication rates and results. He turned 70 years old this year, but his energy is the same as when he was 50. He operates every day, two to three cases a day, he travels to several countries for congresses, he regularly goes to China to operate on patients, and he has many plans for the future. One year ago I was in his home talking with his lovely wife (Mahschid). She "complained" that he was working as hard as ever. I asked her if he was happy and she answered: "Very happy!" This man is a shining example for future generations of neurosurgeons.

I want especially to thank two people who have made possible the success of this project. The first is my secretary, Mrs. Marli Uchida; she was tireless in contacting all of the authors, organizing the chapters, and helping with the editorial review. The second is Mrs. Stephanie Benko from Springer, Heidelberg (Germany). She worked in a very efficient and professional manner, giving us the essential support to realize this project. Finally, I would like to dedicate this book to all patients around the world who have been, or will be helped by the teachings of Madjid Samii.

**Ricardo Ramina**

"Samii's Essentials in Neurosurgery" is a unique book in its conception. It represents a compilation of 33 chapters written by more than 40 distinguished international neurosurgeons from 10 different countries. This book is covering almost all areas of the modern neurosurgery of the brain, skull base, spine and peripheral nerves including radiosurgery. The chapters are distributed along the book not thematically as usual, but as a novelty, according to the countries where the authors are acting. Each chapter of this book contains a range of information which represents the author's particular view of that field of neurosurgery. However, although living and working in five different continents around the world, all authors have one point mutual: they all have enjoyed at least part of their neurosurgical education with Madjid Samii in Hannover in some period of the last 30 years.

Madjid Samii started his neurosurgical carrier about four decades ago. He benefited himself from the high neurosurgical education of an advanced and prestigious centre at that time, the Department of Neurosurgery at the University of Mainz, directed by Professor Kurt Schürmann. Samii's neurosurgical life was profoundly affected by exceptional developments in several fields of medicine of the last four decades, such as increasing knowledge on anatomy and physiology of the nervous system, and on pathophysiology and outcome of neurological diseases. Major technological advances of operating microscope, computed tomography, magnetic resonance tomography, ultrasound aspirator, intraoperative monitoring, neuronavigation and radiosurgery have deeply changed the treatment strategies in neurosurgery over the last de-

cades. Whereas rapidly using all technological advances Samii's art of neurosurgery remained always focused on the patient's issues. His philosophy can be summarized as being open-minded for multi-disciplinary strategies and for the introduction of new technologies, while maintaining neurosurgery as simple as possible.

The idea to publish this book appeared recently. In 2002, a group of friends and former pupils of Professor Samii founded an international medical society called "Madjid Samii Congress of International Neurosurgeons (MASCIN)". Aim of MASCIN is to revive and give continuity to Samii's ideas on different fields of neurosurgery. He deeply influenced the education of a large number of neurosurgeons all over the world, who are today leading several neurosurgical fields in different countries. The present book "Samii's Essentials in Neurosurgery" represents the summary of MASCIN spirit. In fact, because the single most fundamental aspect of surgical neurology is the systematic assessment of patient's neurological state, the neurosurgeon has played one of the most important roles in the development of the entire field of this neuroscience.

We would like to thank the numerous authors for their encouraging response and remarkable contributions. We thank Springer with Stephanie Benko for the exceptional work. During the preparation of this book it was a great pleasure to get contact to many "old friends" around the world.

**The Editors**

# Contents

# List of Contributors

**Marcus André Acioly**
Department of Neurosurgery
Eberhard-Karls University Hospital
72076 Tübingen
Germany

**Paulo Henrique Aguiar**
Hospital das Clínicas of São Paulo Medical School
Department of Neurology
University of São Paulo
Sao Paulo
Brazil

**Antonio Nogueira Almeida**
Hospital das Clínicas of São Paulo Medical school
Department of Neurology
University of São Paulo
Sao Paulo
Brazil

**Hans-Werner Bothe**
Department of Neurosurgery
Westfälische Wilhelms-Universität
Albert-Schweitzer-Strasse 33
D-48149 Münster
Germany

**Gavin W. Britz**
Department of Neurological Surgery
University of Washington
Seattle, WA 98105
USA

**Roger Schimdt Brock**
São Paulo Epilepsy Center
DFV Neuro
São Paulo
Brazil

**Alessandro Ciampini**
Institute of Neurosurgery
Catholic University School of Medicine
L.go Agostino Gemelli, 8
00168 Rome
Italy

**Rogerio Santos Clemente**
Department of Neurosurgery
Neurological Institute of Curitiba
Curitiba
Brazil

**Jose Erasmo Dal 'Col Lucio**
São Paulo Epilepsy Center
DFV Neuro
São Paulo
Brazil

**Gustavo Adolpho de Carvalho**
Silvestre Hospital and Clinic Bambina
Rua Bambina 56 salas 105–107
Botafogo – CEP 22251-050
Rio de Janeiro
Brazil

**Luca Denaro**
Institute of Neurosurgery
Catholic University School of Medicine
L.go Agostino Gemelli, 8
00168 Rome
Italy

**Francesco Doglietto**
Institute of Neurosurgery
Catholic University School of Medicine
L.go Agostino Gemelli, 8
00168 Rome
Italy

**Yvens Barbosa Fernandes**
Department of Neurosurgery
University of Campinas
Campinas
Brazil

**Eduardo Fernandez**
Institute of Neurosurgery
Catholic University School of Medicine
L.go Agostino Gemelli, 8
00168 Rome
Italy

**Eliana Garzon**
São Paulo Epilepsy Center
DFV Neuro
São Paulo
Brasil

**Basavaraj Ghodke**
Department of Neurological Surgery
and Radiology
University of Washington
Seattle, WA 98105
USA

**Michael Hinojosa**
Department of Neurosurgery
Clinic San Borja and Clinic El Golf
Lima
Peru

**Peter Jannetta**
WPAHS Hospital
East Wing Office Building
420 East North Avenue
Suite 302
Pittsburgh PA 15212
USA

**Alexander Klein**
Department of Stereotactic
and Functional Neurosurgery
Neurocentre
Albert-Ludwigs-University of Freiburg
79106 Freiburg
Germany

**Petra M. Klinge**
International Neuroscience Institute
Rudolf-Pichlmayr-Str.4
30625 Hannover
Germany

**André Giacomelli Leal**
Department of Neurosurgery
Neurological Institute of Curitiba
Curitiba
Brazil

**Liverana Lauretti**
Institute of Neurosurgery
Catholic University School of Medicine
L.go Agostino Gemelli, 8
00168 Rome
Italy

**Joao Jarney Maniglia**
Department of Neurosurgery
Neurological Institute of Curitiba
Curitiba
Brazil

**Tobias Alecio Mattei**
Department of Neurosurgery
Neurological Institute of Curitiba
Curitiba
Brazil

**Cordula Matthies**
Department of Neurosurgery
Klinikum Hannover – Nordstadt
Hannover Medical School
30169 Hannover
Germany

**Luciana Midori Inuzuka**
São Paulo Epilepsy Center
DFV Neuro
São Paulo
Brazil

**Makoto Nakamura**
Department of Neurosurgery
Hannover Medical School
Carl-Neuberg-Str. 1
30625 Hannover
Germany

**Sabareesh K. Natarajan**
Department of Neurological Surgery
University of Washington
Seattle, WA 98105
USA

**Maurício Coelho Neto**
Department of Neurosurgery
Neurological Institute of Curitiba
Curitiba
Brazil

**Guido Nikkhah**
Laboratory of Molecular Neurosurgery
Dept. Stereotactic Neurosurgery – Neurocentre
University Hospital of Freiburg
Breisacher Str. 64
79106 Freiburg i.Br.
Germany

**Jorge Rizzato Paschoal**
Department of Neurosurgery
University of Campinas
Campinas
Brazil

**Ricardo Ramina**
Neurological Institute of Curitiba, Curtiba, Brazil
Pontifical Catholic University of Parana
Postgraduate Course in Surgery, Curitiba, Brazil
R. Jeremias Maciel Perretto 300
80210-310 Curitiba
Brazil

**Steffen K. Rosahl**
Department of Neurosurgery
HELIOS Klinikum
Nordhaeuser Str. 74
99089 Erfurt
Germany

**Florian Roser**
Department of Neurosurgery
University of Tübingen
Hoppe-Seyler-Str. 3
72076 Tübingen
Germany

**Fernando Schmidt**
Av. Mauricio Cardoso
833 sala 310
Hamburgo Velho
Novo Hamburgo
Rio Grande do Sul
Brazil

**Robert Schönmayr**
Department of Neurosurgery
HSK Wiesbaden
Ludwig-Erhard-Str. 100
65199 Wiesbaden
Germany

**Laligam N. Sekhar**
Harborview Medical Center
UW Medicine, Dept. of Neurosurgery
325 Ninth Avenue
Box 359924
Seattle, WA 98104-2499
USA

**Ramin Shahidi**
Image Guidance Laboratories
Stanford University
Palo Alto, CA 94305
USA

**Erasmo Barros Silva Jr**
Pontifical Catholic University of Parana
Postgraduate Course in Surgery
Curitiba
Brazil

**Marcos Tatagiba**
Department of Neurosurgery
Eberhard-Karls University Hospital
72076 Tübingen
Germany

**Eduardo Vellutini**
Praça Amadeu Amaral,
27–7 Andar
São Paulo
Brazil 01327-010

**Jan Vesper**
Department of Stereotactic and Functional
Neurosurgery
Neurocentre
Albert-Ludwigs University of Freiburg
79106 Freiburg
Germany

**Ronaldo Vosgerau**
Department of Neurosurgery
Neurological Institute of Curitiba
Curitiba
Brazil

**Klaus R.H. von Wild**
Medical Faculty of the Westphalia Wilhelm's University
Münster
Professor of Neurorehabilitation and Reengineering
of Brain and Spinal Cord Lesions, International
Neuroscience Institute
30625 Hannover
Germany

# I   Madjid Samii's Curriculum Vitae

# Madjid Samii, M.D., Ph.D. Curriculum Vitae

Madjid Samii was born in Tehran on June 19, 1937 and is of Iranian and German nationality. He is married to Mahschid Samii (since 1961) and they have two children. His hobbies after neurosurgery include music and golf. Professor Samii graduated in medicine and biology from the University of Mainz, Federal Republic of Germany, in 1963. He completed his training at the Neurosurgical Clinic of the University of Mainz in 1970 under Professor Dr. Kurt Schurmann. During his residency period, his scientific work resulted in a monograph on pneumoencephalotomography, experimental work on brain edema and experimental research on the surgical reconstruction of peripheral nerve lesions. In 1970 he was nominated Associate Professor and Vice Director of the Neurosurgical Clinic of the University of Mainz. He was also in charge of pediatric neurosurgery. In 1971 he became Professor of Neurosurgery. In that same year he instigated an annual course to teach his experiences in microsurgery.

## Important Dates and Facts of his Career

| | |
|---|---|
| 1977 | Nominated director of the neurosurgical clinic, Nordstadt Hospital in Hannover. |
| 1977 | He established the first microneurosurgical training laboratory in Germany. |
| 1979 | Cofounder of the Skull Base Study Group. |
| 1983 | First Medical World Telecommunication Conference (over the five continents). |
| 1986 | Call for the Chair of Neurosurgery at University of Leiden, The Netherlands. |
| Sept. 1987 | Olivecrona Lecture, Karolinska Institute, Stockholm, Sweden. |
| Dec. 1987 | Call for the Chair of Neurosurgery, University of Mainz. |
| April 1988 | Call for the Chair of Neurosurgery, Hannover School of Medicine (MHH). Accepted. |
| May 1988 | *Federal Republic of Germany Merit Cross First Class Award from the President of the Federal Republic of Germany for the scientific and practical development of neurosurgery and special efforts for the international scientific cooperation in this field. |
| 1988 | ⁺Award of the Prize of Science of Lower Saxony |
| 1988 | Award of Honorary Professor by the Medical School of Military Academy, Beijing, China. |
| 1988 | Keith Professorship University of Toronto, Canada. |
| 1986–1988 | President of the International Society of Skull Base Study Group |
| 1989 | President of the German Society for Plastic and Reconstructive Surgery. |
| 1989 | Visiting Professor for life at Medical Faculty of University of California (UCLA) Los Angeles, USA, and Visiting Director of the Skull Base Center at Neurosurgical Clinic of UCLA. |
| 1989 | Guest of Honor at the Second Annual Neurosurgery in the Rockies Meeting at the University of Colorado, Denver, Colorado, USA. |
| 1989 | Obrador Lecture and Medal, Madrid, Spain. |
| 1989 | Penfield Lecture, Banff, Canada. |

| | |
|---|---|
| 1990–1992 | Re-election as President of the International Skull Base Study Group. |
| 1989 | Sano Lecture, Tokyo, Japan. |
| 1991 | Founder Member and first President of the German Society of Skull Base Surgery. |
| 1991 | Founder Member and first President of Neurobionics Foundation Hannover. |
| 1991 | Founder President of the Board of Trustees of the Foundation AWD Children's Aid, Hannover. |
| 1991 | Jamieson Memorial Lecture and Medal, Australia. |
| 1991 | Guest of Honor of the North American Skull Base Society. |
| 1992 | Traffic Security Award Non disputare, sed agere by the Traffic Guard of Lower Saxony. |
| 1992 | Lars Leksell Lecture, Charlottesville, USA. |
| 1992 | President of International Skull Base Society. |
| 1992 | President of the First International Skull Base Congress. |
| 1992 | Award of Honorary Professor by Medical School of University of Uruguay. |
| 1993 | Honorary Member of the Academia Nacional de Medicina of Brazil. |
| Sept. 1993 | The first Edward Laws Jr. M.D. Lecture, George Washington University, Washington D.C. |
| 1994 | Honorary Citizenship of the City Rosario, Argentina. |
| 1994 | Doctor Honoris Causa (Honorary Doctor) awarded by Catholic University Rio Grande do Sul, Porto Alegre, Brazil. |
| 1994 | President elect of the German Society of Neurosurgery. |
| 1994 | Honorary President of the German Society of Skull Base Surgery. |
| 1994 | Award of Honorary Professor by Peruvian University Cayetano Heredia, Lima, Peru. |
| 1995 | Member of Board of Trustees "EXPO 2000 Hannover". |
| 1995 | Award of Honorary Professor by the National University, Lima, Peru. |
| 1995 | President of the German Society of Neurosurgery 1996–1998. |
| Since 1996 | Chairman of the Neurosurgical Departments at MHH (since 1996) and Klinikum Hannover Nordstadt (since 1977). |
| 1995 | Sir Charles Balance Memorial Lecture and Medal, London, UK. |
| July 1997 | President of the World Federation of Neurosurgical Societies (WFNS), 1997–2001. |
| May 1998 | Award of Honorary Professor by the Pontificia Universidad Javeriana, Bogotà, Colombia. |
| June 1998 | Award of the "Aristoteles Gold Medal" by the University of Thessaloniki, Greece. |
| March 1999 | Award of Honorary Professor of Neurosurgery by The University of Alexandria, Egypt. |
| April 1999 | The Sixth Annual Loyd C. Megison, Jr. Visiting Professorship, Louisiana State University Medical Center, Shreveport, Louisiana, USA. |
| April 2000 | Award of Courtesy Professor in the Department of Neurological Surgery at the University of Florida College of Medicine, Gainesville, USA. |
| July 2000 | President of the International Neuroscience Institute (INI). Inauguration on July 21, 2000. |
| July 2000 | Congress President of the "World Congress on Medicine and Health" July 21–August 20, 2000, Hannover. |
| August 2000 | Award of Doctor Honoris Causa of the University of Antioquia, Medellin, Columbia. |
| Sept. 2000 | European Lecture for Neurosurgery, Opio-Nice, France. |
| Nov. 2000 | Guest of Honor at the Third International Skull Base Congress, Foz do Iguacu, Brazil. |
| Dec. 2000 | Award of the Rudolf Frey Prize for extraordinary achievements in the field of pain therapy. |
| June 2001 | Honorary President of the German Society for Computer- and Robot-Assisted Surgery (CURAC). |

| | |
|---|---|
| Sept. 2001 | Honorary President of the WFNS. |
| 2001 | Guest of Honor during the 50-year anniversary of the Italian Society of Neurosurgery. |
| January 2002 | Award of Honorary Professor by Harbin Medical University, China |
| June 19, 2002 | Award of the Decoration in Gold to celebrate Professor Samii's 65th birthday and his 25th anniversary as a neurosurgeon in Hannover by the Traffic Guard of Germany. |
| June 19, 2002 | Award from the Brazilian Society of Neurosurgery. |
| March 2003 | Honorary President during the Winter Congress of the Italian Society of Neurosurgery, Madonna di Campiglio, Italy. |
| April 2003 | John L. Kemink, M. D. Memorial Lecture, University of Michigan, USA. |
| April 2003 | The Richard C. Schneider Lecture, American Association of Neurological Surgeons, San Diego, USA. |
| 2003 | Inauguration of his statue in the public garden of the capital city of Gilan in Resht, Iran in acknowledgement of his life's work. |
| 2003 | In recognition of Professor Samii's 25-year chairmanship of the Neurosurgical Clinic, City of Hannover, the lecture hall of the hospital has been dedicated to his name (Madjid Samii-Auditorium) |
| 2003 | McLaughlin-Gallie Visiting Professorship of the Royal College of Physicians and Surgeons of Canada with the award of $10,000. For the first time since 1960, this prize was given to a German and worldwide to a neurosurgeon. |
| 2003 | Paul C. Bucy Award for outstanding contributions to neurosurgical education by the University of Chicago, USA. |
| July 2004 | Nomination as President of the China International Neuroscience Institute at the Capital University of Medical Sciences in Beijing, China. |
| Sept. 7, 2004 | First Honorary Ring of the City of Hannover (Garbsen) for outstanding contribution to the fame of the city worldwide. |
| Oct. 1, 2004 | Honorary Membership of the Austrian Society of Neurosurgery during the 40th Annual General Meeting of the society in Vienna, Austria. |
| Oct. 21, 2004 | Honorary Membership and Medal of Recognition of the Polish Society of Neurosurgery by the occasion of the 50th Anniversary of the society in Krakow, Poland. |
| Nov. 2004 | Guest of Honor at the Fourth International Skull Base Congress, Sydney, Australia. |
| Nov. 25, 2004 | Nomination as Honorary Professor by the Capital University of Medical Sciences in Beijing, China. |
| Nov. 25, 2004 | In recognition of his worldwide contribution to skull base surgery, the new established skull base training center at the XuanWu University Hospital of the Capital University of Medical Sciences in Beijing, China has been dedicated to Professor Samii (Samii Skull Base Surgery Training Center). |
| Apr. 24, 2005 | "Walk of Fame", Hannover (Garbsen). |
| May 2005 | Honorary president of the Seventh Congress of the European Skull Base Society/13th Congress of the German Society of Skull Base Surgery. |
| May 18, 2005 | Kurt Schürmann Lecture of the German Society of Skull Base Surgery, Fulda, Germany. |
| Nov. 11, 2005 | Honorary Membership of the Bangladesh Society of Neurosurgeons. |
| Dec. 2005 | Honorary Member of the Society of Nervous System Surgery in Istanbul, Turkey. |
| 2005 | Founding Chair of the Accreditation Committee for WFNS Board of Neurosurgery. |
| June 2006 | Honorary Member of the Association of Russian Neurosurgeons in Moscow, Russia. |
| June 29, 2006 | Matson Memorial Lecture, Harvard University of Boston, USA. |
| 2006 | Honorary member of the Charity Society for School Constructions in Iran |
| 2006 | In recognition of Professor Samii's worldwide achievement, two schools in Isfahan and Rasht, Iran were named after him (Prof. Madjid Samii School). |

| 2006 | Guest of Honor of the Brazilian Society of Neurosurgery at the 26th Brazilian Congress of Neurosurgery, Florianópolis, Brazil. |
| Nov. 13, 2006 | Iranian scientific award "Chrehayeh Mandegar" for medicine 2006, Teheran, Iran. |

Professor Samii has given more than 1000 lectures as Invited and/or Honored Guest of numerous national and international congresses and is an author of over 450 scientific papers and 15 books concerning the central and peripheral nervous systems.

## Present Activities

President of the INI at Otto-von-Guericke University
President of the Chinese INI.
Chairman (retired) of the Neurosurgical Departments of MHH and Klinikum Hannover, Nordstadt.
Regular Lectures Chair of Neurosurgery at MHH.
Visiting Professor of Neurosurgery at various universities.

**Professor Samii is a Member of the editorial or advisory boards of the following medical journals:**
Acta Neurochirurgica Editorial Board
African Journal of Neurosurgical Sciences Editorial Board
Archives of Iranian Medicine Editorial Board/International Board of Consultants
Chinese Journal of Minimally Invasive Neurosurgery Editorial Advisory Board
Chirurgia Neurologica Editorial Board
Critical Reviews in Neurosurgery Editorial Committee (former chairman)
Hong Kong Neuroscience Foundation Charitable Trust Editorial Board
Journal of Operative Techniques in Neurosurgery Editorial Board
Journal of Reconstructive Microsurgery Advisory Board
Journal of Skull Base Surgery Editor Emeritus
Maghreb Journal of Neurosurgery Honorary Board Member
(Morocco-Algeria-Tunisia)
Neuroanatomy Editorial Board
Neurochirugia Comité Editorial Internacional
Neurocirugía-Neurocirurgia Editorial Advisory Board
(Spanish-Portuguese Journal of Neurosurgery)
Neurological Research Associate Editor
Neurosurgical Focus Reviewer
Neurosurgery International Liaison and Advisory Panel
Pan Arab Neurosurgical Journal Advisor
Russian Neurosurgery Editorial Board
Surgical Neurology Editorial Board
Surgical and Radiologic Anatomy Advisor
Türkiye Klinikleri Journal of Medical Sciences Advisory Board
Turkish Neurosurgery and Türk Nörosirürji Dergisi International Advisory Board
Ukrainian Journal of Minimally Invasive and Editorial Board
Endoscopic Surgery

**Professor Samii is a member of the following Medical Societies:**
Deutsche Gesellschaft für Neurochirurgie
German Society of Neurosurgery
Deutsche Gesellschaft für Schädelbasischirurgie
German Society of Skull Base Surgery
Deutsche Gesellschaft für Neuroradiologie
German Society of Neuroradiology

Deutsche Gesellschaft für Unfallheilkunde
German Trauma Society
Deutsche Gesellschaft für Plastische und Wiederherstellungs-Chirurgie e.V.
German Society of Plastic and Reconstructive Surgery
Deutsche Gesellschaft für Computer- und Roboterassistierte (Founding Member)
Chirurgie e.V. (CURAC; Honorary President)
German Society for Computer- and Robot-assisted Surgery
Gesellschaft zum Studium des Schmerzes für Deutschland, Österreich und die Schweiz e.V.
German-Austrian-Swiss Society for the Study of Pain
European Joseph Society (Facial-Plastic and Reconstructive Surgery)
European Council of the European Skull Base Society (1995)
Sunderland Society (Founding Member)
WFNS
Accreditation Committee for WFNS Board of Neurosurgery (Founding Chair)
Neurosurgery
WFNS Skull Base Committee (Chairman)
WFNS Peripheral Nerve Surgery Committee
WFNS Training Committee
International Skull Base Society (Founding Member and Past President)
International Society of Reconstructive Microsurgery (Founding Member)
International Society of Pituitary Surgeons
Skull Base Study Group (Founding Member and Past President)
Academia Eurasiana Neurochirurgica
World Academy of Biomedical Technologies (Founding Member)
Deutsche Gesellschaft für Hals-Nasen-Ohren-Heilkunde, Kopf- und Hals-Chirurgie
(German Society of ENT Therapeutics, Head and Neck Surgery; Corresponding Member)
Argentine Academy of Neurosurgery (Corresponding Member)
Argentine Society of Neurosurgery (Honorary Member)
Argentine Society of Neurosciences (Corresponding Member)
Bangladesh Society of Neurosurgeons (Honorary Member)
Brazilian National Academy of Medicine (Honorary Member)
Brazilian Society of Neurosurgery (Corresponding Member)
Brazilian Society of Skull Base Surgery (Honorary Member)
Sociedade Brasileira de Neurocirurgia (Honorary Member)
Bolivian Neurosurgical Society (Corresponding Member)
Canadian Society of Neurosurgery (Honorary Member)
Chilean Society of Neurology, Psychiatry, and Neurosurgery (Honorary Member)
Colombian Society of Neurosurgery (Honorary Member)
Dutch Society of Skull Base Surgery (Honorary Member)
The Hong Kong Neurosurgical Society (Honorary Member)
The Neurological Society of India (Honorary Member)
Iranian National Academy of Medicine (Honorary Member)
Iranian Society of Neurosurgery (Honorary Member)
Italian Society of Neurosurgery (Honorary Member)
Gruppo di Microneurochirurgia del Periferico, Italy (Honorary President)
Japanese Society of Neurosurgery (Honorary Member)
Peruvian Academy of Surgery (Honorary Member)
Peruvian Society of Neurosurgery (Honorary Member)
Portuguese Society of Neurosurgery (Honorary Member)
Romanian Society of Neurosurgery (Honorary Member)
Romanian Academy of Medical Sciences (Honorary Member)
Scandinavian Society of Neurosurgery (Corresponding Member)
Society of Nervous System Surgery (Honorary Member)
Spanish and Portuguese Society of Neurosurgery (Corresponding Member)
Neurosurgical Society R.O.C. Taiwan (Honorary Member)
Turkish Neurosurgical Society (Honorary Member)

Society of Neurological Surgeons USA (Honorary Member)
The American Academy of Neurological Surgery (Corresponding Member)
American Association of Neurological Surgeons (AANS) (Honorary Member)
Adjunct Subcommittee on International Associate (Member)
Membership of the AANS
American Society for Reconstructive Microsurgery (Corresponding Member)
The Western Neurosurgical Society USA (Honorary Member)
Sociedad de Neurologia y Neurocirugia del Uruguay (Honorary Member)
Latin American Federation of Neurosurgery (First Honorary Member)
Central European Neurosurgical Society (CENS) (First Honorary Member)
Austrian Society of Neurosurgery (Honorary Member)
Polish Society of Neurosurgery (Honorary Member)
Bangladesh Society of Neurosurgery   (Honorary Member)
Association of Russian Neurosurgeons (Honorary Member)

## Explanatory Notes

*Federal Republic of Germany Merit Cross First Class: Awarded by the President for "outstanding services and achievements in the interest of the German people and the effort made to stimulate national and international cooperation in the field of neurosurgery".

Annually, the president of Germany selects a few people throughout the country who have contributed exceptionally to their profession with outstanding work. On the day corresponding to the founding of the Federal Republic of Germany, the president celebrates this event in his residence in Bonn and personally awards the Merit Cross.

+The Lower Saxony Prize 1988 for Science for "the dedication, work, achievements and research in the field of neurosurgery". Every year, the Government of Lower Saxony honors one scientist among all sciences with the Prize of Lower Saxony for Science. An unbiased commission from all branches of public and social life proposes, based on their work, achievements, and dedication, selects the candidate who has excelled in his field over national boundaries, and presents him/her to the State Governor. It is therefore a very significant event that this prize is given to the medical field among all sciences. The award ceremony is hosted by the Governor, Minister of Science, and several hundred outstanding local and national personalities. During the ceremony, the biography of the recipient is highlighted and the event receives full coverage by the media.

# II  Technologic Developments

# The Virtual Operating Field – How Image Guidance can Become Integral to Microneurosurgery

**1**

Steffen K. Rosahl and Ramin Shahidi

## Contents

## 1.1
### Introduction

In neurosurgery, layers of soft tissue, bone, and parenchyma conceal vital structures, landmarks, and the targeted lesion. Guiding an approach to a lesion with the help of computed tomography (CT), magnetic resonance imaging (MRI), or ultrasound images of the anatomy of a patient enables avoidance of accidental damage and the definition of a clear surgical corridor in individually uncharted territory. Today, surgical image guidance based on three-dimensional (3D) volumetric data has become part of the routine in most neurosurgical centers around the world.

There is a concurrent trend in medical disciplines toward augmenting interventions by virtual reality, the envisioned ideal being a virtual stereoscopic view on the surgical field and beyond before the first cut and throughout the operation [14, 23, 35]. Image-based, stereoscopic virtual reality models are used to plan surgical procedures and for teaching purposes in neurosurgery and temporal bone dissection [11, 17, 19, 20, 34, 38, 41]. However, image guidance in neurosurgery, synonymously termed "neuronavigation," has yet to become an integral part of most neurosurgical procedures. While this would be desirable considering the need to anticipate functional and morphological obstacles in the surgical path in individual cases, there are several prerequisites that will have to be met before navigation in neurosurgery will come to be seen as ordinary as navigation in today's automobiles. This chapter briefly explores the history and current development in the field and offers an outlook into the future of neurosurgical image guidance.

## 1.2
### History

The history of neuronavigation can be traced back to the roots of stereotaxis with a Cartesian coordinate system devised by Clarke and Horsley at the beginning of the last century [1]. Image-guided frameless stereotaxis became feasible through the integration of high-speed computers in the 1990s. The first clinical trials were accompanied by concerns about spatial accuracy and ease of application of the technology in the operating theater. Hardware and software were designed by various research groups and even with the first commercially available systems, data transfer, segmentation of morphological structures, and registration procedures were cumbersome and time consuming. Bone-anchored fiducials under local anesthesia often had to be applied a day before surgery, and scanning protocols for CT had to be adjusted to meet the requirements of the specific navigation system. The acquired data had to be saved to digital tapes or magneto-optical discs, and often tedious pre-processing ensued in order to reformat files to make them readable for the system.

Today, the accuracy of most image-guidance systems, as assessed by target registration error, is well documented and usually acceptable with mean values below 2 mm [4, 16, 22, 29, 33, 44, 48], except for targets located remote to the fiducials used for registration or cases where very few fiducials are valid [46]. MRI images can be corrected for object-induced and spatial distortion [40, 45]. Adhesive skin markers and surface registration have replaced bone-anchored fiducials for most intracranial procedures. Data transfer is made by local area networks that connect workstations in the operating theater directly with those in the radiology department. Workflow control allows for intuitive use of the navigation software, making the setup in the operating room fast and easy.

## 1.3
## State of the Art

Three-dimensional stereoscopic guidance has been developed with the goal of allowing the surgeon to explore radiological imaging information in situ [10, 12, 13, 23] by overlaying an image onto the microscopic view. It still has a long way to go with computation capacity, accuracy [24], and visual perception of depth in 3D images [15].

However, with improving image quality, coregistration of various image modalities, and 3D volumetric image rendering in real-time, image guidance today is capable of providing nonstereoscopic, color-coded models that match closely the individual anatomy of the real surgical field and relieves the surgeon of the task of mental reconstruction of tri-axial images on a routine basis [3, 35, 39].

Although ultrasound is being employed increasingly for image guidance [2, 6, 18, 21, 30, 36, 42, 43], MRI (1.5 and 3 Tesla), CT, and CT angiography remain the primary imaging technologies to create volumetric data sets.

CT is usually performed in the axial orientation with a slice thickness of 1 mm and an ultra-high algorithm. For arterial and venous CT angiography in tumor patients, the first bolus of 40 ml intravenous contrast medium is sufficient to visualize enhancing tumors. For vessel depiction, it may be followed by a further 60 ml, administered at a fast rate, after an individual delay determined by a bolus test [47].

Today, MRI is usually performed on 1.5 Tesla or 3 Tesla scanners. A higher field strength is superior for functional imaging, but imaging is also more prone to motion artifacts, especially in regions around the brainstem.

Axial T1-weighted 3D magnetization prepared rapid gradient echo (MPRAGE; TR/TE/T1 11.08/4.3/300 ms, flip angle 15°, band width 130 Hz/pixel, effective slice thickness 1 mm, pixel size 1.2×0.9 mm) with or without intravenous contrast medium (0.1 mmol/kg body weight gadolinium-DTPA) are usually sufficient for MRI guidance. This sequence is acquired in just over 7 min minutes.

For improved imaging of the temporal bone and the cortical surface in the temporal fossa, an axial T2-weighted constructive interference in steady state (CISS) sequence (TR/TE/flip angle 17/8.08ms/70°ms, effective slice 0.7 mm pixel size 0.6×0.45 mm acquisition time 7 min 51 s) has been applied in selected cases, especially when the lesion is located in a cistern or in the ventricles. Data can be transferred to an image-guidance system via a local area network or passed onto the system using portable storage media. Navigation software should be capable of rendering high-resolution, pseudo-3D images that can be interactively rotated in real time.

There is no limitation for image guidance with respect to the pathologies involved. Even in an extensive subdural hematoma, it may be helpful in placing several burr holes at precisely determined locations.

The decision making for the surgical strategy including the approach and the stepwise exclusion of the lesion is usually designed by the surgeon in advance. However, in some cases, image guidance may be employed to modify and adapt these strategies to avoid approach-related morbidity or to define an optimal surgical corridor. The

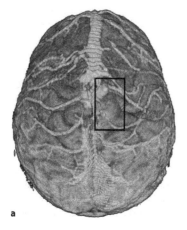 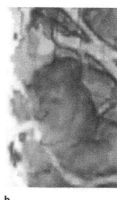 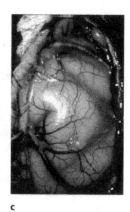

a                                        b                                    c

Fig. 1 **a** "Helicopter view" of the lesion and the motor areas for the left (*green*; pushed anteriorly) and right foot (*pink*) in a three-dimensional (3D) rendering created from magnetization prepared rapid gradient echo sequences and functional magnetic resonance imaging (fMRI) on the image-guidance system. **b** The virtual operating field (VOF, "driver seat view") showing the cortical surface and veins, the lesion, and the adjacent motor areas (*shaded*). Note that the latter two are exclusively seen in the VOF, but not in the real field. **c** Only the veins and the cortical surface can be recognized after the parasagittal craniotomy. Image injection of the VOF with a tumor outline and functionally significant areas can greatly enhance the real operating field in cases like this

segmentation and the creation of volumes of interest from the imaging data containing the landmark anatomical structures in the surgical path will usually be carried out by the neurosurgical team and only occasionally by an experienced neuroradiologist. A virtual "fly through" or "fly around" movie may be generated to simulate the major surgical steps in the planned procedure using the individual imaging data of the patient ("helicopter view", Fig. 1a). Again, the surgical strategy may be adjusted whenever an improved surgical approach could be derived from these visualizations.

Several volumes of interest may be selected and color-coded to create a volumetric image that contains all of the anatomical landmarks that would also appear in the real operating field. This image – the "virtual operating field" (VOF) – on advanced image-guidance systems can be interactively rotated to match the orientation of the real surgical field, as seen through the microscope (Fig. 1). Surfaces may gradually be rendered translucent in the image to allow a view of the lesion in relation to more superficial morphologic landmarks (Figs. 1–3, "driver seat view"). The VOF should ideally be zoomed to the size of the real microscopic field, and both views may be displayed on a

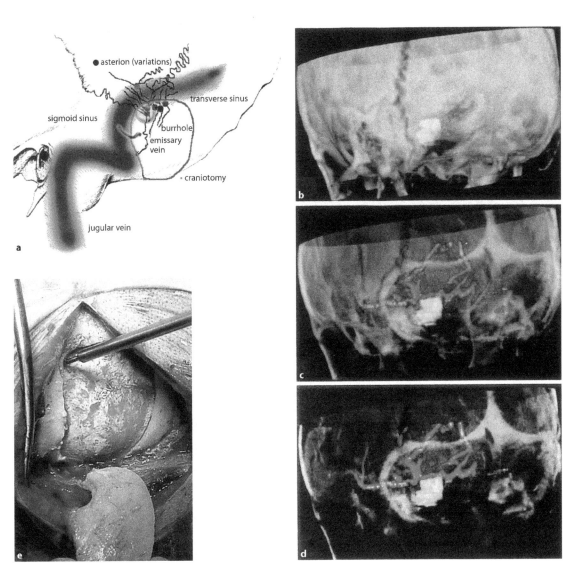

Fig. 2 **a** Anatomical landmarks for the lateral suboccipital approach. Note the variability of the location of the asterion around the sinus transition. **b** 3D rendering of the bone sutures of the posterior fossa with the navigation system. **c,d** Gradual transparency modulation of the bone allows for a look through the posterior fossa. The borders of the venous sinuses (*pink*) become clearly visible so that they can be used as landmarks themselves, replacing the asterion as a historical landmark. The circle of Willis is also shown in the images (*blue*). **e** After a burr hole has been placed just below the transverse-sigmoid junction, an osteoplastic lateral suboccipital craniotomy is carried out

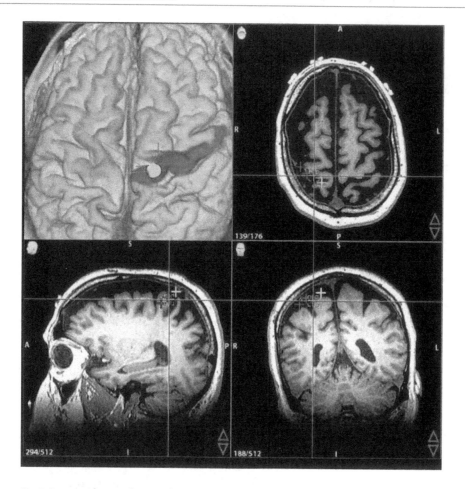

Fig. 3 Image guidance with 3D renderings (upper left) and tri-axial MRI in a patient with intractable thalamic pain during implantation of a motor cortex stimulator. The visualization of the cortical surface with its gyri and sulci is clearly superior in the volumetric 3D rendering. The motor strip has been segmented manually based on fMRI images of the patient. The virtual probe points – just as the real one – to a previously defined electrode location

video monitor or in the ocular of the surgical microscope simultaneously. Depending mostly on the quality of the imaging data and the level of the human computer interface (intuitive software, computer skills of the surgeon), image rendering may take between 15 min and 2 h.

In the operating room, the patient's head is registered either with five to ten adhesive skin fiducials and a pointing probe (which may be substituted by the microscope in some settings), or with a device and algorithm for surface detection. Most systems today are based on infrared transmission employing a camera for detection of a digital reference frame and the instruments (Fig. 4).

The digital reference frame may be attached to the head holder, to the operating table, or directly to the head of the patient. It is kept visible by the camera by draping it with a transparent bag or by mounting it sterile on an appropriate extension. After registration, a quick check should be performed to assess the accuracy of the reg-

istration by targeting a well-defined landmark (e.g., the nasion or the outer ear canal).

The quality of VOF images related to their closeness to reality will obviously depend on the quality of the primary data set. A contrast-enhanced target located adjacent to the bone and targets located in the middle fossa or at the craniocervical junction may pose difficulties because of decreased tissue contrast and MRI distortion. Also, due to the smaller sulci and the lesser amount of cerebrospinal fluid contained in the subdural space, it is usually harder to depict the surface of the temporal lobe cortex in 3D renderings.

The surgical approach is facilitated by VOF images by showing hidden landmarks like the transverse and sigmoid sinus in a retrosigmoid route (Fig. 2). Gradual modulation of the opacity of surfaces in VOF images allows for visualization of hidden anatomical structures, and for relating those structures to more superficial land-

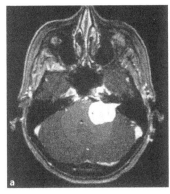
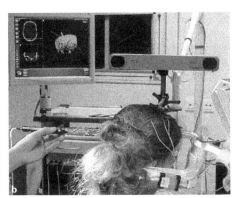
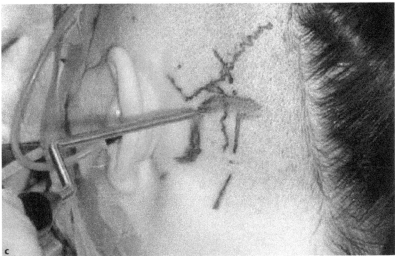
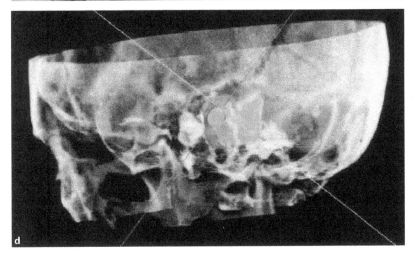

Fig. 4 **a** Gadolinium-enhanced, T1-weighted axial MRI of a vestibular schwannoma on the left side. The primary data for image-guidance in this particular case were obtained from both a MRI and spiral computed tomography. **b** Semisitting position of the patient for the retrosigmoid approach. The infrared camera of the image-guidance system is placed low on the side of the lesion so that it can "see" the probe. **c** The course of the transverse and sigmoid sinuses and the bone sutures meeting at the asterion have been drawn to the skin with a surgical marker. **d** Corresponding image on the navigation screen with the virtual probe pointing to the transverse sigmoid transition

marks that were already within the surgeon's view (like the asterion in Figs. 2 and 4).

With 3D renderings there is no need for the surgeon to mentally reconstruct the surgical anatomy from two-dimensional scans. Compared to tri-axial two-dimensional images, orientation is significantly faster and more comprehensive with VOF images (Figs. 1–3). This becomes more apparent when irregular-shaped structures like the dural sinuses, the basal arterial circulation, the bone of the skull base, tumor borders, and the cortical surface are involved or when the operating field was rotated into an unusual orientation [35].

The advantages of image guidance multiply when functional and/or histological characteristics are added to a VOF. Figure 3 shows how functional image-guidance aids can be in the placement of epidural electrodes for motor cortex stimulation in intractable pain. The morphological outline of the precentral gyrus can be easily and safely traced in 3D images if functional data are available. Precise electrode implantation with this guidance is greatly facilitated, even with the dura remaining closed throughout the procedure [5].

Similar advantages have been reported for subdural placement of electrode grids in patients with epilepsy, for detection of the origin of focal seizure activity [25, 37].

Some brain tumors, even though they reach the surface of the cerebral cortex, do not show any demarcation to normal brain parenchyma (Figs. 1 and 5).

However, if a tumor is well delineated on T2-weighted MRI (Fig. 5), its outline can be mapped or overlaid onto the cortical surface in a VOF. This is especially useful if the tumor is located adjacent to a functionally eloquent area and, therefore, resection has to be restricted precisely to the tumor limits in order to avoid intolerable morbidity. Functional imaging provides further information that would not be available in the real surgical field without neuronavigation (Fig. 1).

The functional anatomy can be shifted or distorted by the tumor. This is especially important when fiber tracking by diffusion tensor imaging is employed. The pyramidal tract may be considerably displaced and then returned to its normal position as tumor resection progresses. Under these circumstances of major brain shift, MRI scans acquired prior to the procedure would not be reliable during surgery. It has been shown that intraoperative functional MRI is feasible with the same protocols that are used outside the operating theater. The combination of neuronavigation and intraoperative functional MRI offers additional safety in these cases [8, 26–28]. Multimodal imaging may also improve the reliability of

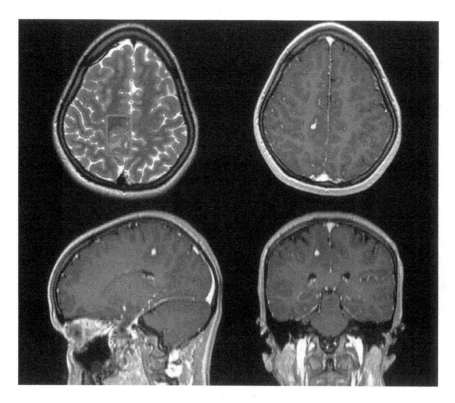

Fig. 5 An infantile desmoganglioma in the right postcentral region of a 14-year-old patient. The T2-weighted MRI (upper left comer) shows that the lesion centers around a sulcus. In the depth, nodular contrast-enhancement in T1-weighted images points to a histologically dubious portion of the tumor

functional information, especially with respect to the language areas of the cortex [7].

Zooming in the virtual images in order to enlarge the detail to the size of the surgical field reduces the amount of information presented at a time to the required minimum, steadying the surgeon's focus of attention (Fig. 1).

Individual, patient-specific anatomy can be visualized in the VOF down to a resolution of about 2 mm for well-delineated structures. In general, all morphological structures that are readily discernable in primary imaging data can be also detected in virtual 3D models of the surgical situs. Using image fusion techniques, bony surfaces, embedded vessels, and different types of soft tissue along the surgical path, both in front of and beyond the lesion, can be identified in a single image, which in turn can be rotated to match the view through the microscope onto the real surgical field.

Stereoscopic images are not obtained as easily, but they have the decisive advantage of conveying information on depth along the $z$-axis [9, 10, 16, 32, 38], which can only be captured in tri-axial images with volumetric pseudo-3D rendering.

Smaller and less discernable structures, such as most cranial nerves, are not well delineated in routine images. Electrophysiological monitoring is still by far the most effective tool for early identification of the cranial nerves.

## 1.4
## Outlook

Microneurosurgery depends on 3D, stereoscopic information on the surgical field delivered through the microscope. A "virtual microscope" operating in 3D space that uses stereoscopic radiographic images of the patient's anatomy would be an ideal instrument to plan these procedures and to obtain on-line information beyond the operating field during surgery. While several problems remain to be resolved [15, 24, 31], true 3D imaging, on a routine basis will probably be performed by taking advantage of stereoscopy in the future.

Overlay of a VOF that virtually matches the surgical field will certainly augment the surgeon's capacities. While anatomical knowledge and experience still remain the most crucial factors affecting the surgical result, virtual reality can provide additional information about elements in the operative field that are beyond the superficial layer and invisible through the operating microscope.

Although now in extensive clinical use, image guidance still is often perceived as an intrusion into the operating room [31]. In our experience, image guidance is best accepted when additional preparation time is minimal and the VOF is adjusted to the size and orientation of the real surgical field containing relevant landmarks without redundant information.

The following list is a brief compilation of essential prerequisites that, according to the literature and to our own experience,, will have to be met in order to turn image guidance into an integral part of most microneurosurgical procedures.

1. Accuracy: Image guidance needs to be precise. Geometric distortions in imaging procedures have to be corrected before the data are taken to the operating room.
2. Easy and speedy applicability: Imaging, data transfer, segmentation, intraoperative setup, and registration combined should require minimal additional time.
3. Image fusion: Multimodal images must be easily co-registered and combined in a single image.
4. Truly stereoscopic 3D images: Stereoscopic visualization improves perception and enhances the ability to understand complex 3D anatomy.
5. Interactivity: The practical benefit of 3D display is increased considerably when the size and orientation of the VOF corresponds to the real microscopic view of the surgical field. Different perspectives of the field (driver's seat view, helicopter view) should be optional. With respect to the limitation of the VOF, less may often be more, since the surgeon will only appreciate relevant information on the surgical field in view under the microscope.
6. Transparency: The possibility of seeing through surfaces by gradually rendering them translucent is advantageous, since landmarks at different depths along the surgical path can be correlated to one another.
7. Integration of the functional characteristics of tissue: Data from functional MRI, including fiber tracking by diffusion tensor imaging as well as, for example, positron emission tomography, electroencephalography, magnetoencephalography, and spectroscopy, should all be made available in images used for intraoperative guidance.
8. Intraoperative correction for tissue shift: In procedures involving major mass extraction or massive drainage of cerebrospinal fluid, an intraoperative update of the images by MRI, CT, ultrasound, or surface tracking should be available.
9. High spatial image resolution: While spatial resolution on MRI has increased over the years, it is difficult to discern objects smaller than 2 mm in size. Since spatial resolution and tissue contrast are crucial for the creation of true 3D images that match the view provided by microscopic magnification, this is an issue that will have to be addressed in the future.

Image guidance based on 3D images will never substitute precise anatomical knowledge and surgical experience, because systematic and accidental technical errors occur and the depiction of anatomical detail is limited by the resolution of imaging techniques. There is little doubt, however, that the VOF will become a very real part of the microsurgical situs and it is hard to see why the two should not be intimately entwined in the near future.

## 1.5
# Summary

Image guidance in neurosurgery – the technique of guiding an approach to a lesion with the help of computed tomography (CT), magnetic resonance imaging (MRI), or ultrasound images of the anatomy of an individual patient – is no longer a novelty. Accuracy validation has been established and advances in both hardware and software have rendered the technology user-friendly and almost intuitive in routine applications. Image acquisition, data transfer, and intraoperative patient registration take only a few minutes to accomplish. The whole procedure is noninvasive and in many surgical approaches, there is no particular need to compensate for brain shift.

Still, image-guidance in neurosurgery (neuronavigation) has not yet evolved into such an omnipresent instrument (e.g., like the microscope), although it does have similar potential considering the constant desire to see beyond tissue barriers in the surgical path in an ever variable, individual, anatomical environment.

In order to be successful, neurosurgeons must develop a thorough comprehension of complex, three-dimensional (3D) anatomy. Current radiological methodology – namely tomography – for everyday purposes has reduced the dimensions available in a single image to two, leaving the surgeon to mentally reconstruct a 3D structure from two-dimensional images in multi-axial planes.

There is a clear discrepancy between today's radiological routines and the challenges of surgical practice described in what could be called "the two-dimensional dilemma." This dilemma is being dissolved only slowly and gradually, but it is obvious that neurosurgery, with its dependence on spatial visual orientation, would be among the specialties that will take the helm in leading medicine into a new era of 3D image guidance.

Technologically, it is already possible to reconstruct a virtual, true 3D model of the operating field with translucent surface modulation and an optional "fly-through" video mode to the target structure from tomographic or ultrasound images. This model can be enhanced by CT–MRI image fusion and by adding functional characteristics, obtained from functional imaging or neurophysiological studies, to the morphology. Complex anatomical structures like the cortical surface, the tortuous course of cerebral vessels, or the outline of the paranasal sinuses can be easily visualized in such a model and recognized by the surgeon at a glance. Comprehension is greatly facilitated as compared to routine mental reconstruction of tri-axial images. It is also possible to simulate depth in a stereoscopic version of such a virtual operating field (VOF) and to zoom in and out according to the magnification of the microscope. The technology of tomorrow will allow for higher spatial resolution to capture very small objects (like small vessels) in the image.

Once stereo images like this can be projected into the microscope and overlaid onto the real operating field, in the view of the surgeon, without requiring much additional effort, image guidance is likely to become an integral part of most microneurosurgical procedures. Supported by sound anatomical knowledge, creating a VOF for any given surgical approach in an individual patient can greatly enhance the capabilities of a neurosurgical team.

## References

1. Alexander E III, Maciunas RJ (1999) Advanced Neurosurgical Navigation. Thieme, New York
2. Bonsanto MM, Metzner R, Aschoff A, et al (2005) 3D ultrasound navigation m syrinx surgery - a feasibility study. Acta Neurochir (Wien) 147:533–540
3. Dey D, Gobbi DG, Slomka PJ, et al (2002) Automatic fusion of freehand endoscopic brain images to three-dimensional surfaces: creating stereoscopic panoramas. IEEE Trans Med Imaging 21:23–30
4. Doshi PK, Lemmieux L, Fish DR, et al (1995) Frameless stereotaxy and interactive neurosurgery with the ISG viewing wand. Acta Neurochir Suppl 64:49–53
5. Gharabaghi A, Hellwig D, Rosahl SK, et al (2005) Volumetric image guidance for motor cortex stimulation: integration of three-dimensional cortical anatomy and functional imaging. Neurosurgery 57:114–120
6. Gronningsaeter A, Lie T, Kleven A, et al (2000) Initial experience with stereoscopic visualization of three-dimensional ultrasound data in surgery. Surg Endosc 14:1074–1078
7. Grummich P, Nimsky C, Pauli E, et al (2006) Combining fMRI and MEG increases the reliability of presurgical language localization: a clinical study on the difference between and congruence of both modalities. Neuroimage 32:1793–1803
8. Hastreiter P, Engel K, Soza G, et al (2003) Remote computing environment compensating for brain shift. Comput Aided Surg 8:169–179
9. Henn JS, Lemole GM Jr, Ferreira MA, et al (2002) Interactive stereoscopic virtual reality: a new tool for neurosurgical education. Technical note. J Neurosurg 96:144–149
10. Hernes TA, Ommedal S, Lie T, et al (2003) Stereoscopic navigation-controlled display of preoperative MRI and intraoperative 3D ultrasound in planning and guidance of neurosurgery: new technology for minimally invasive image guided surgery approaches. Minim Invasive Neurosurg 46:129–137
11. Hinckley K, Pausch R, Downs JH, et al (1997) The props-based interface for neurosurgical visualization. Stud Health Technol Inform 39:552–562
12. Jannin P, Bouliou A, Journet E, et al (1996) A ray-traced texture mapping for enhanced virtuality in image-guided neurosurgery. Stud Health Technol Inform 29:553–563

13. Jannin P, Fleig OJ, Seigneuret E, et al (2000) A data fusion environment for multimodal and multi-informational neuronavigation. Comput Aided Surg 5:1–10

14. John NW (2002) Using stereoscopy for medical virtual reality. Stud Health Technol Inform 85:214–220

15. Johnson LG, Edwards P, Hawkes D (2003) Surface transparency makes stereo overlays unpredictable: the implications for augmented reality. Stud Health Technol Inform 94:131–136

16. King AP, Edwards PJ, Maurer CR Jr, et al (1999) A system for microscope-assisted guided interventions. Stereotact Funct Neurosurg 72:107–111

17. Kockro RA, Serra L, Tseng-Tsai Y, et al (2000) Planning and simulation of neurosurgery in a virtual reality environment. Neurosurgery 46:118–135

18. Kolstad F, Rygh OM, Selbekk T, et al (2006) Three-dimensional ultrasonography navigation in spinal cord tumor surgery. Technical note. J Neurosurg Spine 5:264–270

19. Larsen OV, Haase J, Ostergaard LR, et al (2001) The Virtual Brain Project –development of a neurosurgical simulator. Stud Health Technol Inform 81:256–262

20. Li Y, Brodlie K, Phillips N (2002) Real-time soft tissue modeling for web-based surgical simulation: Surface Chain Mail. Stud Health Technol Inform 85:261–267

21. Lindseth F, Kaspersen JH, Ommedal S, et al (2003) Multimodal image fusion in ultrasound-based neuronavigation: improving overview and interpretation by integrating preoperative MRI with intraoperative 3D ultrasound. Comput Aided Surg 8:49–69

22. Lindseth F, Lango T, Bang J, et al (2002) Accuracy evaluation of a 3D ultrasound-based neuronavigation system. Comput Aided Surg 7:197–222

23. Miller A, Alien P, Fowler D (2004) In-vivo stereoscopic imaging system with 5 degrees-of-freedom for minimal access surgery. Stud Health Technol Inform 98:234–240

24. Mitchell P, Wilkinson ID, Griffiths PD, et al (2002) A stereoscope for image-guided surgery. Br J Neurosurg 16:261–266

25. Morris K, O'Brien TJ, Cook MJ, et al (2004) A computer-generated stereotactic "Virtual Subdural Grid" to guide resective epilepsy surgery. AJNR Am J Neuroradiol 25:77–83

26. Nimsky C, Ganslandt O, Buchfelder M, et al (2006) Intraoperative visualization for resection of gliomas: the role of functional neuronavigation and intraoperative 1.5 T MRI. Neurol Res 28:482–487

27. Nimsky C, Ganslandt O, Fahlbusch R (2006) Implementation of fiber tract navigation. Neurosurgery 58:ONS 292–303

28. Nimsky C, Ganslandt O, Kober H, et al (1999) Integration of functional magnetic resonance imaging supported by magnetoencephalography in functional neuronavigation. Neurosurgery 44:1249–1255

29. Nimsky C, Grummich P, Sorensen AG, et al (2005) Visualization of the pyramidal tract in glioma surgery by integrating diffusion tensor imaging in functional neuronavigation. Zentralbl Neurochir 66:133–141

30. Pailatrom H, Hartov A, Mclnerney J, et al (1999) Coregistered ultrasound as a neurosurgical guide. Stereotact Funct Neurosurg. 73:143–147

31. Peters TM (2000) Image-guided surgery: from X-rays to virtual reality. Comput Methods Biomech Biomed Engin 4:27–57

32. Peters TM, Henn CJ, Munger P, et al (1994) Integration of stereoscopic DSA and 3D MRI for image-guided neurosurgery. Comput Med Imaging Graph 18:289–299

33. Rachinger J, von Keller B, Ganslandt O, et al (2006) Application accuracy of automatic registration in frameless stereotaxy. Stereotact Funct Neurosurg. 84:109–117

34. Ribas GC, Bento RF, Rodrigues AJ Jr (2001) Anaglyphic three-dimensional stereoscopic printing: revival of an old method for anatomical and surgical teaching and reporting. J Neurosurg 95:1057–1066

35. Rosahl SK, Gharabaghi A, Hubbe U, et al (2006) Virtual reality augmentation in skull base surgery. Skull Base 16:59–66

36. Rygh OM, Cappelen J, Selbekk T, et al (2006) Endoscopy guided by an intraoperative 3D ultrasound-based neuronavigation system. Minim Invasive Neurosurg 49:1–9

37. Sebastiano F, Di Gennaro G, Esposito V, et al (2006) A rapid and reliable procedure to localize subdural electrodes in presurgical evaluation of patients with drug-resistant focal epilepsy. Clin Neurophysiol 117:341–347

38. Serra L, Kockro R, Goh LC, et al (2002) The DextroBeam: a stereoscopic presentation system for volumetric medical data. Stud Health Technol Inform 85:478–484

39. Shahidi R, Bax MR, Maurer CR Jr, et al (2002) Implementation, calibration and accuracy testing of an image-enhanced endoscopy system. IEEE Trans Med Imaging 21:1524–1535

40. Skare S, Andersson JL (2005) Correction of MR image distortions induced by metallic objects using a 3D cubic B-spline basis set: application to stereotactic surgical planning. Magn Reson Med 54:169–181

41. Stredney D, Wiet GJ, Bryan J, et al (2002) Temporal bone dissection simulation – an update. Stud Health Technol Inform 85:507–513

42. Trobaugh JW, Trobaugh DJ, Richard WD (1994) Three-dimensional imaging with stereotactic ultrasonography. Comput Med Imaging Graph 18 :315–323

43. Unsgaard G, Rygh OM, Selbekk T, et al (2006) Intra-operative 3D ultrasound in neurosurgery. Acta Neurochir (Wien) 148:235–253

44. Walton L, Hampshire A, Forster DM, et al (1996) Accuracy of stereotactic localization using magnetic resonance imaging: a comparison between two- and three-dimensional studies. Stereotact Funct Neurosurg 66:49–56

45. Wang D, Doddrell DM, Cowin G (2004) A novel phantom and method for comprehensive 3-dimensional measurement and correction of geometric distortion in magnetic resonance imaging. Magn Reson Imaging 22:529–542

46. West JB, Fitzpatrick JM, Toms SA, Maurer CR, Jr, Maciunas RJ (2001) Fiducial point placement and the accuracy of point-based, rigid body registration. Neurosurgery 48:810–816

47. Wilkinson EP, Shahidi R, Wang B, et al (1999) Remote rendered 3D CT angiography (3DCTA) as an intraoperative aid in cerebrovascular neurosurgery. Comput Aided Surg 4:256–263

48. Winder RI, McKnight W, McRitchie 1, Montgomery D, Wulf J (2006) 3D surface accuracy of CAD generated skull defect contour. Stud Health Technol Inform 119:574–576

# Potential and Limitations of Chronic High-Frequency Deep-Brain Stimulation in Parkinson's Disease

**2**

Jan Vesper and Guido Nikkhah

## Contents

## 2.1
## Introduction

Various stimulation techniques have been employed for treating neurologic disorders since the 1950s [5, 10, 12–16, 19, 21, 23–25, 27, 29, 32, 37, 38, 40, 53, 54, 56, 57, 65, 67–69]. However, lesional procedures were the predominant therapeutic strategy for permanently interrupting conduction pathways, although they were associated with many permanent side effects. Not until the 1980s were devices developed that, similar to pacemakers, allow for continuously stimulating central nervous structures. Such stimulation systems were initially used as spinal cord stimulators in treating chronic pain or spastic disorders. Stimulators for influencing deep areas of the brain or cranial nerves were developed in the late 1980s. Initial experience with treating tremor was gained with continuous stimulation of the ventrolateral thalamus [27, 28, 31, 34, 39, 41, 43, 46, 48, 52, 55, 58, 59, 60, 63, 67]. The components of the neurostimulation system were first tested in scientific studies and, since their certification, have been used by many centers. Since the introduction of deep-brain stimulation (DBS), the indications for this procedure have been extended from treating tremor to akinesia, rigidity, and dystonia [1–4, 6–8, 11 ,18 ,20 ,22, 23, 26, 30, 33–36, 42, 44, 45, 47, 49–52, 57, 62, 64, 66, 68, 70]. Different targets are used for stimulation with the

subthalamic nucleus (STN), playing a key role in treating patients with extrapyramidal motor disorders such as Parkinson's disease.

## 2.2
## Patient Selection and Surgical Technique

DBS was performed in patients with extrapyramidal movement disorders not sufficiently responding to conservative management. Patients with Parkinson's disease were eligible for DBS only if the residual action of levodopa (L-DOPA) still had a notable effect on motor symptoms in the on-state. Patients with multisystem atrophies and with late-stage parkinsonism not showing any effect on L-DOPA administration were excluded. Severe dementia was likewise regarded as a contraindication to surgery. The majority of patients treated by DBS suffered from akinetic rigid forms of Parkinson's disease. In patients with essential tremor, Parkinson tremor, but also in those with cerebellar tremor, the ventral intermediate nucleus (VIM) was used as the target of stimulation. Patients with therapy-resistant types of dystonia (generalized primary and secondary forms) were selected for DBS according to their resistance to drug treatment. However, the indication for surgery was finally based on the impairment of the individual patient's quality of life rather than the scores achieved on the rating scales for individual symptoms. The target of DBS was the STN in 117 patients with a predominance of akinetic rigid symptoms, the VIM of the thalamus in 62 patients with tremor-dominant disorders, and the globus pallidus internus (GPI) in 18 patients with Parkinson's disease (Fig. 1). Surgery was performed in two sessions. In the first step, deep-brain electrodes (models 3387, 3389, Medtronic, Minneapolis, MN, USA) were implanted under local anesthesia after planning on the basis of computed tomography and stereotactic target calculation. The final target was calculated intraoperatively using both neurophysiological techniques and a fusion of various imaging modali-

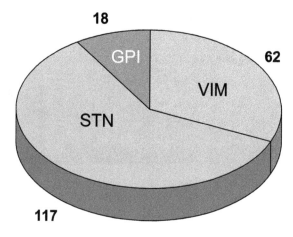

**18**

GPI

**62**

VIM

STN

**117**

Fig. 1 Patients (*n*=197) for deep-brain stimulation. *STN* Sub-thalamic nucleus, *VIM* ventral intermediate nucleus, *GPI* globus pallidus internus

ties. However, final target selection most crucially relies on the results of intraoperative test stimulation, showing both the efficiency of stimulation and the occurrence of adverse effects. If the effects were found to be satisfactory, the electrodes were not connected to an external stimulator. After confirmation of successful stimulation, the final pacemaker was implanted in a second intervention under general anesthesia immediately, either infraclavicularly for unilateral stimulation (Soletra, Medtronic) or abdominally for bilateral stimulation (Kinetra™, Medtronic). The stimulation parameters were adjusted telemetrically in the course of the following 4 weeks (Table 1). The clinical effect was apparent immediately in cases of tremor and rigidity, and occurred within the first few hours of setting or resetting of the stimulator in patients with other symptoms. Tremor reduction was determined using the Essential Tremor Rating Scale (ETRS), and akinetic rigid symptoms were assessed on the Unified Parkinson's Disease Rating Scale (UPDRS) [17]. Assessment of dystonia was done by means of the Burke-Fahn-Marsden Dystonia Rating Scale (BFMDRS) [9].

Statistical evaluation of the results was done by multivariate analysis using the one-way ANOVA rank sum test (Sigmastat 1.0, Jandel Scientific, Chicago, IL, USA).

## 2.3
## Motor Outcome and Complications

Suppression of tremor was similarly successful for resting and postural tremor as well as for action-intention tremor. The etiology of the tremor did not affect the effectiveness of DBS, although other symptoms persisted in multiple sclerosis patients (Fig. 2). The motor symptoms in Parkinson patients also improved significantly (Fig. 3). The Parkinson patients were assessed both "on" and "off" medication as well as "on" and "off" stimulation. Surgery-related adverse events in the form of transient disorientation during bilateral STN stimulation occurred in 16 patients (13%). In two of them (1.8%), the symptoms persisted for some time and required treatment with antipsychotic drugs. Infections were seen in five patients (2.5%). In these cases, the stimulation systems had to be removed and were reimplanted after 6 months. The positive effect of stimulation could be restored in all patients. Intracerebral hemorrhages occurred in two patients. One of them developed permanent contralateral hemiplegia, the other resulted in a permanent neuropsychological deficit.

| Parameter | VIM | GPI | STN |
|---|---|---|---|
| Frequency | 144 | 156 | 133 |
| Pulse width (µs) | 196 | 203 | 98 |
| Amplitude (V) | 2.9 | 3.1 | 3.1 |
| Output (µA) | 83 | 140 | 58 |
| Impedance (Ω) | 1290 | 740 | 997 |

Table 1 Parameter settings for deep-brain stimulation. *VIM* Ventral intermediate nucleus, *GPI* globus pallidus internus, *STN* subthalamic nucleus

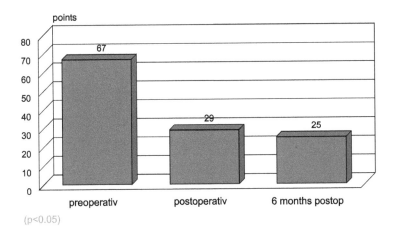

(p<0.05)

Fig. 2  Tremor scale according to Fahn [9] in all patients, significant differences between pre- and postoperative state (*p*<0.001, Wilcoxon's signed-rank test)

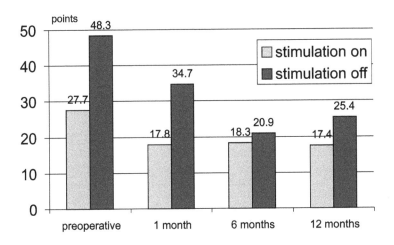

Fig. 3  Unified Parkinson's Disease Rating Scale (UPDRS) scores (medication on; *p*<0.001)

## 2.4
## Discussion

DBS has been shown to be effective in treating the motor symptoms in patients with extrapyramidal movement disorders. Tremor of different origin was suppressed by stimulation of the VIM and STN alike. VIM stimulation and assessment using the ETRS were found to be suitable for essential tremor and cerebellar tremor [66]. Stimulation of the STN should be aimed at in Parkinson patients with tremor as the predominant manifestation because of potential progression of the other motor symptoms, on which VIM stimulation would have no effect. The Parkinson patients were assessed by means of the UPDRS. They showed significant and permanent improvement in

part III of the scale (motor score). Their quality of life also improved considerably on a long-term basis.

Chronic DBS has led to a renaissance of functional neurosurgery. Numerous procedures have been performed in recent years to treat patients with extrapyramidal movement disorders. New methods have decisively improved the targeting accuracy and success rates of stereotactic interventions, and led to new indications for such procedures [61].

The effectiveness of DBS has been confirmed in numerous controlled studies. Adverse events or severe complications are rare. With the advances made in neurophysiologic techniques and imaging modalities, the targets in the basal ganglia can be determined even more reliably. The patients' quality of life is improved ef-

percent (%)

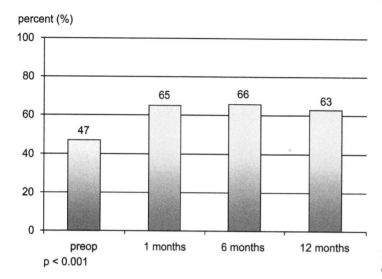

Fig. 4 Activities of daily living scores according to Schwab-England [60]

fectively and permanently. A German multicenter study is currently investigating a potential neuroprotective effect of DBS and its role in the early period of Parkinson's disease.

The indication for DBS may be extended to other neurological disorders such as epilepsy, as suggested by some promising case reports. Studies aimed at investigating this indication in larger patient groups are being prepared.

## 2.5
## Summary and Conclusion

The developments in DBS techniques have let to a significant advancement in the treatment of extrapyramidal motor symptoms. Both tremor and rigidity as well as akinesia can be permanently suppressed by introducing a high-frequency current into different basal ganglia nuclei in diseases like Parkinson's and essential tremor.

Continuous DBS is performed by means of stereotactically implanted quadripolar electrodes in the ventrolateral thalamus, the GPI, or the STN. The current for electrostimulation is supplied by a pulse generator that is implanted subcutaneously in the infraclavicular region in a second procedure (Soletra/Itrel II for unilateral stimulation, Kinetra for bilateral stimulation, Medtronic, USA). The generator is implanted after correct positioning of the electrodes, and their effectiveness has been confirmed by external stimulation. In order to demonstrate the potentials and limitation of DBS in Parkinson disease, the results of 110 patients of our center are provided that were treated with DBS and followed up using standardized rating scales before and after surgery (UPDRS, BFMDRS, and ETRS) [9, 17].

Extrapyramidal symptoms like tremor, rigidity, akinesia, and dystonia are efficiently suppressed by DBS. Fur-

ther studies are ongoing to explore the potential of DBS in treating other types of movement disorders.

Functional neurosurgery has regained significance with the advent of new treatment strategies for various neurological disorders. Continuous high-frequency stimulation effectively and permanently suppresses symptoms of extrapyramidal movement disorders such as tremor, rigidity, akinesia, and dystonia.

## References

1.  Agid Y (1999) Continuous high frequency stimulation of deep brain structures in brain pathology. Brain Res Bull 50:475

2.  Alterman RL, Reiter GT, Shils J, Skolnick B, Arle JE, Lesutis M, Simuni T, Colcher A, Stern M, Hurtig H (1999) Targeting for thalamic deep brain stimulator implantation without computer guidance: assessment of targeting accuracy. Stereotact Funct Neurosurg 72:150–153

3.  Aziz TZ, Bain PG (1999) Deep brain stimulation in Parkinson's disease. J Neurol Neurosurg Psychiatry 67:281

4.  Bejjani BP, Damier P, Arnulf I, Papadopoulos S, Bonnet AM, Vidailhet M, Agid Y, Pidoux B, Cornu P, Dormont D, Marsault C (1998) Deep brain stimulation in Parkinson's disease: opposite effects of stimulation in the pallidum. Mov Disord 13:969–970

5.  Benabid AL (1999) History of stereotaxis. Rev Neurol (Paris) 155:869–877

6.  Benabid AL, Benazzouz A, Hoffmann D, Limousin P, Pollak P (1998) Long-term electrical inhibition of deep brain targets in movement disorders. Mov Disord 13 Suppl 3:119–125

7.  Brown RG, Dowsey PL, Brown P, Jahanshahi M, Pollak P, Benabid AL, Rodriguez-Oroz MC, Obeso J, Rothwell JC (1999) Impact of deep brain stimulation on upper limb akinesia in Parkinson's disease. Ann Neurol 45:473–488

8. Burchiel KJ, Anderson VC, Favre J, Hammerstad JP (1999) Comparison of pallidal and subthalamic nucleus deep brain stimulation for advanced Parkinson's disease: results of a randomized, blinded pilot study . Neurosurgery 45:1375–1382

9. Burke RE, Fahn S, Marsden CD, Bressman SB, Moskowitz C, Friedman J (1985) Validity and reliability of a rating scale for the primary torsion dystonias. Neurology 35:73–77

10. Bushnell MC, Marchand S, Tremblay N, Duncan GH (1991) Electrical stimulation of peripheral and central pathways for the relief of musculoskeletal pain. Can J Physiol Pharmacol 69:697–703

11. Caparros-Lefebvre D, Blond S, N'guyen JP, Pollak P, Benabid AL (1999) Chronic deep brain stimulation for movement disorders. Adv Tech Stand Neurosurg 25:61–136

12. Christiaens JL (1980) Neurosurgery for cancer pain. Bull Cancer 67:222–224

13. Davis KD, Tasker RR, Kiss ZH, Hutchison WD, Dostrovsky JO (1995) Visceral pain evoked by thalamic microstimulation in humans. Neuroreport 6:369–374

14. Dieckmann G, Witzmann A (1982) Initial and long-term results of deep brain stimulation for chronic intractable pain. Appl Neurophysiol 45:167–172

15. Duncan GH, Bushnell MC, Marchand S (1991) Deep brain stimulation: a review of basic research and clinical studies. Pain 45:49–59

16. Ebel H, Rust D, Tronnier V, Boker D, Kunze S (1996) Chronic precentral stimulation in trigeminal neuropathic pain. Acta Neurochir (Wien) 138:1300–1306

17. Fahn S, Elton, R (1987) Members of the UPDRS Development Committee. In: Fahn S, Marsden CD, Calne DB, Goldstein M (eds) Recent Developments in Parkinson's Disease. Macmillan Health Care Information, Florham Park, NJ, pp 153–163, 293–304

18. Fields JA, Troster AI (2000) Cognitive outcomes after deep brain stimulation for Parkinson's disease: a review of initial studies and recommendations for future research. Brain Cogn 42:268–293

19. Frank F, Frank G, Gaist G, Galassi E, Sturiale G, Fabrizi A (1982) Deep brain stimulation in the treatment of chronic pain syndromes. Riv Neurobiol 28:309–316

20. Ghika J, Villemure JG, Fankhauser H, Favre J, Assal G, Ghika-Schmid F (1998) Efficiency and safety of bilateral contemporaneous pallidal stimulation (deep brain stimulation) in levodopa-responsive patients with Parkinson's disease with severe motor fluctuations: a 2-year follow-up review. J Neurosurg 89:713–718

21. Gybels J, Kupers R (1990) Deep brain stimulation in the treatment of chronic pain in man: where and why? Neurophysiol Clin 20:389–398

22. Hubble JP, Busenbark KL, Wilkinson S, Penn RD, Lyons K, Koller WC (1996) Deep brain stimulation for essential tremor. Neurology 46:1150–1153

23. Iacono RP, Linford J, Sandyk R (1987) Pain management after lower extremity amputation. Neurosurgery 20:496–500

24. Katayama Y, Fukaya C, Yamamoto T (1997) Control of poststroke involuntary and voluntary movement disorders with deep brain or epidural cortical stimulation. Stereotact Funct Neurosurg 69:73–79

25. Keay KA, Bandler R (1998) Vascular head pain selectively activates ventrolateral periaqueductal gray in the cat. Neurosci Lett 245:58–60

26. Koller WC, Lyons KE, Wilkinson SB, Pahwa R (1999) Efficacy of unilateral deep brain stimulation of the VIM nucleus of the thalamus for essential head tremor. Mov Disord 14:847–850

27. Krack P, Benazzouz A, Pollak P, Limousin P, Piallat B, Hoffman D, Xie J, Benabid AL (1998) Treatment of tremor in Parkinson's disease by subthalamic nucleus stimulation. Mov Disord 13:907–914

28. Krack P, Poepping M, Weinert D, Schrader B, Deuschl G (2000) Thalamic, pallidal, or subthalamic surgery for Parkinson's disease? J Neurol 247:II122–II134

29. Krainick JU, Thoden U (1976) Methods of pain modulation by electrical stimulation. Langenbecks Arch Chir 342:75–81

30. Krause M, Fogel W, Heck A, Hacke W, Bonsanto M, Trenkwalder C, Tronnier V (2001) Deep brain stimulation for the treatment of Parkinson's disease: subthalamic nucleus versus globus pallidus internus. J Neurol Neurosurg Psychiatry 70:464–470

31. Krauss JK, Mohadjer M, Nobbe F, Mundinger F (1994) The treatment of posttraumatic tremor by stereotactic surgery. Symptomatic and functional outcome in a series of 35 patients. J Neurosurg 80:810–819

32. Kumar K, Wyant GM (1985) Deep brain stimulation for alleviating chronic intractable pain. Can J Surg 28:20–22

33. Kumar R, Dagher A, Hutchison WD, Lang AE, Lozano AM (1999) Globus pallidus deep brain stimulation for generalized dystonia: clinical and PET investigation. Neurology 53:871–874

34. Kumar K, Kelly M, Toth C (2000) Deep brain stimulation of the ventral intermediate nucleus of the thalamus for control of tremors in Parkinson's disease and essential tremor. Stereotact Funct Neurosurg 72:47–61

35. Kumar R, Lozano AM, Kim YJ, Hutchison WD, Sime E, Halket E, Lang AE (1998) Double-blind evaluation of subthalamic nucleus deep brain stimulation in advanced Parkinson's disease. Neurology 51:850–855

36. Kumar R, Lozano AM, Sime E, Halket E, Lang AE (1999) Comparative effects of unilateral and bilateral subthalamic nucleus deep brain stimulation. Neurology 53:561–566

37. Kumar K, Toth C, Nath RK (1997) Deep brain stimulation for intractable pain: a 15-year experience. Neurosurgery 40:736–746

38. Laitinen LV, Bergenheim AT, Hariz MI (1992) Ventroposterolateral pallidotomy can abolish all parkinsonian symptoms. Stereotact Funct Neurosurg 58:14–21

39. Lenz FA, Jaeger CJ, Seike MS, Lin YC, Reich SG, DeLong MR, Vitek JL (1999) Thalamic single neuron activity in patients with dystonia: dystonia-related activity and somatic sensory reorganization. J Neurophysiol 82:2372–2392

40. Levy RM, Lamb S, Adams JE (1987) Treatment of chronic pain by deep brain stimulation: long term follow-up and review of the literature. Neurosurgery 21:885–893

41. Limousin-Dowsey P, Pollak P, Van Blercom N, Krack P, Benazzouz A, Benabid AL (1999) Thalamic, subthalamic nucleus and internal pallidum stimulation in Parkinson's disease. J Neurol 246:II42–II45

42. Lopiano L, Rizzone M, Bergamasco B, Tavella A, Torre E, Prozzo P, Valentini MC, Lanotte M (2001) Deep brain stimulation of the subthalamic nucleus: clinical effectiveness and safety. Neurology 56:552–554

43. Marjama-Lyons J, Koller W (2000) Tremor-predominant Parkinson's disease. Approaches to treatment. Drugs Aging 16:273–278

44. Mobin F, De Salles AA, Behnke EJ, Frysinger R (1999) Correlation between MRI-based stereotactic thalamic deep brain stimulation electrode placement, macroelectrode stimulation and clinical response to tremor control. Stereotact Funct Neurosurg 72:225–232

45. Montgomery EB Jr (1999) Deep brain stimulation reduces symptoms of Parkinson disease. Cleve Clin J Med 66:9–11

46. Ohye C, Shibazaki T, Hirato M, Kawashima Y, Matsumura M (1990) Strategy of selective VIM thalamotomy guided by microrecording. Stereotact Funct Neurosurg 54–55:186–191

47. Olanow CW, Brin MF, Obeso JA (2000) The role of deep brain stimulation as a surgical treatment for Parkinson's disease. Neurology 55:S60–S66

48. Ondo W, Almaguer M, Jankovic J, Simpson RK (2001) Thalamic deep brain stimulation: comparison between unilateral and bilateral placement. Arch Neurol 58:218–222

49. Ondo W, Jankovic J, Schwartz K, Almaguer M, Simpson RK (1998) Unilateral thalamic deep brain stimulation for refractory essential tremor and Parkinson's disease tremor. Neurology 51:1063–1069

50. Pierantozzi M, Mazzone P, Bassi A, Rossini PM, Peppe A, Altibrandi MG, Stefani A, Bernardi G, Stanzione P (1999) The effect of deep brain stimulation on the frontal N30 component of somatosensory evoked potentials in advanced Parkinson's disease patients. Clin Neurophysiol 110:1700–1707

51. Pinter MM, Alesch F, Murg M, Seiwald M, Helscher RJ, Binder H (1999) Deep brain stimulation of the subthalamic nucleus for control of extrapyramidal features in advanced idiopathic parkinson's disease: one year follow-up. J Neural Transm 106:693–709

52. Pinter MM, Murg M, Alesch F, Helscher RJ, Binder H (1999) Does deep brain stimulation of the nucleus ventralis intermedius affect postural control and locomotion in Parkinson's disease? Mov Disord 14:958–963

53. Plotkin R (1982) Results in 60 cases of deep brain stimulation for chronic intractable pain. Appl Neurophysiol 45:173–178

54. Ray CD, Burton CV (1980) Deep brain stimulation for severe, chronic pain. Acta Neurochir Suppl (Wien) 30:289–293

55. Rezai AR, Lozano AM, Crawley AP, Joy ML, Davis KD, Kwan CL, Dostrovsky JO, Tasker RR, Mikulis DJ (1999) Thalamic stimulation and functional magnetic resonance imaging: localization of cortical and subcortical activation with implanted electrodes. Technical note. J Neurosurg 90:583–590

56. Richardson DE (1995) Deep brain stimulation for the relief of chronic pain. Neurosurg Clin N Am 6:135–144

57. Rosenfeld JV (2001) Deep brain stimulation is superior to ablative surgery for Parkinson's disease: moderator's view. J Clin Neurosci 8:293–294

58. Schulder M, Sernas T, Mahalick D, Adler R, Cook S (1999) Thalamic stimulation in patients with multiple sclerosis. Stereotact Funct Neurosurg 72:196–201

59. Schuurman PR, Bosch DA, Bossuyt PM, Bonsel GJ, van Someren EJ, de Bie RM, Merkus MP, Speelman JD (2000) A comparison of continuous thalamic stimulation and thalamotomy for suppression of severe tremor. N Engl J Med 342:461–468

60. Schwab RS, England AD Jr (1969) Projection technique for evaluating surgery in Parkinson's disease. In: Gillingham FJ, Donaldson IML (eds) Third Symposium on Parkinson's Disease, Royal College of Surgeons in Edinburgh, May 20–22, 1968. Livingstone, Edinburgh, pp 152–157

61. Siegfried J, Lazorthes Y, Sedan R (1980) Indications and ethical considerations of deep brain stimulation. Acta Neurochir Suppl (Wien) 30:269–274

62. Starr PA, Vitek JL, Bakay RA (1998) Ablative surgery and deep brain stimulation for Parkinson's disease. Neurosurgery 43:989–1013

63. Taha JM, Janszen MA, Favre J (1999) Thalamic deep brain stimulation for the treatment of head, voice, and bilateral limb tremor. J Neurosurg 91:68–72

64. Tasker RR (1998) Deep brain stimulation is preferable to thalamotomy for tremor suppression. Surg Neurol 49:145–153

65. Tasker RR, Vilela FO (1995) Deep brain stimulation for neuropathic pain. Stereotact Funct Neurosurg 65:122–124

66. Vesper J, Funk T, Kern BC, Wagner F, Straschill M, Brock M (2000) Thalamic deep brain stimulation: present state of the art. Neurosurg Q 4:252–260

67. Watanabe S, Kakigi R, Koyama S, Hoshiyama M, Kaneoke Y (1998) Pain processing traced by magnetoencephalography in the human brain. Brain Topogr 10:255–264

68. Wihl G, Volkmann J, Allert N, Lehrke R, Sturm V, Freund HJ (2001) Deep brain stimulation of the internal pallidum did not improve chorea in a patient with neuro-acanthocytosis. Mov Disord 16:572–575

69. Yamamoto M, Kachi T, Igata A (1995) Pain-related and electrically stimulated somatosensory evoked potentials in patients with stroke. Stroke 26:426–429

70. Yoon MS, Munz M (1999) Placement of deep brain stimulators into the subthalamic nucleus. Stereotact Funct Neurosurg 72:145–149

# Proliferation Behaviour of Meningiomas

**3**

Florian Roser

## Contents

## 3.1
## Introduction

Although generally considered benign, the biological behaviour of meningiomas varies considerably. The microscopic histopathological classification of the World Health Organization (WHO) cannot entirely predict the clinical behaviour of these tumours [23]. Between 7 and 32% of benign meningiomas recur after total resection, and between 19 and 50% (or more) after subtotal removal [10, 18]. Quantifying the proliferative potential may help to predict the biological behaviour of individual tumours of comparable histology. The prognostic significance of various proliferative indices in meningiomas has already been assessed, and it has been suggested that the tumour proliferative potential can predict the patient's clinical course [2, 16, 20, 33, 36, 39, 42, 44]. The nuclear antigen Ki-67 expressed by proliferating cells has become available for routinely processed paraffin sections [7, 13]. The Mib-1 antibody detects an epitope on the Ki-67 antigen, a nuclear protein present only during active phases of the cell cycle (G1, S, G2 and M). The higher incidence of meningiomas among women, their behaviour during pregnancy and the reported epidemiological link between meningiomas and breast carcinomas have led to the assumption that sex steroid hormones influence the growth of meningiomas [29, 35]. Supported by promising results in breast cancer therapy, new chemotherapeutic approaches based on hormone manipulation have been tested in meningioma patients [26]. Decisions regarding patient management therefore rely on a variety of clinical, radiological and pathological prognosticators, as the clinical behaviour of meningiomas with a tendency to recur led to the assumption that meningiomas cannot be classified as a benign entity, despite their pathological classification.

## 3.2
## Materials and Methods

A total of 1766 meningiomas were treated on from 1979 to 2002 at the Neurosurgical Department, Klinikum Hannover, Nordstadt, Germany. All of these tumours were analysed according to the current WHO classification. Five hundred and eighty-eight paraffin blocks of 554 patients with intracranial meningiomas, operated at the Neurosurgical Department between 1990 and 2000, were randomly retrieved from the archives of the Department of Pathology for immunohistochemical analysis. All of these patients were followed for a median of 74 months or until death. The material included 20 patients with neurofibromatosis type-2 (NF-II) disease (for a total of 28 tumours).

Meningioma subtypes were defined according to the new WHO classification. Immunohistochemistry was performed with paraffin sections using Anti-Mib-1 and Anti-human progesterone receptor (PR) 1A6. For Ki-67, the area of densest staining ("hot spot") was searched for and counting was performed in 10 contiguous fields. The average of the results in these fields determined the proliferative index (LI). The PR status was determined by a semi-quantitative scoring scale according to the immunoreactive score (IRS) of Remmele et al., with respect to staining intensity and percentage of positive tumour cells [46]. Tumours with an IRS of 2 and more were considered receptor positive (Table 1).

## 3.3
## Results

The mean Mib-1 LI in male patients was 5.8%, whereas that of female patients was 3.9%; patients with NF-II showed a significantly higher mean Ki-67 LI (6.2%). The Ki-67 LI in WHO grade I tumours was significantly lower than in WHO grades II (atypical) and III (anaplastic) tumours ($p<0.0001$), but not within the subclassifications of WHO grading (meningotheliomatous 3.3%, fibrous

Table 1 Evaluation of progesterone receptor (PR) staining (according to Remmele et al. [30]). *IRS* Immunoreactive score

| Progesterone receptor status | | | |
|---|---|---|---|
| [a]IRS= | Staining intensity | × | Percentage of positive cells |
| | 0 = absent | | 1 = <10% |
| | 1 = weak | | 2 = 10–50% |
| | 2 = moderate | | 3 = 51–80% |
| | 3 = strong | | 4 = >80% |

[a]An IRS of >2 is considered PR positive

3.9%, transitional 2.9%, psammomatous 1.1%, angiomatous 3.0%, clear cell 0.7% or microcystic meningiomas 4.4%; Table 2). First-time-treated meningiomas had a mean Ki-67 LI of 3.9%, versus 6.9% in recurrent meningiomas ($p<0.0001$). Ki-67 LI increased from the initial tumour operation to its second, third, and in five cases to its fourth local recurrence. There was a transformation from benign to atypical meningioma from the second to third local recurrence in 16% of the cases, whereas no dedifferentiation from WHO grade I to type III or WHO grade II to WHO grade III has been seen (Fig. 1). Significantly

lower PR expression in WHO grades II (atypical) and III (anaplastic) meningiomas, compared to WHO grade I meningiomas.

Excluding WHO grades II and III meningiomas, as well as partially resected meningiomas for survival analysis, in WHO grade I and SI resected meningiomas, no significant difference in survival according to different mean Ki-67 LI nor PR status has been found. Combining two factors of proposed prognostic significance in benign meningiomas – LI (Ki-67 LI<4% vs. ≥4%) and PR-Status (negative vs. positive) – a significant decreased recurrence free survival could be shown for negative PR status and Ki-67 LI ≥4% (Fig. 2).

For proliferation and PR status analysis, multiple age groups for each gender were examined (<40 years, 41–55 years, 56–70 years, and >70 years), but no significant differences were found between them (Fig. 3). No relationship between the calcifications, meningioma subtype or LI could be established. Although recurrent meningiomas exhibit higher proliferation rates in general, no age dependency has been seen (Table 3).

## 3.4
## Discussion

Meningiomas are mostly benign tumours that do not usually invade the brain parenchyma. The WHO grading system, which aims to describe different types of tumour,

Table 2 World Health Organization (WHO) grading of 1766 meningiomas operated between 1979 and 2002

| WHO Grading | Young (<70 years) n=1544 | | Aged (≥70 years) n=222 | |
|---|---|---|---|---|
| | Female n=1088 | Male n=456 | Female n=162 | Male n=60 |
| **I** | 92.2% (1424) | | 91.9% (204) | |
| Meningotheliomatous | 63.8% (694) | 58.6% (267) | 54.9% (89) | 58.3% (35) |
| Fibrous | 13.1% (142) | 11.2% (51) | 13.6% (22) | 8.3% (5) |
| Transitional | 11.0% (120) | 8.1% (37) | 11.1% (18) | 8.3% (5) |
| Psammomatous | 5.2% (57) | 2.6% (12) | 11.1% (18) | 10.0% (6) |
| Other types | 2.2% (24) | 4.4% (20) | 1.9% (3) | 5.0% (3) |
| **II** | 6.4% (99) | | 7.2% (16) | |
| Atypical (including clear cell, secretory) | 4.0% (43) | 12.3% (56) | 6.8% (11) | 8.3% (5) |
| **III** | 1.4% (21) | | 0.9% (2) | |
| Anaplastic | 0.7% (8) | 2.9% (13) | 0.6% (1) | 1.7% (1) |

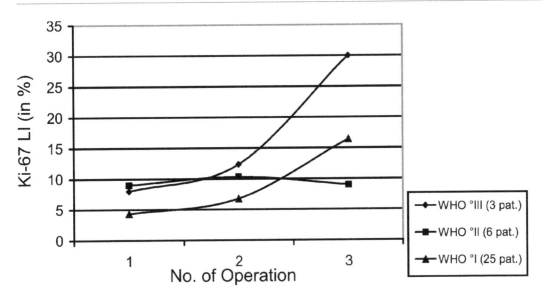

Fig. 1 Individual proliferation in local recurrence of meningioma patients. *WHO* World Health Organization, *pat.* Patients, *LI* proliferative index

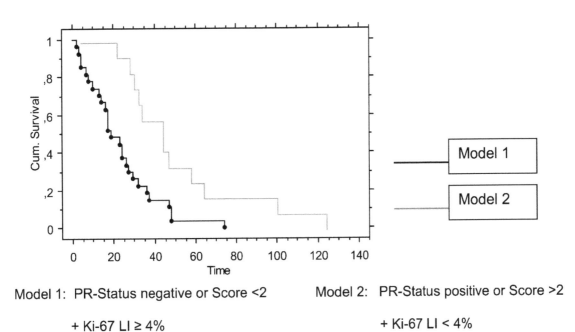

Model 1:  PR-Status negative or Score <2        Model 2:  PR-Status positive or Score >2

+ Ki-67 LI ≥ 4%                                         + Ki-67 LI < 4%

Fig. 2 Recurrence free survival II. Kaplan-Meyer cumulative hazard plot for new recurrence. A model of two prognostic factors considering prognosis in totally removed meningiomas (Simpson I +II). The time scale is months. *PR* Progesterone status

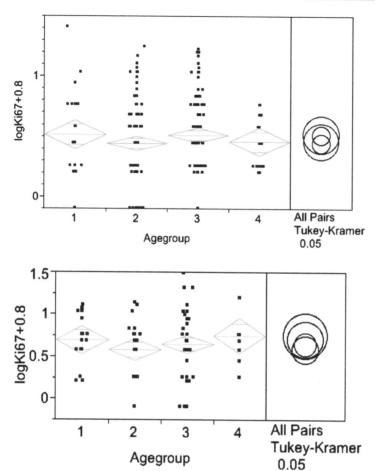

Fig. 3 Statistical analysis of Ki-67 distribution in different age groups: 1=<40 years, 2=41–55 years, 3=56–70 years, 4=>70 years) and separated according to gender (females on the left, males on the right)

frequently fails to determine the clinical behaviour of meningiomas. Even in cases of complete removal according to the Simpson classification, the chance of recurrence is high [53]. Pathological specimens in those cases do not show either atypical features or histopathological signs of increased biological activity. Proliferation markers like BrdU or AgNOR have been used to describe the clinical course in meningioma patients [25, 52]. New biochemical markers like topoisomerase II-α, telomerase or apop-

totic fragmentation reflect meningioma behaviour when considered in conjunction with morphological grading, but they all describe the biological activity in atypical and anaplastic meningiomas better than predicting the recurrence potential in benign meningiomas [11, 28, 31]. Several authors have demonstrated the reliability of the Mib-1 monoclonal antibody, which stains the Ki-67 antigen, in analysing meningioma growth and recurrence [2, 34, 38, 39, 44, 48, 50]. Møller and Braendstrup separated

Table 3  T-test values of recurrent versus non-recurrent meningiomas in the two age groups, with respect to their proliferation status (Ki-67)

| Aged – no recurrence n=38 | 0.41 | Aged – recurrence n=3 |
|---|---|---|
| 0.31 | | 0.31 |
| Young – no recurrence n=314 | 0.02 | Young – recurrence n=30 |

different resection grades and histology before survival analysis in 25 cases and could not give any significant prediction with Ki-67 immunohistochemistry as well [36]. Abramovich and Prayson reported the absence of a significant difference in proliferation in 59 meningioma patients that had been radically operated, recognising a clear overlap in the index range between the groups [2]. On the contrary, Ohta et al. showed a correlation with recurrence-free interval in 42 patients, but the follow-up time was 60 months and the statistics were performed without dividing the meningiomas according to the WHO classification [42]. Perry et al. showed values for interpretation of borderline atypical meningiomas in 425 meningiomas through multivariate analysis [44]: brain invasion, mitosis count >3/10 and a mean Ki-67 LI >4.2% correlated with decreased recurrent-free survival. Matsuno et al. and Nakasu et al. reported a 3.2% and 3% cut-off point, respectively, for higher recurrence tendency [34, 39]. However, 20–50% of the recurrent meningioma group were atypical, and all non-recurrent meningiomas were WHO grade I. Survival analysis was performed taking all patients together without dividing for surgical resection or histological grade. The small number of patients in each group and the uneven distribution of histological grades might have additionally influenced the mean LI and the survival analysis. Failing to separate different histopathological and resection grades exposed these studies to the criticism that Ki-67 may simply describe a well-known phenomenon, in other words that more aggressive histology and less aggressive regression correlate with shorter disease-free survival times.

The LI value did not show any differences concerning sex or age analysis, but NF2 patients showed significant higher levels. This may reflect differences in molecular biology between sporadic and NF2 meningiomas and may be related to an earlier onset, multiplicity or more aggressive behaviour of NF2 tumours [3]. The LI in 45 atypical and 12 anaplastic meningiomas in the Nordstadt series was higher than in benign meningiomas, and reflects the aggressive histopathology described as increased vascularity and mitosis, a loss of architectural pattern, prominent nucleoli, nuclear polymorphism and necrosis [1, 17].

Although embolisation of meningiomas has been performed for many years as an preoperative adjunct to reduce tumour vascularity and facilitate surgical excision, it may potentially cause an erroneous diagnosis of a high-grade lesion due to the fact that it may produce tumour necrosis. Increase in MIB-1 labelling indices in those tumours exhibiting necrotic foci has been demonstrated, but it did not have any prognostic significance [41, 43].

Genetic alterations can explain biologic progression. Next to chromosome 22 anomalies, deletions of the short arm of chromosome 1 have previously been described as the most frequent alterations detected by cytogenetic analysis of meningiomas. Deletion of 1p, and therefore enzyme activity loss of tissue non-specific alkaline phosphatase, has been proposed to be associated with the development of atypical and anaplastic meningiomas [4]. The frequency of loss of heterogeneity on chromosomes 1p, 10q and 22 increases with tumour grade, which would support the concept that aggressive meningiomas develop through tumour progression [37]. Attempts were also made to predict recurrence in benign meningiomas, combining cytogenetics and histology through a multimodal approach [21].

The significant correlation of high vascularity and high Ki-67 LI suggest the neoangeogenetic capability of meningiomas and might account for higher proliferation in these tumours, as reflected by Ki-67 [5]. Meningioma cells inherit the capability to induce vessel formation via a paracrine mechanism, involving molecules like vascular endothelial growth factor (VEGF) and VEGF receptors.

Elevated proliferative activity in recurrent meningiomas throughout the histological grouping has been shown [2, 34, 36, 39, 42]. A decrease in the LI has only been reported by Madsen and Schroder [30]. Caution is recommended when using the LI as the sole prognostic indicator or as a substitute for morphological diagnosis due to the overlap in each group (WHO grade I mean Ki-67 LI 0–30%, WHO grade II mean Ki-67 LI 3–35% or WHO grade III mean Ki-67 LI 5–58%) [19, 24, 27]. This might be due to the heterogeneity of biologic activity within the tumour tissue. Proliferating cells in all histological grades were found to be distributed heterogeneously throughout the tumour, especially in recurrences [42]. It is debatable that the focal accumulation of proliferation may affect tumour recurrence for the "highest-area" counting method. The highest-area counting method is preferred to minimise missing of focal accumulation of biological activity within the meningioma tissue, as recommended by Nakasu et al. [39]. This is an important issue when considering modern neurosurgical techniques, where only small parts of tumour with unknown precise location of the tissue reach the pathologist's hands. Indeed, it is debatable whether recognised areas of high mitotic activity in meningiomas determined with either counting method, reflect the proliferation status of the whole tumour.

A substantial number of patients inherit mean Ki-67 LI of 1% with recurrence times ranging from 11 to 148 months. Therefore, a cut-off value over which a tumour becomes suspicious cannot be given. Precise values from different laboratories are not applicable to other institutions because of differences in methodology, counting procedures and interpretation of the results as reflected by the relatively wide range of initial and recurrent Ki-67 LI determined by several investigators.

The role of steroid hormones in the progression of meningiomas remains a matter of controversy. Several studies, which included meningiomas of all grades, suggested a more favourable prognosis for PR-positive meningiomas [8, 14, 15] with high PR status being associated with lower recurrence rates and vice versa [12, 49]. However, these studies frequently included meningiomas with different resection grades and histological subtypes.

Hsu and colleagues suggested that only a combination of three proposed prognostic factors for survival, that is WHO grade, LI and PR status, should be used to predict meningioma recurrence [15]. However, their model was tested containing atypical and malignant meningiomas and therefore did not demonstrate the true influence of PR status on survival. The focus of interest should be benign borderline cases where additional information is needed for prognostic considerations. Studying the prognostic factors strictly among benign meningiomas, statistical evidence for the influence of PR status on survival was found only in combination with the proliferation marker Ki-67. However, no relationship between PR status and variables like age, tumour location, first-time resection versus re-operation, and histological subtype has been found in the literature, including the latest studies. Data in the literature suggest a female preponderance in PR expression; however, these studies included a substantial number of atypical and malignant meningiomas [9, 12, 22, 51]. These meningiomas are mostly devoid of PRs and are more often found among male patients. After excluding atypical and malignant cases, no gender-related difference in PR expression could be found. Therefore, the previously reported gender-related difference might be due to particular selection criteria, which produced an inhomogeneous patient population.

Previous studies on the human endometrium have shown that progesterone plays a role in neovasculogenesis. High levels of PRs in meningiomas may indicate a similar situation. However, Fewings et al. [12] and Roser et al. [49] suggested that progesterone inhibits angiogenesis by enhancing the production of thrombospondin-1, an angiogenesis inhibitor. It is difficult to draw conclusions from these data, as the PRs in meningiomas are non-functional in the majority of cases [6]. Moreover, our observations come from a clinical and histopathological analysis and may well reflect a multifactorial situation, with progesterone being only one variable in the process of tumour vascularisation.

However, the PR status alone cannot be used to predict behaviour in benign meningiomas and should not influence the decision about follow-up intervals and therapeutic strategies. Moreover, Matsuda et al. demonstrated that the antitumoural effect of antiprogesterone agents on meningiomas, both in vitro and in vivo, exists regardless of the tumour's PR status, suggesting that the antitumoural effect is mediated by other pathways [32]. This was supported by Verheijen and co-workers, who suggested that PR-like proteins do not have a biological function and may lead to the overestimation of the PR status for clinical purposes [54].

In an analysis of Ki-67 LI and PR status in spinal versus intracranial meningiomas, the former was found to be higher in spinal disease (the latter being almost identical) [47]. These findings were compared with recurrence-free survival at follow up to determine if a relationship between these two biological indicators and clinical behaviour of the tumours could be seen. However, recurrence-free survival after total tumour resection was found to be similar in both patients groups. The data suggest that spinal meningiomas differ from their intracranial counterpart in terms of proliferation as measured by the Ki-67 LI; however, they display similar clinical behaviour and PR status. The discrepancy between the Ki-67 LI and recurrence rates cannot be fully explained on the basis of the present data.

The variety and distribution of benign meningioma subtypes is age independent, with the exception of a higher percentage of psammomatous meningiomas among older patients [50]. Phillipon et al. have suggested the higher percentage of calcified psammomatous meningiomas as a reason for lower recurrence rates in meningiomas [45]. Indeed, we found a significantly higher percentage of psammomatous meningiomas in the elderly, but a relationship between psammomatous bodies and intratumoural calcification could not be established. Moreover, psammomatous meningiomas did not display lower proliferation rates than other benign subtypes. Proliferation rates and PR status, useful biological indicators of tumour activity, are age independent [50]. Survival measurements showed comparable outcome in the both age groups within benign meningiomas. Different growth rates in different age groups cannot be explained by means of these two parameters alone.

Ongoing tissue research studies should focus on the growth behaviour of benign meningiomas to characterise specific alterations that could provide us with new diagnostic and prognostic criteria as a rational basis for treatment. The unsolved situation of clinically aggressive benign meningiomas (despite radiotherapy) should lead us to new concepts like chemotherapeutic agents, which might play a role as radiosensitisers [40].

In histopathological borderline cases, with some but not convincing aspects of atypia, the Ki-67 LI, combined with the routine histopathological workup can provide more insight into the behaviour of a meningioma, particularly in the presence of high vascularity, low PR status, subtotal resection and recurrence. PR status in combination with the LI can be a useful prognostic tool for benign meningiomas. High scores of Ki-67 are worrisome and should lead to a closer follow up for evidence of recurrent tumour, but the confidence in a high LI should not interfere the decisions for treatment plans, as some authors recommend.

## References

1.  Abramovich CM, Prayson RA (1998) MIB-1 labeling indices in benign, aggressive, and malignant meningiomas: a study of 90 tumors. Hum Pathol 29:1420–1427
2.  Abramovich CM, Prayson RA (1999) Histopathologic features and MIB-1 labeling indices in recurrent and nonrecurrent meningiomas. Arch Pathol Lab Med 123:793–800

3. Antinheimo J, Haapasalo H, Haltia M, et al (1997) Proliferation potential and histological features in neurofibromatosis 2-associated and sporadic meningiomas. J Neurosurg 87:610–614

4. Bello MJ, de Campos JM, Vaquero J, et al (2000) High-resolution analysis of chromosome arm 1p alterations in meningioma. Cancer Genet Cytogenet 120:30–36

5. Bitzer M, Opitz H, Popp J, et al (1998) Angiogenesis and brain oedema in intracranial meningiomas: influence of vascular endothelial growth factor. Acta Neurochir (Wien) 140:333–340

6. Blankenstein MA, Verheijen FM, Jacobs JM, et al (2000) Occurrence, regulation, and significance of progesterone receptors in human meningioma. Steroids 65:795–800

7. Boker DK, Meurer H, Gullotta F (1985) Recurring intracranial meningiomas. Evaluation of some factors predisposing for tumor recurrence. J Neurosurg Sci 29:11–17

8. Brandis A, Mirzai S, Tatagiba M, et al (1993) Immunohistochemical detection of female sex hormone receptors in meningiomas: correlation with clinical and histological features. Neurosurgery 33:212–217

9. Carroll RS, Glowacka D, Dashner K, et al (1993) Progesterone receptor expression in meningiomas. Cancer Res 53:1312–1316

10. Crompton MR, Gautier-Smith PC (1970) The prediction of recurrence in meningiomas. J Neurol Neurosurg Psychiatry 33:80–87

11. Falchetti ML, Pallini R, Larocca LM, et al (1999) Telomerase expression in intracranial tumours: prognostic potential for malignant gliomas and meningiomas. J Clin Pathol 52:234–236

12. Fewings PE, Battersby RD, Timperley WR (2000) Long-term follow up of progesterone receptor status in benign meningioma: a prognostic indicator of recurrence? J Neurosurg 92:401–405

13. Gerdes J, Becker MH, Key G, et al (1992) Immunohistological detection of tumour growth fraction (Ki-67 antigen) in formalin-fixed and routinely processed tissues. J Pathol 168:85–86

14. Gursan N, Gundogdu C, Albayrak A, et al (2002) Immunohistochemical detection of progesterone receptors and the correlation with Ki-67 labeling indices in paraffin-embedded sections of meningiomas. Int J Neurosci 112:463–470

15. Hsu DW, Efird JT, Hedley-Whyte ET (1997) Progesterone and estrogen receptors in meningiomas: prognostic considerations. J Neurosurg 86:113–120

16. Hsu DW, Efird JT, Hedley-Whyte ET (1998) MIB-1 (Ki-67) index and transforming growth factor-alpha (TGF alpha) immunoreactivity are significant prognostic predictors for meningiomas. Neuropathol Appl Neurobiol 24:441–452

17. Jaaskelainen J, Haltia M, Servo A (1986) Atypical and anaplastic meningiomas: radiology, surgery, radiotherapy, and outcome. Surg Neurol 25:233–242

18. Jellinger K, Denk H (1974) Blood group isoantigens in angioblastic meningiomas and hemangioblastomas of the central nervous system. Virchows Arch A Pathol Anat Histol 364:137–144

19. Karamitopoulou E, Perentes E, Diamantis I and Maraziotis T (1994) Ki-67 immunoreactivity in human central nervous system tumors: a study with MIB 1 monoclonal antibody on archival material. Acta Neuropathol (Berl) 87:47–54

20. Karamitopoulou E, Perentes E, Tolnay M, et al (1998) Prognostic significance of MIB-1, p53, and bcl-2 immunoreactivity in meningiomas. Hum Pathol 29:140–145

21. Ketter R, Henn W, Niedermayer I, et al (2001) Predictive value of progression-associated chromosomal aberrations for the prognosis of meningiomas: a retrospective study of 198 cases. J Neurosurg 95:601–607

22. Khalid H (1994) Immunohistochemical study of estrogen receptor-related antigen, progesterone and estrogen receptors in human intracranial meningiomas. Cancer 74:679–685

23. Kleihues P, Burger PC, Scheithauer B (1993) The new WHO classification of brain tumors. Brain Pathol 3:255–268

24. Kolles H, Niedermayer I, Schmitt C, et al (1995) Triple approach for diagnosis and grading of meningiomas: histology, morphometry of Ki-67/Feulgen stainings, and cytogenetics. Acta Neurochir (Wien) 137:174–181

25. Kunishio K, Ohmoto T, Matsuhisa T, et al (1994) The significance of nucleolar organizer region (AgNOR) score in predicting meningioma recurrence [see comments]. Cancer 73:2200–2205

26. Lamberts SW, Tanghe HL, Avezaat CJ, et al (1992) Mifepristone (RU 486) treatment of meningiomas. J Neurol Neurosurg Psychiatry 55:486–490

27. Langford LA, Cooksley CS, DeMonte F (1996) Comparison of MIB-1 (Ki-67) antigen and bromodeoxyuridine proliferation indices in meningiomas. Hum Pathol 27:350–354

28. Langford LA, Piatyszek MA, Xu R, et al (1997) Telomerase activity in ordinary meningiomas predicts poor outcome. Hum Pathol 28:416–420

29. Lieu AS, Hwang SL, Howng SL (2003) Intracranial meningioma and breast cancer. J Clin Neurosci 10:553–556

30. Madsen C, Schroder HD (1997) Ki-67 immunoreactivity in meningiomas – determination of the proliferative potential of meningiomas using the monoclonal antibody Ki-67. Clin Neuropathol 16:137–142

31. Maier H, Wanschitz J, Sedivy R, et al (1997) Proliferation and DNA fragmentation in meningioma subtypes. Neuropathol Appl Neurobiol 23:496–506

32. Matsuda Y, Kawamoto K, Kiya K, et al (1994) Antitumor effects of antiprogesterones on human meningioma cells in vitro and in vivo. J Neurosurg 80:527–534

33. Matsuno A, Fujimaki T, Sasaki T, et al (1996a) Clinical and histopathological analysis of proliferative potentials of recurrent and non-recurrent meningiomas. Acta Neuropathol (Berl) 91:504–510

34. Matsuno A, Nagashima T, Matsuura R, et al (1996b) Correlation between MIB-1 staining index and the immunoreactivity of p53 protein in recurrent and non-recurrent meningiomas. Am J Clin Pathol 106:776–781

35. Michelsen JJ, New PF (1969) Brain tumour and pregnancy. J Neurol Neurosurg Psychiatry 32:305–307

36. Moller ML, Braendstrup O (1997) No prediction of recurrence of meningiomas by PCNA and Ki-67 immunohistochemistry. J Neurooncol 34:241–246

37. Muller P, Henn W, Niedermayer I, et al (1999) Deletion of chromosome 1p and loss of expression of alkaline phosphatase indicate progression of meningiomas. Clin Cancer Res 5:3569–3577

38. Nakaguchi H, Fujimaki T, Matsuno A, et al (1999) Postoperative residual tumor growth of meningioma can be predicted by MIB-1 immunohistochemistry. Cancer 85:2249–2254

39. Nakasu S, Li DH, Okabe H, et al (2001) Significance of MIB-1 staining indices in meningiomas: comparison of two counting methods. Am J Surg Pathol 25:472–478

40. Nathoo N, Barnett GH, Golubic M (2004) The eicosanoid cascade: possible role in gliomas and meningiomas. J Clin Pathol 57:6–13

41. Ng HK, Poon WS, Goh K, et al (1996) Histopathology of post-embolized meningiomas. Am J Surg Pathol 20:1224–1230

42. Ohta M, Iwaki T, Kitamoto T, et al (1994) MIB1 staining index and scoring of histologic features in meningioma. Indicators for the prediction of biologic potential and postoperative management. Cancer 74:3176–3189

43. Paulus W, Meixensberger J, Hofmann E, et al (1993) Effect of embolisation of meningioma on Ki-67 proliferation index. J Clin Pathol 46:876–877

44. Perry A, Stafford SL, Scheithauer BW, et al (1998) The prognostic significance of MIB-1, p53, and DNA flow cytometry in completely resected primary meningiomas. Cancer 82:2262–2269

45. Philippon J, Cornu P, Grob R, et al (1986) Les meningiomes recidivantes. Neurochirurgie 32:54–62

46. Remmele W, Stegner HE (1987) [Recommendation for uniform definition of an immunoreactive score (IRS) for immunohistochemical estrogen receptor detection (ER-ICA) in breast cancer tissue]. Pathologe 8:138–140

47. Roser F, Nakamura M, Bellinzona M (2006) Proliferation potential of spinal meningiomas. Eur Spine J 15:211–215

48. Roser F, Samii M, Ostertag H, et al (2004a) The Ki-67 proliferation antigen in meningiomas. Experience in 600 cases. Acta Neurochir (Wien) 146:37–44

49. Roser F, Nakamura M, Bellinzona M, et al (2004b) The prognostic value of progesterone receptor status in meningiomas. J Clin Pathol 57:1033–1037

50. Roser F, Nakamura M, Ritz R, et al (2005) Proliferation and progesterone receptor status in benign meningiomas are not age dependent. Cancer 104:598–601

51. Schrell UM, Adams EF, Fahlbusch R, et al (1990) Hormonal dependency of cerebral meningiomas. Part 1: Female sex steroid receptors and their significance as specific markers for adjuvant medical therapy. J Neurosurg 73:743–749

52. Shibuya M, Hoshino T, Ito S, et al (1992) Meningiomas: clinical implications of a high proliferative potential determined by bromodeoxyuridine labeling. Neurosurgery 30:494–497

53. Simpson D (1957) The recurrence of intracranial meningiomas after surgical treatment. J Neurol Neurosurg Psychiatry 20:22–39

54. Verheijen FM, Donker GH, Viera CS, et al (2002) Progesterone receptor, bcl-2 and bax expression in meningiomas. J Neurooncol 56:35–41

# Neural Transplantation and Restoration of Motor Behaviour in Parkinson's Disease

**4**

Alexander Klein and Guido Nikkhah

## Contents

## 4.1

## Introduction

Neurotransplantation has become one of the most fascinating and promising fields in developmental neuroscience in recent times. As there are no efficient therapeutic strategies to stop ongoing neurodegeneration as it takes place in, for example, Parkinson's disease (PD) or Huntington's disease (HD), the transplantation of neurons seems to be the only alternative therapy to drug-based treatment in order to rewire neuronal circuits. Other ablative (e.g. palliodotomy) or technical (e.g. deep-brain stimulation) neurosurgical approaches exist and can partially stop the neurological deterioration of the diseases. However, none of them (including the drug-based therapies) can prevent further progression of the neurodegenerative processes; they can only act as a symptomatic re-lief instead of a restorative tool to heal the diseases. That is why there is an urgent need for further development of cell replacement strategies, which have the potential not only to restore the lost neuronal pathways, but also to provide long-lasting beneficial effects for patients with neurodegenerative diseases.

Different from the peripheral nervous system or other organs of the body (e.g. the skin), after birth the central nervous system (CNS) rapidly looses the potential of self-renewal and other intrinsic regenerative processes. This is one of the main burdens in developmental neuroscience and remains a great challenge in neurorestoration research. Overcoming this problem would enhance the importance of novel therapies for replacing lost function in the CNS and would help to become a standard protocol in the treatment of, for example, HD or PD.

The field of neurotransplantation research can look back on a fascinating, fast and breath-taking development during the past three decades. Finding the optimal cell resources and optimising the best neurosurgical approaches with which to inject the cells into the brain have given scientists intriguing insights into the understanding of brain-repair mechanisms and into the developmental and anatomical organisation of the cerebrum. The search for the best cell sources and the functional integration into the host brain has become two of the most interesting features in neurorestoration. Embryonic and adult stem cells and foetal progenitor cells have been used in various experimental conditions in vivo and in vitro. Much success has been achieved in the field of turning undifferentiated cells into a desired neuronal phenotype in cell culture experiments, and functional improvements could be observed in animal models after transplanting those cells. Nevertheless, there is much still to do with regard to optimising the current protocols, since stem cells have been discussed critically in terms of ethical concerns and in terms of tumour growth.

However, some clinical trials using foetal progenitor cells in PD patients have emphasised the importance and promising aspects of neurotransplantation. Many transplanted patients have shown a significant improvement in their motor skills. Clinicians and researchers still argue about the benefit of those studies (unwanted side effects occurred in a few studies), but there is rising hope that one day, scientists will find a way to introduce a standard restorative therapy for patients suffering from neurodegenerative diseases.

In this chapter, the development of neurotransplantation in experimental and clinical paradigms will be reviewed and an overview of the underlying mechanisms and principles in neurotransplantation will be given as an example of the effects of transplants on motor behaviour in PD.

## 4.2
## Parkinson's Disease

PD is one of the most common neurodegenerative, age-associated diseases caused by the pathological loss mainly of the dopaminergic (DAergic) cells in the nigrostriatal pathway. The cardinal symptoms of PD are rigidity, bra-

dykinesia, akinesia, tremor and postural imbalance. During the course of PD, not only do motor impairments occur, but also dementia [63], depression, apathy [11] and cognitive deficits [71, 78].

The aetiology of PD remains unknown, whereas the pathology of the idiopathic PD has been well investigated. Viral infections or inflammation, exposure to environmental toxins (e.g. pesticides), traumatic events or even hereditary transmission can cause parkinsonian-like symptoms [17, 33, 44, 53, 60, 61, 62, 65, 66]. All of the aforementioned causes of PD result in the degeneration of DAergic neurons within the basal ganglia (BG) circuitry (Fig. 1). The collapse of the dopamine (DA) system elicits a secondary, extranigral cascade of the degeneration of other transmitter systems and of particular areas of the cerebrum, for example the locus coeruleus (noradrenaline), the dorsal raphe (serotonergic), the nucleus basalis Meynert (cholinergic) and parts of the limbic system such as the entorhinal cortex, the hippocampus and the amygdala [64, 122].

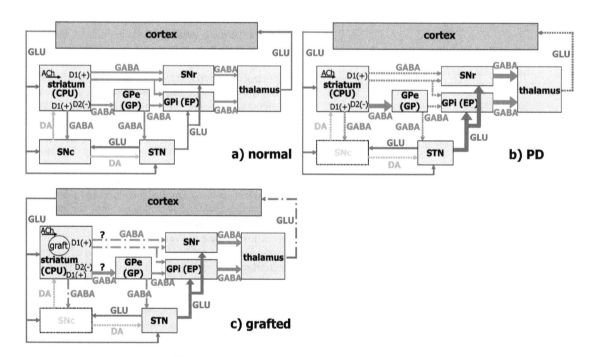

Fig. 1a–c Schemes of the dorsal loop of the basal ganglia (BG). **a** The BG circuitry in the normal brain. **b** The BG with degeneration of dopaminergic (DAergic) neurons in the substantia nigra pars compacta (SNc) and with reduced dopamine (DA) activity in the striatum, which finally leads to a decreased output of the thalamus to the cortex. **c** The BG circuitry in a parkinsonian brain plus an ectopic graft of nigral DAergic cells in the striatum. *Dashed lines* indicate reduced activity (the more dashes, the less activity); *thick arrows* show a hyperactivity of neurons (the thicker the arrow, the greater the activity). Abbreviations in brackets are derived from rodent nomenclature. Modified from Schmidt [122]. For more details see text. *PD* Parkinson's disease, *Glu* glutamate, *GABA* gamma-aminobutyric acid, *Ach* acetylcholine, *CPU* caudate putamen unit, *Gpe* globus pallidus externus, *GP* globus pallidus (in rodents), *GPi* globus pallidus internus, *EP* entopeduncular nucleus, *STN* subthalamic nucleus, *SNr* substantia nigra pars reticulata, *D1, D2* dopamine receptors

## 4.3
## DA, the BG and Motor Behaviour

The BG consist of a group of subcortical nuclei (Fig. 1) that are connected to each other via complex projections and functional loops [3, 4]. They are in close contact with the cortex, from which they receive their afferent glutamatergic (GLUergic) input. The main functions of the BG are to generate target-oriented motor patterns, complex motor behaviour (e.g. skilled limb movements, reaching-for-food movements) and cognitive processes such as habit learning [54, 55, 93, 122]. The nuclei are located in:

1. The telencephalon including the dorsal portion of the striatum (in primates: the putamen and nucleus caudatus; in rodents: the caudate putamen unit, CPU), the ventral portion of the striatum and the nucleus accumbens (Nac).
2. The diencephalon including the globus pallidus externus (GPe; in rodents: the globus pallidus, GP), the globus pallidus internus (GPi; in rodents: entopeduncular nucleus, EP), the ventral pallidum (VP) and the subthalamic nucleus (STN).
3. The mesencephalon including the substantia nigra pars reticulata (SNr), the substantia nigra pars compacta (SNc) and the ventral tegmental area (VTA).

The BG includes two functionally different circuitries: the dorsal motor loop and the ventral limbic loop. The dorsal motor loop, which is the main target area for functional restoration and motor pattern analysis in the neurorestoration research, builds a network consisting of the cortex (i.e. afferent corticostriatal neurons), the dorsal portion of the striatum, pallidal structures, the SNc (area 9, origin of the DAergic neurons, which mainly degenerate during the course of PD) and SNr, the thalamus and the feedback projections back to the cortex. The ventral limbic loop consists of the prefrontal cortical afferents, the Nac, the VTA (area 10, also the origin of DAergic cells, which are less affected by the neuropathological mechanisms of PD), the VP, the thalamus, limbic and associative areas such as the amygdala and the hippocampus, and feedback projections back to the prefrontal cortex.

As mentioned earlier, the DAergic neurons of the SNc are affected primarily by neurodegeneration during the course of PD. This leads to a reduced DA activity in the striatum, which itself remains fully innervated by the GLUergic afferents from the cortex [3, 4, 45, 54, 55, 122]. Consequently, an imbalance between the GLUergic and the DAergic transmitter systems occurs, which in turn leads to a relative overactivity of the GLUergic neurons. This finally causes inhibition of the thalamus, which is the output structure of the BG, and a reduced transmission back to the cortex. This decreased signal, which is generated by the BG network, is the main reason for the impaired motor pattern in PD.

The rationale why DAergic neurons degenerate in idiopathic PD is not known. These neurons are more vulnerable and lose their function more easily than neurons of other transmitter systems [60]. There is a natural age-associated degeneration of DAergic neurons (5% cell loss per decade; [45]). Parkinsonian symptoms occur when there is at least a loss of 50% of all nigral DAergic neurons, which is equivalent to a 70–80% loss of DA activity in the striatum [45]. There are differences within the DAergic neuron population in the way the neurons are affected by PD-associated degeneration: melanin-containing DAergic neurons (SNr and SNc) degenerate by 84% on average, whereas the non-melanin-containing DAergic neurons (VTA) degenerate only by 43–48% on average [60, 65, 66].

The molecular mechanisms of the degenerative processes are still under debate. A combination of many factors contributes to the loss of DAergic cells: oxidative stress, mitochondrial dysfunction, excitotoxicity and apoptosis are some of the main factors in the cascade of neurodegeneration (for review see Dunnett and Bjorklund [40]).

## 4.4
## Therapeutic Strategies to Treat PD

Currently there are no therapies that can stop the degenerative processes involved in PD and restore impaired motor patterns. The main therapeutic approach is still the drug-based therapy, which tries to substitute the loss of DA in the striatum (see below). However, new approaches have been made to counteract the parkinsonian symptoms, especially at later stages of the disease, including deep-brain stimulation [5, 80, 114], continuous apomorphine infusion via mini pumps [108], and – most strikingly – the neurotransplantation of foetal DAergic cells.

### 4.4.1
### Drug-Based Therapy

The classical therapy of treating PD is a symptomatic one: the substitution of DA by the DA precursor molecule 3,4-dihydroxy-L-phenylalanine (L-DOPA). This drug-based method was introduced in the 1960s and is still the gold standard for the treatment of PD [10, 32]. L-DOPA a naturally occurring metabolite in the synthesis of catecholamines, and it is converted to DA by the enzyme DOPA-decarboxylase. A major handicap of the L-DOPA therapy is that during the treatment phase, which may last some years, some patients develop severely disabling side effects: abnormal involuntary movements (motor fluctuations, dyskinesias) and psychiatric disturbances [2, 78, 87]. The rationale behind the dyskinesias has not been fully understood, but it is suggested that the intermittent application of L-DOPA is correlated with the occurrence of these side effects [8, 24, 56, 110, 111]. As a consequence, the drug-based therapy nowadays starts with DA agonists and other drugs (e.g. inhibitors of the enzyme monoamine oxidase B, or N-methyl-D-aspartate antagonists), which support the transmitter balance in the BG circuitry, and only later during the course of PD is L-DOPA administered in small amounts [110]. However, no matter which time L-DOPA is introduced into the antiparkinsonian therapy, the negative side effects of L-DOPA occur in the course of time and outweigh the functional benefits, so that there is a need for other less harmful therapeutic approaches.

## 4.5
## Clinical Neurotransplantation

Since the late 1980s, several open-label clinical trials and recently two placebo-controlled studies have been performed, and in total more than 250 PD patients have received transplants of human foetal DAergic tissue worldwide [81, 140]. The performance of human clinical trials is based on experimental research in primates and rodents. These experiments prove that foetal DAergic grafts are able to survive transplantation, can reinnervate the DA-depleted striatum and foster motor improvement (for more information and references see "4.6 Experimental Neurotransplantation", below).

The first step of transferring the experimental data into clinical studies was to perform open-label clinical trials. The results were very promising because the grafts survived and integrated into the host striatum, and the transplanted cells expressed a DAergic phenotype. Furthermore, the transplanted patients showed a significant improvement in motor function as measured by the Unified PD Rating Scale, and the amount of their daily drug intake could be significantly reduced (for review see [19, 57, 73–76, 81–83, 106, 107, 133, 140]). These effects could be observed in some patients over a period of more than 10 years. The results of open-label clinical trials included the unpreventable placebo effects in patients and the bias of the investigators [50, 51, 123]. So the next step was the establishment of placebo-controlled clinical trials, which have recently been carried out by Freed et al. [47] and Olanow et al. [103].

Surprisingly, the outcome of these first double-blind studies was disappointing: the functional improvement as seen in the first open-label studies could not be repeated and, even worse, several patients (15–57%) developed severe side effects such as abnormal involuntary movements (dyskinesias). Interestingly, in the study of Freed et al. [47] the younger patients (<60 years) showed a significant improvement, but in total (including all patients) there was no effect on the overall performance.

Winkler et al. [140] comprehensively analysed and compared the results of both study designs (open-label vs. placebo-controlled). They described fundamental differences between these two approaches, which make it even more difficult to compare the results of those study designs, and which make it unlikely that the results of the placebo-controlled trials, which were worse than those of the open-label trials, were due mainly to the avoidance of the placebo effect. Therefore, the discrepancy in the two methodologies of how to perform the clinical studies may have been crucial for the disappointing outcome of the placebo-controlled trials. For example, patients of the placebo-controlled studies were not immunosuppressed at all, or only for a short period of time, and consequently post mortem data suggested that there was a strong immune response ongoing, which was not the case in the first open-label trials, where the patients were immunosuppressed for life. Finally, Winkler et al. [140] concluded that the double-blind clinical studies "provide the first observations of graft-induced improvements that are distinguishable from the placebo effect", and that the transplantation procedure itself, the tissue handling and storage, the immunosuppressive treatment and the selection of patients must be improved and standardised. Taking these suggestions into consideration, Winkler et al. [140] claim that "cell transplantation can be developed into a safe and efficacious restorative therapy for advanced, although not too seriously affected, PD patients". However, to promote the progress of the neurotransplantation therapy, intensive experimental research is required, and the ethical issues that arise from the use of foetal tissues must be solved. Finding alternative cell sources and a sufficient in vitro propagation of cells will remain an important challenge for the future.

## 4.6
## Experimental Neurotransplantation

The success of the clinical trials – as described above – would not have been possible without (and still depends on) intensive research in animal models of neurodegenerative diseases and neurotransplantation. The quest for optimised cell sources and better cell survival, and the search for less trauma-causing surgical techniques are still ongoing and are the basis for this fascinating field of research.

### 4.6.1
### The Unilateral 6-Hydroxydopamine Model of PD

There are several animal models to simulate the symptoms of human PD. The main objectives of all

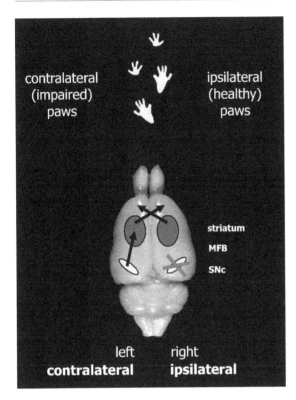

Fig. 2 Lateralisation of the rat brain induced by the unilateral injection of 6-hydroxydopamine (6-OHDA) into the medial forebrain bundle (MFB). In this example it is assumed that the left paw is the preferred one, which is why 6-OHDA is infused into the right MFB (the left body side is controlled by the right hemisphere and vice versa), and the DAergic transmission in the nigrostriatal pathway is interrupted. From now on, this hemisphere is considered to be the ipsilateral (lesioned) one. The preferred paw is now contralateral to the lesioned side. On the ipsilateral side, all DAergic neurons degenerate in the SNc after the injection of 6-OHDA into the MFB. The contralateral nigrostriatal DAergic pathway remains fully intact

these animal models are the mesencephalic DAergic neurons of the substantia nigra (SN) and the analysis of impaired motor function. The neurodegeneration can be induced presynaptically (reversible: reserpine model, irreversible: MPTP-, 6-OHDA models) and postsynaptically (reversible: injection of neuroleptika). Rigidity, bradykinesia and akinesia are the most obvious symptoms in all of them. One of the main criteria for approving an animal model of PD is the severity of the lesion-induced parkinsonian symptoms becoming

less severe when the classical (drug-based) antiparkinsonian therapy (with L-DOPA) is applied (for review see [28, 122]).

One of the most common animal models is the unilateral 6-OHDA medial forebrain bundle (MFB) lesion rat model [28, 69, 128]. In this model, the nigrostriatal DAergic system of only one hemisphere is destroyed (Figs. 2 and 3). The other (contralateral) side serves as an internal control for behavioural evaluation and for morphological analyses of the brain. Another characteristic of 6-OHDA

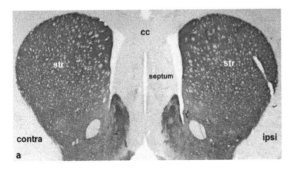

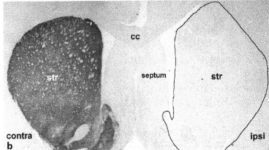

Fig. 3a,b Tyrosine hydroxylase (TH) staining for control rats and unilaterally 6-OHDA-lesioned rats. Both pictures show a brain section at +1.0 from bregma: **a** Control brain with no surgery at all. Both hemispheres are clearly stained for TH in the striatum. **b** Unilateral MFB 6-OHDA lesion: no TH staining and complete DA depletion on the ipsilateral (right) hemisphere. *contra* Contralateral, *ipsi* ipsilateral, *str* striatum, *cc* corpus callosum

MFB lesions is the full depletion of DA in the striatum. In the case of intrastriatal grafts, all cells and fibres found in the striatum are believed to be derived from the donor tissue, since there is no background signal from the host after the MFB lesion.

### 4.6.1.1

### Effects of Unilateral MFB 6-OHDA Lesions on Motor Behaviour

Motor impairments are the most prominent symptoms in hemiparkinsonian rats. The animals develop behavioural asymmetries (hemispatial neglect of the side of their body that is contralateral to the lesion, and turning biases away from this side) and impairments in locomotion, gait and posture [21, 91, 119, 121, 129, 135]. But most importantly, the rats develop severe impairments in their skilled forelimb use of the paw that is contralateral to the lesion (for review see [92, 94, 95, 104, 131, 136, 137]. It has been demonstrated that the DAergic system in particular contributes to the execution of skilled limb movements [137]. Interestingly, there are minor impairments on the ipsilateral side of the lesioned rats, but to a smaller degree than on the contralateral side, indicating that not all fibres of the motor system cross from one hemisphere to the other and that some neurons project to the ipsilateral side (for review see [136]). However, in the rat model of PD, most impairments do not appear unless 80–90% of the nigrostriatal system is destroyed [20, 59, 143].

For the assessment of impaired motor behaviour of rats in neurodegenerative disease models, many different tests have been developed that evaluate either spontaneous behaviour or drug-induced behaviour. The tests that are concerned with spontaneous behaviour analyse (skilled) forelimb movements (e.g. reaching-for-food movements) or full body movements (forelimb/hindlimb coordination). The former include the Montoya staircase test [94], the single pellet reaching test [89, 134], the stepping test [104, 120], and the lever-pressing test [84]; and the latter include the ladder rung walking test [90] and the footprint analysis [91, 34].

### 4.6.2

### Neurotransplantation in the Unilateral Rat Model of PD

On the basis of the hemiparkinsonian rat model and the assessments of the motor deficits after 6-OHDA lesions (see below), the research into neurotransplantation in PD was established by Bjorklund and Stenevi [12] and Perlow et al. [105], when their first studies disclosed that functional improvement could be achieved after grafting ventral mesencephalon (VM)-derived tissue in animal re-

cipients. These were the first successful trials after a long history of defeats in the field of neurotransplantation [13]. The initial publications in 1979 gave a big impetus to the use of grafting cells in models of neurodegenerative diseases. The early studies of functional restoration after 6-OHDA lesions focussed on graft integration and survival, and on transplantation techniques. It was demonstrated that the DAergic grafts partially reinnervate the striatum, that they are able to release DA (the release is controlled by cortical afferent synaptic connections) and that they are able to connect downstream to striatal (host) neurons via new synapses [29, 31, 39, 48, 88, 112, 113, 127, 132]. At the molecular level, the expressions of the upregulated enkephalin-RNA, D2-receptor-RNA and GAD67-mRNA within the reinnervated areas of foetal striatal DAergic grafts are nearly normalised. Other changes, such as the lesion-induced downregulation of substance P, are less affected [26, 27, 30, 138]. The aforementioned effects are clearly dependent on the degree of DAergic reinnervation in the CPU. Therefore, a complete reinnervation of the striatum affected by PD remains the main objective of brain research, and it is assumed that grafting of DAergic cells must become more effective at the behavioural and molecular levels.

It is important to notice that all recent transplantation approaches to adult brains are based on an ectopic cell transplantation concept (see Fig. 1 and [141]). This means that in an adult environment in the cerebrum, the newly generated axonal fibres of the injected neurons do not find their way to their targets if homotopically transplanted. The grafts have only limited fibre outgrowths of about 2–3 mm. In the case of nigrostriatal degeneration, the DAergic VM-derived cells would not rewire the striatum if they were transplanted into the SN (the distance between the SN and striatum is too long).

A modest reinnervation of the nigrostriatal pathway is possible only if cells are transplanted into the SN in a neonatal environment or by using so-called "bridge grafts" [7, 96, 98, 141]. That is why investigating the molecular mechanisms and gene expressions in the young postnatal brain are thought to be the future keys to any functional restorative therapy. Except for two small areas in the hippocampus and the subventricular zone, there is no adult neurogenesis in the brain; in fact, the adult tissue in the CNS is adverse to any neuronal fibre outgrowth (most obviously seen in spinal cord lesions that lead to irreversible motor impairments). Therefore, creating a neonatal environment in the adult host tissue might be crucial for a complete restoration of the degenerated neuronal pathways. Several attempts to change the environment in the adult brain are currently under investigation:
1. Applying neuronal growth factors (via injections or by gene therapy: [6, 22].
2. Blocking surface proteins that are repellent to neuronal growth cones [58, 124].

3. By transplanting cells in two steps, firstly transplantation to create a neonatal environment, and secondly transplantation to rewire neuronal circuits (Hackl et al. 2007, unpublished observations).

But as long as the molecular mechanisms underlying adult neuroregeneration are still under debate [46, 86, 102, 124], ectopic transplantation serves as a valuable alternative for functional restoration. It remains, however, a suboptimal solution in order to restore long distance connections in the brain. Nevertheless, the grafts do form synaptic connections within the host tissue, the release of DA is controlled by cortical afferents, and a partial functional restoration may occur.

The stereotactic transplantation technique of injecting cells into the brain has also changed over the years: at the beginning, monoamine-rich solid pieces of the VM were grafted into the CPU, the lateral ventricle, or into cortical cavities [12, 126]. Poor functional restoration and surgery-related trauma were the driving force to develop new neurotransplantation techniques. Bjorklund et al. [15] established the cell suspension technique, which has become the "hallmark protocol" of cell preparation and

implantation. Nikkhah et al. [100] further optimised this protocol and introduced glass capillaries for the infusion of single-cell suspensions (Fig. 4). This technique caused fewer traumata than the earlier-used metal cannula. The use of the so-called microtransplantation approach resulted in better functional integration, graft survival and enhanced reliability of survival of the graft (fewer differences in the survival rates of grafted cells). The new technique offered the option of injecting multiple deposits of DAergic cells into the entire DA-depleted striatum and/ or SN [95, 97, 101, 104, 139].

Many behavioural tests have been carried out to monitor graft-related changes in motor behaviour. The intrastriatal transplantation of foetal DAergic cells after unilateral 6-OHDA lesion improves not only drug-induced asymmetry (induced by amphetamine and apomorphine; for review see [18]), but also basic elements of spontaneous behaviour such as spontaneous circling and sensorimotor neglect [14, 41, 42, 85, 99].

The functional restoration of skilled forelimb use is more difficult to achieve. The first studies did not show any improvement of motor pattern of the forepaws – despite the obvious improvement in, for example, drug-induced

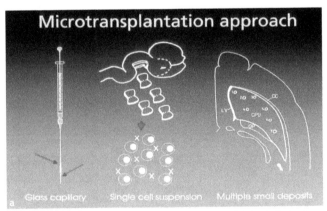

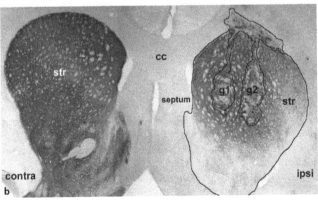

Fig. 4 **a** Schematic description of the microtransplantation approach as published by Nikkhah et al. [100]. **b** TH (rate-limiting enzyme involved in the metabolism of DA; often used to visualise lesion and graft effects) staining in unilaterally lesioned rats with two grafts of embryonic day 14 ventral mesencephalon-derived cells (g1 and g2). *LV* Lateral ventricle

rotation [1, 42, 85, 94, 99]. With the introduction of the microtransplantation approach [100], the injection of multiple deposits of DAergic cells could partially restore the complex grasping behaviour of PD rats [104, 115, 116]. Current results show that partial restoration is achievable. However, a more detailed and qualitative analysis of motor pattern has revealed that the partial recovery might be enhanced by compensatory mechanisms rather than

by a "true" restoration of the original sensorimotor behaviour [70]. These results clearly emphasise the demand for a complete and specific restoration of the degenerated nigrostriatal pathway to achieve functional recovery.

Recent research in the field of neurotransplantation focuses on optimising the surgery protocols and the functional outcome. The investigation into unwanted graft-related side effects such as abnormal involuntary move-

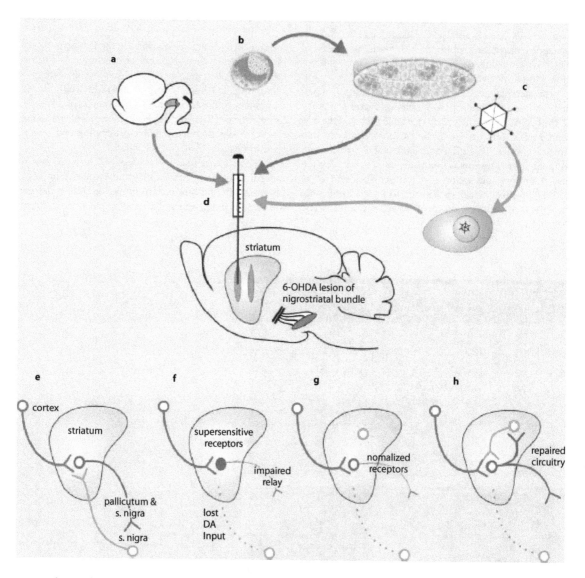

Fig. 5 Scheme of different cell sources and the principles of restoration in the 6-OHDA-lesioned brain (modified from Fricker-Gates and Dunnet [49]). a Dissected and dissociated primary embryonic or foetal neurons. b Embryonic stem (ES) cells derived from mouse or human blastocytes expanded in vitro. c Cells engineered to secrete deficient gene products, such as catecholamine-synthesising enzymes or growth factors. d In each case, the prepared cells were implanted into the brain. e Normal corticostriatopallidal communication is modulated in the striatum by DA inputs from the substantia nigra. f PD or experimental lesions destroy DA inputs, resulting in a loss of regulation of striatopallidal and striatonigral outputs and a supersensitivity of intrinsic striatal DA receptors. g Secretory grafts (c) can normalise receptor supersensitivity and tonic striatal throughput, but do not restore functions that are dependent on dynamic DA modulation. h Grafted ES cells (b), like primary neurons (a), restore intrinsic striatal connections and yield a more complete profile of functional recovery

ments and dyskinesias are in the focus of the researchers [24, 25, 77, 140]. Specific training and an enriched environment have proven to promote neurogenesis in adult mammals and to be beneficial in the development of the grafts in the host brain [16, 35–38, 67, 130]. Furthermore, new cell sources – other than foetal tissues – must be made available, as the transplantation of foetal cells causes considerable ethical problems [49]. Many studies (Fig. 5) have made use of embryonic stem (ES) cell lines [79, 117], stem cells from umbilical cord blood [9, 142], adult stem cells [52, 118] or cells that are genetically engineered in vitro as alternative cell sources for grafting [23, 43].

Not only is cell source an issue to be discussed in the field of neurorestoration research, but also the final phenotype of the in-vitro-harvested and then transplanted DAergic cells. As mentioned earlier, there are morphological and anatomical differences between the DAergic cells of the SNc (A9) and the VTA (A10), which make the A10 cells more resistible and less vulnerable to neurodegenerative processes (for reasons not yet known). Recent attempts to proliferate and differentiate DAergic neurons in vitro provide not only a high amount of DA-positive neurons, but also a high amount of region-specific DAergic neurons, which should help to rewire the lost nigrostriatal projections [109, 125].

The use of ES cells has been very controversially discussed during recent years. Much success has been achieved in cultivating and proliferating those cells [79]. Turning undifferentiated omnipotent ES cells into a DAergic phenotype to a considerable and sufficient amount is difficult, and scientists still try to find the optimal cell culture conditions. Another major concern of the use of ES cells is the potential tumour growth. As soon as (undifferentiated) ES cells are transplanted in vivo, they continue proliferating, which finally leads to severe tumour growth. In contrast, foetal grafts have never been observed to trigger any tumour-like formations. So there must be a time window in which ES cells can still proliferate and after which ES cells lose their omnipotency (becoming "only" multipotent) and their proliferative capacity. Nevertheless, as the transplanted foetal neurons are ontogenetically older, those grafts show a limited graft survival and more foetal tissue is necessary to achieve a functional restorative effect. In order to better control those cells in vivo predifferentiation protocols have been established to avoid the transplantation of immature cells that are still able to proliferate. In vivo experiments showed beneficial effects in an animal model of PD [68], but a recent study [117] suggests that those results should be interpreted more carefully, and it reports a still ongoing proliferative activity of cells in the graft core. So, ES cells remain a fascinating tool for transplantation and in particular for neurorestoration, because they have the capacity to differentiate in many different tissues of the body, but their use is not yet accepted for clinical trials, and more research is needed.

## 4.7
# Summary

In conclusion, it can be stated that the technique of neurotransplantation remains a promising therapeutic tool to restore sensorimotor function in PD, but it needs to be optimised, and many additional factors such as physiotherapy, supporting drug therapy, different cell sources, pretreatment of cells and neuroprotection have to be taken into consideration. The combination of all will help to find the optimal therapy for PD and, potentially, also for other neurodegenerative diseases. All in all, neurotransplantation will continue being a restorative methodology, and more research is needed to identify the mechanisms that could stop the ongoing neurodegeneration during the course of PD, and to clarify the underlying pathology of this condition.

## References

1. Abrous DN, Torres EM, Dunnett SB (1993) Dopaminergic grafts implanted into the neonatal or adult striatum: comparative effects on rotation and paw reaching deficits induced by subsequent unilateral nigrostriatal lesions in adulthood. Neuroscience 3:657–668

2. Ahlskog JE, Muenter MD (2001) Frequency of levodopa-related dyskinesias and motor fluctuations as estimated from the cumulative literature. Mov Disord 3:448–458

3. Albin RL, Young AB, Penney JB (1989) The functional anatomy of basal ganglia disorders. Trends Neurosci 10:366–375

4. Albin RL, Young AB, Penney JB (1995) The functional anatomy of disorders of the basal ganglia. Trends Neurosci 2:63–64

5. Ardouin C, Pillon B, Peiffer E, Bejjani P, Limousin P, Damier P, Arnulf I, Benabid AL, Agid Y, Pollak P (1999) Bilateral subthalamic or pallidal stimulation for Parkinson's disease affects neither memory nor executive functions: a consecutive series of 62 patients. Ann Neurol 2:217–223

6. Behrstock S, Ebert A, McHugh J, Vosberg S, Moore J, Schneider B, Capowski E, Hei D, Kordower J, Aebischer P, Svendsen CN (2006) Human neural progenitors deliver glial cell line-derived neurotrophic factor to parkinsonian rodents and aged primates. Gene Ther 5:379–388

7. Bentlage C, Nikkhah G, Cunningham MG, Bjorklund A (1999) Reformation of the nigrostriatal pathway by fetal dopaminergic micrografts into the substantia nigra is critically dependent on the age of the host. Exp Neurol 1:177–190

8. Bezard E, Brotchie JM, Gross CE (2001) Pathophysiology of levodopa-induced dyskinesia: potential for new therapies. Nat Rev Neurosci 8:577–588

9. Bicknese AR, Goodwin HS, Quinn CO, Henderson VC, Chien SN, Wall DA (2002) Human umbilical cord blood cells can be induced to express markers for neurons and glia. Cell Transplant 3:261–264

10. Birkmayer W, Hornykiewicz O (2001) The effect of 1-3,4-dihydroxyphenylalanine (L-DOPA) on akinesia in parkinsonism (1961). Wien Klin Wochenschr 113:851–854

11. Birkmayer W, Riederer P (1985) Die Parkinson-Krankheit: Biochemie, Klinik, Therapie. Springer, Wien, New York

12. Bjorklund A, Stenevi U (1979) Reconstruction of the nigrostriatal dopamine pathway by intracerebral nigral transplants. Brain Res 3:555–560

13. Bjorklund A, Stenevi U (1985) Intracerebral neural grafting: a historical perspective. In: Bjorklund A, Stenevi U (eds) Neural Grafting in the Mammalian CNS. pp Elsevier, Amsterdam, pp 3–14

14. Bjorklund A, Dunnett SB, Nikkhah G (1994) Nigral transplants in the rat Parkinson model. Functional limitations and strategies to enhance nigrostriatal reconstructions. In: Dunnet SB, Bjorklund A (eds) Functional Neural Transplantation. Raven, New York, pp 47–69

15. Bjorklund A, Stenevi U, Schmidt RH, Dunnett SB, Gage FH (1983) Intracerebral grafting of neuronal cell suspensions. II. Survival and growth of nigral cell suspensions implanted in different brain sites. Acta Physiol Scand Suppl 522:9–18

16. Brown J, Cooper-Kuhn CM, Kempermann G, van Praag H, Winkler J, Gage FH, Kuhn HG (2003) Enriched environment and physical activity stimulate hippocampal but not olfactory bulb neurogenesis. Eur J Neurosci 10:2042–2046

17. Brown AM, Deutch AY, Colbran RJ (2005) Dopamine depletion alters phosphorylation of striatal proteins in a model of Parkinsonism. Eur J Neurosci 1:247–256

18. Brundin P, Duan WM, Sauer H (1994) Functional effects of mesencephalic dopamine neurons and adrenal chromaffin cells grafted to the rodent striatum. In: Dunnet B, Bjorklund A (eds) Functional Neural Transplantation. Raven, New York, pp 9–46

19. Brundin P, Pogarell O, Hagell P, Piccini P, Widner H, Schrag A, Kupsch A, Crabb L, Odin P, Gustavii B, Bjorklund A, Brooks DJ, Marsden CD, Oertel WH, Quinn NP, Rehncrona S, Lindvall O (2000) Bilateral caudate and putamen grafts of embryonic mesencephalic tissue treated with lazaroids in Parkinson's disease. Brain 123:1380–1390

20. Calne DB, Zigmond MJ (1991) Compensatory mechanisms in degenerative neurologic diseases. Insights from parkinsonism. Arch Neurol 4:361–363

21. Carli M, Evenden JL, Robbins TW (1985) Depletion of unilateral striatal dopamine impairs initiation of contralateral actions and not sensory attention. Nature 6004:679–682

22. Carlsson T, Bjorklund T, Kirik D (2007) Restoration of the striatal dopamine synthesis for Parkinson's disease: viral vector-mediated enzyme replacement strategy. Curr Gene Ther 2:109–120

23. Carlsson T, Winkler C, Burger C, Muzyczka N, Mandel RJ, Cenci A, Bjorklund A, Kirik D (2005) Reversal of dyskinesias in an animal model of Parkinson's disease by continuous L-DOPA delivery using rAAV vectors. Brain 128:559–569

24. Carlsson T, Winkler C, Lundblad M, Cenci MA, Bjorklund A, Kirik D (2006) Graft placement and uneven pattern of reinnervation in the striatum is important for development of graft-induced dyskinesia. Neurobiol Dis 3:657–668

25. Cenci MA, Hagell P (2005) Dyskinesia and Neural Grafting in Parkinson's Disease. Kluver Academic/Plenum, New York

26. Cenci MA, Campbell K, Bjorklund A (1993) Neuropeptide messenger RNA expression in the 6-hydroxydopamine-lesioned rat striatum reinnervated by fetal dopaminergic transplants: differential effects of the grafts on preproenkephalin, preprotachykinin and prodynorphin messenger RNA levels. Neuroscience 2:275–296

27. Cenci MA, Campbell K, Bjorklund A (1997) Glutamic acid decarboxylase gene expression in the dopamine-denervated striatum: effects of intrastriatal fetal nigral transplants or chronic apomorphine treatment. Brain Res Mol Brain Res 1:149–155

28. Cenci MA, Whishaw IQ, Schallert T (2002) Animal models of neurological deficits: how relevant is the rat? Nat Rev Neurosci 7:574–579

29. Chkirate M, Vallee A, Doucet G (1993) Host striatal projections into fetal ventral mesencephalic tissue grafted to the striatum of immature or adult rat. Exp Brain Res 2:357–362

30. Chritin M, Savasta M, Mennicken F, Bal A, Abrous DN, Le Moal M, Feuerstein C, Herman JP (1992) Intrastriatal dopamine-rich Implants reverse the increase of dopamine D2 receptor mRNA levels caused by lesion of the nigrostriatal pathway: a quantitative in situ hybridization study. Eur J Neurosci 7:663–672

31. Clarke DJ, Brundin P, Strecker RE, Nilsson OG, Bjorklund A, Lindvall O (1988). Human fetal dopamine neurons grafted in a rat model of Parkinson's disease: ultrastructural evidence for synapse formation using tyrosine hydroxylase immunocytochemistry. Exp Brain Res 1:115–126

32. Cotzias GC, Van Woert MH, Schiffer LM (1967) Aromatic amino acids and modification of parkinsonism. N Engl J Med 7:374–379

33. Dale RC, Church AJ, Surtees RA, Lees AJ, Adcock JE, Harding B, Neville BG, Giovannoni G (2004) Encephalitis lethargica syndrome: 20 new cases and evidence of basal ganglia autoimmunity. Brain 127:21–33

34. de Medinaceli L, Freed WJ, Wyatt RJ (1982) An index of the functional condition of rat sciatic nerve based on measurements made from walking tracks. Exp Neurol 3:634–643

35. Dobrossy MD, Dunnett SB (2003) Motor training effects on recovery of function after striatal lesions and striatal grafts. Exp Neurol 1:274–284

36. Dobrossy MD, Dunnett SB (2004) Environmental enrichment affects striatal graft morphology and functional recovery. Eur J Neurosci 1:159–168

37. Dobrossy MD, Drapeau E, Aurousseau C, Le Moal M, Piazza PV, Abrous DN (2003) Differential effects of learning on neurogenesis: learning increases or decreases the number of newly born cells depending on their birth date. Mol Psychiatry 12:974–982

38. Dobrossy MD, Le Moal M, Montaron MF, Abrous N (2000) Influence of environment on the efficacy of intrastriatal dopaminergic grafts. Exp Neurol 1:172–183

39. Doucet G, Murata Y, Brundin P, Bosler O, Mons N, Geffard M, Ouimet CC, Bjorklund A (1989) Host afferents into intrastriatal transplants of fetal ventral mesencephalon. Exp Neurol 1:1–19

40. Dunnett SB, Bjorklund A (1999) Prospects for new restorative and neuroprotective treatments in Parkinson's disease. Nature 6738:A32–A39

41. Dunnett SB, Bjorklund A, Schmidt RH, Stenevi U, Iversen SD (1983) Intracerebral grafting of neuronal cell suspensions. V. Behavioural recovery in rats with bilateral 6-OHDA lesions following implantation of nigral cell suspensions. Acta Physiol Scand Suppl 522:39–47

42. Dunnett SB, Whishaw IQ, Rogers DC, Jones GH (1987) Dopamine-rich grafts ameliorate whole body motor asymmetry and sensory neglect but not independent limb use in rats with 6-hydroxydopamine lesions. Brain Res 1:63–78

43. Eslamboli A, Georgievska B, Ridley RM, Baker HF, Muzyczka N, Burger C, Mandel RJ, Annett L, Kirik D (2005) Continuous low-level glial cell line-derived neurotrophic factor delivery using recombinant adeno-associated viral vectors provides neuroprotection and induces behavioral recovery in a primate model of Parkinson's disease. J Neurosci 4:769–777

44. Farrer MJ (2006) Genetics of Parkinson disease: paradigm shifts and future prospects. Nat Rev Genet 4:306–318

45. Fearnley JM, Lees AJ (1991) Ageing and Parkinson's disease: substantia nigra regional selectivity. Brain 114:2283–2301

46. Fouad K, Klusman I, Schwab ME (2004) Regenerating corticospinal fibers in the Marmoset (*Callitrix jacchus*) after spinal cord lesion and treatment with the anti-Nogo-A antibody IN-1. Eur J Neurosci 9:2479–2482

47. Freed CR, Greene PE, Breeze RE, Tsai WY, DuMouchel W, Kao R, Dillon S, Winfield H, Culver S, Trojanowski JQ, Eidelberg D, Fahn S (2001) Transplantation of embryonic dopamine neurons for severe Parkinson's disease. N Engl J Med 10:710–719

48. Freund TF, Bolam JP, Bjorklund A, Stenevi U, Dunnett SB, Powell JF, Smith AD (1985) Efferent synaptic connections of grafted dopaminergic neurons reinnervating the host neostriatum: a tyrosine hydroxylase immunocytochemical study. J Neurosci 3 603–616

49. Fricker-Gates RA, Dunnett SB (2002) Rewiring the Parkinsonian brain. Nat Med 2:105–106

50. Fuente-Fernandez R, Ruth TJ, Sossi V, Schulzer M, Calne DB, Stoessl AJ (2001) Expectation and dopamine release: mechanism of the placebo effect in Parkinson's disease. Science 5532:1164–1166

51. Fuente-Fernandez R, Stoessl AJ (2002) The placebo effect in Parkinson's disease. Trends Neurosci 6:302–306

52. Gage FH, Coates PW, Palmer TD, Kuhn HG, Fisher LJ, Suhonen JO, Peterson DA, Suhr ST, Ray J (1995) Survival and differentiation of adult neuronal progenitor cells transplanted to the adult brain. Proc Natl Acad Sci U S A 25:11879–11883

53. Gasser T (2005) Genetics of Parkinson's disease. Curr Opin Neurol 4:363–369

54. Graybiel AM (1995) Building action repertoires: memory and learning functions of the basal ganglia. Curr Opin Neurobiol 6:733–741

55. Graybiel AM (2000) The basal ganglia. Curr Biol 14: R509–R511

56. Guigoni C, Dovero S, Aubert I, Li Q, Bioulac BH, Bloch B, Gurevich EV, Gross CE, Bezard E (2005) Levodopa-induced dyskinesia in MPTP-treated macaques is not dependent on the extent and pattern of nigrostrial lesioning. Eur J Neurosci 1:283–287

57. Hagell P, Schrag A, Piccini P, Jahanshahi M, Brown R, Rehncrona S, Widner H, Brundin P, Rothwell JC, Odin P, Wenning GK, Morrish P, Gustavii B, Bjorklund A, Brooks DJ, Marsden CD, Quinn NP, Lindvall O (1999) Sequential bilateral transplantation in Parkinson's disease: effects of the second graft. Brain 122:1121–1132

58. Harel NY, Strittmatter SM (2006) Can regenerating axons recapitulate developmental guidance during recovery from spinal cord injury? Nat Rev Neurosci 8:603–616

59. Hefti F, Melamed E, Sahakian BJ, Wurtman RJ (1980) Circling behavior in rats with partial, unilateral nigro-striatal lesions: effect of amphetamine, apomorphine, and DOPA. Pharmacol Biochem Behav 2:185–188

60. Hirsch E, Graybiel AM, Agid YA (1988) Melanized dopaminergic neurons are differentially susceptible to degeneration in Parkinson's disease. Nature 6180:345–348

61. Hirsch E.C, Hoglinger G, Rousselet E, Breidert T, Parain K, Feger J, Ruberg M, Prigent A, Cohen-Salmon C, Launay JM (2003) Animal models of Parkinson's disease in rodents induced by toxins: an update. J Neural Transm Suppl 65:89–100

62. Hirsch EC, Hunot S, Damier P, Faucheux B (1998) Glial cells and inflammation in Parkinson's disease: a role in neurodegeneration? Ann Neurol 3:S115–S120

63. Jellinger K (1974) Pathomorphologie des Parkinson-Syndroms. Aktuel Neurol 1:83–98

64. Jellinger KA (1991) Pathology of Parkinson's disease. Changes other than the nigrostriatal pathway. Mol Chem Neuropathol 3:153–197

65. Jenner P (2003) Oxidative stress in Parkinson's disease. Ann Neurol 53:S26–S36

66. Jenner P, Olanow CW (1998) Understanding cell death in Parkinson's disease. Ann Neurol 3:S72–S84

67. Kempermann G, Gast D, Gage FH (2002) Neuroplasticity in old age: sustained fivefold induction of hippocampal neurogenesis by long-term environmental enrichment. Ann Neurol 2:135–143

68. Kim JH, Auerbach JM, Rodriguez-Gomez JA, Velasco I, Gavin D, Lumelsky N, Lee SH, Nguyen J, Sanchez-Pernaute R, Bankiewicz K, McKay R 2002. Dopamine neurons derived from embryonic stem cells function in an animal model of Parkinson's disease. Nature 6893:50–56

69. Kirik D, Rosenblad C, Bjorklund A (1998) Characterization of behavioral and neurodegenerative changes following partial lesions of the nigrostriatal dopamine system induced by intrastriatal 6-hydroxydopamine in the rat. Exp Neurol 2:259–277

70. Klein A, Metz GA, Papazoglou A, Nikkhah G (2007) Differential effects on forelimb grasping behavior induced by fetal dopaminergic grafts in hemiparkinsonian rats. Neurobiol Dis (in press)

71. Knowlton BJ, Squire LR (1995) Remembering and knowing: two different expressions of declarative memory. J Exp Psychol Learn Mem Cogn 3:699–710

72. Knowlton BJ, Mangels JA, Squire LR (1996) A neostriatal habit learning system in humans. Science 5280:1399–1402

73. Kordower JH, Freeman TB, Chen EY, Mufson EJ, Sanberg PR, Hauser RA, Snow B, Olanow CW (1998) Fetal nigral grafts survive and mediate clinical benefit in a patient with Parkinson's disease. Mov Disord 3:383–393

74. Kordower JH, Freeman TB, Olanow CW (1998) Neuropathology of fetal nigral grafts in patients with Parkinson's disease. Mov Disord 13:88–95

75. Kordower JH, Freeman TB, Snow BJ, Vingerhoets FJ, Mufson EJ, Sanberg PR, Hauser RA, Smith DA, Nauert GM, Perl DP (1995) Neuropathological evidence of graft survival and striatal reinnervation after the transplantation of fetal mesencephalic tissue in a patient with Parkinson's disease. N Engl J Med 17:1118–1124

76. Kordower JH, Rosenstein JM, Collier TJ, Burke MA, Chen EY, Li JM, Martel L, Levey AE, Mufson EJ, Freeman TB, Olanow CW (1996) Functional fetal nigral grafts in a patient with Parkinson's disease: chemoanatomic, ultrastructural, and metabolic studies. J Comp Neurol 2:203–230

77. Lane EL, Winkler C, Brundin P, Cenci MA (2006) The impact of graft size on the development of dyskinesia following intrastriatal grafting of embryonic dopamine neurons in the rat. Neurobiol Dis 2:334–345

78. Lang AE, Lozano AM (1998) Parkinson's disease. Second of two parts. N Engl J Med 16:1130–1143

79. Lee SH, Lumelsky N, Studer L, Auerbach JM, McKay RD (2000) Efficient generation of midbrain and hindbrain neurons from mouse embryonic stem cells. Nat Biotechnol 6:675–679

80. Limousin P, Krack P, Pollak P, Benazzouz A, Ardouin C, Hoffmann D, Benabid AL (1998) Electrical stimulation of the subthalamic nucleus in advanced Parkinson's disease. N Engl J Med 16:1105–1111

81. Lindvall O, Hagell P (2000) Clinical observations after neural transplantation in Parkinson's disease. Prog Brain Res 127:299–320

82. Lindvall O, Brundin P, Widner H, Rehncrona S, Gustavii B, Frackowiak R, Leenders KL, Sawle G, Rothwell JC, Marsden CD (1990) Grafts of fetal dopamine neurons survive and improve motor function in Parkinson's disease. Science 4942:574–577

83. Lindvall O, Rehncrona S, Brundin P, Gustavii B, Astedt B, Widner H, Lindholm T, Bjorklund A, Leenders KL, Rothwell JC (1990) Neural transplantation in Parkinson's disease: the Swedish experience. Prog Brain Res 82:729–734

84. MacRae PG, Spirduso WW, Wilcox RE (1988) Reaction time and nigrostriatal dopamine function: the effects of age and practice. Brain Res 451:139–146

85. Mandel RJ, Brundin P, Bjorklund A (1990) The Importance of graft placement and task complexity for transplant-induced recovery of simple and complex sensorimotor deficits in dopamine denervated rats. Eur J Neurosci 10:888–894

86. Markus TM Tsai SY, Bollnow MR, Farrer RG, O'Brien TE, Kindler-Baumann DR, Rausch M, Rudin M, Wiessner C, Mir AK, Schwab ME, Kartje GL (2005) Recovery and brain reorganization after stroke in adult and aged rats. Ann Neurol 6:950–953

87. Marsden CD (1990) Parkinson's disease. Lancet 8695:948–952

88. Mendez I, Elisevich K, Flumerfelt B (1991) Dopaminergic innervation of substance P-containing striatal neurons by fetal nigral grafts: an ultrastructural double-labeling immunocytochemical study. J Comp Neurol 1:66–78

89. Metz GA, Whishaw IQ (2000) Skilled reaching an action pattern: stability in rat (*Rattus norvegicus*) grasping movements as a function of changing food pellet size. Behav Brain Res 2:111–122

90. Metz GA, Whishaw IQ (2002) Cortical and subcortical lesions impair skilled walking in the ladder rung walking test: a new task to evaluate fore- and hindlimb stepping, placing, and co-ordination. J Neurosci Methods 2:169–179

91. Metz GA, Tse A, Ballermann M, Smith LK, Fouad K (2005) The unilateral 6-OHDA rat model of Parkinson's disease revisited: an electromyographic and behavioural analysis. Eur J Neurosci 3:735–744

92. Miklyaeva EI, Castaneda E, Whishaw IQ (1994) Skilled reaching deficits in unilateral dopamine-depleted rats: impairments in movement and posture and compensatory adjustments. J Neurosci 11:7148–7158

93. Mink JW, Thach WT (1993) Basal ganglia intrinsic circuits and their role in behavior. Curr Opin Neurobiol 6:950–957

94. Montoya CP, Astell S, Dunnett SB (1990) Effects of nigral and striatal grafts on skilled forelimb use in the rat. Prog Brain Res 82:459–466

95. Nikkhah G, Bentlage C, Cunningham MG, Bjorklund A (1994) Intranigral fetal dopamine grafts induce behavioral compensation in the rat Parkinson model. J Neurosci 6:3449–3461

96. Nikkhah G, Cunningham MG, Cenci MA, McKay RD, Bjorklund A (1995) Dopaminergic microtransplants into the substantia nigra of neonatal rats with bilateral 6-OHDA lesions. I. Evidence for anatomical reconstruction of the nigrostriatal pathway. J Neurosci 5:3548–3561

97. Nikkhah G, Cunningham MG, Jodicke A, Knappe U, Bjorklund A (1994) Improved graft survival and striatal reinnervation by microtransplantation of fetal nigral cell suspensions in the rat Parkinson model. Brain Res 633:133–143

98. Nikkhah G, Cunningham MG, McKay R, Bjorklund A (1995) Dopaminergic microtransplants into the substantia nigra of neonatal rats with bilateral 6-OHDA lesions. II. Transplant-induced behavioral recovery. J Neurosci 5:3562–3570

99. Nikkhah G, Duan WM, Knappe U, Jodicke A, Bjorklund A (1993) Restoration of complex sensorimotor behavior and skilled forelimb use by a modified nigral cell suspension transplantation approach in the rat Parkinson model. Neuroscience 1:33–43

100. Nikkhah G, Olsson M, Eberhard J, Bentlage C, Cunningham MG, Bjorklund A (1994) A microtransplantation approach for cell suspension grafting in the rat Parkinson model: a detailed account of the methodology. Neuroscience 1:57–72

101. Nikkhah G, Winkler C, Roedter A, Samii M (2000) Microtransplantation of nigral dopamine neurons: a "step-by-step" recipe. In: Dunnett SB, Baker G (eds) NeuroMethods: Cell and Tissue Transplantation in the CNS. Humana, Totowa, pp 207–231

102. Oertle T, van der Haar ME, Bandtlow CE, Robeva A, Burfeind P, Buss A, Huber AB, Simonen M, Schnell L, Brosamle C, Kaupmann K, Vallon R, Schwab ME (2003) Nogo-A inhibits neurite outgrowth and cell spreading with three discrete regions. J Neurosci 13:5393–5406

103. Olanow CW, Goetz CG, Kordower JH, Stoessl AJ, Sossi V, Brin MF, Shannon KM, Nauert GM, Perl DP, Godbold J, Freeman TB (2003) A double-blind controlled trial of bilateral fetal nigral transplantation in Parkinson's disease. Ann Neurol 3:403–414

104. Olsson M, Nikkhah G, Bentlage C, Bjorklund A (1995) Forelimb akinesia in the rat Parkinson model: differential effects of dopamine agonists and nigral transplants as assessed by a new stepping test. J Neurosci 5:3863–3875

105. Perlow MJ, Freed WJ, Hoffer BJ, Seiger A, Olson L, Wyatt RJ (1979) Brain grafts reduce motor abnormalities produced by destruction of nigrostriatal dopamine system. Science 4393:643–647

106. Peschanski M, Defer G, N'Guyen JP, Ricolfi F, Monfort JC, Remy P, Geny C, Samson Y, Hantraye P, Jeny R (1994) Bilateral motor improvement and alteration of L-dopa effect in two patients with Parkinson's disease following intrastriatal transplantation of foetal ventral mesencephalon. Brain 117:487–499

107. Piccini P, Brooks DJ, Bjorklund A, Gunn RN, Grasby PM, Rimoldi O, Brundin P, Hagell P, Rehncrona S, Widner H, Lindvall O (1999) Dopamine release from nigral transplants visualized in vivo in a Parkinson's patient. Nat Neurosci 12:1137–1140

108. Poewe W, Wenning GK (2000) Apomorphine: an underutilized therapy for Parkinson's disease. Mov Disord 5:789–794

109. Pruszak J, Sonntag KC, Aung MH, Sanchez-Pernaute R, Isacson O (2007) Markers and methods for cell sorting of human embryonic stem cell-derived neural cell populations. Stem Cells (in press)

110. Rascol O, Brooks DJ, Korczyn AD, De Deyn PP, Clarke CE, Lang AE (2000) A five-year study of the incidence of dyskinesia in patients with early Parkinson's disease who were treated with ropinirole or levodopa. 056 Study Group. N Engl J Med 20:1484–1491

111. Rascol O, Payoux P, Ory F, Ferreira JJ, Brefel-Courbon C, Montastruc JL (2003) Limitations of current Parkinson's disease therapy. Ann Neurol 53:S3–S12

112. Rioux L, Gaudin DP, Bui LK, Gregoire L, DiPaolo T, Bedard PJ (1991) Correlation of functional recovery after a 6-hydroxydopamine lesion with survival of grafted fetal neurons and release of dopamine in the striatum of the rat. Neuroscience 1:123–131

113. Rioux L, Gaudin DP, Gagnon C, Di Paolo T, Bedard PJ (1991) Decrease of behavioral and biochemical denervation supersensitivity of rat striatum by nigral transplants. Neuroscience 1:75–83

114. Rodriguez-Oroz MC, Obeso JA, Lang AE, Houeto JL, Pollak P, Rehncrona S, Kulisevsky J, Albanese A, Volkmann J, Hariz MI, Quinn NP, Speelman JD, Guridi J, Zamarbide I, Gironell A, Molet J, Pascual-Sedano B, Pidoux B, Bonnet AM, Agid Y, Xie J, Benabid AL, Lozano AM, Saint-Cyr J, Romito L, Contarino MF, Scerrati M, Fraix V, Van Blercom N (2005) Bilateral deep brain stimulation in Parkinson's disease: a multicentre study with 4 years follow-up. Brain 128:2240–2249

115. Rodter A, Winkler C, Samii M, Nikkhah G (2000) Complex sensorimotor behavioral changes after terminal striatal 6-OHDA lesion and transplantation of dopaminergic embryonic micrografts. Cell Transplant 2:197–214

116. Roedter A, Winkler C, Samii M, Walter GF, Brandis A, Nikkhah G (2001) Comparison of unilateral and bilateral intrastriatal 6-hydroxydopamine-induced axon terminal lesions: evidence for interhemispheric functional coupling of the two nigrostriatal pathways. J Comp Neurol 2:217–229

117. Roy NS, Cleren C, Singh SK, Yang L, Beal MF, Goldman SA (2006) Functional engraftment of human ES cell-derived dopaminergic neurons enriched by coculture with telomerase-immortalized midbrain astrocytes. Nat Med 11:1259–1268

118. Sanai N, Tramontin AD, Quinones-Hinojosa A, Barbaro NM, Gupta N, Kunwar S, Lawton MT, McDermott MW, Parsa AT, Manuel-Garcia VJ, Berger MS, Alvarez-Buylla A (2004) Unique astrocyte ribbon in adult human brain contains neural stem cells but lacks chain migration. Nature 6976:740–744

119. Schallert T, Hall S (1988) 'Disengage' sensorimotor deficit following apparent recovery from unilateral dopamine depletion. Behav Brain Res 1:15–24

120. Schallert T, De Ryck M, Whishaw IQ, Ramirez VD, Teitelbaum P (1979) Excessive bracing reactions and their control by atropine and L-DOPA in an animal analog of Parkinsonism. Exp Neurol 1:33–43

121. Schallert T, Upchurch M, Lobaugh N, Farrar SB, Spirduso WW, Gilliam P, Vaughn D, Wilcox RE (1982) Tactile extinction: distinguishing between sensorimotor and motor asymmetries in rats with unilateral nigrostriatal damage. Pharmacol Biochem Behav 3:455–462

122. Schmidt WJ (2000). Zur Verhaltensbiologie der Parkinson-Krankheit. Neuroforum 6:229–234

123. Shetty N, Friedman JH, Kieburtz K, Marshall FJ, Oakes D (1999) The placebo response in Parkinson's disease. Parkinson Study Group. Clin Neuropharmacol 4:207–212

124. Simonen M, Pedersen V, Weinmann O, Schnell L, Buss A, Ledermann B, Christ F, Sansig G, van der PH, Schwab ME (2003) Systemic deletion of the myelin-associated outgrowth inhibitor Nogo-A improves regenerative and plastic responses after spinal cord injury. Neuron 2:201–211

125. Sonntag KC, Pruszak J, Yoshizaki T, van Arensbergen J, Sanchez-Pernaute R, Isacson O (2007) Enhanced yield of neuroepithelial precursors and midbrain-like dopaminergic neurons from human embryonic stem cells using the bone morphogenic protein antagonist noggin. Stem Cells 2:411–418

126. Stenevi U, Bjorklund A, Svendgaard NA (1976) Transplantation of central and peripheral monoamine neurons to the adult rat brain: techniques and conditions for survival. Brain Res 1:1–20

127. Strecker RE, Sharp T, Brundin P, Zetterstrom T, Ungerstedt U, Bjorklund A (1987) Autoregulation of dopamine release and metabolism by intrastriatal nigral grafts as revealed by intracerebral dialysis. Neuroscience 1:169–178

128. Ungerstedt U (1968) 6-Hydroxy-dopamine induced degeneration of central monoamine neurons. Eur J Pharmacol 1:107–110

129. Ungerstedt U, Arbuthnott GW (1970) Quantitative recording of rotational behavior in rats after 6-hydroxy-dopamine lesions of the nigrostriatal dopamine system. Brain Res 3:485–493

130. van Praag H, Kempermann G, Gage FH (2000) Neural consequences of environmental enrichment. Nat Rev Neurosci 3:191–198

131. Vergara-Aragon P, Gonzalez CL, Whishaw IQ (2003) A novel skilled-reaching impairment in paw supination on the "good" side of the hemi-Parkinson rat improved with rehabilitation. J Neurosci 2:579–586

132. Vuillet J, Moukhles H, Nieoullon A, Daszuta A (1994) Ultrastructural analysis of graft-to-host connections, with special reference to dopamine-neuropeptide Y interactions in the rat striatum, after transplantation of fetal mesencephalon cells. Exp Brain Res 1:84–96

133. Wenning GK, Odin P, Morrish P, Rehncrona S, Widner H, Brundin P, Rothwell JC, Brown R, Gustavii B, Hagell P, Jahanshahi M, Sawle G, Bjorklund A, Brooks DJ, Marsden CD, Quinn NP, Lindvall O (1997) Short- and long-term survival and function of unilateral intrastriatal dopaminergic grafts in Parkinson's disease. Ann Neurol 1:95–107

134. Whishaw IQ, Pellis SM (1990) The structure of skilled forelimb reaching in the rat: a proximally driven movement with a single distal rotatory component. Behav Brain Res 1:49–59

135. Whishaw IQ, Tomie JA (1988) Food wrenching and dodging: a neuroethological test of cortical and dopaminergic contributions to sensorimotor behavior in the rat. Behav Neurosci 1:110–123

136. Whishaw IQ, O'Connor WT, Dunnett SB (1986) The contributions of motor cortex, nigrostriatal dopamine and caudate-putamen to skilled forelimb use in the rat. Brain 109:805–843

137. Whishaw IQ, Woodward NC, Miklyaeva E, Pellis SM (1997) Analysis of limb use by control rats and unilateral DA-depleted rats in the Montoya staircase test: movements, impairments and compensatory strategies. Behav Brain Res 89:167–177

138. Winkler C, Bentlage C, Cenci MA, Nikkhah G, Bjorklund A (2003) Regulation of neuropeptide mRNA expression in the basal ganglia by intrastriatal and intranigral transplants in the rat Parkinson model. Neuroscience 4:1063–1077

139. Winkler C, Bentlage C, Nikkhah G, Samii M, Bjorklund A (1999) Intranigral transplants of GABA-rich striatal tissue induce behavioral recovery in the rat Parkinson model and promote the effects obtained by intrastriatal dopaminergic transplants. Exp Neurol 2:165–186

140. Winkler C, Kirik D, Bjorklund A (2005) Cell transplantation in Parkinson's disease: how can we make it work? Trends Neurosci 2:86–92

141. Winkler C, Kirik D, Bjorklund A, Dunnett SB (2000) Transplantation in the rat model of Parkinson's disease: ectopic versus homotopic graft placement. Prog Brain Res 127:233–265

142. Yan WH, Cao MD, Liu JR, Xu Y, Han XF, Xing Y, Wang JZ (2005) Effects of EGF and bFGF on expression of microtubule-associated protein tau and MAP-2 mRNA in human umbilical cord mononuclear cells. Cell Biol Int 2:153–157

143. Zigmond MJ (1994) Chemical transmission in the brain: homeostatic regulation and its functional implications. Prog Brain Res 100:115–122

# Preservation and Restitution of Auditory Function in Neurofibromatosis Type 2

**5**

Cordula Matthies

Contents

## 5.1

## Background

Neurofibromatosis type 2 (NF2) is defined by bilateral vestibular schwannomas; 86% of patients suffer from additional spinal tumours, schwannomas and meningiomas and, in rare cases, also gliomas and ependymomas. Furthermore, most patients present with additional cranial meningiomas or even meningiomatosis of the sinuses. As a consequence, these patients are at risk of bilateral deafness, facial and motor nerve palsies and para- or tetraparesis. Fifty-eight percent of affected patients become symptomatic before the age of 20 years, but first manifestation at over 40 years is possible. About 50% exhibit a familial history of NF2, while the other 50% have a new mutation.

In NF2, different to sporadic schwannomas, cure from a specific tumour cannot be achieved, as even in radical resection, due to the nature of the disease, a recurrence can occur at any site of a preserved nerve and at much higher rate and speed. Especially young patients below 20 and even 30 years of age present much faster growth patterns and a far more active tumour biology. As a rule, the largest schwannomas are be found in the youngest patients. Furthermore, in a large clinical study carried out at Hannover Nordstadt Hospital on 200 NF2 patients, the tumour–nerve relationship in NF2 was considerably different from that in sporadic schwannoma patients. In 25% of the cases, the tumor consisted of several schwannomas originating from several nerves such as the vestibular, facial and caudal cranial nerves. Nerve fascicles had undergone tumorous change and were impossible to differentiate from the tumour.

The progress experienced in unilateral vestibular schwannoma surgery has initiated a completely different approach to the clinical fate of patients with NF2. Two major goals have been formulated with respect to vestibular schwannomas: (1) adequate brainstem decompression from life-threatening tumours and (2) Preservation or restitution of as much useful function as possible.

For most patients, facial nerve function and at least unilateral hearing are of utmost importance. This chapter will focus on auditory function. The vast experience gathered by Madjid Samii in sporadic schwannomas and his persistent activity in hearing preservation surgery has meant that a large number of patients have sought his advice and asked for his personal expertise and surgery.

Preservation of function in NF2 remains far more difficult than in sporadic tumours, and any preserved function could be threatened by further tumour growth from the same or a neighbouring nerve. However, as a result of the evolution of functional microsurgery, cases with successful nerve preservation have occurred at a rate of 29% (Table 1), offering to the individual a completely different life perspective: the chance to finish school, continue their education and studies and develop professional skills and activity.

Along with this progress, there was a longstanding non-interest in hearing implants. However, the experience of tumour recurrence and growth over 5–10 years with a slow, but continuous decrease of the auditory function has raised a further challenge to surgeons to adopt this option for these patients.

Over a period of 16 years, patients with NF2 have received a specific evaluation, counselling and therapy at Hannover Nordstadt Hospital, resulting in a large cohort of data and experiences within the NF2 Study Group; some of the most important are presented here.

## 5.2
## Special Pre-Conditions for Vestibular Schwannomas in NF2

As mentioned above, vestibular schwannomas in NF2 are in most cases larger than average and grow at a faster rate, with about 67% of patients with large T4 tumours at first presentation. Auditory function and tumour growth do not correlate with each other; quite often there is bad hearing on one side, with a small or medium-sized tumour and normal hearing on the other side, with a large brainstem compressive tumour. There might be as well similar quality of hearing on either side and similar tumour size.

In the case of a brainstem compressive tumour, microsurgical decompression is the first-line treatment since the

Table 1 Auditory function in 195 tumour operations in 145 neurofibromatosis type 2 patients. Audiometric hearing loss calculated as the mean at 1–3 kHz. *SDS* Speech discrimination score

| Auditory function | Pre-operative | Post-operative |
|---|---|---|
| H1 (0–20 dB, 100–95% SDS) | 54 | 8 |
| H2 (21–40 dB, 90–70% SDS) | 26 | 13 |
| H3 (41–60 dB, 65–35% SDS) | 24 | 7 (29%) 36 |
| H4 (61–80 dB, 30–10% SDS) | 22 | 8 |
| H5 (>80 dB) | 69 | 159 |

first priority is saving the patient's life. Otherwise, neurological function and quality of life are the parameters of decision. By analysing auditory brainstem responses and quality of hearing on either side, the side with the highest chance for hearing preservation can usually be identified. Audiometric hearing should be good or useful (H1, H2), with up 40 dB loss and with useful speech discrimination of 70% or more. In auditory brainstem response (ABR) testing, all ABR components must be registered and I–III interpeak latency increase should be below two standard deviations. Furthermore, better chances are can be anticipated, the shorter the patient is symptomatic and the shorter the period of nerve compression.

## 5.3
## Development of Auditory Function

At presentation to the neurosurgeon, 33% of ears in NF2 patients are already deaf (Fig. 1). Of those hearing ears, about 67% will become deaf via surgery – life-rescuing surgery in most cases. The average age of deafness in these cases is 26 years. In 29% of patients, some hearing function will be retained at an average age of 27 years and be conserved for up to 14 years (Fig. 1). In those ears observed over time, possibly because of residual hearing function, deafness developed by a "natural course" on average by the age of 29 years.

## 5.4
## Special Considerations of Preservation of Auditory Nerve Function in NF2 Vestibular Schwannomas

In view of the tremendous difficulty and the tremendous need to preserve at least unilateral hearing in NF2, Samii decided and tried in selected cases to achieve hearing preservation by subtotal tumour resection. The microsurgical principles are as follows:

With the patient in the semi-sitting position after retrosigmoid suboccipital craniotomy, cerebrospinal fluid is drained from the basal cistern and light cerebellar retraction is carried out. The tumour in the cistern is at first not touched, but the internal auditory canal is drilled open under meticulous monitoring with repeated breaks. The intrameatal tumour is enucleated and is mobilised away from the nerves. In cases of serious ABR deterioration, intrameatal dissection is stopped, ABR recovery is awaited and extrameatal tumour enucleation is performed. In most cases, the extrameatal tumour part will be largely or completely removed while the dissection close to the porus and at the intrameatal portion may be critical. As long as the ABR show fast recovery during the short breaks from microsurgical activity, further dissection my be tried; if recovery is shown to be slower or incomplete,

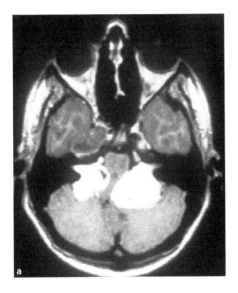

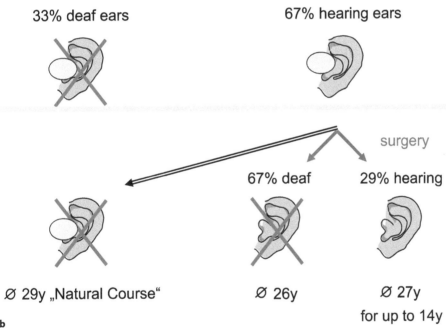

Fig. 1 **a** Bilateral Schwannomas in neurofibromatosis type 2 (NF2) With serious compression of the brainstem. **b** Auditory function in NF2 at presentation to the neurosurgeon

then the tumour resection should be stopped in order to conserve hearing. Nonetheless, secondary deterioration and hearing loss within the first hours or 2 weeks after surgery may occur. In critical cases, the local and systemic administration of vasoactive substances seems to be beneficial [1].

In a series of 23 patients, this technique was successful in 15 cases (65%; Table 2). This method requires detailed patient information and counselling beforehand. In pa-

tients in whom auditory function is of great importance, early surgery at good starting conditions must be recommended; in case of a tumorous nerve change or very sensitive ABR, the subtotal technique with bony decompression of the cranial nerves increases the chances of functional preservation.

Long-term follow-up showed that these patients kept some useful function for several years, in general over 10 years, and in some individual cases over 14 years.

Table 2 Bilateral vestibular schwannomas. Auditory function in 23 incomplete resections. *Preop* Preoperative, *Post-op* post-operative, *HL* hearing level

| Case no. | Year of surgery | Size (mm) | Preoperative HL (dB) | SDS (%) | Post-operative HL (dB) | SDS (%) |
|---|---|---|---|---|---|---|
| 1 | 1986 | 30×20 | 1 | 100 | 35 | 90 |
| 2 | 1987 | 35×25 | 2 | 100 | 50 | 70 |
| 3 | 1989 | 30×20 | 30 | 80 | 33 | 80 |
| 4 | 1990 | 25×20 | 5 | 100 | 60 | 70 |
| 5 | 1990 | 40×40 | 43 | 80 | 28 | 90 |
| 6 | 1991 | 25×20 | 6 | 100 | 18 | 100 |
| 7 | 1991 | 35×20 | 7 | 100 | – | – |
| 8 | 1992 | 35×20 | 6 | 95 | – | – |
| 9 | 1992 | 30×20 | 3 | 100 | – | – |
| 10 | 1993 | 15×10 | 10 | 100 | 25 | 90 |
| 11 | 1993 | 20×15 | 7 | 100 | 72 | 35 |
| 12 | 1993 | 20×20 | 1 | 100 | 22 | 100 |
| 13 | 1993 | 40×30 | 32 | 90 | – | – |
| 14 | 1993 | 20×18 | 27 | 90 | 45 | 80 |
| 15 | 1994 | 10×5 | 1 | 85 | 25 | 80 |
| 16 | 1994 | 15×15 | 1 | 100 | 36 | 100 |
| 17 | 1994 | 20×10 | 7 | 90 | 11 | 90 |
| 18 | 1994 | 50×40 | 55 | 60 | – | – |
| 19 | 1995 | 20×15 | 40 | 65 | 46 | 50 |
| 20 | 1997 | 15×13 | 20 | 100 | – | – |
| 21 | 1997 | 20×12 | 15 | 90 | – | – |
| 22 | 1997 | 7×5 | 6 | 100 | 11 | 100 |
| 23 | 1998 | 28×25 | 46 | 100 | – | – |

Function also remained useful in a case of tumour regrowth over a long period thanks to decompression of the internal auditory canal.

However, vestibular schwannomas in NF2 show recurrence usually after 4–8 years and cause, among other problems, secondary deafness on previously preserved functional ears. Other patients become deaf early on during their illness. Many of these patients are interested in undergoing auditory implantation, a cochlea implant or an auditory brainstem implant (ABI).

## 5.5
## Cochlea Implants in NF2

A few conditions predispose patients to successful cochlea implant therapy. NF2 patients with rather small tumours and sudden complete hearing loss are likely to have a failure of their cochlea function. Furthermore, patients with serious amplitude decrease of component I and of the electrocochleography potential during surgery may have cochlea failure, but a still functioning auditory nerve. By promontory stimulation testing, positive cochlear nerve function can be identified and the option for a cochlea implant can be formulated.

A cochlear implant may enable the patient to regain very useful auditory function; however, if a tumour is still present, and especially if it is infiltrative, cochlear implant function will deteriorate over time. If the tumour is a meningioma, the quality and stability of cochlear implant function might be superior to the schwannoma situation, even in a relatively large tumour. The general rule that cochlear implant function is always superior to brainstem implant function does not hold true for all NF2 patients.

are designed to be laid onto the brainstem surface of the cochlear nucleus. The very first ABI models contained only two electrodes and were applied by Hitselberger and colleagues at the House Ear Institute in 1979. Several companies producing ABIs have developed different shapes with platinum iridium platelet-shaped electrodes in a silicone carrier. Two models have been used for the Hannover patients, the Nucleus Device, which contains a magnet and which can be removed temporarily under local anaesthesia to perform a magnetic resonance imaging, MRI, scan) or the magnet-free Clarion Device (Fig. 2).

## 5.6
## ABIs in NF2

ABIs make use of the same technology as cochlea implants, but they contain a different kind of electrode and

## 5.6.1
## Pre-Conditions to ABIs in NF2

If the patient has a personal interest in hearing and understanding and undertakes efforts in lip-reading, these

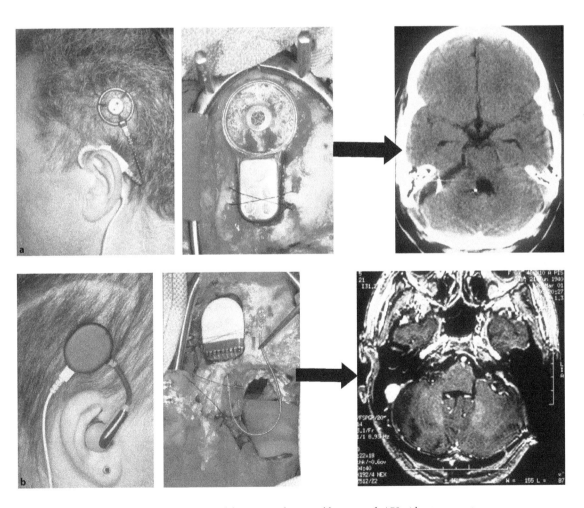

Fig. 2a,b  Auditory brainstem implant (ABI) models. **a** ABI with removable magnet. **b** ABI without a magnet

are favourable factors with regard to the chances of re-learning some hearing. Besides, it is sensible to plan the ABI surgery at a rather stable period of the NF2 disease, whereas it is disadvantageous to decide upon it when there is multiple tumour progression and a necessity to undergo several operations anyway.

The individual risks have to be analysed and weighed against the possible chances of success and usefulness of the implant. Some patients are far more affected by spinal cord compression and impending paraparesis or by multiple caudal cranial nerve palsies.

A further specific indication to ABI may be impending visual loss. Most NF2 patients have long-standing visual deficits due to retinal disease and may use only one eye for communication and reading. If that eye is endangered by a skull base or intraorbital tumour, in most cases meningioma, then an ABI should be implanted early on to enable hearing learning along with some lip reading as long as it is still possible.

Before a definite decision on implantation, each candidate receives a cranial and spinal MRI for staging and comparison with control images of the fore-going years.

Patient counselling must include the prognosis based on previous experiences. Patients may expect that they will receive some noise perception, that speech recognition and understanding by lip reading will be improved by ABI and that the increase in comprehension varies from 5% to 40%. Patients will also be notified that some may be non-responders, especially after previous radiosurgery, and that technical failure of an ABI can occur spontaneously or after trauma.

## 5.6.2
## Operative Technique of ABI in NF2

With the patient in the semi-sitting position, the lateral suboccipital approach is performed for tumour resection as well as for ABI placement. After resection of the tumour, a narrow retractor blade is used to retract the cerebellum over the lateral recess. The latter may be identified by the flocculus and the choroid plexus. In numerous cases there will be additional schwannomas of the caudal cranial nerves; these nerves are extremely sensitive and tolerate only partial tumour resection. If there is extensive tumour formation at this side, the ABI might be better placed on the contralateral side.

The cerebellum needs to be lifted to expose the most lateral part of the floor of the fourth ventricle. Here, the brainstem is completely white, whereas just above at the entrance an arterial branch of the inferior cerebellar artery will be found. This accompanies the cochlear and glossopharyngeal nerves as they course to and from the brainstem. In most patients the cochlear nerve will no longer be found, and the facial nerve is the next superior to be identified. By following cranial nerves VII, VIII and IX, the cochlear nucleus can be safely found within the lateral recess (Fig. 3). A test electrode is placed and by electrostimulation, electrical ABRs (E-ABRs) are searched for (Fig. 4). Once these E-ABRs can be recorded at the majority of electrodes and from the lateral to the medial end of the electrode carrier, a decision is taken for implantation of the definite ABI. At first the otorhinolaryngological surgeon drills out the implant bed at

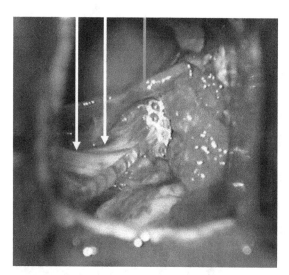

Fig. 3 Anatomy of the lateral brainstem area. The cochlear and glossopharyngeal nerves (*white arrows*) and inferior cerebellar artery branch (*blue arrow*) indicate the route to the lateral recess where the ABI is placed and fixed with fibrin plaster

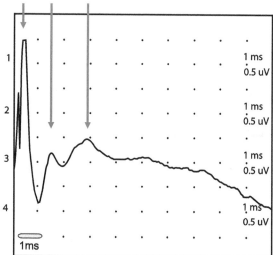

Fig. 4 Electric auditory brainstem responses (E-ABRs) recorded during ABI positioning. Example E-ABR (#2 AA): at 16.2 Hz, 300 µA, 150 µs. Recorded by Dr. C. Frohne and Professor Dr. T. Lenarz (Department of Otolaryngology, Hannover Medical School, Germany) at interdisciplinary surgery of patient #21

the occipital retroauricular area and fixes of the transfer device. Then the neurosurgeon exchanges the test electrode for the definite electrode; after electrophysiological testing for E-ABRs, for exclusion of any side effects of the motor cranial nerves and long tracts, the ABI position is fixed with some fibrin plaster or Gelfoam® sponge. The ABI cable to the transducing system is handled with care and integrated into the dura closure.

## 5.7
## Postoperative Management and Rehabilitation

After surgery and before extubation, these NF2 patients are tested for caudal cranial nerve palsies in view of the manipulation in that area. In some patients, a temporary tracheostomy might be necessary. In general recovery from this surgery is good and similar to that for other types of cerebellopontine angle surgery.

After a period of recovery of 4–6 weeks, the patient is re-admitted so that his implant device can be activated and for programming of a speech processor. The first tests of all electrodes are performed in the intensive care unit with anaesthesiology prepared for any kind of cardiac or respiratory disturbances on brainstem stimulation. The programming of the device has to be carried out with much patience, as it is essential to identify the frequencies perceived by the patient and to give time to recognise various types of sound by somebody with perhaps longstanding deafness. Once the number and site of useful electrodes are identified, the intensity of stimula-

Table 3  Nordstadt series of auditory brainstem implant (*ABI*) surgery. *RadioS* Radiosurgery, *L* left, *R* right, *ext*

| Patient | | Age (years) | Tumour | Side | Tumour, ABI | Previous surgery/RadioS |
|---|---|---|---|---|---|---|
| 1 | TL | 29 | 15 mm T2 | L | 07.05.96 | 09.86 |
| 2 | AA | 51 | 45 mm T4a | R | 25.07.96 | 83 ext, 12.94 |
| 3 | MP | 24 | 37 mm T4b | R | 07.11.96 | – |
| 4 | BC | 25 | 37 mm T4a | L | 07.96 | 81 ext, 85 |
| 5 | TK | 31 | 50 mm T4b | L | 03.97 | 11.96 |
| 6 | JP | 34 | 34 mm T4 | R | 04.05.98 | 84 ext |
| 7 | HP | 49 | 27 mm T3b | L | 23.10.98 | 92 ext |
| 8 | CW | 43 | 30 mm T4a | L | 05.11.98 | 90 ext |
| 9 | AJ | 33 | 49 mm T4b | L | 15.03.99 | 91 ext, RadioS |
| 10 | EL | 32 | 32 mm T4a | R | 03.05.99 | 87 |
| 11 | RF | 61 | 46 mm T4b | L | 07.07.99 | –, RadioS |
| 12 | WF | 54 | 11 mm T1 | R | 29.11.99 | – |
| 13 | ME | 25 | 42 mm T4a | R | 05.07.99 | – |
| 14 | RR | 60 | 8 mm T1 | L | 01.00 | 12.99 |
| 15 | MS | 15 | 35 mm T4a | L | 11.07.00 | – |
| 16 | AH | 21 | 30 mm T4a | R | 12.07.00 | – |
| 17 | SSt | 45 | 18 mm T2 | R | 25.07.00 | 01.93 ext |
| 18 | BK | 18 | 41 mm T4b | L | 20.07.01 | – |
| 19 | AB | 20 | 38 mm T4b | L | 29.10.01 | – |
| 20 | SL | 26 | 45 mm T4b | R | 11.01 | 93 |
| 21 | SK | 32 | 40 mm T4a | R | 22.11.02 | –, RadioS |
| 22 | EH | 43 | 42 mm T4b | R | 22.11.02 | 01 |

tion may be adjusted and some training is commenced. Adaptations to the individual programme and training sequences are repeated at 1- to 3-month intervals in the 1st year and at longer intervals in the 2nd and 3rd years.

## 5.8
## Results of ABI Surgery

### 5.8.1
### Patients

An interdisciplinary team of neurosurgeons, otolaryngologists and electrical engineers performed a series of 25 ABI implantations in 22 patients (Table 3); 14 of these patients had been operated on that same side before, 7 by the Hannover Team with initial hearing preservation. Three patients had undergone previous radiosurgery and 17 patients suffered from large brainstem-compressive tumours (T4).

### 5.8.2
### Surgical Complications

One patient had a haemorrhage in the posterior fossa, which was immediately revised, and the patient's further course was uneventful with fast recovery and very good ABI result. A technical defect occurred after 1 year in another patient, who reported intermittent dysesthesia; therefore the ABI was removed and at surgery, extreme scarring and involvement of the ABI became apparent. The patient had had radiosurgery before.

In two patients, implant dislocation was diagnosed. The first patient with good intraoperative E-ABR showed only side effects with tingling in his leg at first ABI activation; after revision and repositioning there were no side effects and good auditory function. The second patient with ABI dislocation experienced no sound impression on activation and was found to have a floating electrode carrier; further revision was planned.

### 5.8.3
### Audiological Results

The audiological results are summarised by Fig. 5. In a speech-tracking test with continuously read text, patients understand 5–30% by pure visual mode (only lip-reading). This understanding is increased by 10–50% with the aid of audiological ABI perception. Most patients showed improvement over time. There are a few patients with no or a very poor response, namely those who have undergone radiosurgery. There were two patients with major visual deficits, one of who died due to sudden very severe disease progression; in these cases, hearing training was impaired as a result of their poor vision.

Furthermore, intraoperative deformed E-ABRs were a negative predictive factor, whereas nicely formed E-ABR components III and V were very positive predictors. In the case of absent E-ABRs, an ABI was not and would not be implanted according to the philosophy of this team.

## 5.9
## Conclusions

Along with functional microsurgery being developed for skull base lesions in general and being applied for patients with NF2, their chances for a longer survival and

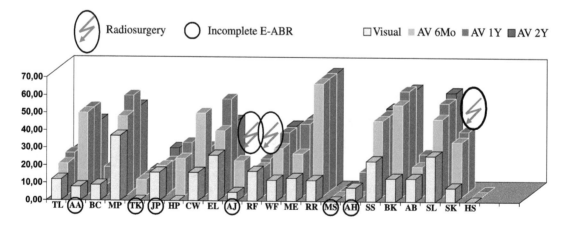

Fig. 5 Nordstadt series of ABI surgery: results. Correct speech recognition in the speech-tracking test tested for pure visual and audiovisual (AV) mode. Improvement in some patients is obvious after 6 months (6Mo), but may continue for over 2 years. Critical predictive factors are poor electrical ABRs (E-ABR) and previous radiosurgery

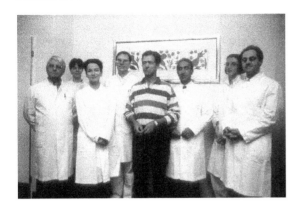

Fig. 6 The interdisciplinary Hannover team for ABI, which comprises neurosurgeons, otolaryngologists and electrical engineers, with a patient (fifth from the left)

for improved quality of life are increased significantly. The chances of preserving some useful auditory function for at least some years means a fundamental difference to a patient's life; the possibility of restoring some hearing even in cases of loss of natural hearing is a further positive stimulus. This prevents these patients from withdrawal from society and facilitates them taking an active part in all decision-making. After some period of struggle, most NF2 patients take an impressively positive attitude towards their fate and decide for an unbelievable active life. It is impressive to learn how these patients, despite neurological disturbances, fight in order to get or keep their job and how much enthusiasm they have for organising information and support meetings for other NF2 patients.

Sincere thanks are addressed to the interdisciplinary teams (Fig. 6) at Hannover Nordstadt Hospital and Hannover Medical School. In addition to M. Samii and the author of this chapter, the Hannover Neurofibromatosis Study Group comprised K. Kniese, S. Thomas, M. Tatagiba and P. Vorkapic. The Auditory Brainstem Implant Group included neurosurgical co-workers, by neurosurgical technical assistants, Mrs E. Heinrich, and by colleagues from Otolaryngology, T. Lenarz, A. Lesinski-Schiedat, M. Moshrefi, C. Frohne, Mr Battmer and Mr. Gärtner. A special thanks is given to all patients for their interest, feedback and active support of the team's work.

## References

1.   Strauss C, Bischoff B, Neu M, Berg M, Fahlbusch R, Romstock J (2001) Vasoactive treatment for hearing preservation in acoustic neuroma surgery. J Neurosurg 95:771–777

# Restoration of Locomotion in Post-traumatic Paraplegics: The Neurosurgeon's Personal View

**6**

Klaus R. H. von Wild

## Contents

## 6.1 Objective

Research and clinical quality management in neurotraumatology is a multidisciplinary task and challenge for neurosurgeons. Scientific cooperation is targeted to exchange personal knowledge and expertise within a given specific field of neurotrauma (e.g. brain, spinal cord and peripheral nerve lesions). The roots of restorative neurosurgery in traumatology go back to the beginning of modern neurological surgery. Nowadays, traffic accidents and personal violence are the major causes of spinal cord lesions. There are in Europe about 300,000 paraplegics, and in every country there are approximately 1000 new cases per year, with an increasing number of tetraplegics due to the quality of both emergency care and early neurorehabilitation. A completely disrupted spinal cord cannot heal for recovery of motor and sensorial functioning, although many promising treatments in laboratory animal experiments are reported, including stem-cell-injections. No procedure has so far proven to be a standard technique to enhance neurological recovery in humans. The important role of external functional electrical stimulation (FES) for training and functional restoration of paralysed muscles and the impact of early functional rehabilitation for spinal-cord-injured victims, however, are indisputable.

In this report, the author's experience from two international European surgical projects for the restoration of voluntary locomotion of recent years is analysed to identify factors that might have caused the pitfalls, since up to now neither approach has been adopted by the rehabilitation physician or restorative neurosurgeons for voluntary restoration of locomotion in paraplegics, notwithstanding the objectively promising clinical results that have been reported.

## 6.2
## Methods

There follows a review of the author's personal experience when approaching different scientific network activities.

### 6.2.1
### Historical Background

#### 6.2.1.1
#### CALIES European Clinical Network (1989)

CALIES stands for "computer-aided locomotion by implanted electrical stimulation" in paralysed persons (Industry and researchers from France, Italy, The Netherlands, Ireland and Germany).

#### 6.2.1.2
#### The BIOMED I-RAFT (1992)

RAFT stands for "restoration of muscle activity through FES and associated technology" run along with CALIES. SUAW ("stand up and walk") is a European Community scientific research project that was established under the direction of Professor J. Edwards and the late Professor K.R. Krishnan (University of Salford, Manchester, UK); Professor Pierre Rabischong (Montpellier, France) was appointed project coordinator.

#### 6.2.1.3
#### SUAW 2

SUAW 2 followed in 1997, supported by The European Community Project under the Biomed 2 programme Contact BMH4-CT96-1501.P. Again, Professor Rabischong became responsible for the clinical and technical management and coordination. Nine out of 14 technicians were from France, like Bernard Denis (Neuromedics), responsible for the industrial partners, assisted by Pierre Couderc (Neuromedics implant), who was in close contact with Professor Rabischong, who is a specialist in human robotics. Other partners came, for example, from IBM France, Thomson CSF, Paris, Het Roessingh, R. & DFD, Enschede, The Netherlands, and the Germans from the Frauenhofer Institut St. Ingbert, Germany, to produce novel implantable miniaturised bipolar neural and epimysial electrodes. This project ran along with CALIES Association. There were six clinical centres involved (Fig. 1): Copenhagen/Alborg (Denmark), Montpellier (France), Münster/Bad Wildungen (Germany), Bologna/Montecantone (Italy), Enschede (The Netherlands) and Southport (UK)

### 6.2.2
### Learning by Doing

In the early eighties, when the author worked as an Assistant Professor in Consultant Professor Samii's neurosurgical department at the Nordstadt Hospital, Hannover (Germany) from 1977 until 1982, he first met with Professor Pierre Rabischong during their active participation in Professor Samii's first ever skull-base conferences. At the end of 1997 that they met again in Hannover at the newly established Neurobionic foundation under the presidency of Professor Samii. At that time, Professor Rabischong started talking about his SUAW project and, since Professor Samii had resigned, was looking for

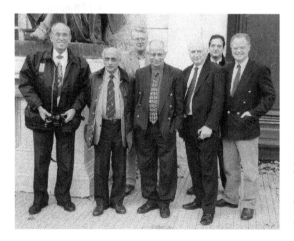

Fig. 1 "Stand up and Walk" (SUAW) international surgical team in front of the Anatomical Institute of the University of Montpelier, 13th December 1998 (from left to right): Giorgio Brunelli (Brescia, Italy), the late Krish Krishnan (Salford, UK), Ole Osgaard (Denmark), Bakulesh Soni (Southport, UK), Pierre Rabischong and Michel Benichou (Montpellier, France) and Hans Van der Aa (Enschede, The Netherlands)

an interested and microsurgically experienced neurosurgeon as the German partner of his team. At the request of Professor Rabischong, the author immediately joined the project, as the SUAW project matched with his focused interest in functional neurorehabilitation and reconstructive neurosurgery (re-engineering). He remained as part of that project until 2002.

## 6.2.3
## Calendar of the Author's Participation in SUAW Preparatory Activities

1. 21st–22nd March 1998, Paris: Workshop on restorative surgical techniques, concept of rehabilitation and research, and biotechnology, with open discussion on technical and ethical issues. The timetable for the first ten patients to be implanted, two in each country, was formulated.
2. 12th–13th December 1998, Montpelier: Centre Propara, Medical Faculty (Fig. 1). All surgeons were experts in hand and plastic reconstructive restorative neurological microsurgery. Presentation of the implant prototypes and the design of the neuroprosthesis box. There was much concern and open questions.
3. 11th–15th February 1999: Cadaver sections for validation of the surgical protocol in Clermont-Ferrand and Montpellier, France (Figs. 2 and 3)
4. 26th–28th March 1999: Further cadaver section and endoscopy in Clermont-Ferrand.

During the workshops, the author got in close touch with Giorgio Brunelli and his own research projects on central nervous system–peripheral nervous system (CNS–PNS) connection (Brunelli's Paradigm, Fig. 4). From that time, as a restorative neurosurgeon, he combined his project with the surgical procedures of spinal cord bypass grafting in Italy.

## 6.2.4
## Building up an International Neurotrauma Network

Research and clinical quality management in neurotraumatology need a multidisciplinary approach that could be a challenging task for neurosurgeons who are interested in re-engineering of brain and spinal cord lesions and early rehabilitation of impaired functioning.

### 6.2.4.1
### Neurotrauma Academies

In 1995 Dr. von Wild founded the Euroacademia Multidisciplinaria Neurotraumatologica (EMN; www.emn.cc), and in 2002 founded the World Academy of Multidisciplinary Neurotraumatology (AMN; www.world-amn.org) for the advancement of neurotraumatology in research, practical application and teaching. Giorgio Brunelli, Honorary Member of EMN and founding Honorary Member of AMN, was the president of the first AMN conference, in conjunction with his fifth international symposium on experimental spinal cord repair and regeneration, and with the third conference of the World Federation of Neurological Societies (WFNS) neurorehabilitation committee in Brescia, Italy, 27th–29th March 2004.

### 6.2.4.2
### Neurological/Neurosurgical Societies

Following the proposal of Dr. von Wild, in 1997 the WFNS established its Committee for Neurorehabilitation, strongly supported by Professor M. Samii, World President of the WFNS. This committee met first at the European Association of Neurosurgical Societies (EANS) congress in Copenhagen, Denmark, in 1999. That committee and its worldwide activities gave way to Professor Yoishi

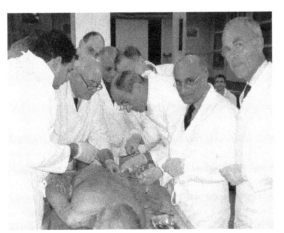

Fig. 2 Cadaver workshop. Clermont Ferrand (France) 29th March 1999. From left to right: Michel Benichou, Pierre Rabischong, Bakulesh Soni, Giorgio Brunelli, the late Krish Krishnan and Klaus von Wild

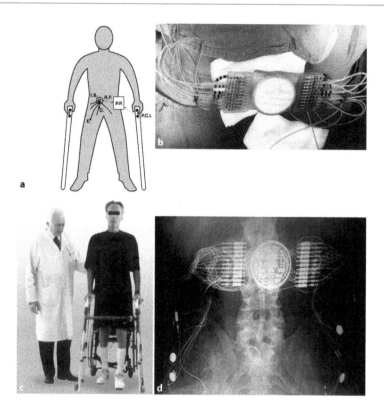

Fig. 3a–d SUAW concept of functional electrical stimulation (FES)-implantable neuroprosthesis. **a** Concept of the SUAW package, implementation of SUAW technical FES package on a patient. *I.S.* implanted stimulator, *C.* connector, *E.* electrode, *P.P.* portable programmer, *R.F.* radio frequency link, *P.C.I.* patient command interface. **b** Neuroprosthesis in situ during implantation into the subcutaneous pouch. Neuromedics implant: 70 mm in diameter , containing the ASCIC chip of 3.9×45 mm size with 70 wire pads bounded to a 9×9 mm ceramic package. There are eight output channels on both sides, monopolar 20 mA, 1.5 kΩ, bipolar 2 mA threshold, which are connected to the electrodes at the end of the implantation procedure under functional stimulation. **c** First patient, Marc M., stood up and walked 2 weeks after implantation with Professor Pierre Rabischong. **d** X-ray SUAW implant in situ (patient Marc M., 6 months after implantation): neuroprosthesis, cables and electrodes subcutaneously in correct place for voluntary FES of the hip muscles to sand up and walk. The neuroprosthesis is still used daily to stand up and walk.

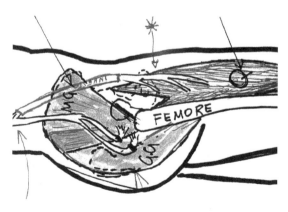

Fig. 4 Brunelli's paradigm. Central nervous system–peripheral nervous system (CNS–PNS) connection: three fascicles from the n. suralis transplant to the receiving muscles were chosen: gluteus maximus for hip extension, gluteus medius for abduction, and stabilisation of the pelvis and quadriceps for hip flexion (in ortostasis) and knee extension (sketch by Giorgio Brunelli in primates)

Katayama, Tokyo, Japan, who followed the author as the chairman, to establish the International Society of Restorative Neurosurgery (ISRN) in 2004, which is linked to the AMN and WFNS. From 1997 until 2003, Dr. von Wild worked as a member of the Scientific Board of Governors of the International Brain injury Association (IBIA), and in 1999 he was appointed chairman of the European Federation of Neurological Societies (EFNS) scientific panel of neurotraumatology. In 2002 the author was elected as a Founding and Executive Board member of the World Federation for Neurorehabilitation (WFNR).

### 6.2.4.3
### Institutions of Excellence

In 2001, Professor von Wild was a Visiting Professor and Consultant at SARAH Rehabilitation Networks, University Brasilia (Brazil), in 2002 at the Armed Force and Rheumatic Rehabilitation Hospital El Agouza Military Hospital, and Spinal Cord Injured Centre, Cairo, (Egypt) and in 2006 at the China Rehabilitation Research Centre, Beijing (China). In 2003 he was made Professor of Neurorehabilitation and Reengineering, at the International Neuroscience Institute, Hannover (Germany), and in 2006 he joined the European Spinal Cord Research Institute (ESCRI), Brescia (Italy), and the Neurobionic Advisory Board in Hannover, Germany.

### 6.3
### Results

Following the permission of the local regional/national ethical committees, surgical procedures were performed in two parallel projects in France and Italy.

### 6.3.1
### SUAW

On 28th September 1999, the first implantation of a neuroprosthesis was performed (Fig. 5; Marc M., 38 years old, paraplegia T7/8 since the age of 9 years following a car accident). The surgical team included Giorgio Brunelli, Michel Benichou and Klaus von Wild; the engineers were P. Couderc, D. Guitaud and Klaus Koch. A Second look operation was performed on 14 February 2000by Michel Benichou and Klaus von Wild, in which the neuroprosthesis was exchanged (Fig. 3b,c) due to electrical problems. The postoperative course and functional follow up was uneventful. Presentation of the SUAW project for final close at the EU, took place in Brussels on 20th March 2000, at which, however, Marc M. was unable to activate his computer in front of the TV and cable crews! Three patients waiting for implantation were also presented. The second patient (Ludovico, 32 years old, 10 years after a motor scooter accident) was implanted according to the

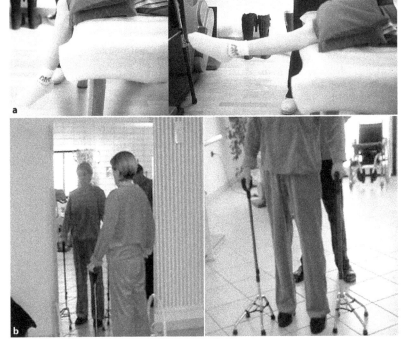

Fig. 5a,b Functional long-term result following CNS–PNS connection. a First patient, Gigliola C., female, 29 years old, 16 months after CNS–PNS connection, first voluntary active extension of both lower limbs occurred via the quadriceps femurs muscle. b Gigliola 2 years after CNS–PNS surgery stands up and walks voluntarily several times a day. She has even been able to climb some steps with the support of two sticks that help her to keep her balance despite complete sensory loss beyond T7

protocol by Giorgio Brunelli, Klaus von Wild and Michel Benichou in Imola, Italy, on 26th July 2000, assisted by Dr. Luisa Monini of Brescia (Italy). A second-look operation was performed in Pisa, Italy, and by another team, to endoscopically replace one slipped femoral electrode. This patient developed a post-operative deep wound infection. Finally, the FES implant with all its cables had to be removed in a third procedure without involvement of the first surgical team

No further implantation followed in one of the other patients who had been prepared in 1999. The author and Giorgio Brunelli were not invited for the meeting of the subsequent SUAW 2 project in Nantes, March 2001. Professor Rabischong and the new group are planning to implant a completely new system (neuroprosthesis, cables, electrodes) in early 2007 (personal communication at the Neurobionic meeting in Hannover, Germany on 16 January 2006). Dr. M. Passover, Colon, gynaecologist and expert in endoscopies of the pelvic region, who was invited and performed the second-look operation in Pisa via endoscopy, left the group immediately after the procedure because of his personal concerns (personal communication, Brescia, Italy, 8th December 2006).

## 6.3.2
### First CNS–PNS Connection

The first CNS–PNS connection (Brunelli's Paradigm, Figs. 6 and 7) to be performed in a human being was carried out for direct neurotisation of the hip muscles with the aid of autologous nerves grafts from the upper (first) motor neurons, in Imola, 20th July 2000. The patient was a 27-year-old lady, Gigliola C., 3 months after complete paraplegia T7 following a car accident (Fig. 5). The chief surgeon was Giorgio Brunelli and the consultant was Klaus von Wild, assisted by Drs. Luisa Monini and Giovanni R. Brunelli. The second patient (Massimo F., 23 years old, male, complete lesion at T7 following a car accident in 2001) was operated in June 2003. The third patient (Vincenzo C., 34 years old, male, paraplegia T7, 8 years after a motorbike accident in 1996) was operated by the same team in January 2004. All CNS–PNS connections were completed uneventfully.

## 6.4
## Discussion

### 6.4.1
### Facts

(Figs. 3, 5 and 6)

#### 6.4.1.1
### Active Participation of the Author for Restorative Neurosurgery in Both Projects

The functional clinical results were as expected and raised the scientific interest of other neurosurgeons. By using the network that has been developed (Fig. 6), both projects were scientifically presented and discussed with neuroscientists, rehabilitation physicians and the public concerning the neurophysiology, biochemistry, surgical reconstructive and physical/psychological pre- and post-operative treatment, and the clinical results on locomotor functioning at neurological, neurosurgical, traumatological, plastic-reconstructive and neurorehabilitative congresses over the last 6 years (e.g. at the World Federation of Neurosurgical Societies, European Association of Neurosurgical Societies, ISRN, European Federation of Neurological Societies, EMN, AMN, Asian Academy for Neurological Surgery, Asian Congress for Neurological Surgeons, Asian Congress for Neurological Surgeons, South American Neurosurgical Society, Baltic Neurosurgical Society, Deutsche Akademie für Neurochirurgie, Deutsche Gesellschaft für Neurotraumatologie und Neurorehabilitation, Deutsche Gesellschaft für Neurorehabilitation and Deutsche Gesellschaft für Plastische und Wiederherstellungschirurgie).

#### 6.4.1.2
### As-is State

To try to convince neuroscientists and rehabilitation physicians to follow both experimental surgical procedures, we decided to perform an international multi-centre prospectively controlled clinical trial on CNS–PNS connections that goes back to 2003–2004.

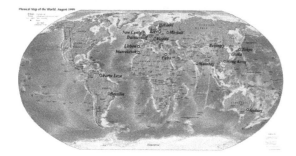

Fig. 6 Physical map of the world with the main places marked where the author has built up a scientific network for advertising both reconstructive neurosurgical procedures for spinal cord injury, SUAW-FES and Brunelli's CNS–PNS paradigm over the last 7 years (1999–2006)

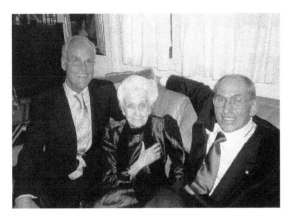

Fig. 7 Professor Rita Levi-Montalcini (Rome, Italy), 1986 Nobel Laureat in Medicine for discovery of growth factors, sitting between Professor Giorgio Brunelli (right) and the author at the Fifth International Symposium on Experimental Spinal Cord Repair, Brescia, Italy, 28th March 2004

### 6.4.1.3
### Drawbacks and Critics

#### SUAW

1. Only two patients instead of ten paraplegics were implanted.
2. Technical complications occurred followed by second-look operations.
3. Mismanagement and a lack of information and trustful cooperation are evident.
4. Technical concerns regarding the electrodes and implants were not disproved.
5. Neuromedics went bankrupt in April 2000. No alternative was ready for implantation.
6. There is an ongoing medical concern of colleagues and partners in neurorehabilitation regarding technology, ethical permission, technical and commercial inspectorate.
7. Economic concern: SUAW not of good repute, too expensive, orthopaedics and physiatrists simply do not see any benefit from voluntary locomotion after paraplegia, while patients otherwise become independent in a wheelchair and are re-socialised; an unbelievably conservative statement.

#### CNS-PNS

Despite the objective results (Figs. 6 and 7) in the first patient (the two others are too fresh to decide on their expected functional improvement) and evidentiary experimental data, well-known neuroscientists and neurologists simply do not believe and/or understand the underlying physiology (personal communication 10 years Neurobionic anniversary at the INI, Hannover, Germany) as it is described in detail by Brunelli et al. [2].

### 6.4.1.4
### Limitation

There was no external audit, and no personal follow-up examination of the patients of both projects by electrophysiological and neuroimaging examinations (e.g. somatosensory-evoked potential, electromyography, motor evoked potential, and functional magnetic resonance imaging).

### 6.4.1.5
### Scientific Reports (PubMed)

SUAW by Professor Pierre Rabischong: four references (without Giorgio Brunelli and Klaus von Wild); Giorgio Brunelli: 11 reports on CNS–PNS connection, not one on SUAW; Klaus von Wild: two references on each project, together with Giorgio Brunelli and Pierre Rabischong.

### 6.4.2
### Concern About Public Relations

Lay Press Media and TV splashed the SUAW story across the media to arouse public interest and scientific information for paraplegic victims in Europe, promoted by Pierre Rabischong (Stern TV in Germany), which raised hope and resulted in hundreds of letters and telephone calls for the author – but in vain!

### 6.4.3
### Author's Concern

The author received much criticism and met with a square refusal. So far it was not possible to convince neuroscientists and orthopaedic specialists around the world to participate actively in restorative surgery for complete spinal cord lesions by demonstrating both surgical restorative concepts and clinical results. Not even those physicians could not believe in CNS–PNS connection who planned with us the prospective study that should be based on their own local/regional structures and possibilities for neurorehabilitation. The Nobel Prize Laureate Professor Rita Levi-Montalcini (Fig. 7), Rome, consequently inspired Giorgio Brunelli and his interdisciplinary Brescia research group to analyse the physiology of their CNS–PNS results with aid of evidentiary gene-biotechnological studies.

## 6.5
## Conclusions

### 6.5.1
### Facts

Both projects were clinically successful regarding restoration of locomotion. Both SUAW and CNS–PNS connection have been demonstrated to enable paraplegics to stand up and to walk voluntarily again. While the neuroprosthesis (Fig. 3) acts immediately post-operatively CNS–PNS connection will take about 2 years for complete functional enervations. SUAW implants bear a technically high risk of infection during the implantation, and the implant is very expensive. The best functional results were achieved by CNS–PNS connection when it was performed within the 1st year after trauma. With both techniques, the patient will need lifelong intensive physical therapy. Patients have otherwise to be healthy and mentally and psychologically absolutely stable and willing to reach the best functional results possible, like our patients Marc M. and Gigliola C. The key issues regarding ethical permission and optimal clinical results remain the expertise of the team and the trust and cooperation of the multidisciplinary specialists for quality management of the project.

### 6.5.2
### Fantasy

The author's opinions turned out to be unrealistic, thinking he would be able to convince rehabilitation physicians, orthopaedic specialists and neurosurgeons to follow the Brunelli paradigm, albeit backed up by objective published scientific data. Neuroscientists and surgeons simply cannot believe or trust in the new biophysiological concept. Irrespective of Pierre Rabischong's excellent international connections, efforts and ongoing announcements, a novel FES neuroprosthesis has not been ready for implantation after 6 years since his first SUAW technical group went into bankruptcy. In addition, no one will pay for the costly implantation in the future, as the economic market is too small and most paraplegics belong to a low socioeconomic group.

### 6.5.3
### Take-Home Message

Research on the restoration of voluntary locomotion in paraplegics is a challenging multidisciplinary task. It needs a realistic experimental approach and trusty international cooperation, independent from economic industrial interests. Involvement of the industry in turn may hinder the grants needed. The International Neurobionic Foundation will hopefully support research into Brunelli's Paradigm and SUAW and our clinical research programs at the International Neuroscience Institute, Hannover in the near future, since surgical restoration of paraplegia is no more a fantasy, but a reality and a challenging fact.

## Bibliography

For a review of the literature regarding SUAW and CNS–PNS connection see:

1. Brunelli GA (2001) Direct neurotization of muscles by presynaptic motoneurons. J Reconstr Microsurg 17:631–636
2. Brunelli G, Spano PF, Barlati S, et al (2002) Glutamatergic reinnervation through peripheral nerve graft dictates assembly of glutamatergic synapses at rat skeletal muscle. PNAS 102:8752–8757
3. von Wild KRH (2001) Neuro-Rehabilitation – a challenge for neurosurgeons in the century 21st Concepts and Visions of the WFNS – Committee on Neurosurgical Rehabilitation. Acta Neurochir (Suppl) 79:3–10
4. von Wild, K, Rabischong P, Brunelli G, et al (2001) Computer added locomotion by implanted electrical stimulation in paraplegic patients (SUAW). Acta Neurochir (Suppl) 79:99–104
5. von Wild K, Brunelli G (2003) Restoration of locomotion in paraplegics with aid of autologous bypass graft for direct neurotisation of muscles by upper motor neurons – the future: surgery of the spinal cord. Acta Neurochir (Suppl) 87:107–112

# III Skull Base

# Surgery of Olfactory Groove Meningiomas

Paulo Henrique Aguiar
and Antonio Nogueira Almeida

## Contents

## 7.1

## Introduction

Olfactory groove meningiomas (OGMs) manifest in the midline over the cribiform plate and frontosphenoidal suture [7,13,17]. These tumours occupy the floor of anterior cranial fossa, extending all the way from the crista galli to the tuberculum sella [4]. However, there are some similarities between posteriorly extending OGMs and tuberculum sella meningiomas (TSMs). The most important feature distinguishing them is the location of the optic nerve in relation to the tumour. OGMs push the chiasm downward and posteriorly as they grow, whereas TSMs elevate the chiasm and displace the optic nerve superolaterally, where the tumour takes up a subchiasmal position.

Spektor et al. [28] reported their experience over a 13-year period with 80 patients who underwent surgical treatment (81 OGM operations). This article describes the different techniques for accessing meningiomas in the olfactory grove. The authors review the potential advantages and disadvantages associated with the use of particular surgical approaches to OGMs, as well as their outcomes and recurrence rates. In their series, the main approaches were through bifrontal craniotomy, the unilateral subfrontal approach, pterional approach with fronto-orbital craniotomy, and via the subcranial approach. Total removal was achieved in 90% of the patients, and subtotal removal in 10%. No operative mortality and no new permanent focal neurological deficit besides anosmia were identified, although 31.3% developed surgery-related complications. The outcomes of these patients prove that proper use of modern microsurgical techniques leads to excellent results. For the increasing number of operations on the anterior fossa in patients with OGMs, the

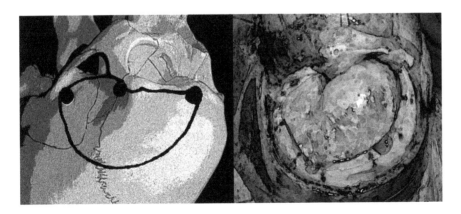

Fig. 1 Depiction of an extended pterional approach in which a larger frontal and temporal exposition is accomplished after craniotomy

selection of the most appropriate approach is especially important. Previous publications have described many surgical management approaches in these tumours. For patients with large or small OGMs, the extended front-opterional approach is preferred (Fig. 1). This approach may achieve full removal while preserving the vascular structures surrounding the tumour. On craniotomy, care is taken at the frontobasal anterior extension in order to reach the midline (falx and crista). The dissection of the sylvian fissure is very important, followed by opening of the carotid and interpeduncular cisterns. These procedures allow the release of cerebrospinal fluid (CSF) and relaxation of the brain, as well as minimise brain retraction. The pterional approach also allows early visualisation of the neurovascular structures and their dissection. Control of the posterior part of the tumour in relation to the most important structures (the optic nerves and internal carotid artery) may be achieved by this approach. Dissection of the anterior cerebral arteries from the capsule may prove difficult because of adherence or encasement. The recurrent artery of Heubner should always be preserved during the dissection. A bifrontal approach is more direct to the tumours; however in our view the late visualisation of the optic nerves and the anterior cerebral complex are disadvantageous points to be considered in choosing this approach [5].

The benign slow growth of these tumours means they frequently reach a large size before detection. Surgical removal of small- to mid-sized tumours is not difficult. Yet, in a significant proportion of patients the meningioma is very large and infiltrates or envelopes surrounding structures, making removal challenging due to strong attachment.

## 7.2
## Preoperative Evaluation

As a rule, patients harbouring OGMs may present with headache, visual loss, seizure, and mental or personality changes, occasionally complaining of spontaneous loss of sense of smell. A detailed neuro-ophthalmologic evaluation should be performed, and a magnetic resonance imaging (MIR) study with gadolinium enhancement is important for the diagnosis. Usually the tumour shows a densely contrast enhancement that pushes the frontal lobe upward and is associated with significant oedema. An angiogram, by means of MRI, could be useful to see the position of the ethmoidal arteries. Preoperative embolisation is not indicated in the majority of cases in our opinion.

## 7.3
## Surgical Anatomy

OGMs present in the midline of the anterior fossa over the cribiform plate of the ethmoid bone, and the area of suture joining this structure and the planum sphenoidale [7,29]. The tumour may involve the area from the crista Galli to the posterior planum sphenoidale and may be symmetric around the midline, or extend predominantly to one side (Fig. 2).

The olfactory nerves are displaced laterally on the surface of smaller tumours and it may be possible to preserve at least one of these nerves. In large tumours, the olfactory tract and cribiform area are destroyed and invaded by the tumour, affecting both nerves. Therefore, olfaction may

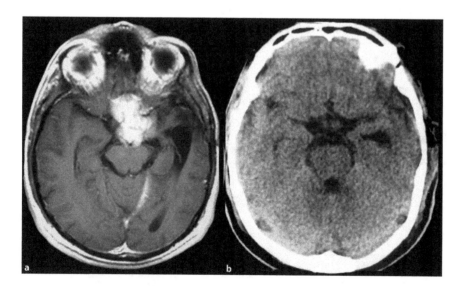

Fig. 2 An olfactory groove meningioma displacing posteriorly the pons (**a**), which was removed completely by a pterional approach (**b**)

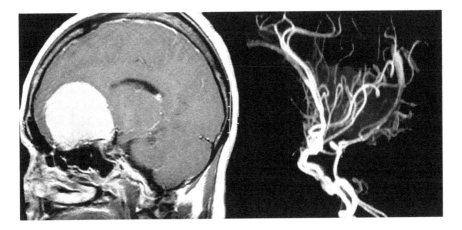

Fig. 3 A large olfactory groove meningioma displacing the anterior cerebral complex seen by magnetic resonance imaging (left) and magnetic resonance angiography (right)

not be salvageable. With large tumours, the optic nerves and chiasm are pushed inferiorly and posteriorly.

The primary blood supply comes from anterior and posterior ethmoid artery branches of the ophthalmic artery, and meningeal artery branches, through the midline of the base of the skull. The A2 segments of the anterior cerebral arteries are displaced posteriorly by the tumour; however, they have a cleavage plane, where brain tissue and arachnoid are present between the two structures (Fig. 3). In large tumours, the capsule of the tumour may envelop the A2 segments of the anterior cerebral artery, making total removal a risky procedure. Frontopolar and other small branches of the anterior cerebral arteries may also be adhered to the posterior and superior tumour capsule.

## 7.4
## Approaches

Many surgical approaches can be applied for tumour removal, although the traditional method is frontal or bifrontal craniotomy with subfrontal approach to the tumour [1, 4, 8, 11, 16, 18, 22, 24, 27, 29, 31]. In some cases, part of the orbit may be removed to improve the frontobasal exposure (Fig. 4). The pterional approach has been advocated by many authors and, in our opinion, is the first choice for small- and mid-sized tumours [1, 5, 12, 20, 25, 30, 33]. Aggressive approaches have been used in OGMs that have expanded into the paranasal sinuses and orbits, including transbasal [6], subcranial [9,23] and fronto-orbital approaches [26], frontal or bifrontal crani-

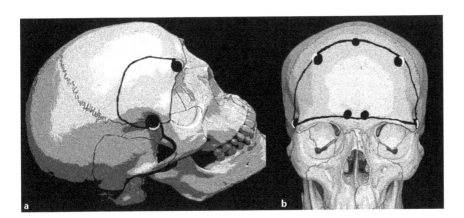

Fig. 4 Craniotomies used to remove olfactory groove meningiomas. The superior arch of the orbit may be removed (a) to accomplish a better frontobasal exposure. Some cases may need a bifrontal approach (b)

otomy being associated with orbital or nasal osteotomies [3,13], and craniofacial resection [10].

### 7.4.1
### Frontotemporal Approach for Small and Mid-Sized Tumours

The patient should be placed in the supine position with the head held in Mayfield three-point fixation or Sugita multiple-point fixation. The head is gently rotated 30° towards the contralateral shoulder. More rotation can be used for anterior tumours, and less for more posterior tumours. The head is flexed slightly to bring the chin towards the ipsilateral clavicle and extended to bring the maxillary eminence to the highest point in the field (Fig. 5).

A curvilinear skin incision is made behind the hairline. The incision begins just anterior to the tragus of the ear and should extend below the zygomatic root to protect the branches of the facial nerve. The incision should be made as close as possible to the tragus of the ear. We should avoid transecting the underlying branches of the superficial temporal artery. The skin flap is folded anteriorly along the pericranium. At the supraorbital ridge, care should be taken to identify and preserve the supraorbital nerve and vessel passing through the supraorbital foramen or notch. As the skin is folded anteriorly, the galea will merge with the superficial layer of the temporalis fascia. A curvilinear incision can be made into the superficial fascia layer at keyhole and continued towards the zygomatic root. Anterior elevation of this fascia and fat pad away from the underlying temporalis muscle avoids injury to the frontalis branch of the facial nerve that runs in this fat plane. The temporalis muscle is elevated as a separate layer and folded anteriorly and inferiorly using fish hooks to expose the supraorbital ridge lateral rim of the orbit.

The craniotomy is accomplished with four burr holes and by means of craniotome, where, as a rule, we use Midas Rex®, with a cut burr. Typically, the dura mater is opened in a C-shaped fashion with its base along the sphenoid ridge. It is folded anteriorly and anchored with stay sutures.

The sylvian fissure is opened with the aid of an operating microscope, either a lateral-to-medial, or a medial-to-lateral overture of the sylvian fissure could be performed. In the lateral-to-medial dissection, the sylvian fissure is then opened using an arachnoid knife, and the dissection is performed superior to the sylvian vein, reflecting the veins with the temporal lobe. Veins crossing the fissure are sacrificed. As the fissure opens, the distal branches of the middle cerebral artery, the M1-bifurcation, and finally the carotid bifurcation can be exposed. Further dissection allows visualisation of the carotid optic triangle and the carotid–oculomotor triangle. On medial-to-lateral dissection of the sylvian fissure, a self-retractor is placed under the frontal lobe to expose the olfactory nerve. Following the surface of the tumour to behind it posteriorly, allows easy identification of the optic nerve and the carotid artery lying laterally to it. The optic carotid cistern and carotid oculomotor cistern generally come into view easily with little retraction. With the use of fine microdissectors, the arachnoid membrane between the optic nerve and frontal lobe is incised and opened. The dissection of this arachnoid continues across the carotid artery to the region of the third nerve, thus opening the optic carotid and carotid oculomotor cisterns. The microsurgical technique consists of dissecting the tumour capsule from the optic nerve in front of and behind the optic nerve in the side view of the surgeon. The frontal lobe is elevated with a retractor and the surface between the tumour and frontal lobe dissected.

The small feeds are also coagulated by means of bipolar forceps and the blood supply occluded along the base and the tumour capsule. The overture in the tumoural capsule should be performed using a knife with a num-

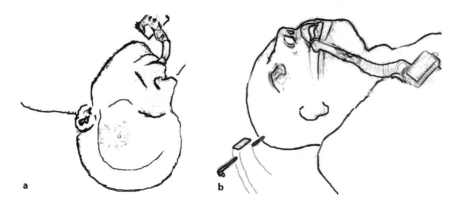

**Fig. 5** Schematic depiction of head positioning: (**a**) frontal view, and (**b**) lateral view (see text for details)

ber 11 blade, and followed by coagulation of the surface. The internal decompression of the tumoural core might facilitate gently pulling the superior portion of the capsule downwards, where with angle forceps we are able to separate the lateral capsule from the brain tissue (frontal lobe) in cleavage tissue plane, dividing the attachments to the frontal lobe as they are encountered. Microdissection must be employed to remove the tumour in piecemeal fashion. The haemostasis should be done with Oxi® or Surgicell®, and bipolar coagulation. The dura mater in the crista galli at the point of tumoural attachment has to be coagulated, the crista galli cut, and drilled by means of a diamond burr. This method allows assessment of the other side of the crista galli, where pieces of tumour could not be exposed. We try to close the skull base dural defect with a pericranium patch retaining the arterial feeding of the graft. External lumbar drainage is left for 5 post-operative days.

## 7.4.2
### Bifrontal Approach for Large Tumours

We recommend bifrontal craniotomy for removal of large tumours. The bifrontal approach permits adequate exposure and allows the surgeon to work on both sides, frontal and temporal, accessing the sylvian fissure. This allows for the preservation of the olfactory nerves; however, in large tumours they are very difficult to keep intact (Fig. 6). The patients should be placed in a supine position, with the head in a neutral position and gently extended toward the floor. After the bifrontal craniotomy using four burr holes, the bone flap is cut with the aid of craniotome Midas Rex® using cutting burrs.

The dura mater is opened in a downward turning C shape, and the sagittal sinus is closed by means of suture or ligation. Both frontal lobes are elevated with retractors in parallel and the interhemispheric fissure is dissected. After drainage of the CSF, we try to dissect the olfactory nerves from bottom to top, up to the olfactory insertion into the bone. In large tumours this proves almost impossible. The microsurgical technique consists of debulking the tumour by means of an ultrasonic aspirator, or by microsurgical instruments. The capsule is turned toward the centre of its debulked area using a tumour punch, and the cleavage plane between the superior portion of the tumour and the inferior portion of the frontal lobe is found and all feedings coagulated by bipolar forceps. The attachment to the crista galli can be explored by a partial resection and coagulating the insertion or drilling the galli crista, and assessing the ethmoidal sinus in order to remove all invaded cavities (Fig. 7). A hipofises curette or tumour forceps can be used to take out the tumour from the ethmoidal cavity. Closure should be in watertight fashion in order to avoid any CSF leakage. We can close the hole in the bone with a piece of bone from the sphenoid wing or a methacrylate graft, and using pericranium or dura substitutes such as polytetrafluoroethylene membrane (Gore Preclude MVP dura substitute, Flagstaff, Arizona, USA) [14, 32]. The large dural defect area can be microsurgically closed watertight. External lumbar drainage is used in the first five post-operative days.

## 7.5
### Complications

Complications should be avoided wherever possible. The microsurgical techniques, intraoperative cranial nerves monitoring, neuroanaesthesiological procedures, along with intensive care improvements have helped the neurosurgeon to decrease the rate of complications nowadays

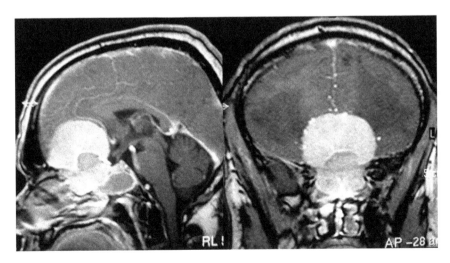

Fig. 6 Large olfactory groove meningioma invading the nasal cavity; a bifrontal approach was employed

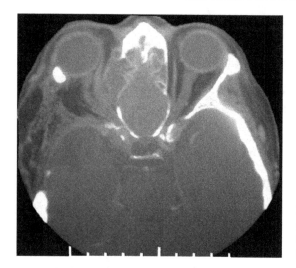

Fig. 7 Computed tomography scan depicting erosion of the cribiform plate by an olfactory groove meningioma. Special care must be taken to avoid post-operative cerebrospinal fluid fistula in such cases

[1, 2, 15, 17, 18, 21, 24, 25, 28]. The most important complications reported in the reviewed literature, and based on our experience are: loss of sense of smell, seizure, CSF rhinorrhoea, infection and medical complications. Occasionally, visual loss might be observed in large tumours due to excessive traction, surgical bed haematoma and hydrocephalus [19]. In patients with large tumours, a frontal lobe syndrome may develop as a result of oedema or cerebral ischaemia. If the patient does not recover promptly from anaesthesia, an immediate computed tomography scan should be done to ascertain the possibility of haematoma, oedema, hydrocephalus, anterior cerebral artery infarction and pneumocephalus (Fig. 8). Post-operative seizure is unusual, but could occur. Post-operative steroids may needed for at least 2 weeks after the surgery.

In large tumours, hypopituitarism and diabetes insipidus can occasionally be observed. If there is an opening into the ethmoid and sphenoid sinus, both should be repaired, and a lumbar drain is inserted and left for almost 5 days. If the leak remains, an endoscopic transnasal approach is performed. If the leak persists, a closure is best accomplished using a transsphenoidal approach.

The main post-operative infections include meningitis, cellulites and bone flap osteomyelitis. Rarely is it necessary to remove the bone flap.

Hydrocephalus may be observed due to venous thrombosis, infection after brain ischemia, haematoma or normal-pressure hydrocephalus in the elderly in the post-operative period. A shunt might be necessary and programmable valves are very useful in these cases.

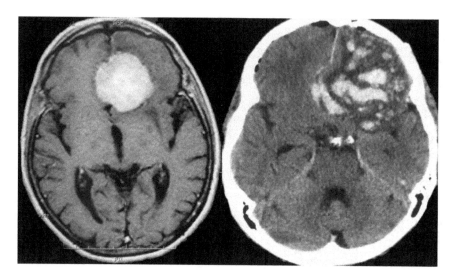

Fig. 8 Post-operative brain contusion due to retraction of the frontal lobe during removal of an olfactory groove meningioma

Medical complications are more common in elderly patients and those with obesity disease who are diabetic or hypertensive and without drug control. In an attempt to prevent thrombophlebitis and pulmonary embolism, pneumatic compression thigh-high air boots should be used throughout the intra- and post-operative period.

## References

1. Aguiar PH, Lourenço DL, Plasencia OZ, et al (2004) Meningiomas del surco olfatorio aspectos clinicos, radiologicos y quirurgicos. Analisis y complicaciones. Rev Child Neurocirugia 22:35–38
2. Andrews BT, Wilson CB (1988) Suprasellar meningiomas. The effect of tumor location on postoperative visual outcome. J Neurosurg 69:523–528
3. Babu R, Barton A, Kasoff SS (1995) Resection of olfactory groove meningiomas: technical note revisited. Surg Neurol 44:567–572
4. Bakay L, Cares HL (1972) Olfactory meningiomas. Report on a series of twenty-five cases. Acta Neurochir (Wien) 26:1–12
5. De Oliveira E, Aguiar PH (2005) Comments in: Spektor S, Valarezo J, Fliss DM, et al (2005) Olfactory groove meningiomas from neurosurgical and ENT perspectives: approaches, techniques, and outcomes. Neurosurgery 57: Operative Neurosurgery Supplement 4:268–280
6. Derome PJ, Guiot G (1978) Bone problems in meningiomas invading the base of skull. Clin Neurosurg 25:435–451
7. Dolenc VV (2003) Elements of the epidural approach to the parasellar space and adjacent regions in the central skull base. In: Dolenc VV (ed) Microsurgical Anatomy and Surgery of the Central Skull Base. Springer, Wien, pp 55–59
8. El Gindi S (2000) Olfactory groove meningiomas: surgical techniques and pitfalls. Surg Neurol 54:415–417
9. Fliss DM, Zucker G, Cohen A, et al (1999) Early outcome and complications of extended subcranial approach to anterior skull base. Laryngoscope 109:153–160
10. Goffin J, Fossion E, Plets C, et al (1991) Craniofacial resection for anterior skull base tumours. Acta Neurochir (Wien) 110:33–37
11. Grisoli F, Diaz-Vasquez P, Riss M, et al (1986) Microsurgical management of tuberculum sellae meningiomas. Results in 28 consecutive cases. Surg Neurol 26:37–44
12. Hassler W, Zentner J (1989) Pterional approach for surgical treatment of olfactory groove meningiomas. Neurosurgery 25:942–947
13. Hentschel S, DeMonte F (2003) Olfactory groove meningiomas. Neurosurg Focus 14:1–5
14. Kitano M, Taneda M (2004) Subdural patch graft technique for watertight closure of large dural defects in extended transsphenoidal surgery. Neurosurgery 54: 653–661
15. Margalit NS, Lesser JB, Moche J, et al (2003) Meningiomas involving the optic nerve. Technical aspects and outcomes for a series of 50 patients. Neurosurgery 53:523–532
16. Obeid F, Al Mefty O (2003) Recurrence of olfactory groove meningiomas. Neurosurgery 53:534–543
17. Ojemann R (1991) Olfactory groove meningiomas. In: Al Mefty O (ed) Meningiomas. Raven, New York, pp 383–392
18. Ojemann RG (1993) Management of cranial and spinal meningiomas. Clin Neurosurg 40:321–383
19. Park CK, Jung HW, Yang SY, et al (2006) Surgically treated tuberculum sellae and diaphragm sellae meningiomas: the importance of short-term visual outcome. Neurosurgery 59:239–243
20. Paterniti S, Fiore P, Levita A, et al (1999) Venous saving in olfactory groove meningioma's surgery. Clin Neurol Neurosurg 101:235–237
21. Puchner MJ, Fischer-Lampsatis RC, Herrmann HD, et al (1998) Suprasellar meningiomas. Neurological and visual outcome at long term follow up in a homogeneous series of patients treated microsurgically. Acta Neurochir (Wien) 140:1231–1238
22. Ransohoff J, Nockels R (1993) Olfactory groove and planum Meningiomas. In: Apuzzo M (ed) Brain Surgery: Complication Avoidance and Management. Churchill Livingstone, New York, pp 177–185
23. Raveh J, Laedrah K, Speiser M, et al (1993) The subcranial approach for fronto orbital and anteroposterior skull base tumours. Arch Otolaryngol Head Neck Surg 119:385–393
24. Samii M, Ammirati M (1992) Olfactory groove meningiomas. In: Samii M (ed) Surgery of the Skull Base: Meningiomas. Springer, Berlin, pp 15–25
25. Schaller C, Veit R, Hassler W (1994) Microsurgical removal of olfactory groove meningiomas via pterional approach. Skull Base Surg 4:189–192
26. Sekhar LN, Tzortzidis F (1999) Resection of tumors by the fronto-orbital approach. In: Sekhar L, de Oliveira E (eds) (1999) Cranial Microsurgery: Approaches and Techniques. Thieme, New York, pp 61–75
27. Solero CL, Giombini S, Morello G (1983) Suprasellar and olfactory groove meningiomas. Report on a series of 153 personal cases. Acta Neurchir (Wien) 67:181–194
28. Spektor S, Valarezo J, Fliss DM, et al (2005) Olfactory groove meningiomas from neurosurgical and ENT perspectives: approaches, techniques, and outcomes. Neurosurgery 57: Operative Neurosurgery Supplement 4:268–280
29. Symon L (1977) Olfactory groove and suprasellar meningiomas. In: Krayenbuhl H (ed) Advances and Technical Standards in Neurosurgery, vol 4. Springer, Vienna, pp 66–91
30. Turazzi S, Cristofori L, Gambin R, et al (1999) The pterional approach for the microsurgical removal of olfactory groove meningiomas. Neurosurgery 45:821–825
31. Tsikoudas A, Martin-Hirsch DP (1999) Olfactory groove meningiomas. Clin Otololaryngol 24:507–509
32. Vinas FC, Ferris D, Kupsky WJ, et al (1999) Evaluation of expanded polytetrafluoroethylene (ePTE) versus polydioxanone (PDS) for the repair of dura mater defects. Neurol Res 21:262–268
33. Yasargil M (1984) Microneurosurgery. Georg Thieme, New York

# Preservation of the Olfactory Tract in Bifrontal Craniotomy

# 8

Paulo Henrique Aguiar and
Antonio Nogueira Almeida

## Contents

## 8.1
### Introduction

The anterior cranial base and the suprasellar and parasellar regions approach and its several methods have been described since 1981 by Suzuki et al. [3, 14, 15]. Extended frontal approaches, however, necessitate removal of the crista galli and sectioning of the olfactory rootlets with the associated risk of anosmia, cerebrospinal fluid (CSF) leak, and the need for complex reconstruction of the frontal floor [11, 12]. Bifrontal craniotomy is the conventional approach to lesions in these locations [10, 11], but its shortcoming has been the damage to the olfactory tract [7].

The preservation of the olfactory tract has been the subject of many studies in extended frontal approaches. Fujiwara et al. [7] and Eriksen et al. [4] reported various cases of anosmia after anterior communicating artery aneurysm surgery. Spetzler et al. [5, 12] modified the technique of handling the cribiform plate to preserve the olfactory unit. Srinivasan et al. [13] described the bifrontal approach that enhanced the exposure of the suprasellar region and minimized manipulation of the optic apparatus and the carotid arteries.

In a previous paper we presented our experience with the use of bifrontal craniotomy in 11 patients with several lesions (e.g., intracerebral schwannoma, craniopharyngiomas, pituitary adenomas, and Rathke cyst). We also reported the complete preservation of olfaction in these patients, who underwent bifrontal craniotomy [1].

With regard to small olfactory groove meningiomas, we prefer the pterional approaches rather than bifrontal craniotomy. The pterional approach has been proved to be enough to reach a complete resection in these tumors [2].

## 8.2
### Operative Technique

With the patient in the supine position, the head is fixed in a three-point head-holder. The skin is incised posterior to the frontal hairline from zygoma to zygoma (Fig. 1) and the scalp and pericranial flaps are reflected anteriorly. Two burr holes are produced on each side on the orbital buttons with a high-speed drill. Through the use of a craniotome, an osteoplastic osteotomy is performed, extending close to the orbital roof anteriorly and along the cranium convexity posteriorly. Both frontal sinus tables are accessed and the mucous membranes are removed. The dura mater is cut parallel to the base and the sagit-

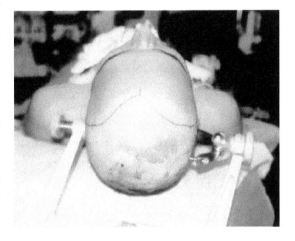

Fig. 1 Case 4. Surgical view of the marked line to be incised

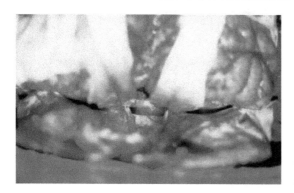

Fig. 2 Case 4. Surgical view under magnification showing the retraction of the frontal poles

tal sinus is ligated and cut at the cecal foramen. Then the falx is transected and the bridging veins are preserved. The frontal poles are retracted, under magnification, using two self-retaining retractors adjusted stepwise (Fig. 2).

The interhemispheric and the bilateral olfactory cisternae are opened in order to drain the CSF and to avoid further retraction. Both olfactory nerves should be dissected symmetrically without coagulation under small bleedings. Surgicell® is enough to stop the small bleedings mainly near the crivous plate of ethmoidal bone. After that, the surgical overview could better show the image of both olfactory nerves and both optic nerves composing a groove enlarged by the tumor. The pseudocapsula of the tumor can be seen through this groove and the dissection between the carotid artery and the pseudocapsula should be performed on both sides. Following this step, a debulking of the tumor should be done, and a piecemeal resection is recommended.

The ultrasonic aspirator may be used with extreme caution. The retraction of bilateral frontal poles should never be strong enough to hurt the pia mater and cause damage to the brain parenchyma [1, 2].

Table 1 Clinical data for 11 patients with preservation of olfactory tract

| Case | Gender | Age (years) | Location | Pathology |
|---|---|---|---|---|
| 1 | M | 24 | Left frontal fossa | Intracerebral schwannoma |
| 2 | F | 54 | Sellar and parasellar | GH pituitary adenoma |
| 3 | F | 35 | Left frontal fossa | Anaplastic glioma |
| 4 | M | 30 | Sellar and parasellar | Craniopharyngioma |
| 5 | M | 35 | Sellar and parasellar | Non secreting pituitary adenoma |
| 6 | M | 36 | Tuberculum sellae | Meningioma |
| 7 | M | 20 | Sellar and parasellar | Craniopharyngioma |
| 8 | M | 5 | Sellar and parasellar | Rathke cyst |
| 9 | F | 61 | Sellar and parasellar | Non secreting pituitary adenoma |
| 10 | F | 63 | Hypothalamus | GBM |
| 11 | F | 52 | Sellar and parasellar | Non secreting pituitary adenoma |

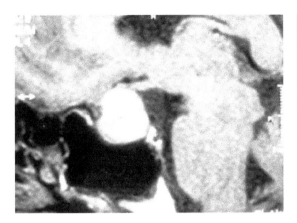

Fig. 3  Case 2. Preoperative magnetic resonance imaging (MRI) of a 54-year-old female with growth-hormone-secreting pituitary macroadenoma

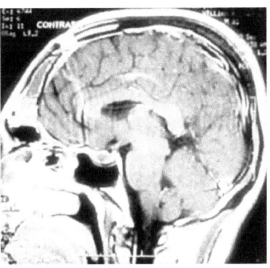

Fig. 4  Case 2. Postoperative MRI of the same 54-year-old female patient as shown in Fig. 3, demonstrating total resection of the tumor

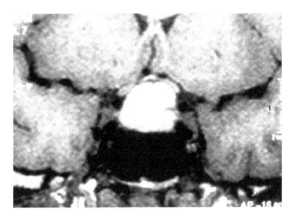

Fig. 5  Case 4. Preoperative MRI of a 50-year-old male with craniopharyngioma

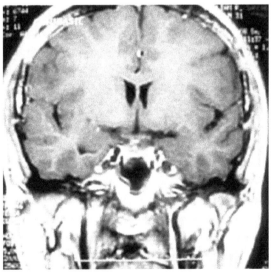

Fig. 6  Case 4. Postoperative MRI of the same 50-year-old male patient as shown in Fig. 5, demonstrating total resection of the tumor

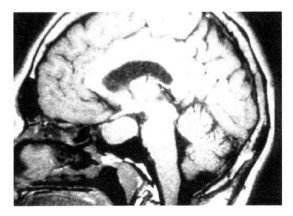

Fig. 7  Case 9. Preoperative MRI of a 61-year-old female with nonfunctioning pituitary adenoma

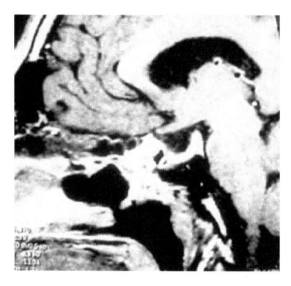

Fig. 8 Case 9. Postoperative MRI of the same 61-year-old female patient as shown in Fig. 7 after total resection of the tumor

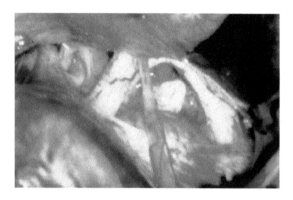

Fig. 9 Case 9. Surgical view showing the olfactory nerve, the optic nerve, and the left carotid artery

## 8.3
## Patient Population

The surgical technique described was applied in the treatment of the 11 patients, as shown in Table 1. Of the 11 patients, 5 were female and 6 were male, with a mean age of 37.7 years (range, 5–63 years). Histological examination revealed four adenomas (Figs. 3, 4, and 7–9), two craniopharyngiomas (Figs. 5 and 6), one glioblastoma, one anaplastic glioma, one meningioma, one Rathke cyst, and one Schwannoma. The symptoms at admission were typical for each pathological condition, and the lesions were totally removed by using a bilateral subfrontal approach. All of these patients were preoperatively evaluated with nonenhanced and enhanced magnetic resonance tomog-

raphy. We evaluated prospectively the clinical findings at the presentation, operative treatment, and outcome of each patient.

In our study there were no deaths or even clinical or surgical complications. We did not register any case of anosmia. A postoperative neurological examination did not reveal new deficits in the 11 patients. They did have their olfactory tract preserved bilaterally. No subjective or objective olfactory disturbance were noted in the follow-up of these 11 patients.

## 8.4
## Discussion

In our opinion, olfaction is an extremely important neurological function, to the point that its damage can impair any individual's quality of life. Olfactory tract damage used to be regarded as the major drawback of bifrontal craniotomy [6, 8, 14]. Knowing that it is fundamental to preserve the anatomy and the function of both olfactory tracts, we strongly recommend the technique described above, which were first reported by Samii et al. [3, 9]

The bilateral subfrontal approach allows a good overview of the sellar, suprasellar, presellar, parasellar and anterior cranial fossa region and permits the complete preservation of olfaction. Bifrontal craniotomy is the ideal approach to various midline lesions of those areas, as sometimes a unilateral extended pterional approach is insufficient for adequate treatment of the lesion. We are aware that this technique requires patience and time, which, in our experience is fully rewarded by its advantages of excellent field exposure and preservation of the olfactory tracts.

From our point of view, we strongly agree with the impressions and findings of Sepehrnia and Knapp [11]. The excellent outcome found in our series as well as that of Sepehrnia and Knapp [11] supports the usefulness of the bilateral subfrontal craniotomy with section of the falx.

## References

1. Aguiar PH, Pulici, Lourenço L, et al (2002) Preservation of the olfactory tract in bifrontal craniotomy. Arq Neuropsiquiatr 60:12–16
2. Aguiar PH, Lourenço DL, Plasencia OZ, et al (2004) Meningiomas del surco olfatorio: aspectos clínicos, radiológicos y quirurgicos. Analisis y complicaciones. Rev Chil Neurocirurgia 22:35–38
3. Bini W, Sepehrnia A, Samii M (1991) Some technical considerations regarding craniopharyngioma surgery: the bifrontal approach. In: Samii M (ed) Surgery of the Sellar Region and Paranasal Sinuses. Springer, Berlin, pp 381–386

4.  Eriksen KD, Boge-Rasmussen T, Kruse-Larsen C (1990) Anosmia following operation for cerebral aneurysms in the anterior circulation. J Neurosurg 72:864–865

5.  Feiz-Erfan I, Han PP, Spetzeler RF (2005) Preserving olfactory function in anterior craniofacial surgery through cribiform plate osteotomy applied in selected patients. Neurosurgery 57:86–92

6.  Fujitsu K, Sekino T, Sakata K, Kawasaki T (1994) Basal interfalcine approach through a frontal sinusostomy with vein and nerve preservation. J Neurosurg 80:575–579

7.  Fujiwara H, Yasui N, Nathal-Vera E, et al (1996) Anosmia after anterior communicating artery aneurysm surgery: comparison between the anterior interhemispheric and basal interhemispheric approaches. Neurosurgery 38:325–328

8.  Pool JL (1961) Aneurysms of the anterior communicating artery: bifrontal craniotomy and routine use of temporary clips. J Neurosurg 18:98–111

9.  Samii M (1981) Olfactory nerve. In: Samii M, Janetta PJ (eds) The Cranial Nerves. Springer, Berlin, pp 69–73

10. Sekhar LN, Nanda A, Sen CN (1992) The extended frontal approach to tumors of the anterior, middle, and posterior skull base. J Neurosurg 76:198–206

11. Sepehrnia A, Knapp U (1999) Preservation of the olfactory tract in bifrontal craniotomy for various lesions of the anterior cranial fossa. Neurosurgery 44:113–117

12. Spetzler RF, Herman JM, Beals S, et al (1993) Preservation of olfaction in the anterior craniofacial approaches. J Neurosurg 79:48–52

13. Srinivasan J, Dailey AT, Berger MS (1999) The bifrontal olfactory nerve-sparing approach to lesions of the suprasellar region in children. Pediatr Neurosurg 30:245–252

14. Suzuki J, Yoshimoto T, Mizoi K (1981) Preservation of the olfactory tract in bifrontal craniotomy for anterior communicating artery aneurysms, and the functional prognosis. J Neurosurg 54:342–345

15. Yasui N, Nathal E, Fujiwara H, et al (1992) The basal interhemispheric approach for acute anterior communicating artery aneurysms. Acta Neurochir (Wien) 118:91–97

# Treatment of Meningiomas Involving the Optic Nerve Sheath

Makoto Nakamura

## Contents

## 9.1

## Introduction

Optic nerve sheath meningiomas (ONSMs) represent one-third of all optic nerve tumors, but they account for only 1–2% of all intracranial meningiomas. Although these tumors are rare, they represent an important clinical entity because if not treated, slow but progressive tumor growth with increasing visual loss will lead to unilateral or even bilateral blindness [38, 44].

The first case of ONSM in a young woman with decreased vision in one eye was probably described by Spry in 1755 [35]. In 1816, Scarpa characterized tumors of the optic nerve including cases of ONSMs, which he treated with surgical excision, but he noted a high rate of orbital recurrence. Optic nerve tumors were not further differentiated until Hudson's classification in 1912, clearly separating ONSMs from optic gliomas [18]. Later on, other authors collected series of patients harboring orbital meningiomas, but no distinction was made between primary optic nerve tumors and secondary meningiomas with intraorbital extension from intracranial sites [26]

until Coston and Friedenwald unequivocally described the primary origin of meningiomas at the optic nerve sheath [10]. Since then, the diagnosis and treatment of primary ONSMs have been reported in small heterogeneous series.

Recent advances in modern neuroimaging now provide detailed orbital imaging in computed tomography (CT) and magnetic resonance imaging (MRI) scans, enabling early diagnosis of even small ONSMs [20, 23, 25, 47].

Over the past decades, treatment strategies for ONSMs changed with the introduction of precise fractionated radiotherapy and stereotactic radiotherapy with preservation of vision, even on long-term follow up [5,24,29,41]. Previous surgical reports in most cases failed to show beneficial advantage over other treatment options with high morbidity in terms of visual loss as well as recurrences due to incomplete removal [12,13,16,45]. However, surgery may still play an important role in the treatment of ONSMs in selected cases.

Our series of ONSMs is based on 24 cases mainly treated surgically between 1981 and 2002 at the Neurosurgical Department of the Nordstadt Hospital, Hannover, Germany.

## 9.2

## Pathologic Anatomy

Primary ONSMs arise from the arachnoidal cap cells surrounding the intracanalicular or intraorbital portion of the optic nerve [36]. They are intimately associated with the nerve and tend to surround the nerve, leading to a concentric thickening. Posterior extension of the tumor into the annulus of Zinn impedes complete resection without compromising the integrity of the optic nerve [36]. Some aggressive ONSMs may also infiltrate the globe or optic nerve.

The location of the tumor along the optic nerve has considerable influence on visual function. Visual deficits in patients with an ONSM at or near the orbital apex are thought to be followed by additional rapid and progressive visual loss [8, 12]. These tumors also have a higher risk of secondary intracranial extension [33], sometimes even with contralateral nerve involvement.

A classification of ONSMs according to their site of origin and growth pattern was recently proposed by Schick et al. [36]. Type I tumors are represented purely intraorbital lesions (Ia – flat extension around the optic nerve, Ib – bulbiform mass around the optic nerve, Ic– exophytic tumor around the optic nerve), type II are intraorbital tumors with intracranial extension through the optic canal or superior orbital fissure (IIa – intraorbital growth through the optic canal, IIb – with growth through the superior orbital fissure or cavernous sinus), and type III are intraorbital tumors with widespread intracranial tumor extension (IIIa – extension to chiasm, IIIb – extension to chiasm, contralateral optic nerve, and planum sphenoidale).

## 9.3
## Clinical Signs and Symptoms

A triad of findings have been considered pathognomonic for ONSMs by Walsh, namely visual loss, optic atrophy, and optociliary shunt vessels [13]. However, the simultaneous occurrence of all three findings in any individual is rather uncommon.

The most frequent presenting symptom of ONSM is loss of visual acuity, which was seen in 96% of reported cases [13]. Visual loss is typically gradual, and decreased color vision is usually an early finding. In a review of 119 reported cases, the mean duration of symptoms prior to presentation was 41.9 months (range 1 month to 17 years) [13]. Visual field defects were documented in 83% of reviewed cases. Among them, peripheral visual field constriction was seen in 35%, central, centrocecal, and paracentral scotomas were noted in 29%, altitudinal defects in 16%, and increased size of the blind spot in 13% [13].

Proptosis usually follows the onset of visual loss and was present in 59% of reviewed patients on initial examination [13]. Proptosis is less frequent in patients harboring intracanalicular ONSMs, since they typically present with visual loss while the tumor is still very small.

Decreased ocular motility was found in 47% of reported cases [13], mostly resulting form mechanical restriction of extraocular muscle function due to a stiffening of the optic nerve sheath. Reportedly, the degree of restriction is often greatest in attempted upgaze [3]. Orbital pain or generalized headache has also been reported in up to 50% of patients in some series [13].

Our mainly surgical series comprised 24 patients with the diagnosis of an ONSM, treated at the Neurosurgical Department of the Nordstadt Hospital, Hannover, Germany during the time period of 1981–2002. Histological confirmation has been obtained in 22 operated cases. The remaining two patients have not undergone surgery and the diagnosis has been made on the basis of typical clinical and radiological features (Table 1).

The presenting symptoms and their duration are detailed in Table 2. Most patients noticed loss of vision as their first symptom and this often preceded the recognition of any proptosis by a year or more. About every fifth patient experienced a more rapid visual loss within 5 months. The clinical findings are outlined in Table 3. Large tumors manifested mainly with proptosis or diplopia, and posteriorly lying tumors with headaches. Patients with presence of proptosis, implying a large tumor mass inside the orbital cavity (type Ib), did not experience stronger visual loss than patients without proptosis. Patients with intraorbital-intracranial extension of

Table 1 Patient data. *ONSM* Optic nerve sheath meningiomas, *M* male, *F* female, *NF-2* neurofibromatosis type 2

| Patients with ONSM | |
| --- | --- |
| Total patients | 24 |
| Mean age at diagnosis | 44.24 years (14–69 years) |
| Gender ratio (M:F) | 3:21 (1:7) |
| Laterality | Left 13, right 9, bilateral 2 |
| NF-2 | 2 patients<br>M:F ratio 1:1<br>Mean age 26.5 years |

Table 2 Presenting symptoms

| Initial symptom | Number | Mean duration (range) |
| --- | --- | --- |
| Visual loss | 13 | 37.3 months (1–96 months) |
| Visual field deficit | 3 | 44.6 months (2–84 months) |
| Diplopia | 2 | 22 months (8–36 months) |
| Protrusio bulbi | 2 | 5.5 months (4–7 months) |
| Lacrimation | 1 | 23 months |
| Orbital pain | 1 | 6 months |
| Periorbital edema | 1 | 6 months |
| Incidental finding | 1 | |

Table 3: Clinical findings

| Clinical findings at presentation | Number of patients | |
|---|---|---|
| Visual loss | Blind | 6 |
| | Light perception | 5 |
| | Acuity of 0.3 | 3 |
| | Acuity of 0.6 | 3 |
| | Acuity of 0.8 | 4 |
| | Normal acuity | 3 |
| Visual field deficit | Quadrant anopsia | 2 |
| | Concentric restriction | 3 |
| | Hemianopsia | 4 |
| | Central scotoma | 7 |
| Proptosis | 10 | |
| Orbital pain | 7 | |
| Diplopia | 5 | |
| Eyelid swelling | 3 | |
| Headaches | 3 | |

ONSM (type IIIa/b) did not experience earlier, progressive, or severe visual loss than patients categorized in other classes. Ophthalmoscopy demonstrated pale and atrophic optic discs in all blind patients and patients with light perception. It was normal in all patients with no loss of vision and decreased vision of 0.6–0.8.

## 9.4
## Radiology

Except for lesions confined to the optic canal, CT can demonstrate enlargement of the orbital optic nerve in the majority of cases; 97–99% of ONSMs were demonstrated on CT scans [13]. Tram-tracking, a radiographic sign in which the denser and thickened optic nerve sheath outlines a central lucency representing the residual optic nerve, is a characteristic finding suggestive of an ONSM.

MRI provides excellent visualization of ONSMs, even in the intracanalicular segment of the optic nerve. It shows a thickening of the nerve with isointense or slightly hyperintense signal intensity compared to normal nerves on T1- and T2-weighted images. Fat-suppression MRI provides improved tissue contrast of orbital structures and accurately represents anatomic borders of the optic nerve, both in the orbit and in the optic canal [13]. When used with contrast administration, fat-suppression

T1-weighted images give superior delineation of the tumor surface adjacent to orbital fat [23].

In our series on CT scan, intraosseous extension of ONSM has been seen either into the medial wall of the orbital cavity extending, therefore, into the ethmoidal cells (one patient) or to the lateral wall producing hyperostosis of the sphenoid ridge (two patients). Calcification occurred in ten patients (42%).

On MRI, an inhomogeneous contrast enhancement particularly evident with fat saturation techniques has been seen in 10 patients (42%) with significant larger tumor volumes. The presence of a nonenhancing optic nerve in the middle of an enhancing tumor, giving evidence of the classical "tram track sign," has been seen in four patients, accounting for 20% (4/20), since the introduction of fat-suppression techniques in magnetic resonance tomography.

## 9.5
## Treatment

The selection of an adequate treatment option for ONSMs remains a matter of debate. Current management of ONSMs includes observation, surgical excision, and/or radiotherapy, depending on the extent of the tumor and the degree and rate of decline in visual impairment [5, 12, 24, 28, 37, 39, 42, 43]. The natural history of this disease is progressive loss of visual acuity, as evidenced by a cohort of patients who underwent observation in several series [5, 13, 14, 21, 29]. Furthermore, if untreated, ONSM can eventually extend intracranially, resulting in seizure, hemiparesis [9, 19, 21] or bilateral blindness, within a few years.

The current literature provides few studies detailing the results from surgical resection. Current treatment protocols indicate surgery for ONSM mainly in blind patients with disfiguring proptosis, intracranial extension, or young patients, where a presumed higher biological activity of the tumor tissue is judged to require immediate surgical intervention [45]. Only very few cases of visual improvement after microsurgical resection of ONSMs have been reported, but the majority describe a decrease of vision through surgery [17, 19, 45] and an association with a high rate of complications, including blindness resulting from central retinal artery occlusion [1, 3, 4, 9, 19, 21, 34] and high rates of local recurrence (>38%) [22]. In reviews of surgical patients treated by Ito et al. [19] and Cristante [11], only 2 of 21 patients who underwent resection had improved vision, although 30% and 62%, respectively, remained with functional visual acuity. Both patients with improved vision had anteriorly located tumors, which tend to grow extradurally, and were more amenable to resection. Single case reports describe surgery for ONSM with benefit only if the location of the meningioma is anterior, close to the globe of the eye bulb [9, 19, 21, 38, 42, 46]. In Kennerdell's series, seven patients with functional acuity preoperatively remained stable for 2–10 years after undergoing subtotal resection, although his group experienced loss of vision in the majority of cases [21]. On the other hand, in 1984 Sibony et al. reported that six out of eight patients improved in either acuity or visual field or both; three of them experienced a decline in visual function 1 year after surgery, but 38% of patients maintained stable acuity over a period of 5 years [38]. Delfini et al. support surgical intervention in patients with symptoms in progress, despite their results of an >80% decline in vision after surgery [12].

Some other reports presented a more favorable outcome after surgery of ONSMs. Verheggen et al. demonstrated an improvement of visual acuity in intracanalicular and intraorbital meningiomas in 89% of their surgically treated cases. They conclude that early surgery improves the chance of preserving visual acuity in cases of ONSM with extradural extension, although there was a high risk of injury to the vessels, cranial nerves, and ocular muscles in the orbital funnel [42].

In a large series presented by Schick and coworkers in 2004, the postoperative visual outcome did not differ significantly from the preoperative vision in 73 surgically treated patients with ONSM. Furthermore, most patients remained stable during a long follow-up period. The authors recommended decompression of the optic canal and resection of intracranial tumor parts prior to adjuvant radiotherapy [36].

In our surgical series, we cannot state categorically that preservation of vision is only achievable in apical ONSMs. We did not experience a correlation between tumor extension and visual loss before and after surgery. Rather, the visual results were most closely related to the duration of visual symptoms, in a way that visual improvement occurred in patients with rapid decline of vision only. This finding concurs with those of Rosenberg et al., who evaluated 20 microsurgically treated patients with ONSM and found a 69% stable or even improved vision postoperatively [32]. However, microsurgical excision of the ONSM with preservation of vascular supply and its pial surroundings of the optic nerve does not imply preservation of vision in all cases, as visual loss might be dependent on tissue consistency, producing various amounts of pressure when encasing the optic nerve, the complicated pial blood supply, and manipulation to the optic nerve producing vasospasm of the optic nerves vasa nervorum.

## 9.6
## Surgical Technique

Regardless of the position of the ONSM in the orbital cavity, standard osteoplastic frontolateral or pterional craniotomies attaining the supra orbital margin of the orbit were performed. Epidural dissection of the orbital roof and removal of the lateral orbital wall are followed by stepwise drilling of the optic canal, after defining the anatomic limits of bone resection as the lower rim of the optic foramen and superior orbital fissure downwards. For types Ib or Ic tumor debulking of the orbital cavity can be performed first. Dural resection borders are the orbital apex anteriorly, in particular the annulus of Zinn at its whole length and the optic nerve sheath. The decompression of the optic nerve in the optic canal is mandatory in cases of intracanalicular ONSMs.

If protrusion of the tuberculum above the line connecting the surface of the nerves as they enter the optic canals is evident, it has to be removed in order to enlarge the transfrontal operative field.

In all cases with intracranial extension of the ONSM, an intradural approach is necessary with opening of the sylvian fissure as the first procedure. The ipsilateral optic nerve and carotid cisterns are identified. In this step, preservation of the small feeding vessels between the carotid artery and the optic nerve is important, which is why we favor irrigation with isothermal Ringer's solution instead of coagulation.

Careful decompression of tumor tissue around the optic nerve is enforced as long as tumor/nerve borders are visible. The dura of the region of the tuberculum sellae and chiasmatic sulcus is carefully inspected for evidence of meningeal tumor infiltration.

If the ONSM infiltrates the optic nerve, resection is limited to the exophytic part. However, in carefully selected cases of type Ia tumors, epineural decompression might be necessary to relieve the pressure of the optic nerve itself. In blind patients with disfiguring painful proptosis, the nerve can be transected and the intraorbital portion is removed.

## 9.7
## Surgical Results

Surgical removal in patients with functional vision was subtotal in all cases. In all blind patients and in one patient with light perception, transection of the optic nerve some distance from the optic chiasm was performed in order to achieve a complete resection of the tumor and prevent tumor growth over the chiasm to the opposite side ($n=7$). The 22 operated patients with ONSM showed no mortality and acceptable low morbidity; 1 patient with frontal hygroma did not need surgical intervention and 2 patients with cerebrospinal fluid fistula were treated effectively with a lumbar drain. The duration of preserved vision for patients with unchanged good vision was longer than 36 month in all cases (36–56 months). Patients with improvements of impaired vision preoperatively harbored types Ib and IIIa tumors and had a stable situation postoperatively for a mean of 60 months (36–96 months). The two patients with a decline of good vision after microsurgery still have functional vision and remained stable for 52 and 212 months, respectively. Overall, 8 out of 16 patients retained or even improved their vision following surgery (Table 4). Two patients lost their postoperative preserved vision due to tumor progression. One patient with neurofibromatosis type 2 needed exenteration of the eye due to massive tumor recurrence 10 years after partial removal. None of the blind patients with total resection and transected optic nerve had either clinical or radiological recurrence of ONSM. Five patients experienced a new lesion of the oculomotor nerve postoperatively, with paresis of the levator palpebrae muscle, which in four of these five cases resolved spontaneously within 8 weeks.

In our series, patients with sudden visual loss (<5 months prior to surgery) showed improvement through surgery, due to decompression of the optic nerve with subtotal resection of the tumor. These patients gained visual function for a mean time of 60 month (36–96 months) with acceptable risk of morbidity and still having the feasibility of radiotherapy in the future.

## 9.8
### Radiotherapy

The invention of highly sophisticated stereotactic radiosurgery or three-dimensional conformal beam fractionated radiotherapy provides increasing evidence for the benefit of radiotherapy in ONSMs [15,24,28,30]. Andrews et al. reported an improvement of vision in 10 of 24 cases (42%), and in 50% of patients, stable visual function was observed after treatment with conventional fractionated stereotactic radiotherapy (LINAC) alone, although the mean follow-up was only 20 month [5]. A comparison of long-term visual outcome by Turbin et al. showed better results for patients treated by conventional multiport or conformal planned delivery of radiotherapy than by surgery plus radiation, surgery alone, or observation during the follow-up period [41]. However, radiotherapy is still associated with relevant treatment-related morbidity (up to 33.3%) like retinopathy, persistent retinitis, dry eye, and neuronal damage to the optic nerve system [2, 6,

27, 29, 41]. Long-term clinical outcome has to give proof of the promising results. To date, however, radiotherapy seems to be a superior treatment modality for patients with excellent vision who deserve treatment or who a experience gradual slow decline in vision [41]. It is also the treatment of choice for recurrent tumors, as surgery for these tumors is mostly devastating with respect to visual function. The appropriate time for therapeutic intervention is still unclear, as follow up of the available case series is limited and these tumors may pursue a stable course for many years, although recent reports demonstrated that early radiotherapy at a stage of mild visual decline has been superior in preservation of vision [29]. However, asymptomatic patients should be observed at close ophthalmological and neuroradiological intervals.

As an additional treatment option in selected cases of multimorbidity or patient's denial of interventional therapies, hydroxyurea has been proposed as chemotherapeutical alternative [7, 31, 40].

## 9.9
### Conclusion

Based on our experience and compared to the standards of newly invented high-precision radiotherapy, we think that surgery still plays a role in the treatment of ONSM with expeditious visual deterioration, in concordance with the work of Andrews et al. [5, 8]. Radiotherapy does not lead to an acute decrease in tumor volume in all cases and therefore cannot be recommended in cases of rapid visual decline, where surgery is indicated to immediately alleviate pressure to visual pathway structures. It should be the goal to resect as much tumor as possible, opening the bony canal to alleviate compression ischemia without manipulation of the optic nerve to minimize visual loss.

Postoperative tumor remnants provide smaller and safer targets for adjuvant radiotherapy. With fat-suppression techniques and high magnetic field MRI, the diagnosis of an ONSM can be sensitive and close to 100%, such that needle biopsy procedures are no longer required for definitive diagnosis [5, 24, 25].

Table 4  Follow up of visual acuity

| Preoperative vision | Improved | No change | Worsened | Stable (months) |
|---|---|---|---|---|
| Good (1.0–0.8) | – | 2 | 2 | 56 (36–72) |
| Impaired (0.6–0.3) | 2 | 4 | 2 | 60 (36–96) |
| Light perception | 1 | – | 4 | – |

Our recommendation for ONSMs includes surgical decompression of the optic nerve in patients with type IIa ONSM and sudden visual decline. For patients with no visual loss in type Ia or IIa, conservative treatment or early three-dimensional conformal beam radiation therapy is recommended. In patients with type Ib ONSM and functional vision, surgical debulking first with adjuvant radiotherapy for tumor remnants surrounding the optic nerve should be considered. Microsurgical intervention still plays a role in cases of intracranial extension of the ONSM (types II and III) when growth can be observed toward the chiasm, or if the carotid artery is going to be encased by the tumor. In these cases, microsurgical removal of the intracranial tumor part with decompression of the nerve sheath and the annulus of Zinn along its whole length, followed by radiotherapy, depending on tumor resection grade and visual function, seems to be the optimal treatment option.

## References

1. Al Mefty O, Holoubi A, Rifai A, Fox JL (1985) Microsurgical removal of suprasellar meningiomas. Neurosurgery 16:364–372

2. Al Mefty O, Kersh JE, Routh A, Smith RR (1990) The long-term side effects of radiation therapy for benign brain tumors in adults. J Neurosurg 73:502–512

3. Alper MG (1981) Management of primary optic nerve meningiomas. Current status – therapy in controversy. J Clin Neuroophthalmol 1:101–117

4. Andrews BT, Wilson CB (1988) Suprasellar meningiomas: the effect of tumor location on postoperative visual outcome. J Neurosurg 69:523–528

5. Andrews DW, Faroozan R, Yang BP, et al (2002) Fractionated stereotactic radiotherapy for the treatment of optic nerve sheath meningiomas: preliminary observations of 33 optic nerves in 30 patients with historical comparison to observation with or without prior surgery. Neurosurgery 51:890–902

6. Capo H, Kupersmith MJ (1991) Efficacy and complications of radiotherapy of anterior visual pathway tumors. Neurol Clin 9:179–203

7. Cassidy LM, Moriarty PA, Griffin JF, et al (1997) Hormonal treatment of bilateral optic nerve meningioma [letter]. Eye 11:566–568

8. Castel A, Boschi A, Renard L, De Potter P (2000) Optic nerve sheath meningiomas: clinical features, functional prognosis and controversial treatment. Bull Soc Belge Ophtalmol 275:73–78

9. Clark WC, Theofilos CS, Fleming JC (1989) Primary optic nerve sheath meningiomas. Report of nine cases. J Neurosurg 70:37–40

10. Coston TO (1936) Primary tumor of the optic nerve: with report of a case. Arch Ophthalmol 15:696–702

11. Cristante L (1994) Surgical treatment of meningiomas of the orbit and optic canal: a retrospective study with particular attention to the visual outcome. Acta Neurochir (Wien) 126:27–32

12. Delfini R, Missori P, Tarantino R, et al (1996) Primary benign tumors of the orbital cavity: comparative data in a series of patients with optic nerve glioma, sheath meningioma, or neurinoma. Surg Neurol 45:147–153

13. Dutton JJ (1992) Optic nerve sheath meningiomas. Surv Ophthalmol 37:167–183

14. Egan RA, Lessell S (2002) A contribution to the natural history of optic nerve sheath meningiomas. Arch Ophthalmol 120:1505–1508

15. Eng TY, Albright NW, Kuwahara G, et al (1992) Precision radiation therapy for optic nerve sheath meningiomas. Int J Radiat Oncol Biol Phys 22:1093–1098

16. Fineman MS, Augsburger JJ (1999) A new approach to an old problem. Surv Ophthalmol 43:519–524

17. Gabibov GA, Blinkov SM, Tcherekayev VA (1988) The management of optic nerve meningiomas and gliomas. J Neurosurg 68:889–893

18. Hudson AC (1912) Primary tumors of the optic nerve. R Ophthalmol Hosp Rep 18:317–439

19. Ito M, Ishizawa A, Miyaoka M, et al (1988) Intraorbital meningiomas. Surgical management and role of radiation therapy. Surg Neurol 29:448–453

20. Kanamalla US (2003) The optic nerve tram-track sign. Radiology 227:718–719

21. Kennerdell JS, Maroon JC, Malton M, et al (1988) The management of optic nerve sheath meningiomas. Am J Ophthalmol 106:450–457

22. Kupersmith MJ, Newall J, Ransohoff J (1989) Optic nerve sheath meningioma. J Neurosurg 71:305

23. Lindblom B, Truwit CL, Hoyt WF (1992) Optic nerve sheath meningioma. Definition of intraorbital, intracanalicular, and intracranial components with magnetic resonance imaging. Ophthalmology 99:560–566

24. Liu JK, Forman S, Hershewe GL, et al (2002) Optic nerve sheath meningiomas: visual improvement after stereotactic radiotherapy. Neurosurgery 50:950–955

25. Mafee MF, Goodwin J, Dorodi S (1999) Optic nerve sheath meningiomas. Role of MR imaging. Radiol Clin North Am 37:37–58, ix

26. Mayer LL (1928) Endothelioma of the orbit: report of a case. Am J Ophthalmol 11:617–622

27. Morita A, Coffey RJ, Foote RL, et al (1999) Risk of injury to cranial nerves after gamma knife radiosurgery for skull base meningiomas: experience in 88 patients. J Neurosurg 90:42–49

28. Moyer PD, Golnik KC, Breneman J (2000) Treatment of optic nerve sheath meningioma with three-dimensional conformal radiation. Am J Ophthalmol 129:694–696

29. Narayan S, Cornblath WT, Sandler HM, et al (2003) Preliminary visual outcomes after three-dimensional conformal radiation therapy for optic nerve sheath meningioma. Int J Radiat Oncol Biol Phys 56:537–543

30. Paridaens AD, van Ruyven RL, Eijkenboom WM, et al (2003) Stereotactic irradiation of biopsy proved optic nerve sheath meningioma. Br J Ophthalmol 87:246–247

31. Paus S, Klockgether T, Schlegel U, et al. (2003) Meningioma of the optic nerve sheath: treatment with hydroxyurea. J Neurol Neurosurg Psychiatry 74:1348–1350

32. Rosenberg LF, Miller NR (1984) Visual results after microsurgical removal of meningiomas involving the anterior visual system. Arch Ophthalmol 102:1019–1023

33. Saeed P, Rootman J, Nugent RA, et al (2003) Optic nerve sheath meningiomas. Ophthalmology 110:2019–2030

34. Sarkies NJ (1987) Optic nerve sheath meningioma: diagnostic features and therapeutic alternatives. Eye 1:597–602

35. Scarpa A (2007) Trattato delle Principali Maletties degli Occhi. Pietro Bizzoni, Pavia

36. Schick U, Dott U, Hassler W (2004) Surgical management of meningiomas involving the optic nerve sheath. J Neurosurg 101:951–959

37. Shimano H, Nagasawa S, Kawabata S, et al (2000) Surgical strategy for meningioma extension into the optic canal. Neurol Med Chir (Tokyo) 40:447–451

38. Sibony PA, Krauss HR, Kennerdell JS, et al (1984) Optic nerve sheath meningiomas. Clinical manifestations. Ophthalmology 91:1313–1326

39. Sleep TJ, Hodgkins PR, Honeybul S, et al (2003) Visual function following neurosurgical optic nerve decompression for compressive optic neuropathy. Eye 17:571–578

40. Thom M, Martinian L (2002) Progesterone receptors are expressed with higher frequency by optic nerve sheath meningiomas. Clin Neuropathol 21:5–8

41. Turbin RE, Thompson CR, Kennerdell JS, et al (2002) A long-term visual outcome comparison in patients with optic nerve sheath meningioma managed with observation, surgery, radiotherapy, or surgery and radiotherapy. Ophthalmology 109:890–899

42. Verheggen R, Markakis E, Muhlendyck H, et al (1996) Symptomatology, surgical therapy and postoperative results of sphenoorbital, intraorbital-intracanalicular and optic sheath meningiomas. Acta Neurochir Suppl (Wien) 65:95–98

43. Whittaker CK (1997) Indications for removal of optic nerve sheath meningioma [letter; comment]. AJNR Am J Neuroradiol 18:396–397

44. Wright JE (1977) Primary optic nerve meningiomas: clinical presentation and management. Trans Am Acad Ophthalmol Otolaryngol 83:617–625

45. Wright JE, McNab AA, McDonald WI (1989) Primary optic nerve sheath meningioma. Br J Ophthalmol 73:960–966

46. Yuceer N, Erdogan A, Ziya H (1994) Primary optic nerve sheath meningiomas. Report of seven cases (clinical neuroradiological, pathological and surgical considerations in seven cases) J Neurosurg Sci 38:155–159

47. Zimmerman CF, Schatz NJ, Glaser JS (1990) Magnetic resonance imaging of optic nerve meningiomas. Enhancement with gadolinium-DTPA. Ophthalmology 97:585–591

# Surgical Management of Tuberculum Sellae Meningiomas

**10**

Makoto Nakamura and Madjid Samii

Contents

## 10.1
## Introduction

Tuberculum sellae meningiomas represent a distinct group of tumors that arise from the tuberculum sellae, chiasmatic sulcus, limbus sphenoidale, or diaphragma sellae and grow in a subchiasmal position. This type of tumor was often mixed with other meningiomas occupying the suprasellar area, although with different dural origin (i.e., the frontobasal dura, anterior clinoid process, medial sphenoidal ridge, or even the olfactory groove). Due to the distinct dural attachment, tuberculum sellae meningiomas grow in such a direction that the optic nerves and chiasm are elevated or displaced with increas-

ing tumor size. According to the literature, tuberculum sellae meningiomas comprise approximately 5–10% of intracranial meningiomas [2, 12, 22, 25, 27, 32].

The first successful removal of a tuberculum sellae meningioma was performed by Cushing in 1916, but it was not reported until 1929 [11]. In 1938, Cushing and Eisenhardt [12] reported on 28 cases of meningiomas of the tuberculum sellae and proposed a classification of four stages according to their size. They used the term suprasellar to describe tumors arising from the dura over the tuberculum sellae. Following this early series, many reports have been published under the rubric of suprasellar meningiomas, which, however, covered tumors arising from different dural origins [1, 3, 6, 8, 9, 13, 19, 21, 24, 32, 33, 37–39]. In some surgical series, authors proposed to label meningiomas of the tuberculum sellae as a separate entity [2, 4, 14–18, 20, 22, 25, 27, 28, 30, 34].

## 10.2
## Pathologic Anatomy

The tuberculum sellae is a slight bony elevation in front of the pituitary fossa measuring several millimeters in height and length. When the tumor is small or moderate in size, the area of attachment is rather small, although the dural attachment may extend anteriorly to the sphenoid limbus or posteriorly involving the diaphragma sellae to the infundibulum. With increasing tumor size, the optic nerves and chiasm become elevated and may produce visual disturbance. Tuberculum sellae meningiomas may invade the bone, causing hyperostosis, but they mostly grow in the subdural compartment and remain outside the arachnoid, as it also observed in other skull-base meningiomas. Growing superiorly, they may displace and stretch the optic nerves in the superolateral direction. One or both nerves may also be enveloped by the tumor. In addition, the internal carotid arteries can be displaced laterally, but to a lesser degree than the optic nerves. Occasionally, they can be totally encased. The tumors may further extend posteriorly into the sella and retrosellar area as well as into the interpeduncular cistern. The pituitary stalk is then displaced posteriorly, along with the basilar artery. In large tumors, the third ventricle and hypothalamus can be compressed causing hydrocephalus. Less commonly, tumors can extend to the cavernous sinus laterally.

## 10.3
## Clinical Presentation

As with meningiomas in other locations, tuberculum sellae meningiomas occur more frequently in women than men with a ratio of 3:1 [13] and predominance in the fourth decade of life [2, 15, 22].

The "chiasmal syndrome" produced by tuberculum sellae meningiomas was noted by Holmes and Sargent in 1927 [2] and later emphasized by Cushing and Eisenhardt [12]. This syndrome includes a primary optic atrophy with asymmetric bitemporal field defects in adult patients showing a normal sella on plain skull x-ray, and has been the classic characteristic presentation. Although the most common pattern of visual disturbance is insidious or gradual vision loss in one eye, followed by gradual visual disturbance in the contralateral eye, these visual symptoms may sometimes be acute or fluctuating [2, 15, 25, 27]. Other symptoms may be headache, mental changes, epilepsy, anosmia, and motor deficits [38]. Despite modern neuroimaging studies, diagnosis may be delayed for up to 2 years from the onset of symptoms [3,20]. Symptoms can be aggravated during pregnancy, and this phenomenon is well documented in the literature [3, 15, 26]. Due to the sellar involvement of the tumor, pituitary structures may be compressed, but reportedly preoperative signs of pituitary insufficiency are uncommon [38, 39].

## 10.4
## Preoperative Evaluation

To fully appreciate the whole extent of the tumor, gadolinium-enhanced magnetic resonance imaging (MRI) is presently the study of choice. MRI provides the most accurate distinction of suprasellar tumors; however, it may still be difficult to differentiate between a suprasellar macroadenoma and a tuberculum sellae meningioma with intrasellar extension. Similar to other intracranial meningiomas, tuberculum sellae meningiomas have a hypo- or isointense signal intensity on T1- and T2-weighted images [29].

Hyperostosis in the parasellar region or tumor calcification is best appreciated with a computed tomography (CT) scan with bone windows in the coronal plane.

Cerebral angiography may provide information concerning displacement of anterior cerebral arteries, which are frequently involved in large tuberculum sellae meningiomas. However, vascular displacement or encasement can be well visualized in MRI or magnetic resonance angiography, and these studies have largely replaced cerebral angiography. The anterior cerebral arteries are most frequently elevated superiorly and stretched; the internal carotid artery may be displaced laterally, or even encased in large tumors.

Similar to other sellar lesions, an ophthalmological evaluation including visual acuity and visual field testing should be performed in every suspected case of tuberculum sellae meningioma. In every tumor with significant intrasellar tumor extension or suspected pituitary dysfunction, an endocrinological assessment should be performed.

## 10.5
## Treatment

The primary goal of treatment for tuberculum sellae meningiomas is total surgical removal including the dural tumor matrix and any part of invaded bone. Due to advances in modern neurosurgical techniques and modern neuroanesthesia, this should be possible in the majority of cases, even for large tumors. Conventional or stereotactic radiation therapy, including stereotactic radiosurgery, is not preferred as the initial therapy for tuberculum sellae meningiomas [2, 22]. However, radiation therapy may serve as an adjuvant treatment for recurrent or residual tumors, which is considered less favorable for radical surgical removal. In particular, those tumors involving the cavernous sinus may be considered for adjuvant radiation therapy to prevent further tumor growth. In our view, preoperative embolization is not a feasible option to prepare for easier surgery for tuberculum sellae meningiomas, as the arterial supply of these tumors are fed primarily via branches of the ophthalmic artery, which could be endangered by this procedure.

Different surgical approaches have been advocated to resect meningiomas of the tuberculum sellae. The unifrontal or bifrontal approach were often performed in earlier macrosurgical [13, 15, 19, 32, 38, 39] and some microsurgical series [2, 3, 6, 16]. The pterional or frontotemporal approach was adopted with the availability of the operating microscope [14, 17, 22]. The frontal or frontolateral approach was preferred in some microsurgical series [1–3, 6, 36].

In our surgical series, all three approaches (frontolateral, bifrontal, and pterional) were used by applying microsurgical techniques to resect these tumors.

## 10.6
## Surgical Technique

### 10.6.1
### Frontolateral Approach

The patient is lying in the supine position on the operating table with the head secured in a Mayfield head holder.

The patient's head is rotated to the contralateral side at a 10–20° angle. The neck is extended with the head above the heart level to facilitate adequate venous drainage during surgery. A slight retroflexion of the head is performed to allow the frontal lobe to move away from the frontal base, resulting in less retraction of the brain during surgery.

For the frontolateral approach, a single burr hole is placed just posterior to the anterior temporal line, using a high-speed drill. The direction of drilling is performed in such a way that opening of the periorbita is prevented. A high-speed craniotome is used to cut a free bone flap medial to the burr hole, as shown in Fig. 1. The lateral border of the frontal sinus has to be considered during craniotomy. The bone flap is usually 2.5 cm (width)×2 cm (height). The inner edge of the supraorbital bone is drilled to optimize the angle to reach the frontobasal area.

When the frontal sinus is entered during craniotomy, the mucosa of the sinus is removed and special attention is paid to ensuring that no remnant of mucosa is left in the lower part of the bone flap. The frontal sinus is tamponaded with iodine-soaked cottonoids and covered adequately.

The dura is opened in a curved fashion with its base toward the supraorbital rim. The next step is to drain cerebrospinal fluid (CSF) by opening of the sylvian fissure. This procedure leads to spontaneous sinking of the frontal lobe, making significant retraction of the frontal lobe unnecessary.

The frontolateral approach provides a more medial view of the clinoid and suprasellar region (Fig. 1)

## 10.6.2
## Bifrontal Approach

The patient is lying in the supine position on the operating table with their head secured in a Mayfield head holder. The skin is cut slightly posterior to the frontal hairline from zygoma to zygoma. The scalp and pericranial flaps are reflected anteriorly. A burr hole is placed on each side of the orbital buttons. A craniotomy is performed extending anteriorly as close as possible to the orbital roof and posteriorly along the convexity of the cranium. The basal line of the craniotomy involves both tables of the frontal sinuses, and the mucous membranes are completely removed. The dura is cut parallel to the base and the sagittal sinus is ligated and cut at the cecal foramen; the falx is transected to open up the operative field (Fig. 2).

## 10.6.3
## Pterional/Frontotemporal Approach

For the pterional approach, operative positioning is similar to the frontolateral approach, but the head is rotated more to the contralateral side (30–40°). A single burr hole is placed at the same location, but the craniotomy is performed more posteriorly, exposing the frontal and temporal lobes with the sylvian fissure and the sphenoid ridge. The lesser wing of the sphenoid is resected to the superior orbital fissure, depending on the tumor size, to allow exposure of the lesion with minimum brain retraction (Fig. 3).

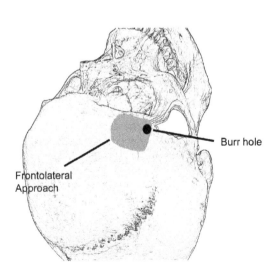

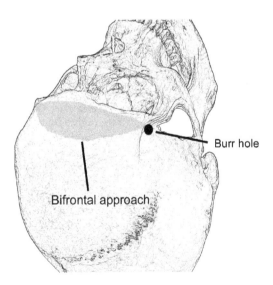

Fig. 1 Frontolateral approach. The craniotomy is performed through a burr hole at the orbital button of the frontal bone behind the anterior temporal line

Fig. 2 Bifrontal approach. The craniotomy is performed through a burr hole at the orbital button of the frontal bone behind the anterior temporal line

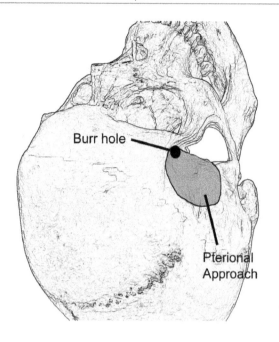

Fig. 3 Pterional approach. The craniotomy is performed through a burr hole at the orbital button of the frontal bone behind the anterior temporal line, extending more to the frontotemporal region compared to the frontolateral approach

## 10.7
## Microsurgical Tumor Resection

When the frontolateral or pterional approach is performed, the ipsilateral optic nerve and the internal carotid artery are first identified. The tumor capsule is opened medial to the ipsilateral optic nerve and the tumor debulked to decompress the optic nerve, using microsurgical techniques. Tumor resection is continued in a piecemeal fashion until the optic chiasm and the contralateral optic nerve is visible. Regardless of the selected surgical approach, it is paramount to avoid injury to the blood supply of the optic apparatus. As the inferior surface of the optic nerve and chiasm receive their blood supply from a group of small arteries, which arise from the medial wall of the internal carotid artery [5], these may not be mistaken as tumor feeders and the use of bipolar coagulation should be restrictive. Special attention has to be paid to the identification and preservation of the optic cistern, also the separation of the layers of the optic cistern and the tumor capsule. To preserve the small arteries supplying the optic nerve and chiasm, it is advisable to leave the tumor capsule until sufficient tumor debulking and preparation have been completed. This will provide a protective plane of dissection for the optic nerves and optic chiasm as well as the perforation vessels. Only when enough space is achieved after tumor removal, the tumor capsule should be removed respecting the arachnoidal plane to the small vessels.

Then the tumor matrix is coagulated and the basal dura resected. In case of hyperostosis or bony tumor involvement, this site is removed with a diamond drill. Tumor resection is completed to the posterior direction, when the pituitary stalk becomes visible and is preserved.

In case of eventual opening of the sphenoid sinus, a pericranial flap or fascia of the temporal muscle with addition of fibrin glue has been used for covering the defect to avoid any postoperative CSF fistula.

The authors' surgical series includes 72 meningiomas arising solely from the tuberculum sellae, treated through three different surgical approaches between 1978 and 2002. Tumors were operated through the frontolateral (1984–2002, $n=30$), pterional/frontotemporal (1982–2002, $n=21$), and bifrontal (1978–1995, $n=21$) approaches. Four of these patients had undergone previous surgeries in other hospitals.

The maximum tumor diameter ranged from 1 to 5 cm, with a mean diameter of 2.8 cm. Tumor size was <3 cm in 39 cases (54.2%) and ≥3 cm in 33 cases (45.8%).

The mean diameter of the tumors was 2.5 cm (1–5 cm) in patients operated using the frontolateral approach, 2.66 cm (1–5 cm) where the pterional/frontotemporal approach was used, and 3.49 cm (1.5–5 cm) in cases where the bifrontal approach was performed. In tumors involving the cavernous sinus, the intracavernous part of the tumors was not radically removed to prevent any new cranial neuropathies (Fig. 4).

## 10.8
## Results

## 10.8.1
## Morbidity and Mortality

The mortality rates for surgery of tuberculum sellae meningiomas ranged from 0% in microsurgical series [14, 31] to even as high as 67% in earlier macrosurgical series [27].

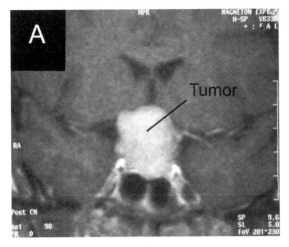
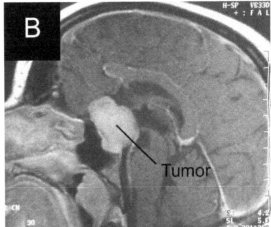
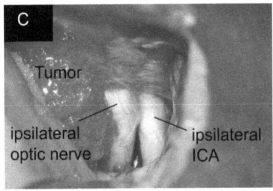
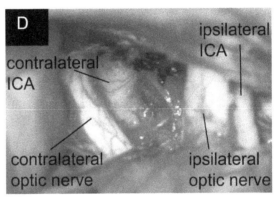
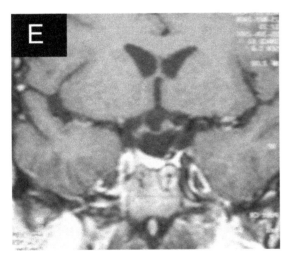

Fig. 4 **a** Tuberculum sellae meningioma on preoperative T1-weighted coronal magnetic resonance imaging (MRI) scan with gadolinium enhancement. **b** Same tumor on preoperative T1-weighted sagittal MRI scan with gadolinium enhancement. **c** Intraoperative view of the tumor through a right frontolateral approach, showing lateral displacement of the ipsilateral optic nerve, which is also partially covered by the tumor. *ICA* Internal carotid artery. **d** After complete tumor removal, the contralateral optic nerve and ICA are visible. **e** Postoperative T1-weighted coronal MRI scan with gadolinium enhancement, confirming total tumor removal

The mortality rates of surgical series published since the year 2000 ranges from 0 to 8.7% [4, 14, 16, 22], including our present series. Concerning our current surgical series, it has to be emphasized that mortality rates were considerably different depending on the selected surgical approach. The mortality rate of the frontolateral and pterional groups was 0%, whereas the mortality rate in patients who underwent bifrontal craniotomy was 9.5%.

Some authors noted the influence of tumor size on surgical outcome for suprasellar meningiomas [6, 15, 23, 39]. Higher mortality rates were reported in patients with tumors larger than 3 cm in diameter compared with mortality rates in patients with smaller tumors. However, others could not confirm this finding in their surgical series [3, 19], and we also cannot support this observation in our series.

In the literature, several potential complications were reported following the removal of tuberculum sellae meningiomas. They have been divided mainly into ophthalmological and nonophthalmological causes.

In a review of suprasellar meningiomas, Finn and Mount [15] found that 20% of survivors had evidence of serious morbidity. The reported nonophthalmological complications of removal of these tumors include diabetes insipidus, CSF fistula (via the frontal sinus or an eroded base of the skull), meningitis, cerebral infarction, or hemorrhage [7, 12, 15, 25, 32, 38, 39]. Diabetes insipidus after removal of a suprasellar meningioma is one of the most frequently reported endocrinological events reported in the literature, with a frequency of 5–33% [2, 10, 13, 15, 25, 39], although we did not observe any case of diabetes insipidus in our series.

Injury of the olfactory nerves was reported more frequently after a subfrontal (unilateral frontal or bifrontal) approach. This observation is also reflected in our series, especially in patients who underwent bifrontal craniotomy. Some authors therefore advocated the pterional approach, which has the advantage of minimizing injury to the olfactory nerves [22].

The occurrence of CSF leakage or infection from frontal sinus transgression was also considered as a disadvantage of the subfrontal approach [22]. However, it has already been shown in the past that violating the frontal sinus does not necessarily lead to serious complications. In early reports, the infection rate was less than 2% [35] and there was no incidence of fatal meningitis. In addition, more recent series did not reveal any severe complications from entering the frontal sinus [2]. In our surgical series, postoperative CSF fistula did not lead to postoperative meningitis with proper precautions.

In our surgical series, the incidence of postoperative brain edema (n=4, after bifrontal craniotomy) and venous brain infarction (n=1, after bifrontal craniotomy) was considerably higher in patients who underwent bifrontal craniotomy. In our experience, these complications have to be ascribed to the routine sectioning of the superior sagittal sinus and draining midline veins when performing the bifrontal approach. As a result of our experience, we can no longer support the previous statement that the anterior third of the superior sagittal sinus can be safely transected without risking serious complications. As a result, the senior author no longer performs the bifrontal approach for resection of tumors in the anterior skull base and sellar region.

## 10.8.2
## Extent of Tumor Resection

The percentage of gross total tumor resection of suprasellar meningiomas ranged from 35 to 100% [1–4, 9, 10, 12, 14–20, 22, 23, 32, 38, 39]. The extent of tumor resection has improved with the advent of modern microsurgery, with a total resection rate of 35–76% in macrosurgical series compared to 58–100% in microsurgical series. Although it as been stressed that complete tumor resection should not be attempted, risking higher morbidity rates, recent microsurgical series (including our series) showed that high rates of complete tumor resection can be performed without increasing morbidity [2, 10, 14, 22].

The rate of total tumor removal (Simpson 1+2) did not differ significantly among the different approaches in our series. In patients operated using the frontolateral approach, total tumor removal (Simpson 1+2) could be achieved in 28 of 30 cases (93.3%). Tumors operated using the pterional or bifrontal approach could be totally resected in 19 of 21 cases (90.5%) in each group. Total tumor removal could be achieved in 66 cases altogether (Simpson 1+2, 91.7%).

Previously, it was often mentioned that the frontolateral approach does not allow the tumors to be attacked from various angles compared to the bifrontal approach; however, we have learned that there is no need to see the tumors from different directions to achieve high rates of total tumor resection.

## 10.8.3
## Visual Outcome

Tuberculum sellae meningiomas most frequently present with visual deterioration before diagnosis. The primary aim of surgery is therefore to achieve improvement, or at least maintenance, of visual function on the same preoperative level.

In macrosurgical series, the rate of visual improvement after surgical resection of a suprasellar meningioma ranged from 40 to 63% [12, 13, 15, 18, 19, 23, 25, 32, 39]. Cushing and Eisenhardt reported a 50% visual improvement rate in 1929 [11]. In later microsurgical series, the improvement rates ranged from 25% to as high as 80% [2–4, 10, 14, 16, 20, 22, 31].

Some authors reported an association between the tumor size and postoperative visual outcome. Rosenstein and Symon [37] reported that tumors smaller than 3 cm had a better visual outcome compared to those larger than 3 cm in diameter. Similar results were found in other series [3, 25] with tumor diameters smaller or larger than 3 [25] or 6 cm [3]. However, other authors reported that tumor size did not affect visual outcome [13, 14]. We found an improvement rate of 71% in small tumors (maximum diameter of <3cm) and 64% in larger tumors (diameter of ≥3 cm) but the difference was not statistically significant.

The duration of visual deterioration before surgery was considered to be one of the main factors influencing visual outcome. Andrews and Wilson [3] reported that patients with duration of visual symptoms less than 6 months had a better chance of postoperative improvement of vision, whereas patients with symptoms longer than 24 months had a higher risk of visual deterioration. Others found a significantly favorable rate of improvement in patients with a history of symptoms less than 2 years compared to those whose symptoms were longer standing [37]. Our results are similar, with a significantly higher improvement rate in patients who had visual symptoms for less than 6 months compared to those who had them for more than 12 months. However, there are reports showing no influence of the duration of symptoms on visual outcome [6].

## 10.8.4
## Tumor Recurrence

In the literature, the recurrence rate for suprasellar meningiomas ranged from 0 to 12% in both macrosurgical and microsurgical series, with a follow up period ranging widely from 3.2 years to 10.6 years. In our surgical series, radiological recurrence with tumor growth after surgery was observed in two patients (2.8%). The mean time to recurrence was 48 months (36–60 months). Surgery due to clinical recurrence (recurrence of symptoms, visual deterioration) was performed in one patient (1.4%) after a time period of 104 months.

The mean follow up time for all patients was 4–238 months (mean 45.3 months, 3.8 years).

Although with modern CT and MRI scanning, recurrent tumors can be detected much earlier compared to in the macrosurgical era, there is no profound difference to earlier studies. Although radiosurgery has been advocated for small residual or recurrent tumors, we prefer surgery in cases of clinical recurrence due to the intimate relationship with the optic nerve and chiasm in these tumors. No patient in our series underwent postoperative radiation or radiosurgery.

## 10.9
## Conclusion

The surgical treatment of tuberculum sellae meningiomas still represents a difficult task for neurosurgeons. Considering the operative morbidity and mortality, the frontolateral and pterional approach provide remarkable improvement compared to the bifrontal approach. These approaches allow quick access to the tumors and are minimally invasive, with less brain exposure, but still enable high rates of total tumor removal.

## References

1. Al Mefty O, Holoubi A, Rifai A, Fox JL (1985) Microsurgical removal of suprasellar meningiomas. Neurosurgery 16:364–372

2. Al Mefty O, Smith RR (1991) Tuberculum sellae meningiomas. In: Al Mefty O (ed) Meningiomas. Raven, New York pp 395–411

3. Andrews BT, Wilson CB (1988) Suprasellar meningiomas: the effect of tumor location on postoperative visual outcome. J Neurosurg 69:523–528

4. Arai H, Sato K, Okuda, et al (2000) Transcranial transsphenoidal approach for tuberculum sellae meningiomas. Acta Neurochir (Wien) 142:751–756

5. Bergland R (1969) The arterial supply of the human optic chiasm. J Neurosurg 31:327–334

6. Brihaye J, Brihaye-van Geertruyden M (1988) Management and surgical outcome of suprasellar meningiomas. Acta Neurochir Suppl (Wien) 42:124–129

7. Chan RC, Thompson GB (1984) Morbidity, mortality, and quality of life following surgery for intracranial meningiomas. A retrospective study in 257 cases. J Neurosurg 60:52–60

8. Chicani CF, Miller NR (2003) Visual outcome in surgically treated suprasellar meningiomas. J Neuroophthalmol 23:3–10

9. Ciric I, Rosenblatt S (2001) Suprasellar meningiomas. Neurosurgery 49:1372–1377

10. Conforti P, Moraci A, Albanese V, et al (1991) Microsurgical management of suprasellar and intraventricular meningiomas. Neurochirurgia (Stuttg) 34:85–89

11. Cushing H, Eisenhardt L (1929) Meningiomas arising from the tuberculum sellae with the syndrome of primary optic atrophy and bitemporal field defects combined with a normal sellae turcica in a middle-aged person. Arch Ophthalmol 1:1–41

12. Cushing H, Eisenhardt L (1938) Suprasellar meningiomas In: Cushing H, Eisenhardt L (eds) Meningiomas: Their Classification, Regional Behaviour, Life History, and Surgical End Results. Charles C. Thomas, Baltimore, pp 224–249

13. Ehlers N, Malmros R (1973) The suprasellar meningioma. A review of the literature and presentation of a series of 31 cases. Acta Ophthalmol Suppl 1–74

14. Fahlbusch R, Schott W (2002) Pterional surgery of meningiomas of the tuberculum sellae and planum sphenoidale: surgical results with special consideration of ophthalmological and endocrinological outcomes. J Neurosurg 96:235–243

15. Finn JE, Mount LA (1974) Meningiomas of the tuberculum sellae and planum sphenoidale. A review of 83 cases. Arch Ophthalmol 92:23–27

16. Goel A, Muzumdar D, Desai KI (2002) Tuberculum sellae meningioma: a report on management on the basis of a surgical experience with 70 patients. Neurosurgery 51:1358–1363

17. Gokalp HZ, Arasil E, Kanpolat Y, et al (1993) Meningiomas of the tuberculum sella. Neurosurg Rev 16:111–114

18. Grant FC (1953) Meningiomas of tuberculum sellae. Am J Ophthalmol 36:715–717

19. Gregorius FK, Hepler RS, Stern WE (1975) Loss and recovery of vision with suprasellar meningiomas. J Neurosurg 42:69–75

20. Grisoli F, Diaz-Vasquez P, Riss M, et al (1986) Microsurgical management of tuberculum sellae meningiomas. Results in 28 consecutive cases. Surg Neurol 26:37–44

21. Halves E, Vogt H (1975) Proceedings: meningiomas of the sellar region. Acta Neurochir (Wien) 31:280–281

22. Jallo GI, Benjamin V (2002) Tuberculum sellae meningiomas: microsurgical anatomy and surgical technique. Neurosurgery 51:1432–1439

23. Jane JA, McKissock W (1962) Importance of failing vision in early diagnosis of suprasellar meningiomas. Br Med J 5296:5–7

24. Jefferson A, Azzam N (1979) The suprasellar meningiomas: a review of 19 years' experience. Acta Neurochir Suppl (Wien) 28:381–384

25. Kadis GN, Mount LA, Ganti SR (1979) The importance of early diagnosis and treatment of the meningiomas of the planum sphenoidale and tuberculum sellae: a retrospective study of 105 cases. Surg Neurol 12:367–371

26. Krenkel W, Frowein RA (1975) Proceedings: Suprasellar meningiomas. Acta Neurochir (Wien) 31:280

27. Kunicki A, Uhl A (1968) The clinical picture and results of surgical treatment of meningioma of the tuberculum sellae. Cesk Neurol 31:80–92

28. Ley A, Gabas E (1979) Meningiomas of the tuberculum sellae. Acta Neurochir Suppl (Wien) 28:402–404

29. Nakamura M, Roser F, Michel J, et al (2003) The natural history of incidental meningiomas. Neurosurgery 53:62–70

30. Ohta K, Yasuo K, Morikawa M, et al (2001) Treatment of tuberculum sellae meningiomas: a long-term follow-up study. J Clin Neurosci 8:26–31

31. Ojemann RG (1980) Meningiomas of the basal parapituitary region: technical considerations. Clin Neurosurg 27:233–262

32. Olivecrona H (1967) The suprasellar meningiomas. In: Olivecrona H, Tönnis W (eds) Handbuch der Neurochirurgie. Springer, Berlin, pp 167–172

33. Puchner MJ, Fischer-Lampsatis RC, Herrmann HD, et al (1998) Suprasellar meningiomas – neurological and visual outcome at long-term follow-up in a homogeneous series of patients treated microsurgically. Acta Neurochir (Wien) 140:1231–1238

34. Raco A, Bristot R, Domenicucci M, et al (1999) Meningiomas of the tuberculum sellae. Our experience in 69 cases surgically treated between 1973 and 1993. J Neurosurg Sci 43:253–260

35. Ray BS (1968) Intracranial hypophysectomy. J Neurosurg 28:180–186

36. Rosenberg LF, Miller NR (1984) Visual results after microsurgical removal of meningiomas involving the anterior visual system. Arch Ophthalmol 102:1019–1023

37. Rosenstein J, Symon L (1984) Surgical management of suprasellar meningioma. Part 2: Prognosis for visual function following craniotomy. J Neurosurg 61:642–648

38. Solero CL, Giombini S, Morello G (1983) Suprasellar and olfactory meningiomas. Report on a series of 153 personal cases. Acta Neurochir (Wien) 67:181–194

39. Symon L, Rosenstein J (1984) Surgical management of suprasellar meningioma. Part 1: The influence of tumor size, duration of symptoms, and microsurgery on surgical outcome in 101 consecutive cases. J Neurosurg 61:633–641

# Sphenoid Wing Meningiomas

**11**

Florian Roser

## Contents

## 11.1
### Introduction

Meningiomas are presumed to account for 15% of brain tumours and are the most common tumours of the sphenoid wing [21, 22]. They are considered to be benign tumours arising from cap cells located in clusters around the arachnoid granulations that exist in relation to neural structures and their foramen. With diverse origins, clinical presentations and surgical management, they all occupy the parasellar region with its complex anatomical boundary zone between orbital and intracranial compartments including the cavernous sinus [32].

Medial sphenoid wing meningiomas (SWMs) present a more difficult problem for neurosurgeons because they invariably involve the anterior visual pathways, arteries of the anterior circulation, and sometimes invade the cavernous sinus. Higher morbidity, mortality, and recurrence rates have been observed in these tumours compared with meningiomas in other locations, and for medial SWMs recurrence is reported as one of the highest for intracranial meningiomas [3, 17, 23].

A higher proportion of SWMs are known to present with intraosseous growth in comparison to meningiomas in other locations. The cause, management and prognosis of these bony changes have been a point of controversy [10, 13, 16]. The differentiation of adjacent hyperostotic bone next to the tumour or infiltrating tumour masses into the sphenoid bone – referred to as intraosseous tumour masses – is necessary and has to be considered when planning the surgical exposure and the surgical goal

(i.e. whether to aim for radical removal or decompression with subsequent radiosurgery). Complete surgical excision is still the benchmark of successful surgery for meningioma; however, there is still an estimated recurrence rate of 20–30% with SWMs involving the sphenoid bone [30, 33].

## 11.2
### Hannover Series

A total of 1800 cases of meningiomas were operated at the Department of Neurosurgery, Klinikum Hannover Nordstadt (Germany) between 1978 and 2002. Among them were 256 SWMs. Among others, we evaluated two distinct entities of SWM: 174 medial SWMs of globoid shape and 82 patients with osseous involvement of SWM. Osseous involvement was determined either due to histological confirmation of tumour infiltration within the sphenoid bone or due to typical radiological features of osseous involvement (e.g. marked hyperostosis, osteolytic changes or intraosseous tumour masses). Patients with neurofibromatosis type 2 (NF-II) disease, associated with multiple intracranial and intraspinal tumours, were excluded from the study because of the confounding effect of multiple tumours.

On the basis of the evaluated pathologies, we proposed an anatomical classification system for the Hannover series of SWMs due to their growth behaviour and their main localisation (Fig. 1).

The collected data were meticulously analysed and studied concerning age, gender, site of tumour origin, presenting symptoms, neurological deficits, radiological appearance, surgical approach and outcome as well as clinical and radiological follow-up findings. At the time of surgery, multiple samples of dural attachment, tumour and affected bone of the sphenoid wing were sent for pathological evaluation. As most of the hyperostotic and obvious tumour-infiltrated bone material was removed by drilling, only a small share of bony tissue reached the pathologist's hands. It underwent microscopic examination, but its evaluation did not affect the surgical procedure directly as the demineralisation process takes days. The extent of tumour resection was classified according to the Simpson classification [36]:

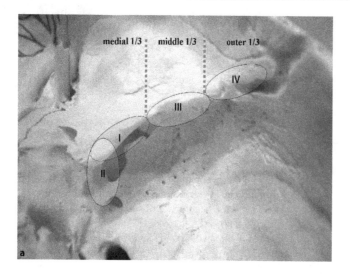

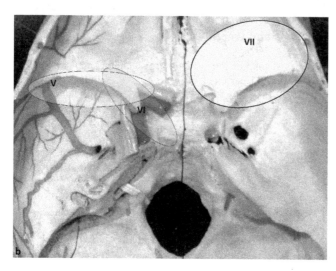

Fig. 1a,b  Classification of sphenoid wing meningioma (SWM). **a** I – Medial SWM without cavernous sinus (CS) involvement; II – medial SWM with CS involvement; III – middle SWM; IV – lateral SWM. **b** V – Osseous SWM without CS involvement; VI – osseous SWM with CS involvement; VII – true intraosseous SWM

1. Grade I: total tumour resection with excision of infiltrated dura.
2. Grade II: total tumour resection and coagulation of dural attachments.
3. Grade III: gross total tumour resection without excising dural attachments or extradural extensions (e.g. infiltrated sinus or bone).
4. Grade IV: subtotal tumour resection.

## 11.3
## Surgical Considerations

Surgery is performed with general anaesthesia, with the aid of an operating microscope and microsurgical instrumentation in all cases. For microsurgical tumour removal, the frontolateral or the pterional approaches are per-

formed (Fig. 2), techniques that are well described elsewhere [8, 31, 32]. For the frontolateral approach, a single burr hole is placed just posterior to the anterior temporal line using a high-speed drill, preventing opening of the periorbita. The frontolateral approach provides a more medial view of the clinoid and suprasellar region and thus early identification of the optic nerve in clinoidal meningiomas. For the pterional approach, the single burr hole is placed at the same location, but the craniotomy is performed more posteriorly, exposing the frontal and temporal lobe with the sylvian fissure and the sphenoid ridge. The lesser wing of the sphenoid is resected to the superior orbital fissure, depending on the tumour size, to allow exposure of the lesion with minimum brain retraction. The superior orbital fissure is similarly unroofed to expose the periorbital fascia, which is only opened in cases of obvious tumour infiltration of intraorbital structures. If

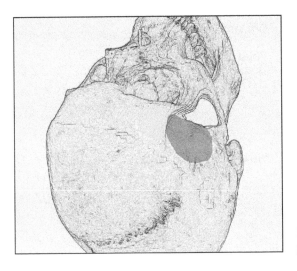

Fig. 2  Approaches to SWM: frontolateral (*yellow*) and standard pterional (*orange*)

there is marked hyperostosis around the optic canal, it is mandatory to first perform a partial clinoidectomy, then unroofing of the optic canal extradurally. The dura of the region of the tuberculum sellae and chiasmatic sulcus is carefully inspected for evidence of meningeal tumour infiltration in order to identify the optic nerve intradurally, and the dural cuff of the optic nerve is incised for a short distance whenever there is evidence of tumour ingrowth. If protrusion of the tuberculum above the line connecting the surface of the nerves as they enter the optic canals is evident, it has to be removed in order to enlarge the transfrontal operative field.

Generally, great caution has to be taken when approaching meningiomas of the medial sphenoid wing because the carotid and middle cerebral arteries may be embedded in the tumour. The dura is opened in a trapdoor fashion, and the tumour is approached through the sylvian fissure. The tumour is visualised laterally from above and a plane of dissection is established between the tumour and the frontal and temporal lobe. The tumour capsule is identified and coagulated. The capsule is then opened, and the tumour is debulked by piecemeal resection with the aid of bipolar coagulation, microscissors, and ultrasonic aspiration. After the tumour has been debulked and branches of the middle cerebral arteries are encountered, the tumour capsule is carefully dissected off the branches of the middle cerebral artery. The tumour resection is continued along these branches proximally to reach the internal carotid artery (ICA), which may be completely embedded in the tumour. In that case, the vessel is microsurgically dissected free of the tumour. Usually, an arachnoidal membrane separates the tumour from the adventitia of the vessels, and microsurgical dissection can be performed without injury to the arteries. Microsurgical dissection along cerebral arteries may lead to visible vasospasm. In this case, local administration of nimodipine or papaverine sponges can be applied to prevent cerebral ischaemia. However, a systematic analysis of the effect of local vasodilator application on post-operative ischaemic events has not yet been performed.

After resection of the tumour, the dural attachment is resected, including hyperostotic bone of the lesser sphenoid wing or the anterior clinoidal process. In tumours involving the cavernous sinus (group II), the intracavernous part of the tumour is not radically removed to prevent any new cranial neuropathies. In cases where only the lateral or superior sinus walls are involved, the wall is peeled off and carefully coagulated. After tumour removal, the dura is reconstructed with fascial grafts. In some cases, a muscle graft is required at the cranial base, augmented with fibrin glue, to achieve as watertight a closure as possible. In some patients, temporary post-operative lumbar drainage may be necessary to prevent a cerebrospinal fluid (CSF) fistula. Bone flaps are repositioned after drilling of hyperostotic bone from the meningioma. Further reconstruction of the orbital roof is not necessary.

11.4
## Operative Results

Figure 3 shows the classification of SWMs according to the predominant symptoms at the time of initial evaluation. The most common symptoms were visual disturbance (highest in groups I and II: 66.7% and 60.9%, respectively) and headaches, regardless of their predominant location. Double vision was a complaint in 30.4% of patients with group II SWMs, compared to only 5.1% in group I. The average length of history of these patients until the first consultation with a physician, ranged from 1 to 360 months, with a mean of 26.45 months, but these figures decreased over the years with frequent and early use of sophisticated diagnostic investigations

| SWM Class | | No. of patients | First symptoms |
|---|---|---|---|
| Group I | 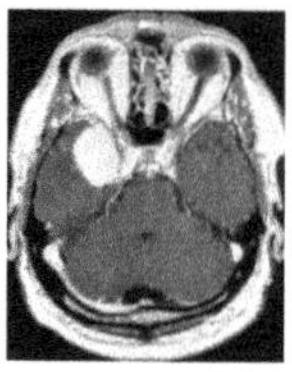 | 39 | Visual distribance Headache |
| Group II | 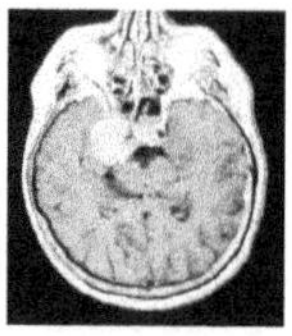 | 69 | Visual distribance Headache |
| Group III | 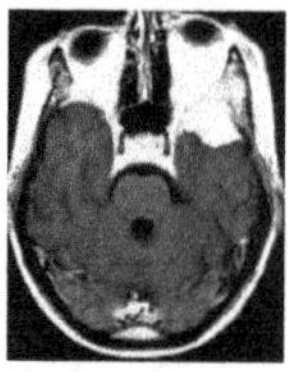 | 19 | Dizziness<br>Seizures |
| Group IV | 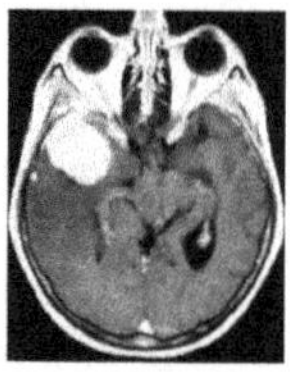 | 30 | Headache<br>Psychological deficit |
| Group V | 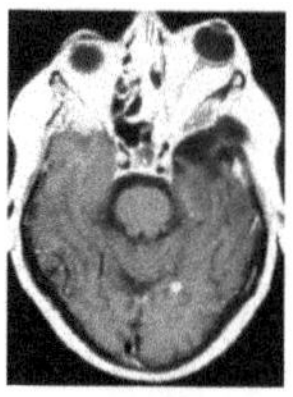 | 35 | Protrusio bulbi Headaches |
| Group VI | 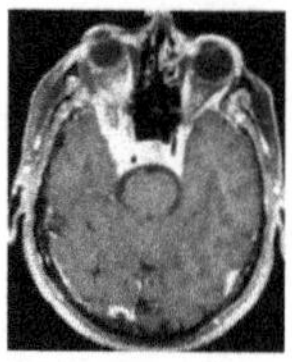 | 6 | Headaches Protrusio bulbi |
| Group VII | 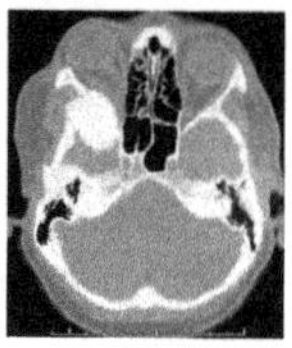 | 23 | Protrusio bulbi Headaches |

Fig. 3 Classification of SWM with their predominant clinical symptoms at the time of diagnosis

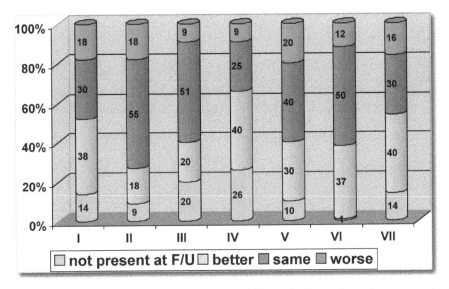

Fig. 4 Alteration of clinical symptoms of SWM in the follow-up (*F/U*) period according to group classification

(1992–2002: 24.07 months, range 1–96 months; 1980–1991: 38.03 months, range 1–360 months).

There was bony involvement in 41% of cases of group I tumours and 42% in group II tumours. The rate of hyperostosis or intraosseous involvement was not different between the groups. Encasement of the ICA and its branches was observed in the majority of cases within the medial SWM (groups I, II and VI). Peritumoural oedema on computed tomography or magnetic resonance imaging (MRI) scans were observed in 22% of SWMs with intraosseous involvement, in 31% of group I and 52% of group II tumours. Tumour calcification was significantly higher in osseous SWMs (41%) than in patients with groups I and II tumours (25.6% and 21.7%, respectively).

In addition, gadolinium-enhanced MRI scans showed enhancement within the bone in the majority of cases, reflecting true intraosseous tumour masses.

Within the follow-up period (51 patients lost; mean of 63 months; range 2–256 months), clinical and radiological recurrence took place. Figure 4 demonstrates how symptoms develop in the post-operative period according to the SWM classification. Recurrence rates were evaluated exclusively for benign meningiomas (Table 1) and were compared to patients without osseous involvement (*n*=174). There were higher recurrence rates for osseous involved meningiomas (30.5%), as total removal in these patients is less likely. The mean time between first treatment and radiological or clinical recurrence was

Table 1 Recurrence behaviour of sphenoid wing meningiomas with osseous involvement, compared to SWM without bone infiltration; World Health Organization group I meningiomas

| Recurrence | Osseous involved SWM | SWM without osseous involvement |
| --- | --- | --- |
| Number of patients | 82 | 174 |
| Number of recurrences | 25 (30.5%) | 20 (11.6%) |
| Grade of resection | | |
| Simpson I + II | 38% | 46% |
| Simpson III + IV | 62% | 52% |
| Mean time of recurrence (in months) | 32.2 (8–153) | 33.8 (5–86) |

Table 2  Clinical course in group VII sphenoid wing meningiomas

| Symptoms | Preoperative (%) | Initial post-operative (%) | Long-term outcome (%) | Time to progress (months) |
|---|---|---|---|---|
| Visual loss | 41 | 27 | 41 | 31.1 |
| Headache | 32 | 9 | 14 | 56.8 |
| Proptosis | 91 | 27 | 36 | 36.1 |
| Orbital pain | 23 | 23 | 5 | |
| Oculomotor palsy | 23 | 23 | 9 | |

Table 3  Morbidity and mortality of the Hannover sphenoid wing meningioma series. *CSF* Cerebrospinal fluid, *MCA* middle cerebral artery, *VP* ventriculoperitoneal

| Morbidity | No. of patients (*n*=228) |
|---|---|
| CSF fistula | 34 |
| Hydrocephalus | 8 (external drainage) |
| | 9 (VP shunt) |
| Cranial nerve deficit | 8 |
| MCA infarction | 8 |
| Post-operative haematoma | 5 |
| Meningitis | 6 |
| Brain oedema | 6 |
| Deep vein thrombosis | 2 |
| **Mortality** | **1 (pulmonary embolism)** |

32 months in World Health Organization (WHO) group I tumours (6–153 months) and 12 months in WHO group II tumours (6–18 months). The course of symptoms in the long-term follow-up is exemplarily demonstrated in group VII SWMs (Table 2): despite radical removal of infiltrated sphenoid bone, the cardinal symptoms of alterations in visual function and proptosis recurred after 31.1 and 36.1 months, respectively. Comparing the microsurgical results of group I and II SWMs, significant differences in resection rates according to the Simpson classification as well as a higher morbidity in visual and oculomotor outcome, resulting in a lower Karnofsky index for group II SWMs has been seen (Fig. 5). The mor-

bidity and mortality rates of the presented cases are displayed in Table 3, which demonstrates that CSF fistula is still the main cause of complications in the early post-operative period and might be the basis for even more complications like meningitis.

## 11.5
## Discussion

When analysing 256 operated patients with SWM, one has to emphasise the heterogeneity among the evaluated groups. We applied a new classification system as we observed that osseous involvement is not restricted to a special group of SWMs, as was proposed by Brotchi and colleagues (Fig. 1). Moreover we found that hyperostosis or intraosseous tumour masses can occur in all kinds of SWM, whether they are of globoid shape or en plaque, or whether they are lateral or invading the cavernous sinus. In addition, the impact of whether the SWM infiltrates the cavernous sinus or not, is of great importance for the approach of the neurosurgeon.

The cause of associated hyperostosis in meningiomas at the sphenoid bone remains a point of controversy – specifically regarding whether this represents a secondary change of the bone without tumour invasion, versus direct infiltration of the bone by tumour [28]. Tumours of this type, which invade through the tough fibrous dura and meander through the marrow spaces, are nevertheless unable to penetrate the delicate fibrous tissue of the arachnoid and the pia, and thus do not invade the brain. The mechanisms by which meningiomas accomplish this extensive invasion of bone are not at all clear: preceding trauma, vascular disturbances, enzymatic reactions or stimulation of osteoblasts have been made responsible for the production of bone by tumour or invasion of tumour in the bone [3, 10, 13, 16, 37]. Furthermore, it has been demonstrated that hyperostosis is a true formation of additional bone; the invasion is therefore not simply a lytic process. Tumour infiltration of the sphenoid bone has been examined histologically and proliferation indices have been determined supporting the conclusion by Pompili et al. [28] and Roser et al. [30] that hyperostosis behaves like a slow-growing tumour and must be removed to ensure cure. The surgical impact of a preoperative known bone involvement is high [6]. Radical removal is fairly achievable, especially in "en plaque" meningiomas or any involvement of the cavernous sinus, although the primary goal should be to completely resect obvious infiltrated bone, when this can be performed with reasonable safety. In addition, the periorbita, which might be infiltrated, should also be explored [27, 30, 33].

Different surgical approaches have been proposed for removal of SWMs, for example an intradural approach for large SWMs not involving the cavernous sinus [38], although this does not account for osseous involved SWMs, were the main target lies extradurally and must be attacked first [7]. The primary advantage of the extradural approach is exposure, provided by selective removal of the sphenoid wing, opening of the optic canal and removing the anterior clinoid for dissection of the tumour adjacent to the proximal intracranial ICA. The additional space provided by the removal of bone leads to control of the dural arterial feeders extradurally and allows minimal retraction intradurally as the tumour and the abnormal dura are removed [11, 22].

The value of cranial-base techniques in managing osseous involved SWM is the improvement of functional outcome. We have seen that the cardinal symptoms, especially in pure intraosseous SWMs, recur despite extensive bone removal (Table 1). Recurrence of proptosis despite a removed sphenoid wing might reflect venous outflow constriction, scar tissue formation or tumour infiltration within the periorbita. Considering the recurrence rates for SWM that have been resected radiographically but are likely to have remaining bony invasion, the challenge for the cranial-base surgeon is to determine, based on long-term follow-up, the degree to which clinical outcome correlates with extensive bony removal. Furthermore, the extent of resection impacts the perioperative morbidity in such a way that repeated surgical interventions for recurrences with minimally invasive approaches and immediate relief of symptoms can be achieved, compared with one-time aggressive removal with the chance of recurrence as well.

"En plaque" SWMs with osseous involvement (groups V and VI), which are characterised more by their clinical and radiological appearance than their histological appearance, present as slow growing, sheet-like or slightly nodular-shaped tumours that are more likely to produce adjacent hyperostosis or even show direct infiltration of the sphenoid wing [9, 14, 33, 39]. This bony change itself produces the clinical symptoms and signs. Complete resection of these SWMs is even more challenging, as they may infiltrate not only the bone, but also the adjacent periorbita or dural sheath of the optic nerve. In our view, repeated surgical decompression with minimally invasive surgery allows for good quality of life in these patients, considering the fact that these tumours are known to be very slow growing.

If an SWM additionally infiltrates the cavernous sinus, resection rates are even lower compared to the achieved resection rates in other locations (Fig. 5). In this respect, it is important to distinguish between meningiomas that are confined to the cavernous sinus and those that involve the cavernous sinus secondarily. The degree of involvement of the ICA, which is also an indicator of the growth behaviour of the tumour, is the major factor in determining the resectability of a meningioma. A more aggressive approach to meningiomas of the cavernous sinus will lead to greater surgical morbidity without the guarantee of a cure. In our experience, a tumour remnant in the cavernous sinus does not impart a major risk to the patient. In these cases cytoreductive surgery in preparation for radiosurgery should be the primary goal [1, 4, 12, 18, 26, 34].

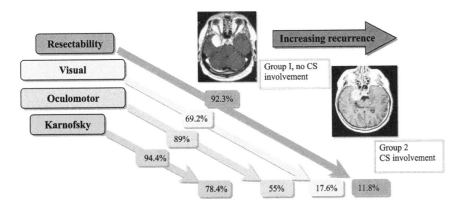

Fig. 5 Comparison of post-operative results in SWM groups I and II. *CS* Cavernous sinus

We have encountered only two cases of medial SWM analogous to type 1 clinoid meningioma as reported by Al-Mefty, in which the tumour adhered to the adventitia of the ICA, lacking a separating arachnoid membrane [2]. Adherence to the adventitia of vessels was otherwise observed only in patients who underwent previous surgeries. It was pointed out that in these cases, the arachnoidal membrane may be violated, and, subsequently, the plane of dissection is lost and the tumour will be in direct contact with the adventitia. Dissecting the tumour becomes difficult, similar to the situation described in type 1 tumours. Our experience is similar to the report by Brotchi and Bonnal, in which, among 82 sphenoidal meningiomas, in only 1 case was a tumoural infiltration of the carotid wall observed [5]. The type 1 tumours were also not encountered by Lee et al. [19]; however, the number of patients in their series of clinoidal meningiomas was limited. In cases of carotid involvement of the SWM, we recognised the inability of preoperative neuroradiological imaging to differentiate between tumour infiltration into the vessel walls, making any resection impossible, and tumour encasement, where careful dissection allows complete tumour removal. In this field, further studies are necessary to achieve a useful prediction of meningioma behaviour through sophisticated imaging.

In the Hannover series, the main factor leading to subtotal tumour resection was cavernous sinus involvement. We therefore classified the medial SWMs according to preoperative radiological evidence of cavernous sinus involvement. In our opinion, the type 3 tumours of Al-Mefty and Ayoubi [2] (originating at the optic foramen) are optic foramen meningiomas with an extension onto the anterior clinoid process and do not represent true clinoidal meningiomas. We have considered meningiomas of the optic foramen as a separate entity and did not include these tumours in the current series.

Previous studies showed that despite radical intracavernous removal of meningiomas, recurrences occur after a relatively short time period. A more aggressive approach to meningiomas involving the cavernous sinus would lead to more surgical morbidity, and it has not been proven that this strategy lowers the long-term recurrence rate compared with more conservative approaches. The current analysis of medial SWMs with cavernous sinus involvement (group II tumours) indeed showed a high recurrence rate of 27.5%, but the mean follow-up period was significantly longer at 79.04 months compared with those in the aforementioned studies. It remains unclear whether recurrences in previously reported surgical series with radical intracavernous tumour removal would reach a similar rate with longer follow up. Because this approach poses a significant additional surgical risk to the patient, we do not share this attitude.

Actual control rates of tumour growth gamma-knife radiosurgery of cavernous sinus meningiomas ranged from 86.4% at 3 years [35] to 92–96.5% at 5 years [15, 20], although tumour volume increase after radiosurgery was also reported, ranging from 6 to 9.5% [15, 20]. Improvement of neurological status after gamma-knife radiosurgery of cavernous sinus meningiomas was reported in 28.6%, 29%, or even 78.5% [25]. Neurological status remained stable in 62%, but deterioration was observed in 9–22.5% [20, 35]. Concerning oculomotor deficits, Roche et al. reported that 27.8% of patients improved, 14.8% recovered, 55.6% remained stable and 1.9% worsened [29]. Obviously, the objective of radiosurgery differs essentially from that of microsurgery because the goal is prevention of tumour progression instead of cytoreduction. However, clinical outcome of remnant cavernous sinus meningiomas treated with gamma knife seems to be superior to microsurgery, and therefore, gamma-knife radiosurgery may be considered as a useful adjunct to microsurgical tumour removal, particularly in group II medial SWMs.

Our strategy for deciding whether gamma-knife radiosurgery should be recommended depends on the availability of preoperative radiological imaging studies, from which the tumour growth potential can be evaluated. In cases of remnant cavernous sinus meningiomas, in which serial preoperative imaging clearly indicates high tumour growth, gamma-knife radiosurgery after a post-operative recovery period is preferred [24]. If preoperative assessment of tumour growth potential is not possible, it is recommended to perform a post-operative MRI control after 6 months to see whether there is any change in the size of the remnant tumour.

In medial SWMs, immediate post-operative improvement of visual function was observed in 56% and vision was preserved at the preoperative level in 44% of patients with group I tumours who were not blind before surgery. Contrary to previous reports by Lee et al. [19], we do not consider that extradural anterior clinoidectomy plays a major role in determining the visual outcome for clinoidal meningiomas. In clinoidal meningiomas, the frontolateral approach allows a more medial view of the clinoid and suprasellar region, and thus early identification of the optic nerve, because it is usually displaced medially and posteriorly by the tumour. In our view, the aforementioned extradural cranial-base approach with clinoidectomy or even more extended resection of the sphenoid bone is not absolutely necessary unless there is radiographic evidence of an associated intraosseous tumour.

11.6
## Conclusion

The surgical treatment of medial SWMs still represents a difficult task for neurosurgeons. Morbidity and mortality rates have improved because of recent advances in microsurgical techniques, but recurrence rates are unquestionably the highest among cranial-base meningiomas. Group I SWMs present a more favourable subgroup with fortunate visual outcome, mostly enabling total resection with low recurrence rates. In group II SWMs, visual outcome is less favourable and radical removal is limited because of cavernous sinus infiltration, with consequential higher recurrence rates. In this subgroup, gamma-knife radiosurgery may serve as a reasonable adjuvant therapy after microsurgery when preoperative imaging studies indicate high tumour growth potential. However, recurrent group II tumours presenting with deteriorating visual function need to undergo microsurgery, and visual function can be preserved at the same preoperative level in the majority of patients.

With respect to clinical appearance, surgical management and recurrence behaviour, osseous involved SWMs reflect a single entity. In cases with involvement of the cavernous sinus, a subtotal but extensive removal combined with bony decompression of the cranial nerves at the superior orbital fissure and optic canal, frequently produces good functional and cosmetic results. Close follow-up intervals in an interdisciplinary manner – involving ophthalmologists, radiologists and neurosurgeons – are necessary to individualise the optimal treatment plan for patients. These lesions require constant surveillance and an attitude that disease control rather than disease cure is the goal.

## References

1. Abdel-Aziz KM, Froelich SC, Dagnew E, et al (2004) Large sphenoid wing meningiomas involving the cavernous sinus: conservative surgical strategies for better functional outcomes. Neurosurgery 54:1375–1383
2. Al Mefty O, Ayoubi S (1991) Clinoidal meningiomas. Acta Neurochir Suppl (Wien) 53:92–97
3. Bonnal J, Thibaut A, Brotchi J, et al (1980) Invading meningiomas of the sphenoid ridge. J Neurosurg 53:587–599
4. Brell M, Villa S, Teixidor P, et al (2006) Fractionated stereotactic radiotherapy in the treatment of exclusive cavernous sinus meningioma: functional outcome, local control, and tolerance. Surg Neurol 65:28–33; discussion 33–24
5. Brotchi J, Bonnal J (1991) Lateral and middle sphenoid wing meningiomas. In: Al Mefty O (ed) Meningiomas. Raven, New York, pp 413–425
6. Brotchi J, Levivier M, Raftopoulos C, et al (1991) Invading meningiomas of sphenoid wing. What must we know before surgery? Acta Neurochir Suppl (Wien) 53:98–100
7. Cook AW (1971) Total removal of large global meningiomas at the medial aspect of the sphenoid ridge. Technical note. J Neurosurg 34:107–113
8. Day JD (2000) Cranial base surgical techniques for large sphenocavernous meningiomas: technical note. Neurosurgery 46:754–759
9. DeMonte F (1996) Surgical treatment of anterior basal meningiomas. J Neurooncol 29:239–248
10. Derome P, Visot A (1993) Osseous lesions of the anterior and middle base. In: Sekhar LN, Janecka IP (eds) Surgery of Cranial Base Tumors. Raven, New York, pp 809–817
11. Dolenc V (1979) Microsurgical removal of large sphenoidal bone meningiomas. Acta Neurochir Suppl (Wien) 28:391–396
12. Dufour H, Muracciole X, Metellus P, et al (2001) Long-term tumor control and functional outcome in patients with cavernous sinus meningiomas treated by radiotherapy with or without previous surgery: is there an alternative to aggressive tumor removal? Neurosurgery 48:285–294
13. Heick A, Mosdal C, Jorgensen K (1993) Localized cranial hyperostosis of meningiomas: a result of neoplastic enzymatic activity? Acta Neurol Scand 87:243–247
14. Honeybul S, Neil-Dwyer G, Lang DA, et al (2001) Sphenoid wing meningioma en plaque: a clinical review. Acta Neurochir (Wien) 143:749–757
15. Iwai Y, Yamanaka K, Ishiguro T (2003) Gamma knife radiosurgery for the treatment of cavernous sinus meningiomas. Neurosurgery 52:517–524
16. Kim KS, Rogers LF, Lee C (1983) The dural lucent line: characteristic sign of hyperostosing meningioma en plaque. AJR Am J Roentgenol 141:1217–1221
17. Konovalov AN, Fedorov SN, Faller TO, et al (1979) Experience in the treatment of the parasellar meningiomas. Acta Neurochir Suppl (Wien) 28:371–372
18. Kurita H, Sasaki T, Kawamoto S, et al (1997) Role of radiosurgery in the management of cavernous sinus meningiomas. Acta Neurol Scand 96:297–304
19. Lee JH, Jeun SS, Evans J, Kosmorsky G (2001) Surgical management of clinoidal meningiomas. Neurosurgery 48:1012–1019; discussion 1019–1021
20. Lee JY, Niranjan A, McInerney J, et al (2002) Stereotactic radiosurgery providing long-term tumor control of cavernous sinus meningiomas. J Neurosurg 97:65–72
21. MacCarty CS (1972) Meningiomas of the sphenoidal ridge. J Neurosurg 36:114–120
22. Maroon JC, Kennerdell JS, Vidovich DV, et al (1994) Recurrent spheno-orbital meningioma. J Neurosurg 80:202–208
23. Mirimanoff RO, Dosoretz DE, Linggood RM, et al. (1985) Meningioma: analysis of recurrence and progression following neurosurgical resection. J Neurosurg 62:18–24
24. Nakamura M, Roser F, Michel J, et al (2003) The natural history of incidental meningiomas. Neurosurgery 53:62–70
25. Nicolato A, Foroni R, Alessandrini F, et al (2002) Radiosurgical treatment of cavernous sinus meningiomas: experience with 122 treated patients. Neurosurgery 51:1153–1159; discussion 1159–1161
26. Pendl G, Schrottner O, Eustacchio S, et al (1998) Cavernous sinus meningiomas – what is the strategy: upfront or adjuvant gamma knife surgery? Stereotact Funct Neurosurg 70:33–40
27. Pompili A, Cacciani L, Cattani F, et al (1997) Intracranial meningiomas in the elderly. Minerva Med 88:229–236
28. Pompili A, Derome PJ, Visot A, et al (1982) Hyperostosing meningiomas of the sphenoid ridge – clinical features, surgical therapy, and long-term observations: review of 49 cases. Surg Neurol 17:411–416

29. Roche PH, Regis J, Dufour H, et al (2000) Gamma knife radiosurgery in the management of cavernous sinus meningiomas. J Neurosurg 93:68–73

30. Roser F, Nakamura M, Jacobs C, et al (2005) Sphenoid wing meningiomas with osseous involvement. Surg Neurol 64:37–43; discussion 43

31. Samii M, Draf W (1989) Surgery of the Skull Base. Springer, Berlin

32. Samii M, Tatagiba M, Monteiro ML(1996) Meningiomas involving the parasellar region. Acta Neurochir Suppl (Wien) 65:63–65

33. Schick U, Bleyen J, Bani A, et al (2006) Management of meningiomas en plaque of the sphenoid wing. J Neurosurg 104:208–214

34. Selch MT, Ahn E, Laskari A, et al (2004) Stereotactic radiotherapy for treatment of cavernous sinus meningiomas. Int J Radiat Oncol Biol Phys 59:101–111

35. Shin M, Kurita H, Sasaki T, et al (2001) Analysis of treatment outcome after stereotactic radiosurgery for cavernous sinus meningiomas. J Neurosurg 95:435–439

36. Simpson D (1957) The recurrence of intracranial meningiomas after surgical treatment. J Neurol Neurosurg Psychiatry 20:22–39

37. Terstegge K, Schorner W, Henkes H, et al (1994) Hyperostosis in meningiomas: MR findings in patients with recurrent meningioma of the sphenoid wings. AJNR Am J Neuroradiol 15:555–560

38. Tomasello F, de Divitiis O, Angileri FF, et al (2003) Large sphenocavernous meningiomas: is there still a role for the intradural approach via the pterional-transsylvian route? Acta Neurochir (Wien) 145:273–282

39. Verheggen R, Markakis E, Muhlendyck H, et al (1996) Symptomatology, surgical therapy and postoperative results of sphenoorbital, intraorbital-intracanalicular and optic sheath meningiomas. Acta Neurochir Suppl (Wien) 65:95–98

# Chordomas and Chondrosarcomas

Marcos Tatagiba
and Marcus André Acioly

## Contents

## 12.1

## Introduction

Primary bone tumors of the skull base are unusual pathologies, mostly chordoma and chondrosarcoma [44]. Their development sends us to the embryological period in which the axial skeleton is formed [21]. The notochord is the initial axial skeletal structure that is progressively involved by the mesodermal tissue and later on replaced by cartilaginous and bone tissues [21]. Remnants of the notochord may remain entrapped by bone [21, 29], particularly in the clivus and sacrum [28, 29, 56]. They are also encountered in the nucleus pulposus [56] or forming a rather distinct intradural clival mass that may be found incidentally at autopsy, namely the ecchordosis physalifora [23]. In addition, focal persistent rests of fetal cartilage may remain unchanged in the skull base during ossification [11, 44].

Chordomas arise from the notochord remnants [7, 21, 23, 29, 43, 44], while the persistent fetal cartilage rests may be the progenitors of chondrosarcomas [11, 27, 44]. Another assumption is the origin of chondrosarcomas from metaplasia of meningeal fibroblasts when occurring outside the skull base [4]. Both chordomas and chondrosarcomas are rare tumors, comprising 0.1–0.2% and 0.02–0.2% of all intracranial tumors, respectively [10, 15, 56, 57].

Chordomas were first described in 1856 by Virchow [7, 23, 43]. Then, Müller proposed the relationship with notochord remnants and Ribbert assigned the term chordoma for the first time [7, 23, 43]. These are slow-growing tumors [28], but they are locally invasive with a great tendency to recur [28, 56]. Chordomas occur mostly in the sacrococcygeal region in 49% of cases followed by the spheno-occipital region (clival) in 36%, and finally in the vertebral region in 15% [21]. Even though they generally arise in the midline, these tumors may develop laterally in the parasellar or petrous bone areas, justified by the distal projections of the cranial notochord to the clinoid process or petrous bone [29, 56].

Chondrosarcomas are primary malignant cartilaginous tumors that share with chordomas the properties of local invasiveness and recurrence [15, 56]. They arise commonly in the temporo-occipital junction/petrous bone (37–66%); however medial seeding is also observed in the clivus (23–28%) and in the spheno-ethmoid complex (6–14.6%) [27, 44].

Several series have studied both pathologies together because they share similar clinical, radiological, and even histological features, as well as surgical treatment [9, 15, 17, 56, 57]. However, the distinction between these entities is clinically relevant in that current data have showed a better outcome for chondrosarcomas [10, 17, 27, 44]. Therefore, this distinction seems reasonable and should be promoted. Herein, these entities are tackled didactically together; nevertheless their particular features will be discussed separately.

## 12.2
## Pathology

### 12.2.1
### Chordoma

The origin of chordomas from the notocord remnants is encouraged by their similar histological, immunohistochemical, and ultrastructural features [22, 23]. Chordomas consistently involve the clivus [28, 29, 56], presenting as spheno-occipital masses [28, 29] that grow in or around the spheno-occipital synchondrosis [21]. Ventral extensions produce a distinct nasopharyngeal mass [28, 29]. Tumors involving the rostral end of the clivus present as sellar or parasellar masses [28, 29], while tumors arising at the caudal end involve the foramen magnum [28, 29]. Chordomas may have lateral extensions or may arise exclusively from the petrous bone, presenting as petrosal masses [28, 29].

They are soft grayish masses with a smooth or lobulated surface [21, 56]. Although they appear encapsulated in soft tissues, this distinction is not present in invaded bone [21]. Chordomas are highly locally invasive, infiltrating the bone along its lines of least resistance [21, 56]. The osteolytic features occur due to the presence of cathepsin K in the tumor fronts [20]. Cathepsin K is a member of papaine family of cysteine proteases and is thought to have an important participation in osteoclast bone resorption [42].

Thus, the hallmark of the disease is to present extradurally [56], although exclusively intradural cases have been reported anecdotally [28, 41, 56]. Intradural extensions, on the other hand, are a common feature among chordomas, their potential pathogenesis being a matter of discussion [41]. Indeed, they may invade the dura mater after intradural approaches [56].

Microscopically, chordomas are characterized by large, polygonal cells with abundant eosinophilic cytoplasm [22] or vacuolated physaliferous cells filled with intracytoplasmic mucin [21, 22, 28, 56]. The nuclei may vary from a small and dense hyperchromatic to large and vacuolated patterns [22, 56]. The tumor is arranged in lobules created by the intralesional fibrous septum [21, 28, 37, 38, 56]. These fibrous septa are believed to be a tumor–host interaction caused by the tumor in the bone trabeculae and soft tissues [37]. Thus, the lobules are arranged with sheets of physaliferous cells embedded in a pool of mucin [21, 56, 22]. It is worth noting that the loss of the lobulated pattern due to invasion of the fibrous septa, as well as the production of the mucoid matrix,

indicate later stages in the tumorigenesis [38, 39]. In addition, the loss of the lobular growth might depict an adverse outcome in chordomas [38].

Although necrosis and mitotic figures were described as infrequent [21, 28, 56], another study has found them in all types of chordomas [22]. Typically, chordomas are subclassified into conventional, chondroid, and dedifferentiated variants [21, 24]. The conventional type comprises tumors with lobular appearance embedded in a mucoid matrix and characteristic cellular arrangements [21, 22]. The chondroid type was initially described by Heffelfinger in 1973 [21] with the assumption that they would have a better outcome, an assumption that was not corroborated by current studies [9, 11, 22, 44, 56]. It is characterized by foci of conventional type enmeshed with hyaline cartilage [21, 22]. Although the chondroid chordomas may resemble low-grade chondrosarcomas [13, 32] due to the cartilaginous tissue, these tumors show areas typical of classic chordomas [44]. The dedifferentiated type is a highly malignant form with sarcomatous features [44], mostly in the sacrococcygeal region [21], which is poorly responsive to treatment [21, 56]. The role of irradiation in the pathogenesis of the dedifferentiated type is still unknown [21, 56].

Hoch et al. [22] described the cellular and poorly differentiated types. The cellular type shows a highly cellular pattern without extracellular mucoid matrix or lobular appearance, while in the poorly differentiated type, the typical presentation of chordomas is totally absent, lacking the high-grade sarcoma areas of the dedifferentiated type [22]. Chordomas rarely present metastatic dissemination [21, 56], although this is observed in up to 40% of cases at autopsy [28]. In children under 5 years, on the other hand, metastases occur in up to 57.9% of patients [22].

Chordomas and chondrosarcomas present specific pathological appearances that allow an accurate diagnosis [44]. However, they have common characteristics that may introduce a diagnostic dilemma [21, 28, 44]. The distinction of such pathologies is nowadays mandatory because of the clear difference in their biological behavior [44]. The use of immunohistochemical markers is useful in this differentiation because chordomas stains positively for epithelial markers such as cytokeratin [28] and epithelial membrane antigen [28], which are not evident in the mesodermal-origin chondrosarcomas [28, 44]. Also, chordomas stain positively for vimentin and S-100 protein [22, 56]. In up to 34% of patients in a large series, the original diagnosis of chordoma was changed to that of chondrosarcoma with the aid of immunohistochemistry [44].

### 12.2.2
### Chondrosarcoma

Chondrosarcomas are usually paramedian bone tumors [27, 44, 56], although tumors arising from the basal dura mater or even entirely intradural tumors have also been described [18, 27, 33, 62]. They can be subclassified into conventional or classic (hyaline, myxoid, mixed hyaline/myxoid), clear cell, mesenchymal, and dedifferentiated types [35, 44]. Based on histological examination, these tumors are further grouped into grades I, II, and III according to mitotic rates, nuclear size, cellularity, and extent of cartilaginous matrix [14, 27, 44, 56]. By far the most common is the conventional low-grade type [27, 44].

Conventional chondrosarcomas are composed of hyaline or myxoid cartilages or a mixture from both [44]. They are hypercellular, large-cell tumors within abundant cartilaginous matrix [44, 56]. In the hyaline type, the atypical chondrocytes are arranged in lacunar spaces surrounded by hyaline matrix, while in the myxoid variant, the lacunar spaces are no longer observed and the atypical chondrocytes are embedded into a myxoid matrix [44]. Mesenchymal tumors have a classic biphasic pattern of a chondroid component and a small-cell, undifferentiated, mesenchymal component [30, 56, 62]. Finally, the dedifferentiated type presents with sarcomatous features [56].

The myxoid chondrosarcoma is the most likely to be misdiagnosed as chordoma [44]. In the study of Rosenberg et al. [44], all of the 74 patients (34% of their study) whose tumor was initially classified as chordoma showed a myxoid cartilage matrix [44]. Chondrosarcomas stain positively to vimentin [27] and S-100 protein, but do not stain for epithelial markers [27, 44].

## 12.3
## Clinical Presentation

Chordomas and chondrosarcomas are locally invasive lesions that assume an advanced stage before becoming symptomatically evident. This delay in diagnosis has been significantly reduced due to advances in the fields of neuroimaging, and its widespread use.

Chordomas are typically tumors of the fourth to sixth decades of life [15, 21], occurring almost equally between males and females, with a slight male predominance [9, 15, 22]. They are uncommon in children and adolescents, accounting for less than 5% of cases [22]. Chondrosarcomas develop commonly at the end of the fourth decade of life, with a slight female predominance [27, 44].

The clinical presentation is nonspecific. Generally, the patients present with headaches and diplopia [10, 11, 15, 17, 21, 27]. The symptoms and signs depend on the specific sites of tumor extensions [21, 29]. Chordomas usually arise from the body of the clivus, stretching the sixth cranial nerve and producing the typical clinical presentation of uni- or bilateral abducens nerve paresis [10, 11, 29], a symptom that is also observed in chondrosarcomas [10, 27]. Tumors may extend ventrally, resulting in a nasopharyngeal mass, which accounts for symptoms such as nasal obstruction, epistaxis, and dysphagia [29, 56]. Tumors arising at the superior clivus may cause the development of hypopituitarism or chiasmal compression,

resulting in visual loss [9, 21, 29, 56], whereas tumors located at the inferior clivus may create brainstem compression and hypoglossal paresis [11, 29, 56]. Petrosal extensions may produce symptoms of trigeminal, facial, vestibulocochlear, and caudal cranial nerve dysfunctions [10, 11, 15, 29]. Neck pain may represent spinal instability in patients suffering from tumors in or around the occipital condyles.

## 12.4
## Radiological Features

Patients suffering from chordomas and chondrosarcomas deserve a thorough radiological evaluation in order to plan the best treatment options. Computed tomography (CT) scans provide better visualization of the bone structures, whereas magnetic resonance imaging (MRI) demarcates the tumor, tumor vicinities, and its relationship to adjacent soft structures. Eventually, magnetic resonance or conventional cerebral angiography is required to study the collateral circulation in large tumors that displace or partially encase the intracranial arteries [13]. In addition, a balloon test occlusion may be performed to depict the collateral blood supply in case of permanent vessel occlusion during surgery [35].

CT scans usually show hyper- to isodense lesions [13, 56], but hypodense lesions also may be noted [41, 56]. Alternatively, another authors have observed that 33.3% of tumors were hypodense, 52.4% were isodense, and 14.3% were hyperdense [41]. On contrast-enhanced CT, the tumors also reveal a multifaceted presentation, showing various degrees of enhancement [13, 41, 56]. No enhancement was encountered in 52.4% and mild to strong contrast enhancement was documented in 47.7% of the patients studied by Pamir and Ozduman [41]. Extensive bone destruction is evidenced in almost all cases on bone CT scans [13, 35, 41]. Sclerotic bone reaction, on the other hand, was not documented in any report [13, 41, 56]. Intratumoral calcifications are believed to depict bone sequestra rather than dystrophic calcifications [13, 41], and are represented in the great majority of cases [13, 41, 56].

MRI provides a better delineation of the tumor boundaries owing to the multiplanar capabilities and the tissue contrast [13]. On T1-weighted images, the tumor has intermediate to low intensity in 95.2% of cases [41]. Hyperintense lesions are rarely observed on T1-weighted images [13, 35, 41] and hyperintense foci may represent hemorrhage [35]. Hemorrhagic foci are better noted in gradient-echo images as dark areas [13]. On T2-weighted images, the tumors are typically hyperintense [13, 35, 41, 35], which reflects the high fluid content [13]. Hypointense foci on T2-weighted images may symbolize areas of calcification, hemorrhage, mucous pool, or intratumoral septa (Fig. 1) [13, 35]. Contrast-enhanced images reveal mild to strong enhancement after gadolinium injection in

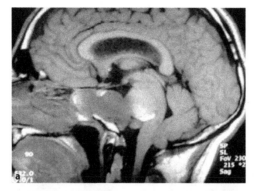

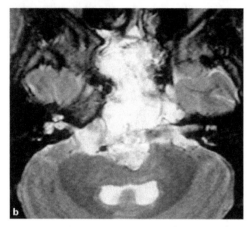

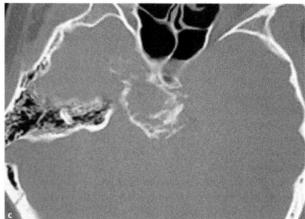

Fig. 1 **a** Sagittal T1-weighted magnetic resonance imaging (MRI) scan depicting a large chordoma causing severe brainstem compression. The tumor is predominantly hypointense, showing some hyperintense foci that might depict focal hemorrhage. **a** Axial T2-weighted MRI scan showing a heterogeneous signal. The hypointense foci may represent calcifications, hemorrhage, mucous pool, or intratumoral septa. **c** Bone computed tomography (CT) scan of a chondrosarcoma revealing the characteristic intratumoral calcifications

almost all cases [13, 35, 41]. Fat-suppression MRI scans are particularly useful to delineate tumor limits, as well as to follow for tumor recurrences [13, 56], particularly after fat-graft skull-base reconstructions [56]. Chordomas and chondrosarcomas cannot be differentiated based exclusively on their radiological features, either on CT or MRI [41, 56].

## 12.5
## Treatment

Chordomas and chondrosarcomas require a multidisciplinary approach due to the complexity of their management [11, 32]. The treatment comprises clinical and radiological observation, biopsy and clinical observation, biopsy and radiotherapy, tumor resection, and surgery followed by radiotherapy [15, 56].

The extent of bone removal has been associated with survival, both long-term and disease-free [2, 9, 17, 56, 59, 61]. However, the origin of such tumors (i.e., those that grow from the bone at the skull base and are intrinsically related to neural and vessel structures) frequently precludes radical tumor removal [12, 17, 24, 40, 60]. In addition, radical tumor resection carries an increased rate of surgical morbidity, although it is advocated by some authors [9, 15, 17, 59, 61].

Whereas local recurrence is the most frequent cause of treatment failure [15, 56], the treatment is nowadays conducted with a multimodal therapy of surgery plus radiotherapy [15, 32, 60], which offers an improvement in patient survival duration in comparison to both methods separately [60]. In this regard, the prognosis of such pathologies has improved noticeably in recent years owing to skull-base microsurgical development and advances in the fields of radiotherapy and neuronavigation (Fig. 2) [1, 13, 32, 61]. However, a standard treatment has yet to be defined.

## 12.5.1
## Surgery

The surgical approaches to chordomas and chondrosarcomas depend principally on the tumor extensions. The tumors may be accessed by anterior, anterolateral, lateral, and posterolateral approaches [47, 56]. Several operative approaches have been used to achieve the clival area, as follows: transfrontal [47], transbasal [29], unilateral subfrontal [29], extended subfrontal [17, 56, 58], transoral [47, 56], midfacial degloving [5, 6, 29, 56], transsphenoidal [29, 47, 56], frontotemporal [10, 17, 56], frontotemporal with fronto-orbitozygomatic osteotomy [1, 56], frontotemporal subtemporal (extended pterional) [46,

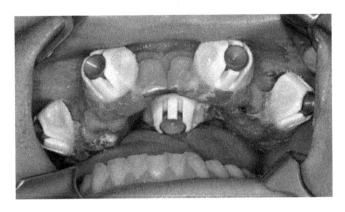

Fig. 2 Photograph of the navigation fiducials used for skull-base surgery navigation

47], subtemporal transpetrous apex [17, 56], petrosal approaches [56], retrosigmoid [47], combined presigmoid-subtemporal (supra- and infratentorial) [45, 46, 49], and far lateral transcondylar (see Chapter 33) or retrocondylar [48], among others. Endoscopic technology may be added to microsurgical techniques. Pure endoscopic resection of these tumors [16, 25] has not been routinely used in our institution.

In general, we use endonasal transsphenoidal approaches [19, 34] for midline clival tumors involving the sphenoid sinus and for palliative debulking. For tumors that project ventrally, we perform transmaxilar-transethmoidal midfacial degloving. Lateral tumor extension toward the petrous apex can be approached from the contralateral side. Transoral approaches are reserved for tumors at the lower clivus and craniocervical transition. The retrosigmoid with or without suprameatal extension [50, 51] and far lateral retrocondylar approaches [48] are used for tumor extension into the cerebellopontine angle and lateral foramen magnum area. These approaches have widely replaced the combined presigmoid-subtemporal (supra- and infratentorial) approach in recent years. The combined approaches are reserved for occasions where large tumors expand into the middle and posterior fossa.

opened basally and reflected superiorly [46, 49]. After releasing the cerebrospinal fluid (CSF), a brain spatula is inserted to retract the temporal lobe, bringing into view the optic nerve, the internal carotid artery, and the anterior structures of the tentorial incisure. Tumors arising laterally are debulked and the hard parts are drilled with a diamond burr, whereas for tumors that expand into the petrous apex, the tentorial margin is opened transversally to improve the surgical view, and the superior petrosal sinus may be coagulated and divided [46, 49]. Care should be taken with the trochlear nerve, which runs together with the free margin of the tentorium. For this reason, the tentorium is opened 1–2 cm behind the trochlear nerve entrance in the cavernous sinus in a medial-to-lateral fashion [49]. For extradural tumors, the cranial base dura is also opened. Further exposure is then gained by drilling part of the petrous apex at Kawase's triangle (Fig. 3). Tumor resection is carried out with extensive bone drilling; however, the objective is to remove as much as possible without jeopardizing the cranial nerves and vessels and so avoid functional losses. When primary dural closure is not achievable, reconstruction is performed with a fascia lata graft or a pedicled temporal muscle flap to cover the defect.

## 12.5.1.1
### Frontotemporal Subtemporal (Extended Pterional) Approach

This approach is suitable for tumors that involve structures of the tentorial incisure and cavernous sinus along with posterior fossa extensions to the cerebellopontine angle. It can be associated or not with an additional orbit-zygomatic technique. A frontotemporal (pterional) craniotomy is performed in which the bone flap is placed more temporally. For extradural tumors, dura is detached from the bone at the middle fossa. Drilling the bone will expose the foramen rotundum and foramen ovale, so exposing the V2 and V3 branches of the trigeminal nerve. The tumor is entered and debulked. If the tumor has intradural extension (e.g., recurrent tumors), the dura is

## 12.5.1.2
### Endonasal Transsphenoidal Approach

The patient is placed supine with the head slightly extended and tilted toward the surgeon. We use the operating microscope from the beginning. With the aid of a hand speculum, the right nostril is entered. After identification of the middle turbinate, we coagulate the septal mucosa at the anterior wall of the sphenoid sinus. The mucosa is incised and a right submucosal tunnel is developed. Then, with the aid of a high-speed drill, the bone septum is drilled to the contralateral side. The septal mucosa on the left side is identified and a contralateral submucosal tunnel is created with a fine dissector. Thus, the anterior wall of the sphenoid sinus is entirely uncovered. The hand speculum is substituted with a self-retain-

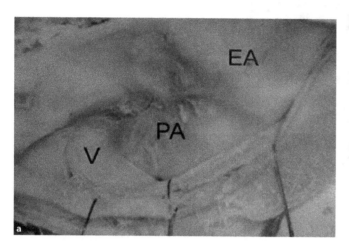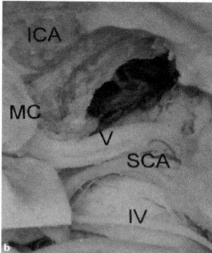

Fig. 3a,b Anatomical dissection of the cranial base detailing the frontotemporal subtemporal (extended pterional) approach to the petrous apex. **a** For tumors arising extradurally, the dura mater of the cranial base is opened, revealing the petrous apex and the trigeminal nerve, as well as the eminence arcuate.

**b** Magnified view of the approach following drilling of Kawase's triangle. Note the superior cerebellar artery joining the trigeminal nerve and the trochlear nerve at the free tentorial edge. *PA* Petrous apex, *V* trigeminal nerve, *EA* eminence arcuate, *SCA* superior cerebellar artery, *IV* trochlear nerve, *MC* Meckel's cave

ing Hardy speculum, retracting the mucosa laterally. The sphenoid sinus is entered after drilling the anterior wall of the sphenoid sinus. The sinus mucosa is resected, with subsequent tumor identification. Eventually, we use the fluoroscopic C-arm control. The tumor is removed as described above. Lateral extensions of the tumor preclude complete removal. After tumor resection, the mucosa and nasal septum are returned by opening a hand speculum in both nostrils. There is no need to suture the mucosa.

### 12.5.1.3

### Retrosigmoid, Retrosigmoid Intradural Suprameatal, and Far Lateral Retrocondylar Approaches

The retrosigmoid approach is used to treat lesions at the lower clivus or petrous bone that extend posteriorly toward the cerebellopontine angle, displacing the brainstem. Whereas the retrosigmoid intradural suprameatal approach is preferred in tumors that have a petrous apex component that traverses to the middle fossa via Meckel's cave (Fig. 4). The operative nuances are depicted in Chapter 14. Tumors arising at the craniocervical junction may be removed using a retrosigmoid approach along with C1 hemilaminectomy (Fig. 5) [48]. Eventually, the posterior third of the occipital condyle is drilled away. Transcondylar approaches are seldom necessary [49].

### 12.5.1.4

### Combined Presigmoid-Subtemporal Approach (Supra- and Infratentorial)

The patient is operated on while in a semisitting position or, eventually, in a park bench position. The head is tilted 30° to the side of the lesion. The preoperative and intraoperative precautions were discussed in the Chapter 14. A skin incision is placed starting 2 cm above and anterior to the ear, running posterior along with the temporal line (Fig. 6). Then, the incision is curved downward, extending in a linear fashion posterior to the mastoid tip. The temporal muscle is reflected anteriorly and inferiorly. A temporal craniotomy is carried to the floor of the middle fossa. The transverse sinus is identified and exposed. A suboccipital craniotomy or craniectomy is then performed under direct view of the transverse and sigmoid sinuses. Thereafter, a presigmoid retrolabyrinthine mastoidectomy is accomplished using a high-speed drill in a posterior to anterior and lateral to medial direction (Fig. 7). When hearing is preserved, care should be taken not to enter the endolymphatic duct, the posterior semicircular canals, or the fallopian canals. The dura incision is carried in a T-fashion, in which supratentorially is temporobasal and infratentorially is presigmoid. The temporal lobe is retracted superiorly after exposure and preservation of the vein of Labbé. The superior petrosal sinus is ligated and transected to the free margin of the tentorium. The

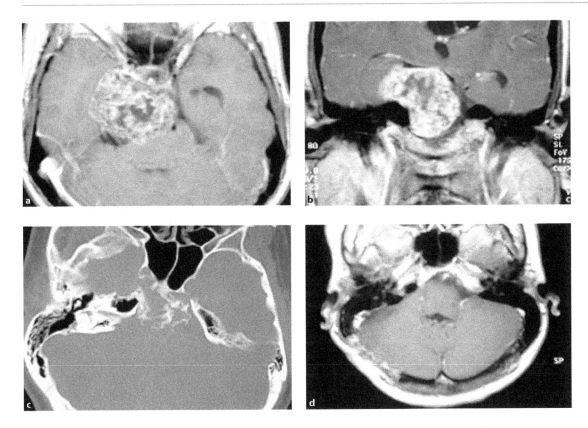

**Fig. 4** Axial (**a**) and coronal (**b**) T1-weighted gadolinium-enhanced MRI scans showing a chondrosarcoma extending into the middle and posterior fossa. **c** Bone window CT revealing the extensive bone destruction. **d** Postoperative axial T1-weighted gadolinium-enhanced MRI scan taken following surgery using the retrosigmoid intradural suprameatal approach (RISA), demonstrating complete tumor removal

trochlear nerve is dissected away from the tentorium and preserved. The cerebellum, together with the sigmoid sinus and the divided tentorial edge, are retracted posteriorly. The tumor is removed as described previously. The dura is closed as usual in a watertight fashion and the air cells are sealed with fibrin glue and a muscle graft. The disadvantages of this approach are that it is time-consuming and carries an increased risk of facial palsy, hearing loss, CSF fistula, and vein of Labbé injury.

## 12.5.2
## Radiotherapy

### 12.5.2.1
### Conventional Radiotherapy

Conventional radiotherapy has been used for decades in the management of chordomas [8]. Nevertheless, inconsistent results have meant that chordomas are now considered to be radioresistant tumors at doses in the range of 45–60 Gy [21, 28, 56]. On the other hand, some studies using escalated radiation doses (>60 Gy) have shown a dose–response relationship for chordomas and chondrosarcomas [3, 12, 52, 56]. Limitations of its use arise as a result of radiotolerance of adjacent normal tissues, such as the brainstem or the visual pathway [12, 40, 52]. Actually, controversy still persists concerning the standard dose and radiation protocol, since available data regarding conventional radiotherapy have revealed no convincing evidence of symptom relief or survival after the delivery of higher doses of radiation [60]. Owing to the uncertainty of responses associated with the risks of clinically late toxicity, other forms of radiotherapy have been studied [8, 15, 40, 52, 56]. In addition, higher doses of radiation may be delivered with other radiation modalities, such as radiosurgery or proton beam radiotherapy [56]. Therefore, some authors no longer recommend conventional radiotherapy in the management of such tumors [56].

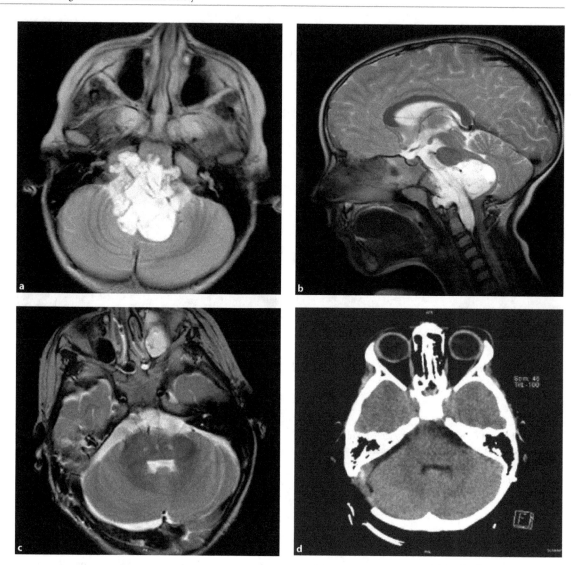

Fig. 5 Axial T2- fluid-attenuated inversion recovery (FLAIR) (**a**) and sagittal T2-weighted (**b**) MRI revealing a large chordoma in a 6-year-old girl. **c**, **d** The tumor was completely removed using a retrosigmoid approach together with a far lateral retrocondylar approach on the right side

## 12.5.2.2
### Stereotactic Radiosurgery

Radiosurgery combines the accuracy of the stereotactic assistance with the advantages of high-dose single-session irradiation [26]. In addition, the steep dose falloff outside the tumor boundaries allow the delivery of higher doses to the tumor volume without exceeding the predicted tolerance levels of the surrounding nervous and vascular structures [8, 26]. Small patient series preclude definitive conclusions [8, 15, 26, 36]; however, it is worth noting that radiosurgery, regardless of whether it is achieved with a linear accelerator or gamma knife, resulted in tumor shrinkage in 45.5–80% of the patients studied [8, 15, 36]. The mean radiation dose ranged from 17–36 Gy [8, 15, 36] and the mean tumor volume ranged from 4.6 to 9.7 ml [15, 36]. Thus, it seems that radiosurgery is a reasonable option for treating small residual or recurrent tumors [8, 15, 36], as well as to deliver a radiation boost to recurrent tumors in previously irradiated patients [26]. Further studies are required to establish the role of radiosurgery in the management of chordomas and chondrosarcomas.

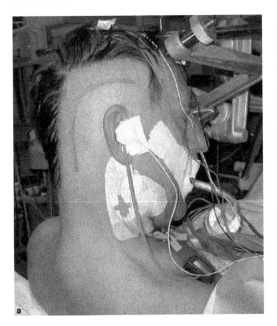
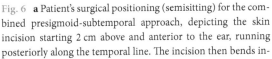
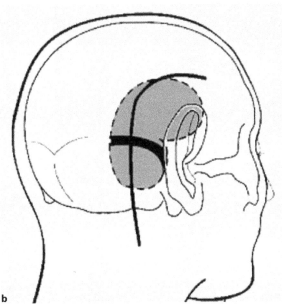

Fig. 6 **a** Patient's surgical positioning (semisitting) for the combined presigmoid-subtemporal approach, depicting the skin incision starting 2 cm above and anterior to the ear, running posteriorly along the temporal line. The incision then bends inferiorly, ending posterior to the mastoid tip. **b** Schematic view of the surgical positioning depicting the temporal and suboccipital craniotomy (*black dotted line*)

### 12.5.2.3
### Heavy Charged Particle Radiotherapy

Heavy particle irradiation, such as protons or carbon ions, provides a higher physical selectivity, leading to improvement of dose delivery and distribution within the tumor, and sparing the normal tissues [40, 52]. These advantages occur due to the steep falloff of the dose at the end of the range, offering a finite range in the tissue (namely the Bragg peak effect) [32, 40, 52]. Several studies have been conducted with proton beam radiotherapy that have provided excellent results for this tool as an adjunctive treatment for skull-base chordomas and chondrosarcomas [24, 40]. These effects were also noted for chordomas in children [22]. Therefore, proton beam radiotherapy remains the method of choice as adjuvant therapy for chordomas and chondrosarcomas [40, 52]. The total dose delivered with this modality ranges from 64.8 to 79.2 CGE (cobalt Gy equivalent) [24]. Tumor size (>25 ml) and optic nerve or chiasm and brainstem involvement limit the target dose, thereby decreasing the local control [24]. The major disadvantages are the high associated costs and limited availability (only a few centers worldwide) [15, 36, 52].

Carbon ions are biologically more effective in comparison to protons [52]. Carbon ion radiotherapy carries with it a low toxicity and is clinically effective treatment that offers high control rates for chordomas and chondrosarcomas [52–55] and is considered an alternative to proton radiotherapy [59]. The mean gross tumor volume treated with carbon ion radiotherapy was 62 ml for chondrosarcomas and 97.6 ml for chordomas, with a median tumor dose of 60 GyE (Gy×relative biologic effectiveness) [52]. Tumor shrinkage was also observed in patients treated with carbon ion radiotherapy [52, 54]. In addition, this modality may be considered for cases of reirradiation in previously irradiated patients [52, 54, 55].

The treatment with heavy particle radiotherapy is not free of clinical toxicity [24, 40, 52–55]; however, relatively few complications have been reported, when considering the high doses delivered and the radiosensitive tissues in the tumor vicinities [40]. Temporal lobe injury [1, 24, 40, 53, 55] and hypopituitarism [24, 40, 53], as well as visual and auditory disturbances [24, 40, 53, 54] have been reported as potential complications of the heavy particle radiotherapy.

### 12.6
### Outcome

The patient's prognosis varies greatly due to the intrinsic biological behavior of the tumor [1, 28]. In this regard,

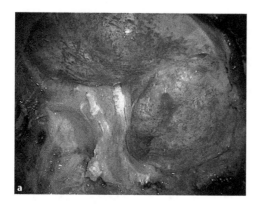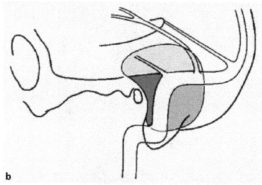

Fig. 7 **a** Intraoperative view of a combined presigmoid-subtemporal approach following temporal craniotomy and sub-occipital craniectomy. **b** Schematic view of the surgical approach showing the bone resection and the venous relationship

Tzortzidis et al. [61] and Lüdemann and Samii [31] commented on a group of slow-growing chordomas that present a better prognosis after radical surgery and presenting delayed recurrence. For this group, Lüdemann and Samii [31] disserted: "The crucial question when treating the latter group is what amount of morbidity has to be taken into account for a radical resection." Gay et al. [17] reported on a series of 60 patients treated surgically. In 67% of cases, they achieved radical or near-total resection and 20% of the patients received postoperative radiotherapy. The recurrence free survival rates at 5 years was 90% for chondrosarcomas and 65% for chordomas. Their series presented 80% of new postoperative cranial nerve deficits and 18% of mortality. Recently, Tzortzidis et al. [61] evaluated the long-term results of radical surgery of chordomas. The patients were followed for a mean period of 96 months [61]. At 10 years, recurrence-free survival was observed in 31% of patients [61]. With regard to primarily operated patients, the 10-year recurrence-free survival was 42% and for reoperation patients, it was 26% [61]. Interestingly, 56% of the patients presented recurrence within 1–36 months [61]. This fact was also observed by other studies, leading some authors to consider early postoperative radiotherapy regardless of the extent of resection [1, 15]. However, the timing for radiotherapy remains controversial [1, 9, 11, 15, 28, 56].

Using proton-beam radiotherapy postoperatively, Hug et al. [24] described actuarial 5-years survival rates of 100% for patients with chondrosarcoma and 79% for patients with chordoma. Whereas the local control rates at 5 years were 75% for chondrosarcomas and 59% for chordomas [24]. Rosenberg et al. [44] reported their experience in 200 chondrosarcomas treated postoperatively with proton-beam radiotherapy. The local control rate at 5 years was 99%, and 98% at 10 years, while the disease-specific survival rates were both 99% [44]. For large tumors, carbon ion radiotherapy incurs progression-free survival rates of 100% for chondrosarcomas and 87% for chordomas at 3 years and overall survival of 100% for chondrosarcomas and 89% for chordomas [54]. This work was updated for low-grade chondrosarcomas revealing actuarial 4 years local control rates of 89.8% and overall survival rates of 98.2% at 5 years [53]. Whether carbon ion radiotherapy is superior to proton beam radiotherapy is not known [53]. Further randomized studies are necessary to prove this improved clinical efficacy of carbon ion radiotherapy over proton beam radiotherapy, as well as the decreased clinical toxicity observed in the former modality [53].

## 12.7
## Current Strategies

The rationale underlying the management of these tumors at our department is the utmost surgical resection, notwithstanding the minimal surgical morbidity, preserving patients' clinical status, and adjuvant carbon ion radiotherapy in cases of residual tumors not scheduled for surgery, or recurrent tumors. Palliative resections are planned in patients with recurrent tumors, and such patients may be considered for reirradiation.

## References

1. Al-Mefty O, Borba LA (1997) Skull base chordomas: a management challenge. J Neurosurg 86:182–189
2. Arnautovic KI, Al-Mefty O (2001) Surgical seeding of chordomas. Neurosurg Focus 10:E7
3. Austin JP, Urie MM, Cardenosa G, Munzenrider JE (1993) Probable causes of recurrence in patients with chordoma and chondrosarcoma of the base of skull and cervical spine. Int J Radiat Oncol Biol Phys 25:439–444

4.  Bahr AL, Gayler BW (1977) Cranial chondrosarcomas. Report of four cases and review of the literature. Radiology 124:151–156

5.  Berghaus A (1990) Midfacial degloving. HNO 38:7–11 (in German)

6.  Berghaus A, Jovanovic S (1991) Technique and indications of extended sublabial rhinotomy ("midfacial degloving"). Rhinology 29:105–110

7.  Boemke F, Joest W (1936) Chordome im Bereich des Schädels. Virchows Arch 297:351–367

8.  Chang SD, Martin DP, Lee E, Adler JR Jr (2001) Stereotactic radiosurgery and hypofractionated stereotactic radiotherapy for residual or recurrent cranial base and cervical chordomas. Neurosurg Focus 10:E5

9.  Colli BO, Al-Mefty O (2001) Chordomas of the skull base: follow-up review and prognostic factors. Neurosurg Focus 10:E1

10. Crockard HA, Cheeseman A, Steel T, Revesz T, et al (2001) A multidisciplinary team approach to skull base chondrosarcomas. J Neurosurg 95:184–189

11. Crockard HA, Steel T, Plowman N, Singh A, et al (2001) A multidisciplinary team approach to skull base chordomas. J Neurosurg 95:175–183

12. Debus J, Schulz-Ertner D, Schad L, Essig M, et al (2000) Stereotactic fractionated radiotherapy for chordomas and chondrosarcomas of the skull base. Int J Radiat Oncol Biol Phys 47:591–596

13. Erdem E, Angtuaco EC, Van Hemert R, Park JS, et al (2003) Comprehensive review of intracranial chordoma. Radiographics 23:995–1009

14. Evans HL, Ayala AG, Romsdahl MM (1977) Prognostic factors in chondrosarcoma of bone: a clinicopathologic analysis with emphasis on histologic grading. Cancer 40:818–831

15. Feigl GC, Bundschuh O, Gharabaghi A, Safavi-Abassi S, et al (2005) Evaluation of a new concept for the management of skull base chordomas and chondrosarcomas. J Neurosurg 102 Suppl:165–170

16. Frank G, Sciarretta V, Calbucci F, Farneti G, et al (2006) The endoscopic transnasal transsphenoidal approach for the treatment of cranial base chordomas and chondrosarcomas. Neurosurgery 59:ONS50–57

17. Gay E, Sekhar LN, Rubinstein E, Wright DC, et al (1995) Chordomas and chondrosarcomas of the cranial base: results and follow-up of 60 patients. Neurosurgery 36:887–897

18. Gerszten PC, Pollack IF, Hamilton RL (1998) Primary parafalcine chondrosarcoma in a child. Acta Neuropathol (Berl) 95:111–114

19. Griffith HB, Veerapen R (1987) A direct transnasal approach to the sphenoid sinus. Technical note. J Neurosurg 66:140–142

20. Haeckel C, Krueger S, Kuester D, Ostertag H, et al (2000) Expression of cathepsin K in chordoma. Hum Pathol 31:834–840

21. Heffelfinger MJ, Dahlin DC, MacCarty CS, Beabout JW (1973) Chordomas and cartilaginous tumors at the skull base. Cancer 32:410–420

22. Hoch BL, Nielsen GP, Liebsch NJ, Rosenberg AE (2006) Base of skull chordomas in children and adolescents: a clinicopathologic study of 73 cases. Am J Surg Pathol 30:811–818

23. Horten BC, Montague SR (1976) Human ecchordosis physaliphora and chick embryonic notochord. A comparative electron microscopic study. Virchows Arch A Pathol Anat Histol 371:295–303

24. Hug EB, Loredo LN, Slater JD, DeVries A, et al (1999) Proton radiation therapy for chordomas and chondrosarcomas of the skull base. J Neurosurg 91:432–439

25. Jho HD, Carrau RL, McLaughlin MR, Somaza SC (1997) Endoscopic transsphenoidal resection of a large chordoma in the posterior fossa. Acta Neurochir (Wien) 139:343–348

26. Kondziolka D, Lunsford LD, Flickinger JC (1991) The role of radiosurgery in the management of chordoma and chondrosarcoma of the cranial base. Neurosurgery 29:38–46

27. Korten AG, ter Berg HJ, Spincemaille GH, van der Laan RT, et al (1998) Intracranial chondrosarcoma: review of the literature and report of 15 cases. J Neurol Neurosurg Psychiatry 65:88–92

28. Lanzino G, Dumont AS, Lopes MB, Laws ER Jr (2001) Skull base chordomas: overview of disease, management options, and outcome. Neurosurg Focus 10:E12

29. Laws ER Jr (1993) Clivus chordomas. In: Sekhar LN, Janecka IP (eds) Surgery of Cranial Base Tumors. Raven, New York, pp 679–685

30. Lichtenstein L, Bernstein D (1959) Unusual benign and malignant chondroid tumors of bone. A survey of some mesenchymal cartilage tumors and malignant chondroblastic tumors, including a few multicentric ones, as well as many atypical benign chondroblastomas and chondromyxoid fibromas. Cancer 12:1142–1157

31. Lüdemann W, Samii M (2006) Patient outcome at long-term follow-up after aggressive microsurgical resection of cranial base chordomas. Neurosurgery 59:230–237

32. Maier W, Lohnstein PU, Rosahl SK, Tatagiba M, et al (2006) Multidisciplinary management of skull base and craniocervical chordoma. Laryngorhinootologie 85:272–278 (in German)

33. Malik SN, Farmer PM, Hajdu SI, Rosenthal A (1996) Mesenchymal chondrosarcoma of the cerebellum. Ann Clin Lab Sci 26:496–500

34. Marquardt G, Yahya H, Hermann E, Seifert V (2004) Direct transnasal approach for pituitary surgery. Neurosurg Rev 27:83–88

35. Meyers SP, Hirsch WL Jr, Curtin HD, Barnes L, et al (1992) Chondrosarcomas of the skull base: MR imaging features. Radiology 184:103–108

36. Muthukumar N, Kondziolka D, Lunsford LD, Flickinger JC (1998) Stereotactic radiosurgery for chordoma and chondrosarcoma: further experiences. Int J Radiat Oncol Biol Phys 41:387–392

37. Naka T, Boltze C, Kuester D, Samii A, et al (2005) Histogenesis of intralesional fibrous septum in chordoma. Pathol Res Pract 201:443–447

38. Naka T, Boltze C, Kuester D, Samii A, et al (2005) Intralesional fibrous septum in chordoma: a clinicopathologic and immunohistochemical study of 122 lesions. Am J Clin Pathol 124:288–294

39. Naka T, Boltze C, Samii A, Herold C, et al (2003) Skull base and nonskull base chordomas: clinicopathologic and immunohistochemical study with special reference to nuclear pleomorphism and proliferative ability. Cancer 98:1934–1941

40. Noel G, Habrand JL, Mammar H, Pontvert D, et al (2001) Combination of photon and proton radiation therapy for chordomas and chondrosarcomas of the skull base: the Centre de Protontherapie D'Orsay experience. Int J Radiat Oncol Biol Phys 51:392–398

41. Pamir MN, Ozduman K (2006) Analysis of radiological features relative to histopathology in 42 skull-base chordomas and chondrosarcomas. Eur J Radiol 58:461–470

42. Patel NP, Mhatre AN, Lalwani AK (2004) Molecular pathogenesis of skull base tumors. Otol Neurotol 25:636–643

43. Podlaha J, Pavlica F (1928) Das bösartige sacrococcygeale Chordom. Ein neuer Fall; pathologisch-anatomische Studie. Virchow Arch 267:363–378

44. Rosenberg AE, Nielsen GP, Keel SB, Renard LG, et al (1999) Chondrosarcoma of the base of the skull: a clinicopathologic study of 200 cases with emphasis on its distinction from chordoma. Am J Surg Pathol 23:1370–1378

45. Samii M, Ammirati M (1988) The combined supra-infratentorial pre-sigmoid sinus avenue to the petro-clival region. Surgical technique and clinical applications. Acta Neurochir (Wien) 95:6–12

46. Samii M, Draf W (1989) Surgery of space-occupying lesions of the lateral middle skull base. In: Samii M, Draf W (eds) Surgery of the Skull Base – An Interdisciplinary Approach. Springer, Berlin Heidelberg, pp 296–358

47. Samii M, Draf W (1989) Surgery of the clivus. In: Samii M, Draf W (eds) Surgery of the Skull Base – An Interdisciplinary Approach. Springer, Berlin Heidelberg, pp 432–460

48. Samii M, Klekamp J, Carvalho G (1996) Surgical results for meningiomas of the craniocervical junction. Neurosurgery 39:1086–1095

49. Samii M, Tatagiba M (2004) Basic principles of skull base surgery. In: Winn HR (ed) Youmans Neurological Surgery. Saunders, Philadelphia, pp 909–929

50. Samii M, Tatagiba M, Carvalho GA (1999) Resection of large petroclival meningiomas by the simple retrosigmoid route. J Clin Neurosci 6:27–30

51. Samii M, Tatagiba M, Carvalho GA (2000) Retrosigmoid intradural suprameatal approach to Meckel's cave and the middle fossa: surgical technique and outcome. J Neurosurg 92:235–241

52. Schulz-Ertner D, Haberer T, Jakel O, Thilmann C, et al (2002) Radiotherapy for chordomas and low-grade chondrosarcomas of the skull base with carbon ions. Int J Radiat Oncol Biol Phys 53:36–42

53. Schulz-Ertner D, Nikoghosyan A, Hof H, Didinger B, et al (2007) Carbon ion radiotherapy of skull base chondrosarcomas. Int J Radiat Oncol Biol Phys 67:171–177

54. Schulz-Ertner D, Nikoghosyan A, Thilmann C, Haberer T, et al (2003) Carbon ion radiotherapy for chordomas and low-grade chondrosarcomas of the skull base. Results in 67 patients. Strahlenther Onkol 179:598–605

55. Schulz-Ertner D, Nikoghosyan A, Thilmann C, Haberer T, et al (2004) Results of carbon ion radiotherapy in 152 patients. Int J Radiat Oncol Biol Phys 58:631–640

56. Sekhar LN, Chanda A, Chandrasekar K, Wright DC (2004) Chordoma and chondrosarcomas. In: Winn HR (ed) Youmans Neurological Surgery. Saunders, Philadelphia, pp 1283–1294

57. Sekhar LN, Pranatartiharan R, Chanda A, Wright DC (2001) Chordomas and chondrosarcomas of the skull base: results and complications of surgical management. Neurosurg Focus 10:E2

58. Sekhar LN, Wright DC (1999) Resection of anterior, middle, and posterior cranial base tumors via the extended subfrontal approach . In: Sekhar LN, De Oliveira E (eds) Cranial Microsurgery – Approaches and Techniques. Thieme, New York, pp 82–90

59. Sen C, Triana A (2001) Cranial chordomas: results of radical excision. Neurosurg Focus 10:E3

60. Tai PT, Craighead P, Bagdon F (1995) Optimization of radiotherapy for patients with cranial chordoma. A review of dose–response ratios for photon techniques. Cancer 75:749–756

61. Tzortzidis F, Elahi F, Wright D, Natarajan SK, et al (2006) Patient outcome at long-term follow-up after aggressive microsurgical resection of cranial base chordomas. Neurosurgery 59:230–237

62. Yassa M, Bahary JP, Bourguoin P, Belair M, et al (2005) Intra-parenchymal mesenchymal chondrosarcoma of the cerebellum: case report and review of the literature. J Neurooncol 74:329–331

# Petroclival Meningiomas: Diagnosis, Treatment, and Results

# 13

Ricardo Ramina, Yvens Barbosa Fernandes, and Maurício Coelho Neto

## Contents

## 13.1
## Introduction

There are several lesions arising in the petroclival region. The most frequent tumor is the petroclival meningioma, followed by chondrosarcomas, chordomas, schwannomas of the cranial nerves V and VII, and other malignant tumors [2, 15, 16, 20, 24]. Vascular lesions like basilar artery aneurysms, arteriovenous malformations, and cavernomas are also found in this region.

Petroclival meningiomas are tumors of the skull base that present a formidable challenge to surgical resection because of their deep location and relationship to vital neurovascular structures. In the majority of the cases they are benign tumors, but may involve or infiltrate the skull base bone, the dura mater, the brainstem, and all important neurovascular structures of this region.

## 13.2
## Definition of the Petroclival Region

In accordance with our concept, the petroclival region comprises the anatomical location of the body of the sphenoid bone, the anterior central portion of the occipital bone, and is bordered on the lateral aspect by the petrous apex. The roof of this space is formed by the petroclival ligaments and the tentorium. This space contains important neurovascular structures that are frequently involved or displaced by the tumor in a variable pattern. The basilar artery with its branches (the anterior inferior and posterior inferior cerebellar arteries, and the perforating branches, superior, cerebellar, posterior cerebral arteries) may be embedded or displaced by the meningioma. The petrosal vein is often displaced posteriorly by the tumor. Cranial nerves III and IV are usually displaced upwardly and the nerve VI is often surrounded by tumor.

Petroclival meningiomas by definition have their origin medial to cranial nerves V, VII, VIII, IX, X, and XI, and reach the tentorium (Fig. 1). They frequently extend to the middle cranial fossa, cavernous sinus, prepontine space, and down to the magnum foramen. These tumors frequently compress the brainstem and may invade the pia mater, making total removal very difficult or impossible without neurologic deficits. Sphenoid ridge, cerebellopontine angle (CPA), and low clivus meningiomas may reach these areas, but are not considered having a petroclival origin (Fig. 1). These lesions usually need different surgical approaches and present distinct surgical difficulties.

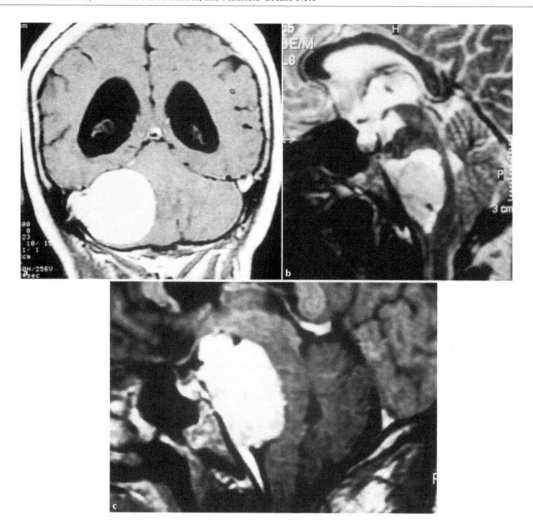

Fig. 1 **a** Cerebellopontine angle meningioma. **b** Low clivus, meningioma. **c** Petroclival meningioma

## 13.3
## History

Posterior fossa meningiomas were classified in 1953 by Castellano and Ruggiero [5], using Olivecrona's series, into five groups: cerebellar convexity, tentorium, posterior surface of the petrous bone, clivus, and magnum foramen. After the development of computed tomography (CT), this classification was revised. Yasargil et al. [27] in 1980 suggested that these tumors arise along the petroclival line, and classified them into clival, petroclival, sphenopetroclival, magnum foramen, and CPA meningiomas. Mayberg and Symon in 1986 [12] published a series using the terminology clival and petrous apical meningiomas. Since this time, the term petroclival meningioma has been used for those tumors in many publications. CPA meningiomas must be excluded from these series because they represent a separate group with different surgical implications. They arise posterior to the

sigmoid sinus, displacing cranial nerves VII, VIII, IX, X, and XI anteriorly. Surgical removal of these lesions is usually easier than in cases of petroclival meningiomas.

## 13.4
## Diagnosis

### 13.4.1
### Clinical Symptoms

Petroclival meningiomas are rare, slow-growing tumors that usually produce clinical symptoms after reaching a large size. According to Bricolo et al. [4], it takes between 2.5 and 4.5 years from the onset of symptoms to establishing the correct diagnosis. This fact delays the treatment. Indication for surgical removal of small tumors is controversial because even small petroclival meningiomas require a major surgical procedure that might increase morbidity, making patients worse after surgery. Clinical symptoms are related to involvement of the cranial nerves, compression of the brainstem and cerebellum, and increases in intracranial pressure. Headache and gait disturbances followed by hearing loss and facial paresthesias are the symptoms most frequently presented by these patients. Symptom progressions are relentless during a long period of time, which may delay diagnosis. The trigeminal nerve (cranial nerve V) is more frequently affected, followed by cranial nerves IX and X. Facial nerve disturbance will occur in 30% of patients. Visual disturbances, cerebellar signs, and somatomotor deficits usually occur late due to progression of the disease. Patients with hydrocephalus, requiring treatment, are rare, because these slow-growing lesions will produce late cerebrospinal fluid (CSF)-pathway occlusion when the tumor has achieved a large size. Characteristically, patients with petroclival meningioma may present good hearing, in contrast to those with severe trigeminal and caudal cranial nerve involvement.

## 13.4.2
## Neuroradiological Evaluation

CT scan examination is useful for evaluation of the bony structures of the skull base. It may reveal bone erosion, hyperostosis, or both. The tumor is usually slightly hyperintense in comparison with the brain tissue and shows strong contrast enhancement. They usually infiltrate the dura mater and present a large implantation (Fig. 2). Calcifications may also be observed. Magnetic resonance imaging (MRI) is the radiological examination that shows very precisely the extension and relationship of the lesion with brainstem, vessels, and the cranial nerves (Fig. 2).

Displacement and compression of normal structures are demonstrated clearly by MRI. In most cases, strong gadolinium enhancement is observed. Signs of dura mater infiltration ("dura tail") may be present. Edema may appear in T2-weighted images, meaning arachnoid invasion. Tumor vascularity and relationships to major vessels are demonstrated by magnetic resonance angiography (MRA). For surgical planning, high-definition MRI studies are of fundamental importance. Four-vessel digital angiography (DSA) shows the vascular supply, displacement, and involvement (narrowing) of the basilar artery and internal carotid artery (ICA) and their branches. These tumors are usually fed by branches of the external carotid artery, and the meningohypophyseal trunk (Bernasconi-Cassinari artery) is enlarged. Hypervascular tumors may be embolized preoperatively with particles or glue.

## 13.5
## Natural History

The natural history of meningiomas is characterized by progressive growth causing compression and involvement of neighboring structures. Van Havenberg et al. [26] studied 21 patients with petroclival meningiomas who were treated conservatively. There was a minimum follow-up of 4 years. They found tumor growth in 76% of cases and clinical impairment in 63%. Jung et al. [9] reported a series of 38 patients with subtotal removal. They followed these patients and found a linear growth of 0.37 cm/year and a volumetric increase of 4.94 cm$^3$/year. These authors reported, however, that 60% of patients showed no clinical signs of disease progression.

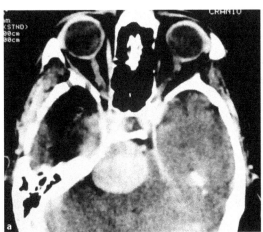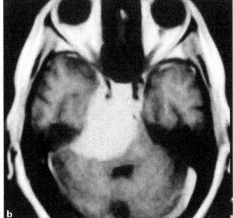

Fig. 2 **a** Computed tomography scan with contrast showing a large petroclival meningioma. **b** Magnetic resonance imaging (MRI) scan with gadolinium enhancement, showing cavernous sinus infiltration

## 13.6
## Management

Surgical removal of large petroclival meningiomas presents the neurosurgeons an enormous challenge. The operative mortality was very high, but is could be reduced by the development of new diagnostic and surgical procedures [4, 7, 10, 13, 19, 26, 27]. In spite of all recent advances in neurosurgery, neuroradiology, and radiotherapy, the morbidity of surgical treatment of large petroclival meningiomas remains high. Management of petroclival meningiomas includes three options: clinical observation, total removal, and subtotal surgical ablation with or without adjunctive therapy.

Clinical observation may be indicated for patients in poor general clinical condition or advanced age. Very small, asymptomatic tumors may be followed with MRI every 6 months. Another reason for conservative management is the patient's refusal to have surgery. According to our experience, removal of small, minimally symptomatic petroclival meningiomas is indicated because these lesions have the best chance of total resection with no mortality or morbidity. With the strategy of "wait and scan" in these cases, the tumor can grow, involve cranial nerves and vessels, and making tumor dissection from these structures impossible.

Radiotherapy and radiosurgery may be indicated as initial treatment or after partial surgical removal. The complications of radiotherapy for lesions in and around the brainstem have been described. Our strategy is to follow patients with subtotal removal with MRI studies every 6 months. Radiotherapy is recommended only when clear signs of tumor growth are demonstrated.

## 13.7
## Surgical Treatment

Total surgical removal is the only treatment that may cure this benign tumor; however, it may cause disability and mortality. The pros and cons of surgery, radiotherapy, and conservative management are discussed thoroughly with the patients before surgery. The main factor limiting radical removal with preservation of involved structures is invasion of the pia mater. These cases have no clear cleavage plane to permit safe the dissection of cranial nerves and vessels. Small, perforating brainstem vessels embedded in the lesion may be damaged during dissection, causing brainstem infarction. In these tumors, a small piece of tumor around these structures is left behind to avoid postoperative deficits. Cavernous sinus invasion may be a cause of subtotal removal.

### 13.7.1
### Selection of Surgical Approach

Choice of surgical approach is usually based on tumor location and extension, involvement of venous structures (Vein of Labbé), and the experience of the surgeon. An additional factor to be considered is the shape of skull. Patients with braquicephalic skull have a shorter anterior–posterior distance to the petrous apex and the middle fossa fronto-orbito-zygomatic approach may be indicated (Fig. 3). Dolicocephalic patients are best suited for petrosal approaches because the lateral distance to the petrous apex is shorter. Larger tumors invading the cavernous sinus with extension into the posterior fossa

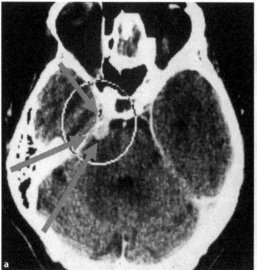
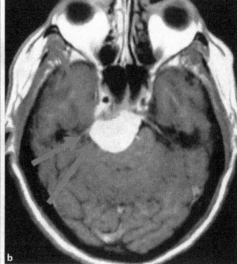

Fig. 3a,b  Distances to the petrous apex. **a** Brachicephalic skull. **b** "Normal" skull

may be removed in two surgeries through different approaches. Elderly patients may tolerate better two short-duration surgeries than one long-duration procedure.

## 13.7.2
## Surgical Approaches

Three main surgical accesses are used: fronto-orbito-zygomatic, petrosal, and retrosigmoid approaches. They may be used as single approach or may be combined.

### 13.7.2.1
### Fronto-orbito-zygomatic Approach

This approach is utilized for petroclival tumors with main extension in the middle fossa involving the cavernous sinus (Fig. 4). The advantages of this access are related to wide exposure of the middle fossa and adequate control of the ICA. This approach does not, however, provide good tumor exposure in the infratentorial midline and within the posterior fossa below cranial nerves VII and VIII, even with opening of the tentorium margin.

### Surgical Technique

The patient is placed in the dorsal decubitus position with the head turned 30° to the opposite side. Intraop-erative monitoring of cranial nerves III, IV, VI, VII, and VIII is performed. A C-shaped preauricular skin incision is made, 1 cm below the zygomatic arch, extending to the frontal area, behind the hairline. The skin flap is turned down at the level the of temporalis fascia, exposing the root of zygomatic arch, temporal-mandibular joint, and lateral orbital rim. The ramus frontalis of the facial nerve is preserved. The temporalis muscle is elevated and a fronto-orbito-temporal craniotomy with the zygomatic arch attached to it, is cut in one piece (Fig. 5a, b). The temporal mandibular joint is opened with preservation of its meniscus. The great sphenoid wing, lateral orbit wall, and base of the middle fossa are removed with a high-speed drill. The foramen ovale, spinosum, and rotundum are identified (Fig. 5c). The middle meningeal artery is co-agulated and cut. The superior orbital fissure is opened. If necessary, the petrous portion of the ICA is exposed after dissection of the great petrosal nerve, medially to the fo-ramen spinosum and Eustachian tube. Usually, we prefer a proximal control of the ICA in the neck. The dura is in-cised and the sylvian fissure is opened wide, exposing the ICA and olfactory, optic, and oculomotor nerves (Fig. 6a, b). Careful dissection of the carotid bifurcation and an-terior and middle cerebral arteries is the next step. These structures are frequently involved by the tumor. In order to preserve these vessels, dissection begins in the nonin-volved portion and dissected from the tumor capsule. The optic canal is drilled out with diamonds burs. After iden-tification and dissection of all neurovascular structures, the tumor in the middle fossa is removed, exposing the

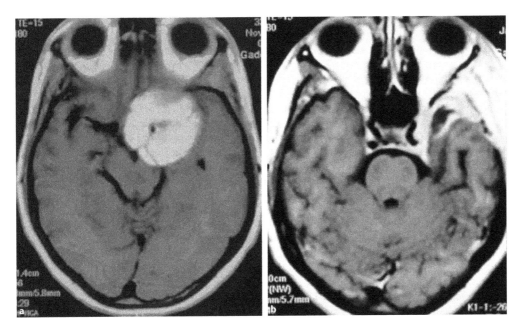

**Fig. 4 a** Preoperative MRI showing petroclival meningioma with main extension in the middle fossa. **b** Postoperative MRI after total removal using the fronto-orbito-zygomatic approach

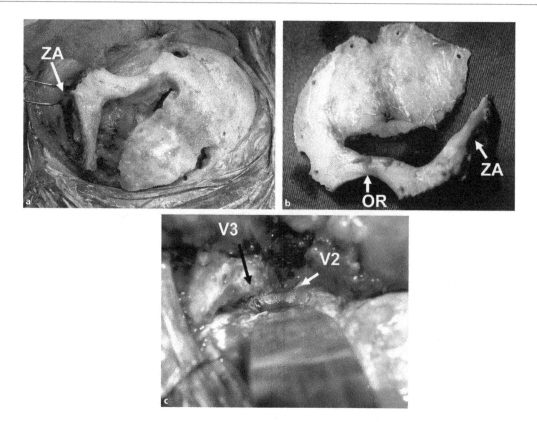

Fig. 5 **a** One-piece craniotomy. **b** Craniotomy flap. **c** Extradural exposition of the second and third branches of the trigeminal nerve. *ZA* Zygomatic arch, *OR* orbital rim, *V2* second branch of the trigeminal nerve, *V3* third branch of the trigeminal nerve

lateral wall of the cavernous sinus. If the cavernous sinus is infiltrated, its lateral wall is opened through a pre- or subtemporal access. A "peeling" of the dura of the lateral wall of cavernous sinus is performed (Fig. 6c). Cranial nerve III and the branches of trigeminal nerve are identified and dissected. The ICA and abducens nerve may be totally involved by the tumor within the cavernous sinus (Fig. 7). Intraoperative micro-Doppler may be useful to identify the ICA. The intracavernous branches of the ICA may be enlarged, feeding the tumor. A high-flow bypass between the external carotid artery and the middle cerebral artery (M2 segment), with a radial artery or saphenous vein graft, is performed if the ICA is to be removed with the lesion (Fig. 8). Tumors with anterior extension into the superior orbital fissure may infiltrate the cranial nerves. The objective of surgery is total tumor removal with preservation of the ICA and cranial nerves II and III. If the tumor capsule is very adherent to these structures without clear arachnoidal plane, or they are infiltrated by the tumor and the nerves are still functioning, a subtotal removal is performed.

Tumor extension within the posterior fossa is removed after opening the tentorium behind the entrance of cra-

nial nerve III in the cavernous sinus. The petrous apex and the posterior clinoid process are removed with diamond burs to enlarge exposure. The basilar artery and its branches and cranial nerves VII and VIII are dissected from the tumor capsule. An adequate surgical exposure is not possible below the level of the internal auditory canal. Tumor exposure in the middle and lower portions of the clivus is not adequate with this approach. After removal of the lesion, the dura mater is closed in watertight fashion and the craniotomy flap is replaced and fixed to the skull. The wound is closed in routine fashion.

### 13.7.2.2
### Petrosal Approach

#### Indication

The petrosal approaches are: presigmoid retrolabyrinthine, presigmoid translabyrinthine, and total petrosectomy. These approaches are used when the lesion is located in the posterior, middle fossa and clivus region (Fig. 9). If the patient has good preoperative hearing, we

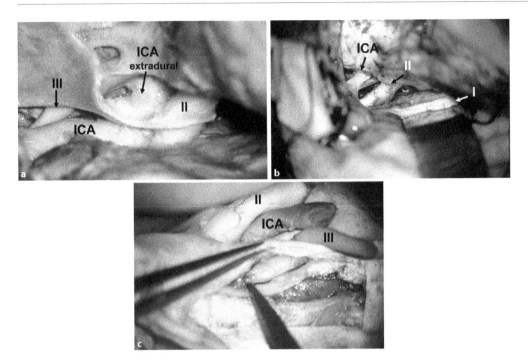

Fig. 6 **a** Anatomical specimen: extradural internal carotid artery exposure. **b** Surgical picture. **c** Anatomical specimen; "peeling" of the cavernous sinus (CS) wall. *ICA* Internal carotid artery, *III* oculomotor nerve, *II* optic nerve

prefer the presigmoid retrolabyrinthine access. When there is no hearing, it is possible to remove the semicircular canals, and this approach is called presigmoid translabyrinthine. For giant tumors crossing the midline in the prepontine region, a more lateral and extensive approach is necessary. These cases are operated through total petrosectomy.

## Surgical Technique

### Presigmoid (Retrolabyrinthine) Approach

Surgery is performed with the patient in the dorsal decubitus position with the head rotated to the opposite side. A semicircular skin incision is made from the temporal region, 4 cm above the zygomatic arch, passing 3 cm

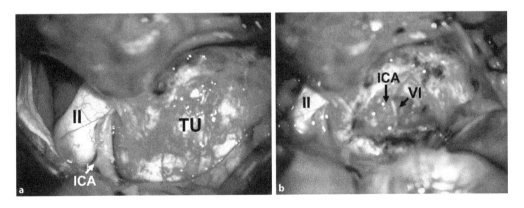

Fig. 7a,b Intraoperative pictures: **a** Tumor within the CS causing bulging of the lateral CS wall and optic nerve. **b** After tumor removal: the ICA and abducens nerve can be seen. *TU* Tumor, *VI* abducens nerve

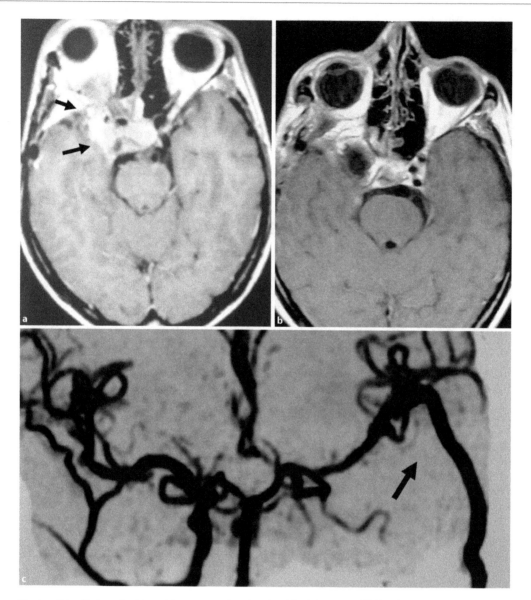

Fig. 8 **a** Petroclival meningioma with cavernous sinus invasion. The ICA is embedded in the tumor (*arrows*). **b** Postoperative MRI after total removal. **c** A high-flow bypass was performed between the external carotid artery and middle cerebral artery with radial artery graft (*arrow*)

behind the ear, extending 2 cm behind the mastoid tip (Fig. 10a, c). To avoid postoperative CSF leak, a skull-base reconstruction technique utilizing fascia/muscle flaps was developed. The temporalis muscle fascia is cut and dissected with the mastoid periosteum, the craniocervical fascia, and the sternocleidomastoid muscle, which is detached from its insertion. These structures form a large vascularized muscle/fascia flap that is rotated back at the end of surgery to cover the entire surgical field. The temporal muscle is dissected in the anterior direction and used to cover the dura mater, as a vascularized muscle, at

the end of the operation. The cortical bone of the mastoid is drilled out, exposing the antrum, tegmen mastoid, and sinus plate. The labyrinth block and the facial nerve canal are identified. These canals are not opened. Two trepanations above and two below the sigmoid sinus are placed and, with a high-speed drill, a craniotomy is cut exposing the middle fossa and the posterior fossa (retrosigmoid) (Fig. 10b, d). The superior petrosal, the sigmoid and the transverse sinuses are exposed. The retrofacial mastoid cells are removed down to the jugular bulb. The dura mater anterior to the sigmoid sinus is exposed. The zy-

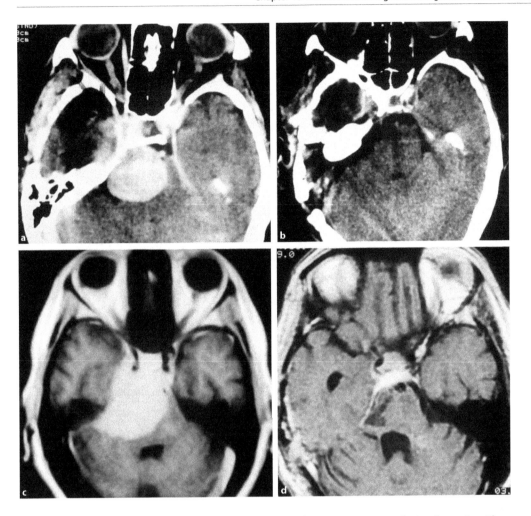

Fig. 9 Preoperative (**a,c**) and postoperative (**b,d**) MRI of petroclival meningiomas removed using the presigmoid approach

gomatic and supralabyrinthine cells are removed, maintaining the semicircular canals and middle ear intact. The superior petrosal sinus is coagulated and ligated between two stitches. The dura mater is incised anterior to the sigmoid sinus and parallel to the middle fossa floor (Fig. 11a). The superior petrosal sinus is cut. The tentorium is severed initially perpendicular to the superior petrosal sinus in a length of 2 or 3 cm, and then medially, parallel to the transverse sinus for an additional 3 cm. This maneuver allows a wide exposure of the cerebellum, separating it from the posterior aspect of temporal lobe like "opening a book." Care should be taken to preserve the vein of Labbé, which has a variable anatomy and usually enters the transverse sinus 10 mm before its junction with the sigmoid sinus. Preoperative evaluation of the venous anatomy is necessary in planning this approach. The tentorium incision is continued up to the incisura where cranial nerve IV is exposed and preserved. Some small,

basal, temporal-lobe bridge veins are coagulated and cut, allowing a wide subtemporal exposure. Two brain spatulas are placed, supporting the temporal lobe and the cerebellum, exposing the entire petroclival region from cranial nerves III to VII and VIII. The trigeminal nerve can usually be seen displaced posterior and superiorly. The tumor is devascularized by bipolar coagulation of its dural insertion. Intracapsular, piecemeal tumor resection using the ultrasonic aspirator is the next surgical step. Tumor debulking allows dissection of the tumor capsule from the nerves, basilar artery, and superior cerebellar and posterior cerebral arteries. The abducens nerve is very thin and fragile (Fig. 11b, c). Dorello's canal is located medially to cranial nerves VII and VIII. This region should be approached only after wide resection of tumor. Tumor extension into the posterior portion of cavernous sinus is resected following the trigeminal nerve. All infiltrated petrous and clivus bone is removed with a diamond

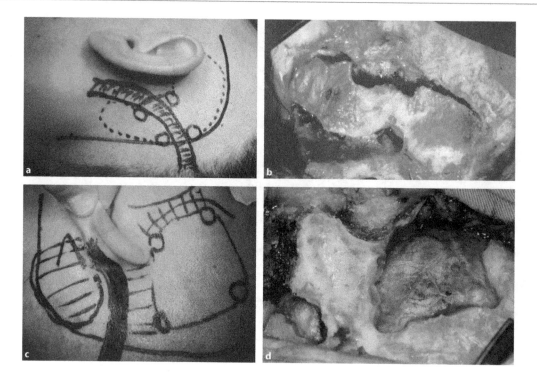

Fig. 10a–d Presigmoid approach. **a,b** Skin incision and craniotomy. **c,d** Skin incision, temporal craniotomy, and retromastoid craniectomy

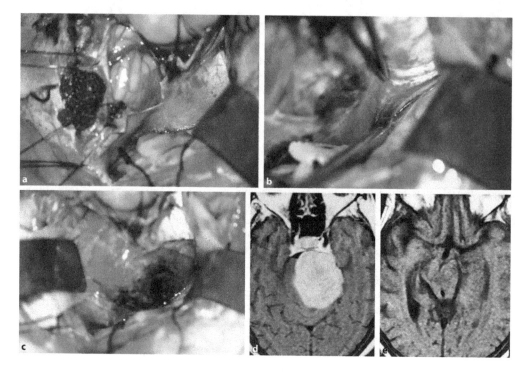

Fig. 11a–e Intraoperative pictures (**a–c**) showing the presigmoid approach. **d,e** Pre- and postoperative MRI scans

drill. After total removal (Fig. 11d, e), the dura mater is closed in watertight fashion or with fascia graft and fibrin glue. The additus and antrum are closed with a muscle plug and the temporalis muscle flap is rotated to cover the entire exposed dura mater. The fascia–muscle flap (temporalis, cranial-cervical fasciae, and sternocleidomastoid muscle) is sutured into its original position, and the skin is closed.

### Presigmoid, Translabyrinthine Approach

This surgical procedure is similar to the anterior approach with additional removal of the labyrinth. Drilling the semicircular canals will add about 1.5 cm in surgical exposure, allowing better visualization of the midline structures. In to our experience, opening the semicircular canals causes deafness.

### Total

With this access, the surgical procedure is initially the same as that for the presigmoid approach, completed with additional removal of semicircular canals and cochlea, and transposition of the facial nerve. The petrous ICA is exposed in its entire course within the petrous bone until its entrance into the cavernous sinus. This approach is especially useful for very large lesions crossing the midline in patients who are already deaf. Facial nerve transposition will cause postoperative facial paralysis, which improves within 3 months after surgery to House and Brackmann [8] grade 1–2. The Eustachian tube is closed with a muscle plug to avoid postoperative CSF fistula. If there is narrow space between the sigmoid sinus and labyrinth in hearing patients and nondominant sigmoid sinus, a trans-sigmoid approach can be used.

#### 13.7.2.3
### Retrosigmoid Approach

### Indications

This access was the most used in our petroclival meningiomas series. It is simple and easy to perform. This approach is indicated when the tumor is located mainly in the posterior fossa with a small extension in the middle fossa and posterior portion of cavernous sinus (Fig. 12).

### Surgical Technique

The dorsal decubitus (mastoid position) with rotation and light lateral extension of the head is used (Fig. 13a). The skin incision starts in the retromastoid region, 5 cm behind the external auditory canal, and extends 2 cm behind the mastoid tip, ending in the upper neck (Fig. 13b).

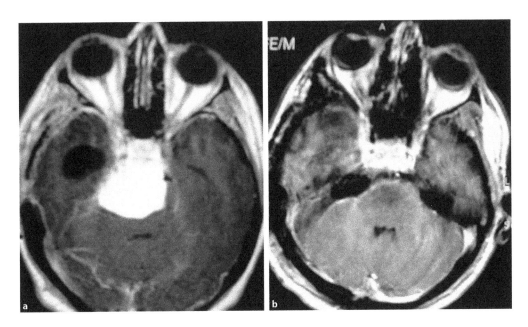

Fig. 12  **a** Preoperative MRI showing a petroclival meningioma. **b** MRI scan demonstrating total removal of the tumor (achieved using the retrosigmoid approach)

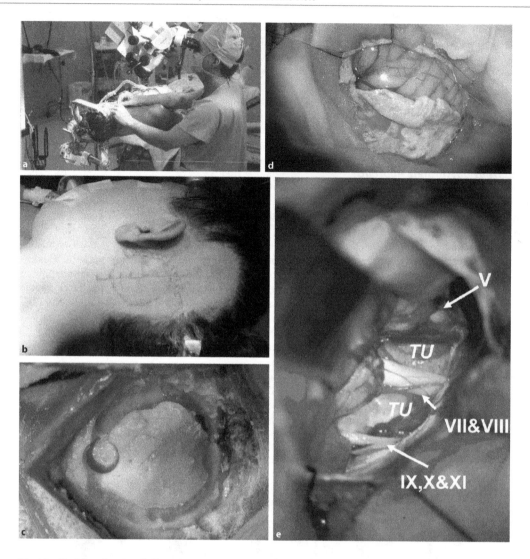

Fig. 13 **a** Position of patient. **b** Skin incision. **c** Craniotomy. **d** Dura opening. **e** Tumor exposure. *V* Trigeminal nerve, *VII* facial nerve, *VIII* cochlear nerve, *IX* glossopharyngeal nerve, *X* vagus nerve, *XI* spinal accessory nerve

Fascia and muscles are cut straight down, exposing the occipital bone, the asterium, and the retromastoid region. A 4-cm-diameter craniotomy is cut exposing the transverse and sigmoid sinuses (Fig. 13c). The mastoid emissary vein is coagulated and cut. The dura mater is incised parallel to the sigmoid sinus (Fig. 13d), the lateral aspect of cerebellum is lightly retracted, and the cerebello-medularis cistern is opened. The lower cranial nerves, VII and VIII, usually lie posterior to the tumor capsule (Fig. 13e). These nerves are often embedded within the tumor, and very careful, monitored dissection must be performed. Cranial nerve V runs in the superior tumor pole or is displaced upward with cranial nerve IV through the free tentorium margin. Cranial nerve VI is

usually located anteriorly or within the tumor. Its identification and dissection is only possible after extensive debulking of the lesion. After coagulation of the dural attachments, intracapsular piecemeal resection between the cranial nerves "windows" is carried out (tentorium-V; V–VII and VIII; VII and VIII–IX, X, XI). Tumor involvement of the basilar artery and its branches as well as the vertebral artery is common. The noninvolved segment of these vessels is first identified and then followed to the involved portions. Dissection of the arachnoidal plane around the vessels and cranial nerves is necessary to preserve these structures. The retrosigmoid approach allows tumor resection from the jugular foramen up to the posterior portion of the cavernous sinus. Middle fossa tumor extensions can be resected by opening the tentorium and drilling the suprameatal tubercule and petrous apex. After total tumor removal, a watertight running dura mater closure is performed. All opened mastoid cells are sealed with muscle graft and fibrin glue. The wound is sutured in the usual fashion and no drain is placed.

## 13.8
## Clinical Material

In the last 16 years, 67 patients with petroclival meningiomas were operated on in our clinic. Gross total tumor removal (Simpson's grade I and II) could be achieved in 36 cases (55%). The postoperative complications in this series are listed in Table 1. There was no operative mortality. One patient died 4 weeks after surgery due to pulmonary embolism and other patient died 6 weeks after surgery due to rupture of an anterior communicating aneurysm. New postoperative cranial nerves deficits were: trigeminal nerve in three patients, abducens nerve in five, facial nerve in six, cochlear nerve in six, and caudal cranial nerves in seven cases. Two patients with large petroclival meningiomas presented with brainstem infarction due to damage to the perforators from the basilar artery. These patients developed postoperative hemiplegia that improved 6 months after surgery in one case; the other patient retained major hemiparesis. There was no CSF leak or meningitis in this series.

## 13.9
## Discussion

Petroclival meningiomas are rare tumors representing a small percentage of posterior fossa meningiomas, which correspond to 10% of all intracranial meningiomas. Total resection of a benign petroclival meningioma may cure the patient. However, surgical removal remains difficult in spite of all advances in skull-base surgery (Table 2).

Tumor size, involvement of the important vessels, cranial nerves, and brainstem, and the biological behavior of these tumors are the main factors in determining the grade of surgical removal and morbidity.

Subtotal removal may be indicated in patients harboring large tumors with few clinical symptoms, to avoid new cranial nerve deficits, which are the most frequent complication of surgery. Residual tumor may grow, requiring further treatment. Samii and Tatagiba [18] and Sekhar et al. [21] observed residual tumor growth in only one of five patients known to harbor a residual tumor. Couldwell et al. [6] noted tumor progression in 12 of 14 patients with clinical or radiographic evidence of residual tumor within the cavernous sinus. They emphasize the importance of this location as a site for recurrence. CT studies give information on bony anatomy and invasion of the skull base, but MRI provides the most valuable information for planning the surgical approach. MRA shows displacement of large vessels and important details about the venous anatomy. DSA is performed when the lesion is seen to be highly vascularized on MRI. It is useful to demonstrate involvement of the main vessels and tumor feeders. An ICA balloon test occlusion is performed when the ICA is involved. Embolization of tumor feeders is performed in selected cases of very highly vascularized tumors. Several approaches have been used to remove these tumors. Tumor location, extension of dural attachments at the skull base, quality of patient's preoperative hearing, and experience of surgeon are the most important factors. The retrosigmoid approach is used mainly for tumors located in the posterior fossa with small extensions into the middle fossa and posterior cavernous sinus. Removal of the suprameatal tubercule and petrous apex enlarges the exposure. The fronto-orbito-zygomatic access is indicated for tumors with the main portion in the middle fossa and small extension into the posterior fossa. An anatomical study performed in our clinic showed that this approach is more suitable for patients with brachicephalic skulls because the distance from the pterion to the petrous apex is shorter than from the petrosal approach [14]. In the beginning of our series the pre-sigmoid approach was used more frequently. Today, for large tumors we prefer to stage the surgical procedure using initially a fronto-orbito-zygomatic approach, and 2 weeks later remove the remnant lesion through a retrosigmoid access. According to our experience, patients tolerate better two short-duration surgeries than a single, long-lasting surgical procedure. Conventional radiotherapy, focused radiosurgical techniques, and radiosurgery have been used as adjuvant therapy for tumor rests or primary treatment for small (up to 3 cm in diameter) petroclival meningiomas. Subach et al. [25] reported a series of 62 patients

Table 1 Surgical complications (67 cases)

| Complications | No. of patients |
|---|---|
| Brainstem stroke/hemiparesis | 2 |
| Postoperative hematoma | 1 |
| New cranial nerve deficits | |
| III | 5 (3 transient) |
| IV | 4 (3 transient) |
| V | 3 (1 transient) |
| VI | 7 (3 transient) |
| VII | 8 (5 transient) |
| VIII | 8 |
| IX, X, XI | 6 (3 transient) |
| Death | 0 |

Table 2   Literature review of series of petroclival meningiomas

| Authors | No. of cases | Resection (%) | Mortality (%) | Morbidity (%) | New cranial nerve deficits (%) |
|---|---|---|---|---|---|
| Yasargil et al. [27] | 20 | 35 | 10 | 30 | 50 |
| Mayberg and Simon [12] | 35 | 26 | 9 | 34 | 54 |
| Al-Mefty et al. [3] | 13 | 85 | | 8 | 31 |
| Hakuba et al. [7] | 8 | 75 | 12 | 38 | 100 |
| Samii et al. [18] | 24 | 71 | | 17 | 46 |
| Bricolo et al. [4] | 33 | 79 | 9 | 18 | 76 |
| Kawase et al. [10] | 42 | 76 | | 12 | 36 |
| Sekhar et al. [21] | 75 | 60 | 3 | 16 | 60 |
| Couldwell et al. [6] | 109 | 69 | 3,7 | 15 | 33 |
| Abdel Aziz et al. [1] | 35 | 37 | | 9 | 31 |
| Present series | | | | | |
| Total | 67 | 55 | 3 | 12 | 33 |
| Small | 12 | 100 | 0 | 0 | 0 |

with petroclival meningiomas treated with radiosurgery. After a follow-up period of 37 months, tumor volumes decreased in 14 (23%), remained stable in 42 (68%), and increased in 5 (8%). Roche et al. [17] treated 32 petroclival meningiomas with gamma-knife surgery (GKS). Twenty-four patients were primarily treated by this method. In a follow-up from 24 to 118 months (mean 52.6 months), they observed no change in tumor volume in 28 cases and a slight decreased in 4 cases. Two patients with larger tumors presented with permanent hemiparesis due to focal pontine infarction. Linskey et al. [11] compared 38 patients treated with GKS with 35 patients treated with surgery (Simpson's grade 1 or 2; resection in 86.1%). In the group treated by GKS, tumor volume was smaller (7.85 cm³) than in the surgical group (44.4 cm³). They concluded that both treatments are safe and effective. According to our experience, surgery should be the treatment of choice for small petroclival meningiomas (up to 3 cm in diameter). These small lesions can be totally removed (Simpson's grade 1) with preservation of the involved structures (Table 2). Surgery gives these patients the only chance of cure from this benign tumor. Radiotherapy may present good results with respect to cranial nerve preservation and control of tumor growth, but all patients remain with a residual tumor that may grow. Development of malignant neoplasms after radiotherapy have been described in the literature [22, 23, 28].

Adjuvant treatment with chemotherapy (hydroxyurea) or hormonal therapy (mifepristone) has been described, but the results were not satisfactory.

## 13.10
## Conclusion

In the majority of cases, petroclival meningiomas are benign lesions. Total resection is the only treatment that may cure these tumors, but may be not possible due to involvement and invasion of the cavernous sinus, cranial nerves, vessels, and pia mater. The size, consistency, and biological behavior of the tumor are other limiting factors. Choice of surgical approach and surgeon experience are very important to achieve good results. In our series, small tumors (up to 3 cm in diameter) obtained the best surgical results. These patients are also more suitable for radiosurgery.

## References

1.  Abdel Aziz KM, Sanan A, van Loveren HR, et al (2000) Petroclival meningiomas: predictive parameters for transpetrosal approaches. Neurosurgery 47:139–152

2. Aguiar PHP, Rotta JM, Pereira CU (2001) Cistos epidermóides cranianos. In: Pereira CU, Aguiar PHP, Ramina R (eds) Cisto Epidermóides Cranianos. Revinter, Rio de Janeiro, pp 53–57

3. Al-Mefty O, Fox JL, Smith RR (1988) Petrosal approach for petroclival meningiomas. Neurosurgery 22:510–517

4. Bricolo AP, Turazzi S, Talachi A (1992) Microsurgical removal of petroclival meningiomas. A report of 33 patients. Neurosurgery 31:813–828

5. Castellano F, Ruggiero G (1953) Meningiomas of the posterior fossa. Acta Radiol 104:1–177

6. Couldwell WT, Fukushima T, Giannotta SL, et al (1996) Petroclival meningiomas: surgical experience in 109 cases. J Neurosurg 84:20–28

7. Hakuba A, Nishimura S, Jang BJ (1988) A combined retroauricular and preauricular transpetrosal-transtentorial approach to clivus meningiomas. Surg Neurol 30:108–116

8. House JW, Brackmann DE (1985) Facial nerve grading system. Otolaryngol Head Neck Surg 93:146–147

9. Jung HW, Yoo H, Paek SH, et al (2000) Long term outcome and growth rate of subtotally resected petroclival meningiomas. Experience with 38 cases. Neurosurgery 46:567–575

10. Kawase T, Shiobara R, Toya S (1994) Middle fossa transpetrosal-transtentorial approaches for petroclival meningiomas: selective pyramid resection and radicality. Acta Neurochir (Wien) 129:113–120

11. Linskey ME, Davis SA, Ratanatharathom V (2005) Relative roles of microsurgery and stereotactic radiosurgery for the treatment of patients with cranial meningiomas: a single-surgeon 4-year integrated experience with both modalities. J Neurosurg 102:59–70

12. Mayberg MR, Symon LD (1986) Meningiomas of the clivus and apical petrous bone: report of 35 cases. J Neurosurg 65:160–167

13. McElveen JT Jr, Dorfman BE, Fukushima T (2001) Petroclival tumors: a synthesis. Otol Clin North Am 34:1219–1230

14. Meneses MS, Moreira AL, Bordignon KC, et al (2004) Surgical approaches to the petrous apex: distances and relations with cranial morphology. Skull Base 14:9–20

15. Ramina R, Coelho Neto M, Fernandes YB, et al (2006) Meningiomas petroclivais diagnóstico, tratamento e resultados. In: Aguiar PHP, Ramina R, Veiga JCE, Tella O Jr (eds) Meningiomas. Diagnóstico e Tratamento Clínico e Cirúrgico. Aspectos Atuais. Revinter, Rio de Janeiro pp 174–184

16. Ramina R, Coelho Neto M, Meneses MS, et al (1997) Management of chordomas and chondrosarcomas of the skull base. Crit Rev Neurosurg 7:141–148

17. Roche PH, Pellet W, Fuentes S, et al (2003) Gamma knife radiosurgical management of petroclival meningiomas results and indications. Acta Neurochir (Wien) 145 883–888

18. Samii M, Tatagiba M (1992) Experience with 36 surgical cases of petroclival meningiomas. Acta Neurochir (Wien) 118:27–32

19. Samii M, Ammirati M, Mahran A, et al (1989) Surgery of petroclival meningiomas: report of 24 cases. Neurosurgery 24:12–17

20. Samii M, Migliori M, Tatagiba M (1995) Surgical treatment of trigeminal schwannomas. J Neurosurg 82:711–718

21. Sekhar LN, Swamy KS, Jaiswal V (1994) Surgical excision of meningiomas involving the clivus: preoperative and intraoperative features as predictos of postoperative functional deterioration. J Neurosurg 81:860–868

22. Shamisa A, Bance M, Nag S, et al (2001) Glioblastoma multiforme occurring in a patient treated with gamma knife surgery: case report and review of the literature. J Neurosurg 94:816–821

23. Shin M, Ueki K, Kurita H, et al (2002) Malignant transformation of a vestibular schwannoma after gamma knife radiosurgery. Lancet 360:309–310

24. Spetzler RF, Hamilton MG, Daspit CP (1994) Petroclival lesions. Clin Neurosurg 41:62–82

25. Subach BR, Lunsford LD, Kondziolka D (1998) Management of petroclival meningiomas by stereotactic radiosurgery. Neurosurgery 42:437–443

26. Van Havenberg T, Carvalho G, Tatagiba M, et al (2003) Natural history of petroclival meningiomas. Neurosurgery 52:55–64

27. Yasargil M, Mortara R, Curcic M (1980) Meningiomas of basal posterior cranial fossa. Adv Tech Stand Neurosurg 7:3–115

28. Yu JS, Yong WH, Wilson D (2000) Glioblastoma induction after radiosurgery for meningioma. Lancet 356:1576–1577

# Retrosigmoid Approach to the Posterior and Middle Fossae

**14**

Marcos Tatagiba
and Marcus André Acioly

## Contents

"Our years of experience treating skull base lesions have allowed us to recognize a number of cases in which the use of extensive skull base procedures does not improve the surgical result and in fact may endanger it."
Samii and Tatagiba [43]

## 14.1
## Introduction

Since the first description of the unilateral approach to the cerebellopontine angle (CPA) in 1903 by Fedor Krause [22, 23], several techniques were developed by Cushing [7], Seiffert [47], Dandy [8–10], House [18, 19], and Fisch [13] among others in order to access the CPA structures. Surgery of the CPA is ruled by three approaches: the transtemporal extradural approach, the transmastoid translabyrinthine approach, and the lateral suboccipital or retrosigmoid approach [37].

The retrosigmoid approach provides a wide exposure of the CPA structures [5, 31, 37, 43, 55] and may be extended inferiorly through the far-lateral transcondylar approach [5] and far-lateral retrocondylar approach [38, 43], or superiorly through the retrosigmoid intradural suprameatal approach (RISA) [31, 44, 45, 49]. Extensive skull-base approaches may greatly increase the surgical morbidity and consequently the risk of postoperative neurological deficits [43]. Therefore, the simple retrosigmoid approach has gained more and more interest [43]:

"Gross, partial or total petrosectomy should be performed only if it is believed that it will facilitate tumor removal, increase surgical completeness, and improve outcome by increasing survival and reducing morbidity." [43]

This is Prof. Samii's philosophy and it has been integrated into our daily practice.

Herein, we discuss the surgical techniques underlying the retrosigmoid approach to the posterior fossa and the to the middle fossa, as well as their clinical applications. The detailed depiction of single pathologies is described elsewhere in this book.

## 14.2
## Preoperative Evaluation

Cranial computed tomography (CT) and/or magnetic resonance imaging (MRI) are performed for all patients enrolled for CPA surgery. For microvascular decompression, the radiological examination is accomplished mainly to rule out secondary causes of neurovascular conflicts such as tumors or arachnoid cysts. MRI is preferred in the evaluation of intrinsic lesions such as multiple sclerosis, as well as in the identification of the offending vessel or vessels.

For the semisitting position, the preoperative evaluation includes functional cervical spine x-rays to exclude cervical instability and a transthoracic echocardiography to confirm a patent foramen ovale. In patients with neurofibromatosis type 2, we usually perform a cervical spine MRI due to associations with another central nervous system tumors.

Pure tone audiogram, speech discrimination, somatosensory evoked potentials (SSEPs), and brainstem audi-

tory evoked potentials (BAEPs) are considered in patients suffering from pathologies in the vicinities of the facial-vestibulocochlear nerve bundle. These patients are classified according to Hannover Classification of hearing conditions and BAEPs [26, 39].

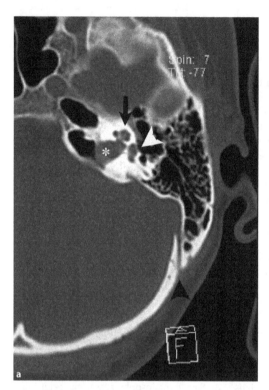
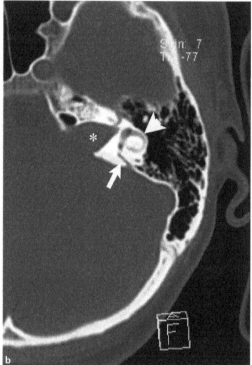
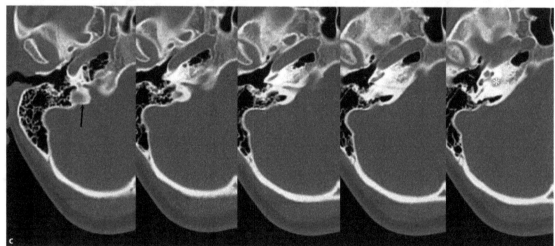

Fig. 1a–c Preoperative thin-slice temporal bone computed tomography (CT) scans. **a** Note the close relationship between the cochlea (*black arrow*), vestibule (*white arrowhead*), and internal auditory canal (*asterisk*). The emissary vein (*black arrowhead*) is seen on its way to the sigmoid sinus. **b** The relationship between the endolymphatic duct (*white arrow*) and the labyrinth structures (*white arrowhead*), and internal auditory canal (*asterisk*). **c** Normal position of the jugular bulb (*black arrow*) 4 mm below the internal auditory canal (*asterisk*)

High-resolution bony CT scans (slice thickness 1 mm) of the petrous bone provide information regarding the position of the labyrinth and endolymphatic duct, as well as the height of the jugular bulb (Fig. 1). This is essential information that will determine the boundaries of the bone resection, particularly in patients scheduled for vestibular schwannoma surgery or RISA. Also, the size of the emissary vein is noted and considered for surgical planning (Fig. 1). For vestibular schwannomas, T2-weighted MRI scans are useful to observe whether the tumor reaches the end of the internal auditory canal (IAC), because the complete filling of the IAC has a negative impact on hearing preservation (Fig. 2).

Cerebral angiography is sometimes required for meningiomas. Less commonly, tumor intravascular embolization is needed to diminish intraoperative bleeding and reduce operative morbidity.

## 14.3
## Retrosigmoid Approach to the Posterior Fossa

### 14.3.1
### Surgical Technique

The operation is carried out with general anesthesia and with the patient in the supine, park-bench, or semisit-

ting position [55]. The semisitting position is the authors' preference. However, the supine position is preferred in cases of microvascular decompression or patent foramen ovale. At surgery, bilateral SSEPs and electrophysiological monitoring of ipsilateral cranial nerves VII and VIII are performed for upper CPA lesions. For large tumors and lower CPA lesions, the electrophysiological records of the caudal cranial nerves are also monitored.

The head is fixed with a Mayfield frame such that a single pin is placed on the side of the lesion around the linea temporalis and anterior to the external auditory canal. Paired pins are also applied around the linea temporalis on the contralateral side. The patient is then placed in a semisitting position with the head hyperextended, turned 30° toward the affected side, and flexed. The legs are raised to or above the level of the heart and the knees are slightly flexed (Fig. 3). Thus, the venous pressure can be raised and therefore the risk of air embolus is reduced. SSEPs are recorded continuously on both sides during the positioning. In the event of changes of latency or amplitude, the surgeon should be warned in order to correct the patient's position. A precordial Doppler device is attached to detect air emboli. Recently, air emboli have been monitored with the aid of transesophageal echocardiography.

The hair is shaved to simplify the identification of the surface anatomy. A slightly curved skin incision is drawn with a skin marker extending superiorly 2 cm behind the pinna, passing through the asterion and terminating

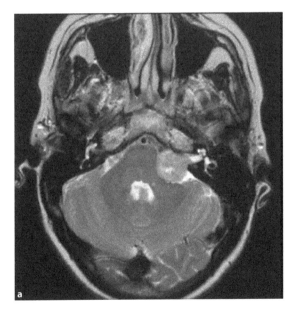 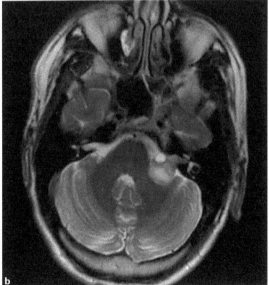

Fig. 2a,b Preoperative T2-weighted magnetic resonance imaging (MRI) scans showing vestibular schwannomas of similar sizes, but with different intrameatal extensions. **a** The tumor does not reach the fundus of the internal auditory canal. Note the collection of cerebrospinal fluid (CSF) between the tumor and the fundus. **b** The tumor reaches the fundus, completely filling the internal auditory canal

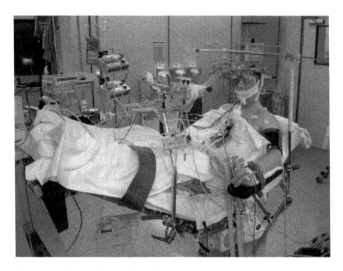

Fig. 3 View of the Mayfield fixation and surgical semisitting position with the legs at the level of the heart

1–2 cm medial to the mastoid tip (Fig. 4). The inferior border of the skin incision depends on the need of caudal extension. No local anesthetic is used. The skin flap is elevated with the periosteum and held with a skin retractor. The neck muscles are divided in line with the skin incision and retracted with a self-retaining Leyla retractor.

The burr hole is made below the asterion and then a suboccipital craniectomy is carried out with rongeurs toward the transverse and sigmoid sinus and the squamous part of the occipital bone. The asterion and the posterior part of the parietomastoid suture allow a good estima-

tion of the extracranial projection of the transition of the transverse–sigmoid sinuses [32], and therefore constitute the superolateral limit of the craniectomy [5, 32] (Fig. 5). Virtual reality in image guidance may also be used to confirm in real time the position of the dural sinuses and their relationship with bone landmarks, thereby facilitating the surgical planning [33]. Usually, a suboccipital craniectomy of about 3–4 cm in diameter is sufficient to approach the CPA.

A high-speed diamond drill is used to expose the borders of the transverse sinus, the transition of the

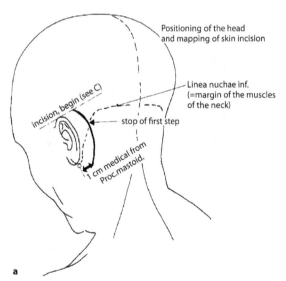

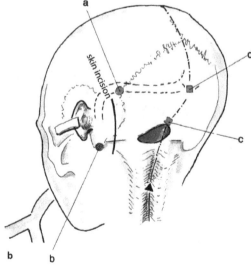

Fig. 4a,b The surface landmarks are examined (courtesy of Professor Wolfgang Seeger). **a** The skin incision extends from 2 cm behind the pinna to 1–2 cm medial to the mastoid tip. *Proc. mastoid.* Mastoid process, inf. inferior. **b** Drawing of the course of the transverse and sigmoid sinus, as well as the transverse–sigmoid sinus transition (*black dotted line*) *a* Asterion, *b* mastoid tip, *c* opisthion, *d* inion

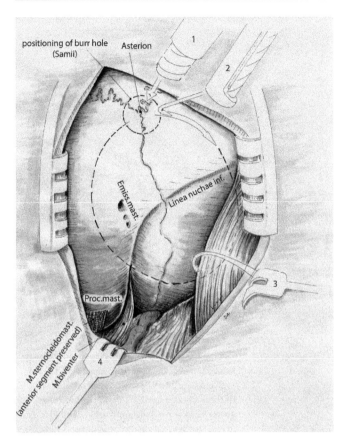

Fig. 5 Note the placement of the burr hole near to the left asterion (*1*) (courtesy of Professor Wolfgang Seeger). The *black dotted lines* correspond approximately to the area of the suboccipital craniectomy. *Emiss. mast.* Mastoid emissary vein, *M. sternodcleidomast.* sternocleidomastoid muscle, *M. biventer* biventer muscle

transverse–sigmoid sinuses, and the sigmoid sinus (Fig. 6). Continuous irrigation provides cooling during drilling. Bone wax is used to pack the mastoid air cells and the emissary vein. Care should be taken with the emissary vein when operating on a patient in the semisitting position because its laceration may precipitate the formation of an air embolus. When a large emissary vein is detected on the preoperative temporal bone thin-slice CT, we prefer to skeletonize the vein with a fine diamond burr and coagulate it under direct view. Smaller craniectomies are accomplished if microvascular decompression is planned, directed to the upper or lower CPA [28, 31, 32, 37].

Supporting armrests are attached to the operating table, providing more comfort and accuracy for the surgeon. The dura is opened in a C-shaped, medially based fashion along the transverse and sigmoid sinus [37, 43] under magnification using an operating microscope. The opening is performed some millimeters away from the sinuses to allow closure [37, 43]. Auxiliary oblique incisions at the angles of the primary incision increase the surgical view [37], but it is not routinely necessary. Three or four tack-up sutures are placed with further increase of the surgical view, thereby reducing the amount of cerebellar retraction required (Fig. 7). Solely upper or lower incisions are performed according to the underlying pathology encountered in the upper or lower CPA, respectively [37].

With a narrow brain retractor and a fine bayonet forceps, the surgeon opens the cerebrospinal fluid (CSF) cisterns. We use cotton strips to protect the cerebellum against lacerations. Thus, CSF is withdrawn, then relaxing the cerebellum (Fig. 8). Further brain relaxation may be achieved with mannitol administered intravenously at the time of skin incision. Thereafter, the brain retractors have a more protective effect without significant compression on the cerebellum. Oblique and smooth movements of the brain spatula on the cerebellum are preferred rather than longitudinal stretching through the facial-vestibulocochlear nerve bundle in order to avoid damage to the vestibulocochlear nerve [17, 26, 51, 54]. In addition, for vestibular schwannoma and upper CPA tumors, smooth movements of the brain spatula are required to prevent the occurrence of trigeminocardiac reflex [14, 16, 21]. The foramen of Luschka and the lateral recess of the fourth ventricle are reached with a slight elevation of the cerebellar flocculus. The subsequent steps are determined for the pathology and are described below.

One advantage of the semisitting position is spontaneous drainage of CSF and blood, which, allied to suction

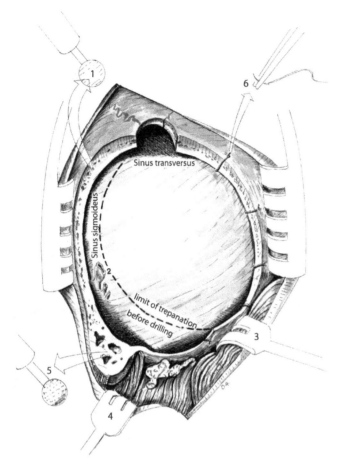

Fig. 6 Schematic view of suboccipital craniectomy before and after the drilling (courtesy of Professor Wolfgang Seeger). The *black dotted line* indicates the limit of bone resection performed with rongeurs. A high-speed diamond drill (*1* and *5*) is used to enlarge the craniectomy, bringing into view the transverse–sigmoid sinus transition, as well as the transverse and sigmoid sinuses

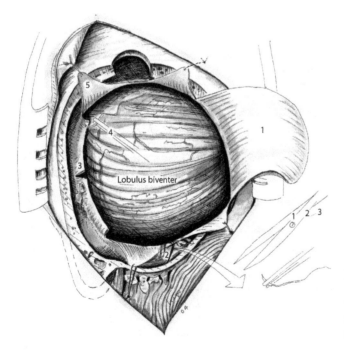

Fig. 7 Schematic view of retrosigmoid approach (courtesy of Professor Wolfgang Seeger) showing the C-shaped dural flap (*1*) and the tack-up sutures (*5*). Small oblique incisions are usually not necessary (*3*)

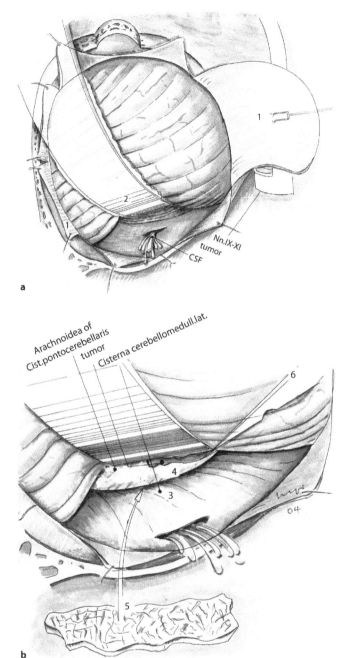

**a**

Arachnoidea of
Cist.pontocerebellaris        Cisterna cerebellomedull.lat.
                      tumor

**b**

Fig. 8 Schematic view representing the opening of the lateral cerebellomedullary cistern (courtesy of Professor Wolfgang Seeger). **a** By elevating the cerebellum using a narrow brain spatula, the surgeon opens the CSF cistern with a fine bayonet forceps. **b** amplified view demonstrating one of the most important steps of the surgical approach. *Nn. IX–XI* Cranial nerves IX–XI, *Cist.* Cisterna, *cerebellomedull. lat.* cerebellomedullaris lateralis

irrigators with saline solution, provides a clean surgical field, thereby reducing the dissection time. At the end of the procedure, jugular vein compression is performed by the anesthesiologist to search for possible venous bleeding, especially if the patient is in the semisitting position. Hemostasis is achieved with the utmost care.

The dural flaps are gathered with single, nonresorbable sutures, and then a continuous suture closes the dural opening in a watertight fashion. A dural patch is seldom needed due to the C-shaped opening. Cranioplasty is performed with methyl methacrylate. The mastoid cells are covered with muscle and fibrin glue. The neck muscles are sutured back, respecting the anatomical layers. No drains are used. A compressive bandage is used after the skin closure.

### 14.3.2
### Clinical Applications

#### 14.3.2.1
#### Microvascular Decompression

Microvascular decompressions at the CPA are performed with the patient in the supine position with the head turned to the contralateral side. After the standard craniectomy and dural opening, the cerebellomedullary cisterns are opened to gain CSF and relax the brain. Cerebellum will collapse a bit so that the brain retractor can be applied without compressing the cerebellum. The brain retractor is placed at the edge of the petrotentorial junction accompanying the superior petrosal sinus for trigeminal nerve decompression. Care should be taken with the petrosal vein. Although some authors advocate its ligature without additional morbidity [28, 31], we prefer to preserve the petrosal vein whenever possible, since closure of the petrosal vein has been related to complications such as cerebellar edema or bleeding [15, 34].

For hemifacial spasm, the lower cranial nerves are identified prior to expose of the facial nerve. Then dissection is done upward toward the brainstem to avoid stretching of the facial-vestibulocochlear nerve bundle. Vascular compression is usually identified at the facial nerve exit zone at the brainstem. Use of an endoscope to assist microsurgery in cases of trigeminal neuralgia or hemifacial spasm may enhance visualization behind the nerves [2, 3, 20].

#### 14.3.2.2
#### Vestibular Schwannoma

The CPA and the tumor are exposed after opening the lateral cerebellomedullary cistern with a fine bayonet forceps, and the cerebellum is slightly lifted with a narrow brain retractor attached to a self-retaining Leyla retractor

(Fig. 9). We prefer initially to open the internal auditory canal (IAC) as a first step to early identify cranial nerves VII and VIII and reduction of intracanalicular pressure [1, 24]. Elevated intracanalicular pressure may impair the blood supply to the cochlear nerve and labyrinth [1, 24]. An ischemic inner ear environment may be further worsened by traction, tumor debulking, or the hypotension precipitated by the trigeminocardiac reflex [16], thus decreasing the chances of hearing preservation. Therefore, the mean arterial blood pressure is maintained around 90 mmHg to avoid the negative impact of the hypotension on auditory function [16].

To open the IAC a C-shaped dural opening of about 1×1 cm is performed based on the posterior lip of the IAC and directed superolaterally. Navigation-guided opening of the IAC was attempted to direct the drilling due to the anatomical variability of the labyrinth structures [35]. We start with a large cutting burr that is progressively replaced for smaller diamond burrs as the IAC is approached (Fig. 10). Irrigation is used for cooling. The roof of the IAC is the best anatomical landmark for removal of the posterior wall [37]. The length of drilling is determined by the preoperative bone-windowed CT, but usually 8 mm is sufficient for adequate exposure of the intrameatal contents. Further drilling increases the risk of damage to the semicircular canals. The IAC dura is opened longitudinally (Fig. 11). Once the tumor is identified, piecemeal debulking is started with microscissors and tumor forceps. A short hook is used to create the arachnoid plane between the tumor and the nerves. Then, a long hook is introduced from medial to lateral to palpate the IAC fundus and to remove the tumor. Pulling the tumor medially is avoided to reduce stretching of the tiny cochlear fibers. En bloc removal is possible for small tumors. The facial nerve is usually displaced anterosuperiorly and the cochlear nerve anteroinferiorly. Monopolar stimulation is frequently used to identify the facial nerve into the IAC (Fig. 12).

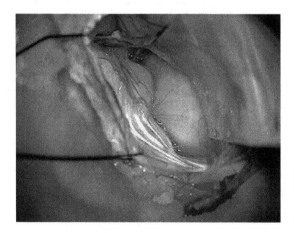

Fig. 9 Intraoperative view of a large vestibular schwannoma (type IVa) demonstration cerebellar retraction with a narrow, curved brain retractor. The petrosal vein is observed on its course to the superior petrosal sinus

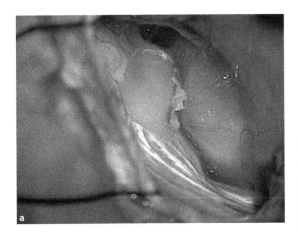

Fig. 10a–b Intraoperative view of the dural incision directed superolaterally, precluding endolymphatic duct injury (courtesy of Professor Wolfgang Seeger). Schematic view of the opening of the internal auditory canal (IAC) by using progressively smaller diamond burrs. The roof of the IAC is an important anatomical landmark guiding the bone removal

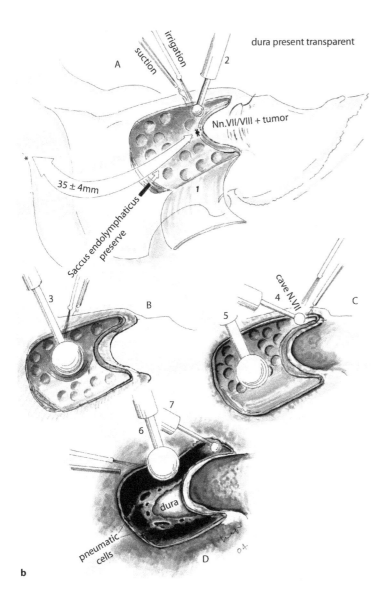

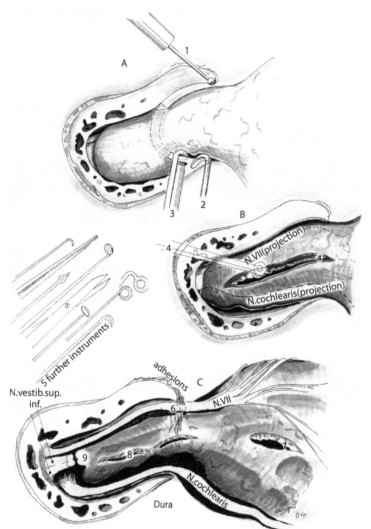

A

1

3    2

B

4    N.VII(projection)    4

N.cochlearis(projection)

5 further instruments

N.vestib.sup.
inf.

adhesions    C

6    N.VII

9    8

N.cochlearis

Dura

Fig. 11 **a** Following bone removal, the tiny
bones attached to the edges of the IAC are
removed by using a small diamond burr
(*1*) or fine hooks (*2*). **b** The dura is opened
longitudinally and tumor debulking is
initiated intrameatally (*4*). **c** Thereafter,
the facial, cochlear and vestibular nerves
are exposed (**c**). Courtesy of Professor
Wolfgang Seeger. *N. vestib. sup.* Superior
vestibular nerve, *inf.* inferior

Thereafter, the dissection is taken toward the CPA.
The tumor capsule is opened and used to develop the
arachnoid plane. The tumor is progressively debulked
with microscissors, tumor forceps, and an ultrasonic
aspirator. When the capsule is relaxed, we use a tumor
forceps to hold the tumor and a fine bayonet forceps to
create the arachnoid plane (Fig. 13). Then, debulking
and dissection are subsequently alternated in a stepwise
manner. In tumors of an extremely soft or too hard consistency, as well as in cystic vestibular schwannomas, the
plane development may be difficult to achieve. The site
of maximal adhesion, normally in the IAC, is dissected at
the end. The branch of the vestibular nerve is transected
and the tumor is removed without jeopardizing the facial and cochlear nerves. To assure the completeness of
removal, an endoscope may be introduced to examine

the IAC fundus and remove eventual tumor remnants
[52].

At the end of the procedure, a short jugular vein compression is performed by the anesthesiologist to verify hemostasis. The IAC is sealed with a piece of muscle and fibrin
glue. The remaining steps were described previously.

**14.3.2.3**

## CPA Meningioma

These meningiomas are classified according to the location of the tumor in relationship to the IAC. The tumors
may arise anteriorly (group 1), involve the IAC (group 2),
superiorly (group 3), inferiorly (group 4), or posteriorly
(group 5) to the IAC [30]. The operative strategies and

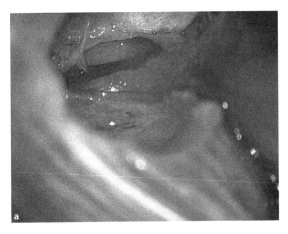

Fig. 12 Intraoperative view following piecemeal tumor debulking. The facial comes into view displaced usually anterosuperiorly (left). Identification of the facial nerve within the IAC through monopolar stimulation is sometimes required (right)

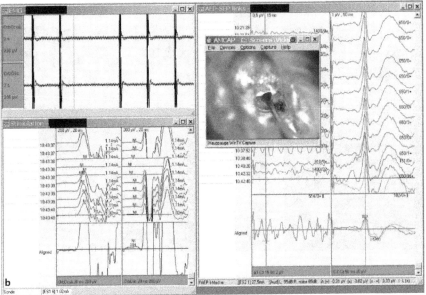

functional facial and cochlear nerve outcomes are different among the groups [30, 43]. After opening of the cerebellomedullary cistern, anterior meningiomas are removed between the cranial nerve bundles, mostly between the trigeminal and facial-vestibulocochlear nerves. For the groups 2–5, the tumors should be debulked and reduced in size to identify these nerves. The IAC is eventually opened in tumors with primary or secondary IAC extension.

The dural attachment is coagulated and resected. Hyperostosis is drilled with a diamond burr in order to ensure complete resection. Also, this region has a rich blood supply and drilling is useful to promote effective hemostasis [37]. Muscle piece and fibrin glue are used to occlude the exposed bone and mastoid cells. The next steps proceed as detailed previously.

## 14.3.2.4
## Epidermoid Cyst

After entering the CPA, a pearly tumor is identified. Epidermoid cysts spread through CSF cisterns encasing the nerve bundles rather than infiltrating or displacing them [11, 29, 46]. The CPA is divided into four compartments, as follows: between the tentorium and the trigeminal nerve; between the trigeminal and facial-vestibulocochlear nerves; between the facial-vestibulocochlear nerve bundle and the lower cranial nerves; below the lower cranial nerves [46]. The cyst is resected in each compartment from the bone toward the brainstem, that is, in a lateral-to-medial direction. Thus, the identification of the cranial nerves is facilitated due to the relatively well-preserved anatomy at the bony entrance [46]. Total tumor removal

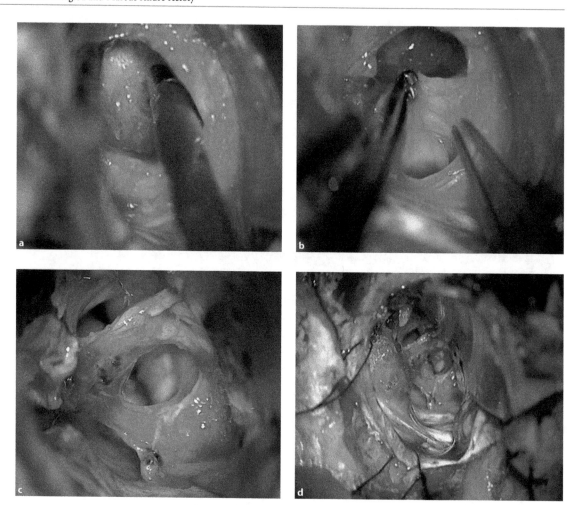

Fig. 13a–d Intraoperative view of a large vestibular schwannoma. The tumor located on the cerebellopontine angle is debulked with ultrasonic aspirator (**a**). While the capsule is relaxed, the arachnoid plane is separated by using two forceps: one tumor forceps to hold the tumor and a fine bayonet forceps to create the plane. Note the lower cranial nerves (**b**). Final aspect following complete tumor resection. The facial, superior vestibular and cochlear nerves are anatomically preserved (**c**). Afterward meticulous hemostasis, the IAC is sealed with a piece of muscle and fibrin glue (**d**)

is attempted; nonetheless, small and adherent capsule remnants could be left, avoiding additional postoperative morbidity. The closure is performed as usual.

### 14.3.2.5
### Other Space-Occupying Lesions

Schwannomas and meningiomas of the jugular foramen, cavernomas of the IAC, aneurysms, ependymomas, plexus papillomas, arachnoid cysts, and metastases, among others can also be removed by the retrosigmoid approach. The surgical technique has the same principles as described in the preceding sections.

### 14.3.2.6
### Auditory Brainstem Implant and Auditory Midbrain Implant

The skin incision is extended superiorly to the parieto-occipital area where the bony bed for the auditory brainstem implant (ABI) receiver is placed. After vestibular schwannoma resection, the microsurgical dissection is directed toward the foramen of Luschka. The choroid plexus, the caudal cranial nerves, and the cerebellar flocculus are used as landmarks. Then, the flocculus is slightly elevated together with the choroid plexus, and the tela choroidea comes into field. It is opened and the lateral recess of the fourth ventricle is entered. Thereafter, the cochlear nuclei are identified bulging from the floor

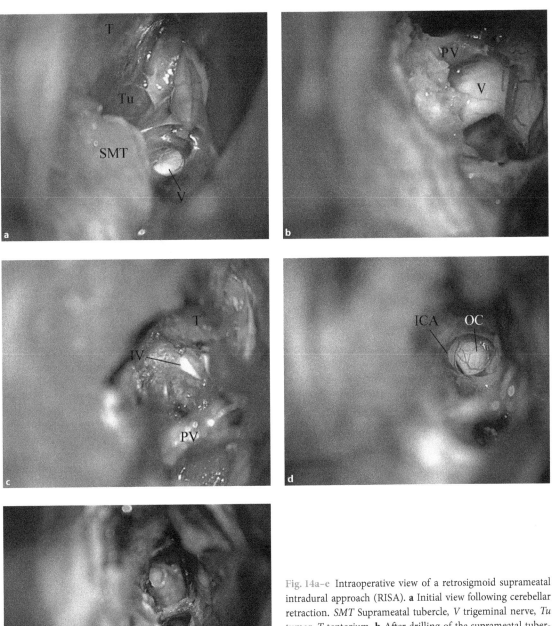

Fig. 14a–e Intraoperative view of a retrosigmoid suprameatal intradural approach (RISA). **a** Initial view following cerebellar retraction. *SMT* Suprameatal tubercle, *V* trigeminal nerve, *Tu* tumor, *T* tentorium. **b** After drilling of the suprameatal tubercle, the trigeminal nerve may be mobilized. *PV* Petrosal vein. **c** Following tentorium splitting, the trochlear nerve (*IV*) is localized at the free tentorial edge. **d** At the completion of tumor resection, the internal carotid artery (*ICA*) and the optic chiasm (*OC*) come into view. **e** Overall view following tumor removal, showing the extent of bone resection and preservation of the petrosal vein

of the fourth ventricle. The electrode array is placed with a fine forceps and inserted into the lateral recess [6]. Multimodal monitoring then takes over to find the optimal ABI positioning [6, 27]. The Dacron mesh of the electrode cable is fixed with fibrin glue to the petrous ridge.

A second-generation brainstem implant has been developed for patients with neural deafness associated with cochlear nucleus damage [25, 36]. The usual indication is presence of neurofibromatosis type 2. The device is called an auditory midbrain implant [25, 36], where a penetrating electrode is placed into the inferior colliculus central nucleus [25, 36]. 'A combined retrosigmoid approach extended with a lateral supracerebellar approach to the inferior colliculus provides sufficient exposure for both procedures.

## 14.4
## RISA to the Middle Fossa

### 14.4.1
### Surgical Technique

The initial steps are similar those described for the retrosigmoid approach to the posterior fossa. After CSF release and cerebellar retraction, additional exposure is gained. The petrosal vein is preserved whenever possible. Large tumors may greatly displace, compress, or encase the petrosal vein. In these cases, a strong collateral venous circulation may allow petrosal vein ligature without additional operative morbidity [45].

Large tumors are typically encountered anterior to the facial-vestibulocochlear nerve bundle, which is displaced inferiorly and posteriorly [45]. Tumor is debulked in its CPA portion with the aid of an ultrasonic aspirator, microscissors, and tumor forceps. After debulking, the dura above the suprameatal portion of the petrous bone is incised and resected. This part of the petrous bone is called the suprameatal tubercle, which blocks the view of the trigeminal nerve and upper clivus [31, 49]. Drilling is performed with a diamond burr under continuous irrigation for cooling. Further drilling is directed toward the dorsolateral portion of the trigeminal nerve. Meckel's cave is reached and entered [4, 45]. Thereafter, the trigeminal nerve may be mobilized laterally and medially, improving the surgical view. Smooth movements are recommended, preventing the occurrence of trigeminocardiac reflex [16, 21]. In addition, the tentorium may be opened, thus increasing the surgeon's working field by the exposure of the posterior part of the middle fossa. The incision is carried out 2 cm away and parallel to the superior petrosal sinus in the direction of the free tentorial edge. Care should be taken with the trochlear nerve near to the free tentorial edge (Fig. 14). With large tumors, the corridor created by their growth allows visualization up to the middle fossa without further cerebellar retraction [45]. Endoscope-assisted RISA provides an

additional view of the anteromedial middle fossa, and sellar and parasellar regions [12].

At the completion of tumor resection, prior to dura closure, jugular vein compression is done by to detect any possible venous bleeding. Muscle pieces and fibrin glue seal the exposed petrous bone. The dura is closed in a watertight fashion. The cranioplasty and closure of the neck muscles and the wound are as standard.

### 14.4.2
### Clinical Application

#### 14.4.2.1
#### Petroclival Meningioma

These tumors may present major extensions into the middle or posterior fossa or grow in a dumbbell fashion [45]. Large tumors that encase the cranial nerves are debulked piecemeal with the aid of an ultrasound aspirator. The dissection is carried out starting from the bone toward the brainstem using the same principles described for epidermoid cysts. En bloc resection is discouraged to prevent damage to the cranial nerves. RISA is accomplished as described above. Opening the tentorium provides exposure of the posterior middle fossa. It is performed with a surgical blade 2 cm away and along the superior petrosal sinus. The incision is then extended toward the free edge of the tentorium with microscissors. The trochlear nerve is dissected and preserved near to the free tentorial edge. The tumor is pulled with fine hooks or curettes, which, allied to the gravitational effect of the surgical positioning (semisitting), promotes an extensive resection including the tentorial dural attachment. Radical tumor removal is achieved with RISA in the majority of patients (Fig. 15) [44, 45]. Extension to the cavernous sinus precludes radical removal through this approach. On the other hand, it is particularly useful in elderly patients in whom decompression is the major surgical goal [45].

#### 14.4.2.2
#### Trigeminal Schwannoma

Trigeminal schwannomas may extend predominantly into the middle fossa (type A), the posterior fossa (type B), in a dumbbell fashion (type C), or extracranially (type D) [42]. RISA is performed when the major tumor bulk is encountered in the posterior fossa with extension to the middle fossa through the Meckel's cave [4]. After the initial exposure, the capsule is opened and the tumor debulked. When the capsule becomes relaxed, a tumor forceps is used to hold the tumor and a fine bayonet forceps separates the arachnoid plane. The surgical steps are similar to those used for removal of vestibular schwannomas. Dissection should be meticulous in order to prevent vascular lesions [42].

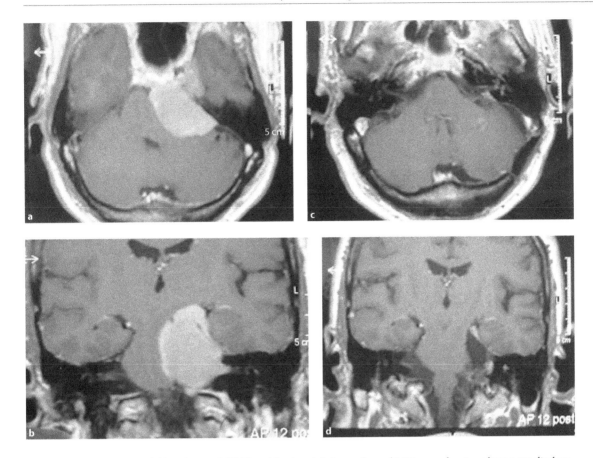

Fig. 15a–d Preoperative axial (**a**) and coronal (**b**) T1-weighted, gadolinium-enhanced MRI scans showing a large petroclival meningioma on the left side. **c,d** The tumor was radically removed following RISA

### 14.4.2.3
### Other Space-Occupying Lesions

Several lesions such as epidermoid cysts, chordomas, chondrosarcomas, and chondromas are also encountered in the petroclival region [4, 45]. The surgical technique is as described previously.

### 14.5
### Complications

The transverse sinus, the sigmoid sinus, or the transition of the transverse-sigmoid sinuses can be damaged during craniectomy. Small lacerations are treated with Surgicel or a muscle piece. Large lacerations demand sinus wall reconstruction. The sinus is exposed under the magnification of the operating microscope and sutured [48].

Cerebellar laceration is prone to occur with the use of brain spatulas. Petrosal vein lacerations are managed with Surgicel and cottonoid pack compression at the superior petrosal sinus, and coagulation at the free end of the vein at the cerebellar surface [28].

In drilling the IAC, the labyrinth can be accidentally damaged. Immediate occlusion can be achieved with bone wax without aspiration at the damaged area [53]. Also, inadvertent avulsion of a high jugular bulb can occur at this stage. In such cases, hemostasis is accomplished with muscle pieces and fibrin glue occlusion while the anesthesiologist promotes jugular vein compression to avoid an air embolus [50]. Cranial nerve disruption, particularly the trochlear nerve when accessing the tentorium, and the facial nerve in large vestibular schwannomas, are repaired primarily with single sutures.

Postoperative CSF leakage is a common complication and is treated with lumbar drainage for 1 week. If the CSF leakage persists for more than 1 week, we prefer to review the wound. Some degree of pneumocephalus may appear on the postoperative cranial CT, mainly after surgery in a semisitting position; no treatment is usually needed. Tension pneumocephalus, on the other hand, deserves treatment through a coronal trepanation followed by air evacuation and filling the subdural space with saline solution.

Cerebellar hemorrhage or ischemia is seldom noted. The management includes anti-edematous measures and, eventually, surgical decompression.

Complete facial nerve paralysis is handled with an hourglass dressing and eye drops [40, 48]. Lid loading with subcutaneous insertion of a platinum plate into the superior eyelid protects against conjunctivitis or corneal ulcerations during recovery of the facial nerve. Hypoglossal facial anastomosis can be performed in patients with severe facial palsy [37, 40]. Lower cranial nerve dysfunctions demand preventive use of a nasogastric tube before extubation to avoid aspiration and consequently pneumonia [41].

## References

1. Badie B, Pyle GM, Nguyen PH, Hadar EJ (2001) Elevation of internal auditory canal pressure by vestibular schwannomas. Otol Neurotol 22:696–700

2. Badr-El-Dine M, El-Garem HF, Talaat AM, Magnan J (2002) Endoscopically assisted minimally invasive microvascular decompression of hemifacial spasm. Otol Neurotol 23:122–128

3. Cappabianca P, Cavallo LM, Esposito F, de Divitiis E, et al (2002) Endoscopic examination of the cerebellar pontine angle. Clin Neurol Neurosurg 104:387–391

4. Cheung SW, Jackler RK, Pitts LH, Gutin PH (1995) Interconnecting the posterior and middle cranial fossae for tumors that traverse Meckel's cave. Am J Otol 16:200–208

5. Clatterbuck RE, Tamargo RJ (2004) Surgical Positioning and exposures for cranial procedures. In: Winn HR (ed) Youmans Neurological Surgery. Saunders, Philadelphia, pp 623–630

6. Colletti V, Fiorino FG, Carner M, Giarbini N, et al (2000) The retrosigmoid approach for auditory brainstem implantation. Am J Otol 21:826–836

7. Cushing H (1917) Tumors of the Nervus Acusticus and the Syndrome of the Cerebellopontine Angle. Saunders, Philadelphia London

8. Dandy WE (1925) An operation for the total removal of cerebellopontine (acoustic) tumours. Surg Gynecol Obst 41:129–148

9. Dandy WE (1934) Removal of cerebellopontine acoustic tumours through a unilateral approach. Arch Surg 29:337–344

10. Dandy WE (1941) Results of removal of acoustic tumours by the unilateral approach. Arch Surg 42:1026–1033

11. De Micheli E, Bricolo A (1996) The long history of a cerebello-pontine angle epidermoid tumour – a case report and lessons learned. Acta Neurochir (Wien) 138:350–354

12. Ebner FH, Koerbel A, Kirschniak A, Roser F, et al (2007) Endoscope-assisted retrosigmoid intradural suprameatal approach to the middle fossa: Anatomical and surgical considerations. Eur J Surg Oncol 33:109–113

13. Fisch U (1976) Chirurgie im inneren Gehörgang und an benachbarten Strukturen. In: Naumann HH (ed) Kopf- und Hals-Chirurgie, vol. 3. Thieme, Stuttgart, New York, pp 457–543

14. Gharabaghi A, Acioly de Sousa MA, Tatagiba M (2006) Detection and prevention of the trigeminocardiac reflex during cerebellopontine angle surgery. Acta Neurochir (Wien) 148:1223

15. Gharabaghi A, Koerbel A, Lowenheim H, Kaminsky J, et al (2006) The impact of petrosal vein preservation on postoperative auditory function in surgery of petrous apex meningiomas. Neurosurgery 59:ONS68–74

16. Gharabaghi A, Koerbel A, Samii A, Kaminsky J, et al (2006) The impact of hypotension due to the trigeminocardiac reflex on auditory function in vestibular schwannoma surgery. J Neurosurg 104:369–375

17. Grundy BL, Lina A, Procopio PT, Jannetta PJ (1981) Reversible evoked potential changes with retraction of the eighth cranial nerve. Anesth Analg 60:835–838

18. House WF (1961) Surgical exposure of the internal auditory canal and its contents through the middle cranial fossa. Laryngoscope 71:1363–1385

19. House WF (1964) Transtemporal bone microsurgical removal of acoustic neuromas. Arch Otolaryngol 80:597–756

20. Jarrahy R, Berci G, Shahinian HK (2000) Endoscope-assisted microvascular decompression of the trigeminal nerve. Otolaryngol Head Neck Surg 123:218–223

21. Koerbel A, Gharabaghi A, Samii A, Gerganov V, et al (2005) Trigeminocardiac reflex during skull base surgery: mechanism and management. Acta Neurochir (Wien) 147:727–733

22. Krause F (1903) Zur Freilegung der hinteren Felsenbeinfläche und des Kleinhirns. Beitr Klein Chir 37:728–764

23. Krause F (1911) Surgery of the Brain and Spinal Cord, vol. II. Rebmann, New York, pp 3–32

24. Lapsiwala SB, Pyle GM, Kaemmerle AW, Sasse FJ, et al (2002) Correlation between auditory function and internal auditory canal pressure in patients with vestibular schwannomas. J Neurosurg 96:872–876

25. Lenarz T, Lim HH, Reuter G, Patrick JF, et al (2006) The auditory midbrain implant: a new auditory prosthesis for neural deafness – concept and device description. Otol Neurotol 27:838–843

26. Matthies C, Samii M (1997) Management of vestibular schwannomas (acoustic neuromas): the value of neurophysiology for evaluation and prediction of auditory function in 420 cases. Neurosurgery 40:919–930

27. Matthies C, Thomas S, Moshrefi M, Lesinski-Schiedat A, et al (2000) Auditory brainstem implants: current neurosurgical experiences and perspective. J Laryngol Otol Suppl 27:32–36

28. McLaughlin MR, Jannetta PJ, Clyde BL, Subach BR, et al (1999) Microvascular decompression of cranial nerves: lessons learned after 4400 operations. J Neurosurg 90:1–8

29. Mohanty A, Venkatrama SK, Rao BR, Chandramouli BA, et al (1997) Experience with cerebellopontine angle epidermoids. Neurosurgery 40:24–30

30. Nakamura M, Roser F, Dormiani M, Matthies C, et al (2005) Facial and cochlear nerve function after surgery of cerebellopontine angle meningiomas. Neurosurgery 57:77–90

31. Rhoton AL Jr (2000) The cerebellopontine angle and posterior fossa cranial nerves by the retrosigmoid approach. Neurosurgery 47:S93–129

32. Ribas GC, Rhoton AL Jr, Cruz OR, Peace D (2005) Suboccipital burr holes and craniectomies. Neurosurg Focus 19: E1

33. Rosahl SK, Gharabaghi A, Hubbe U, Shahidi R, et al (2006) Virtual reality augmentation in skull base surgery. Skull Base 16:59–66

34. Roser F, Ritz R, Koerbel A, Loewenheim H, et al (2005) Peduncular hallucinosis: insights from a neurosurgical point of view. Neurosurgery 57:E1068

35. Samii A, Brinker T, Kaminsky J, Lanksch WR, et al (2000) Navigation-guided opening of the internal auditory canal via the retrosigmoid route for acoustic neuroma surgery: cadaveric, radiological, and preliminary clinical study. Neurosurgery 47:382–388

36. Samii A, Lenarz M, Majdani O, Lim HH, et al (2007) Auditory midbrain implant: a combined approach for vestibular schwannoma surgery and device implantation. Otol Neurotol 28:31–38

37. Samii M, Draf W (1989) Surgery of the internal auditory canal and cerebellopontine angle. In: Samii M, Draf W (eds) Surgery of the Skull Base. An Interdisciplinary Approach. Springer, Berlin Heidelberg, pp 360–409

38. Samii M, Klekamp J, Carvalho G (1996) Surgical results for meningiomas of the craniocervical junction. Neurosurgery 39:1086–1095

39. Samii M, Matthies C (1997) Management of 1000 vestibular schwannomas (acoustic neuromas): hearing function in 1000 tumor resections. Neurosurgery 40:248–262

40. Samii M, Matthies C (1997) Management of 1000 vestibular schwannomas (acoustic neuromas): the facial nerve – preservation and restitution of function. Neurosurgery 40:684–695

41. Samii M, Matthies C (1997) Management of 1000 vestibular schwannomas (acoustic neuromas): surgical management and results with an emphasis on complications and how to avoid them. Neurosurgery 40:11–23

42. Samii M, Migliori MM, Tatagiba M, Babu R (1995) Surgical treatment of trigeminal schwannomas. J Neurosurg 82:711–718

43. Samii M, Tatagiba M (2004) Basic principles of skull base surgery. In: Winn HR (ed) Youman's Neurological Surgery. Saunders, Philadelphia, pp 909–929

44. Samii M, Tatagiba M, Carvalho GA (1999) Resection of large petroclival meningiomas by the simple retrosigmoid route. J Clin Neurosci 6:27–30

45. Samii M, Tatagiba M, Carvalho GA (2000) Retrosigmoid intradural suprameatal approach to Meckel's cave and the middle fossa: surgical technique and outcome. J Neurosurg 92:235–241

46. Samii M, Tatagiba M, Piquer J, Carvalho GA (1996) Surgical treatment of epidermoid cysts of the cerebellopontine angle. J Neurosurg 84:14–19

47. Seiffert A (1937) Zur Operation der Akustikusneurinome. Z. Hals-Nase-Ohrenheilkd 42:237–239

48. Sekhar LN, Tzortzidis F (1999) Retrosigmoid approach to the cerebellopontine angle. In: Sekhar LN, De Oliveira E (eds) Cranial Microsurgery. Approaches and Techniques. Thieme, New York, pp 352–377

49. Seoane E, Rhoton AL Jr (1999) Suprameatal extension of the retrosigmoid approach: microsurgical anatomy. Neurosurgery 44:553–560

50. Shao KN, Tatagiba M, Samii M (1993) Surgical management of high jugular bulb in acoustic neurinoma via retrosigmoid approach. Neurosurgery 32:32–37

51. Sindou MP (2005) Microvascular decompression for primary hemifacial spasm. Importance of intraoperative neurophysiological monitoring. Acta Neurochir (Wien) 147:1019–1026

52. Tatagiba M, Matthies C, Samii M (1996) Microendoscopy of the internal auditory canal in vestibular schwannoma surgery. Neurosurgery 38:737–740

53. Tatagiba M, Samii M, Matthies C, el Azm M, et al (1992) The significance for postoperative hearing of preserving the labyrinth in acoustic neurinoma surgery. J Neurosurg 77:677–684

54. Watanabe E, Schramm J, Strauss C, Fahlbusch R (1989) Neurophysiologic monitoring in posterior fossa surgery. II. BAEP-waves I and V and preservation of hearing. Acta Neurochir (Wien) 98:118–128

55. Yasargil MG (1984) Microneurosurgery, vol. 1. Thieme, New York, pp 238–239

# The Surgical Management of Trigeminal Schwannomas

## 15

Ricardo Ramina, Maurício Coelho
Neto, Yvens Barbosa Fernandes,
André Giacomelli Leal, and
Erasmo Barros da Silva Junior

Contents

## 15.1

## Introduction

Schwannomas originating from the cranial nerves are usually benign, isolated, and slow-growing lesions. They are commonly multiple when associated with neurofibromatosis type 2 (NF2). Schwannomas arising from the trigeminal nerves are the second most common intracranial schwannoma. They are rare, representing 0.8–8% of all intracranial schwannomas [3, 21, 27, 33]. Trigeminal schwannomas (TSs) tend to occur in middle age, with highest incidence being between 38 and 40 years, and are more frequent in women [15, 16, 32]. Patients with TSs present more frequently with symptoms related to the function of the trigeminal nerve, but they can also be asymptomatic. In a recent review of the literature, Samii et al. [30] found trigeminal nerve symptoms in 51% of patients, followed by headache (16%) and diplopia (11%). Prior to the advent of computed tomography (CT) and magnetic resonance imaging (MRI) scans, diagnosis of

TS was difficult. Treatment of choice is radical surgical resection. In 1918, Frazier [8] reported the first removal of a TS. Very high mortality has been associated with surgical treatment prior to the late 1950s [31]. Since this time, several small series [5, 7, 19, 21, 30], and a large series of 111 patients [16] published very good results with very low mortality and morbidity. Different surgical approaches may be used depending on the location and extension of the lesion.

## 15.2

## Surgical Anatomy

The trigeminal nerve emerges from the ventrolateral surface of the pons and runs anteriorly about 1–2 cm [4] through the cerebellopontine cistern, reaching the petrous apex. Vascular structures, such as the petrosal vein and the superior cerebellar artery, present a close relationship with the nerve. Over the petrous apex, with an average of 7 mm from the medial lip of the internal acoustic meatus [18], it forms the triangular portion and Gasserian ganglion, which is involved in a dural deflection forming Meckel's cave, laterally from the cavernous sinus and carotid artery. At the exit of Meckel's cave, the nerve has three branches: the ophthalmic (V1), the maxillary (V2), and the mandibular (V3). These three divisions run under the medial fossa dura and exit the temporal bone through the lateral wall of the cavernous sinus (V1), foramen rotundum (V2), and foramen ovale (V3).

The trigeminal nerve can by divided into three surgical segments: Cisternal (from the brainstem to the petrous apex), intracranial-extradural (from Meckel's cave to the foramens), and extracranial (V1, V2, and V3).

Functionally, the trigeminal nerve has two portions: the "pars compacta" (which will form the triangular portion) carrying the primary afferent fibers, which are responsible for the special sensibility of the face, and the motor root, carrying the branchiomotor fibers to the muscles of mastication.

The motor root runs separately from the "pars compacta", but together with the cranial portion of the nerve.

At the level of Meckel's cave it goes medially and exits the skull with the maxillary nerve.

The intracranial-extradural portions of V2 and V3 are surgically identified using the foramen spinosum as an anatomical landmark. It is located at the sphenoid bone and contains the middle meningeal artery. The foramen ovale is located about 2–5 mm superior and anterior to the foramen spinosum, and the foramen rotundum is about 10–12 mm more superior and medial.

## 15.3
### Classification of Tumor Extension

TSs may origin from the root, ganglion, and peripheral branches. Tumor growing may involve different portions of the trigeminal nerve. Jefferson [14] initially divided these tumors into four groups depending on their anatomic location. These four groups are: posterior fossa (root type), combined posterior fossa-middle fossa (dumbbell type), middle fossa (ganglion type), and peripheral (division type). Samii et al. [30] classified tumor extension according to radiological findings into four types: type A, intracranial tumor predominantly in the middle fossa; type B, intracranial tumor predominantly in the poste-rior fossa; type C, intracranial dumbbell-shaped tumor in the middle and posterior fossa; type D, extracranial tumor with intracranial extension. Our cases were classified according to tumor extension as: type A, predominantly extracranial tumor with small extension in the middle fossa (Fig. 1); type B, intracranial tumor predominantly in the middle fossa with extracranial extension (Fig. 2); type C, tumor in the middle fossa (Fig. 3); type D, tumor in the posterior fossa (Fig. 4); type E, tumor with middle and posterior fossa extensions (Fig. 5); type F, tumor with extracranial and middle and posterior fossa extensions (Fig. 6).

## 15.4
### Clinical Material

This series includes 16 patients treated surgically between 1987 and 2006. Two patients had NF2 with other associated intracranial lesions. One patient presented a posterior communicating aneurysm at the same side of the TS. Prior to 1990, diagnosis and follow-up of patients was done with CT scan. After this period, all patients had pre- and postoperative CT scans and MRI. There were two type A tumors, two type B, four type C, two type D, four

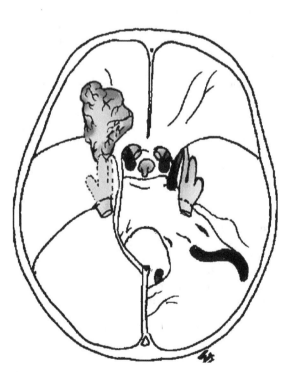
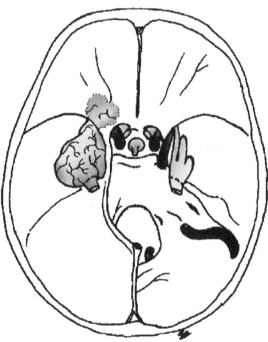

Fig. 1 Large extracranial trigeminal schwannoma with small middle fossa extension (type A)

Fig. 2 Drawing of trigeminal schwannoma with main portion in the middle fossa and small extracranial extension (type B)

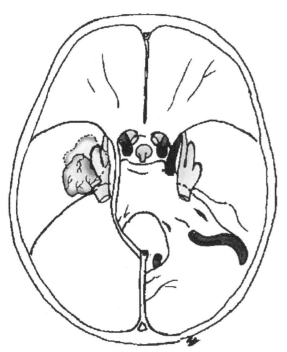

Fig. 3 Middle fossa trigeminal schwannoma (type C)

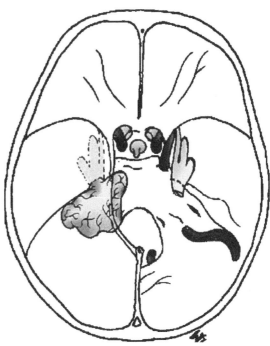

Fig. 4 Schematic drawing showing a posterior fossa trigeminal schwannoma (type D)

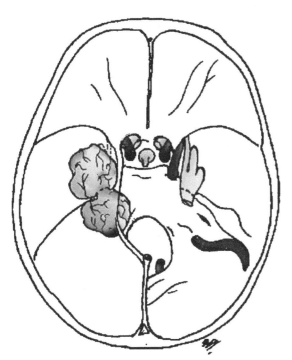

Fig. 5 Drawing of trigeminal schwannoma with middle and posterior fossa extensions (type E)

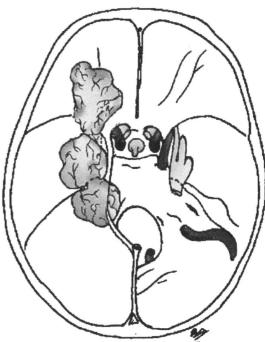

Fig. 6 Schematic drawing showing a trigeminal schwannoma with extracranial, middle and posterior fossa extensions (type F)

type E, and two type F. The cavernous sinus was involved in 12 cases. The size of lesions was: small (<3 cm) in 2, medium (between 3 and 4 cm) in 3, large (<4 cm) in 6, and giants (>4 cm) in 4 cases.

The clinical symptoms in these patients included trigeminal hypesthesia (9 patients), facial pain (8 patients), headache (5 patients), hearing symptoms (3 patients), seizure (3 patients), diplopia (2 patients), ataxia (2 patients), and hemiparesis and increased intracranial pressure with papilledema (1 patient). The extent of resection was confirmed by postoperative imaging in all patients. Total resection was possible in 15 patients. Nearly total removal was performed in one patient with NF2 due to adherences within the cavernous sinus. There was no surgical mortality. Seven patients developed postoperative anesthesia in at least one branch of trigeminal nerve. Trigeminal motor function was preserved in six patients. Two cases developed cerebrospinal fluid (CSF) leak,

which was treated successfully by lumbar fluid drainage. Facial pain was reduced from eight patients to one. Two patients exhibited minimal facial palsy, which improved during the follow-up period. The patient with preoperative hemiparesis showed progressive improvement after surgery. There was one recurrence in a patient with NF2, 5 years after a radical removal of a type C tumor. The recurrent tumor was removed with an uneventful postoperative outcome.

## 15.5
## Surgical Approaches

Choice of surgical approach was influenced by the type of tumor extension. Type A tumors were removed through a transmaxillary (Fig. 7) approach (TM) or TM in combination with a middle fossa extradural approach (EMF).

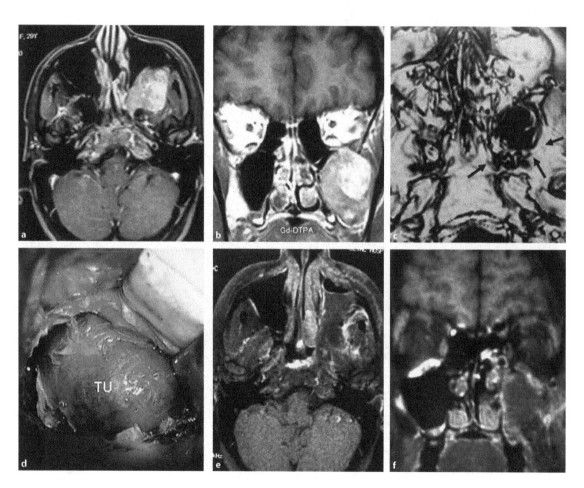

Fig. 7 **a,b** Magnetic resonance imaging (MRI) scan of a large trigeminal schwannoma with main portion in the maxillary sinus (type A). *Gd-DPTA* Gadopentetate. **c** Computed tomography (CT) scan showing enlargement of the foramen rotundum (*arrows*). **d** Surgical picture: transmaxillary approach exposing the tumor (*TU*). **e,f** Postoperative MRI

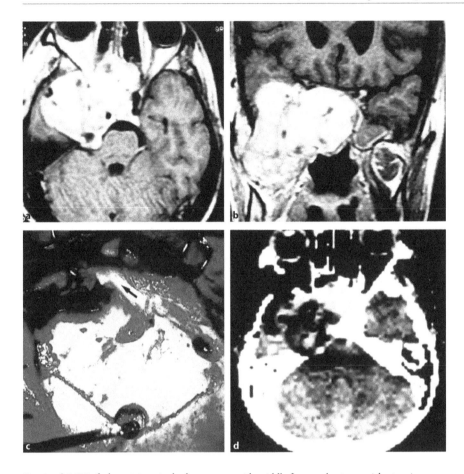

Fig. 8  **a,b** MRI of a large trigeminal schwannoma with middle fossa and extracranial extension (type B). **c** Middle fossa craniotomy. **d** Postoperative CT scan

Type B lesions were approached using a intradural middle fossa approach (IMF) or, when the extracranial tumor was large, IMF in combination with TM (Fig. 8). Type C tumors are removed through the middle fossa. When the lesion was small, the EMF approach was used, and when the tumor was large with intradural extension to the posterior fossa, the IMF approach was used (Fig. 9). Type D and E tumors were resected using presigmoid or retrosigmoid approaches (Figs. 10 and 11). Type F lesions were removed with a combination of the previous approaches (Fig. 12).

### 15.5.1
### The Transmaxillary Approach (Caldwell-Luc Procedure)

This procedure is usually performed in combination with the middle fossa approaches to remove large TSs. It was used as the only surgical approach in our series to remove a large schwannoma within the maxillary sinus with a small extension into the middle fossa and cavernous sinus. This tumor could be totally excised through the TM approach. This procedure is performed under general anesthesia. The gingiva is infiltrated with lidocaine 1% with 1:100,000 epinephrine. A 3-cm incision centered over the canine tooth and first premolar is made. To allow better closure, 1 cm of gingival tissue is left intact above the dentition. Soft tissue and periosteum are elevated from the anterior wall of the maxilla. The infraorbital nerve is identified at its exit from the infraorbital foramen (mid-papillary line). The anterior wall of the maxillary sinus is opened and this opening is enlarged with Kerrinson rongeurs. With the aid of a surgical microscope, the tumor is identified and an intracapsular debulking is performed. Total removal of the maxillary portion and a small portion of the middle fossa and cavernous sinus can be achieved with this approach. The wound is closed with 4-0 absorbable sutures.

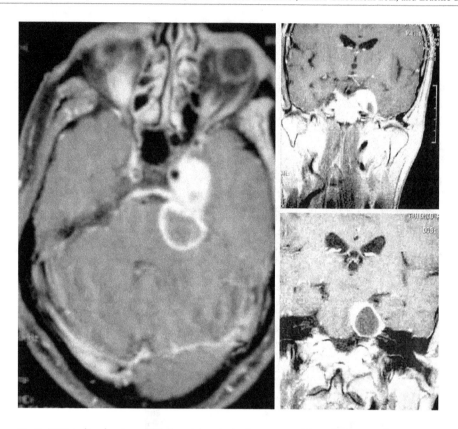

Fig. 9  MRI studies showing middle fossa trigeminal schwannoma with cystic posterior fossa portion (type C)

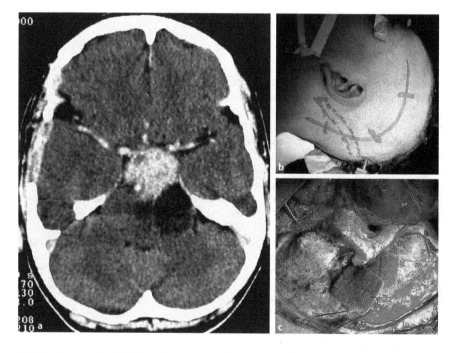

Fig. 10  **a** Preoperative MRI showing a posterior fossa trigeminal schwannoma (type D) with cystic portion. **b** Skin incision. **c** Presigmoid craniotomy

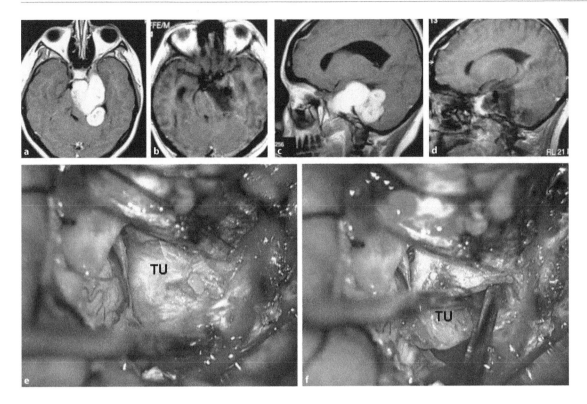

**Fig. 11a–f** Pre- (**a** and **c**) and postoperative (**b** and **d**) MRI scans of a large trigeminal schwannoma (type E) with extension within the middle and posterior fossa. **e** Surgical picture of pre-sigmoid approach for removal of the tumor. **f** Removal of the tumor capsule from the brainstem

### 15.5.2
## The Middle Fossa Zygomatic Approach

The patient is placed in the supine position with the head fixed in a three-pin device and rotated approximately 30° to the opposite side. A C-shaped skin incision is made over the pterium. The temporalis muscle fascia is incised to protect the frontal branch of the facial nerve, and the scalp-fascia flap is reflected anteriorly. The temporalis muscle is retracted inferiorly and posteriorly. A pterional craniotomy is cut. The craniotomy is enlarged to the cranial base of the temporal fossa by removing bone with rongeurs, to obtain a flat viewing angle across the floor of the middle fossa. The dura is dissected and elevated from the middle fossa. The superior orbital fissure is exposed. The middle meningeal artery is coagulated and cut. The second and third branches of the trigeminal nerve are identified. The foramen ovale and foramen rotundum are unroofed with a drill. The dura is elevated from the lateral cavernous sinus wall, exposing extradurally the tumor and the branches of trigeminal nerve. Tumor debulking is performed and the tumor capsule is dissected from intact branches of trigeminal nerve. Radical removal is achieved. Large tumors are approached intradurally. The

sylvian fissure is opened. The optic nerve, internal carotid artery, and cranial nerve III are identified. The lateral cavernous sinus wall is exposed via a temporopolar approach and the tumor removed with preservation as far as possible of the trigeminal nerve fibers. The petrous apex is drilled and the petroclinoidal ligament is cut to expose the posterior fossa portion. The tumor extension within the posterior fossa is totally removed trough this middle fossa approach.

### 15.5.3
## The Retrosigmoid Approach

This approach is performed with the patient in the dorsal (mastoid) position with the head turned to the opposite side with the ipsilateral shoulder elevated. The skin incision is linear and placed 4 cm behind the external auditory canal. The asterium is exposed to determine the position of the junction of the transverse and sigmoid sinuses. A 4-cm craniotomy is performed with the superior and anterior margin bordering the transverse and sigmoid sinuses. The dura is opened parallel to the sigmoid sinus, and CSF is released from the cerebellomedullaris cisterna.

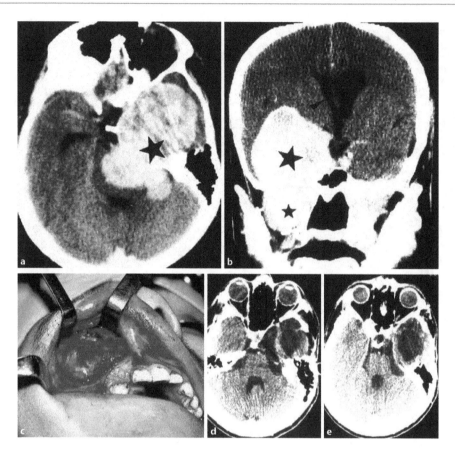

Fig. 12a–e CT scan of a large trigeminal schwannoma (type F) with extensions in the posterior fossa, middle fossa and maxillary sinus (**a,b**; *stars*). **c** Transmaxillary tumor exposure. **d,e** Postoperative CT scans

The cranial nerves IX, X, XI, VII, and VIII are identified. The tumor is exposed close to the tentorium margin. After intracapsular tumor debulking, microsurgical radical removal is performed. Watertight dural closure is carried out, and the craniotomy bone flap is replaced and fixed. All opened mastoid cells are sealed with bone wax to help prevent CSF leaks.

### 15.5.4
### The Presigmoid Approach

The patient is placed in the dorsal (mastoid) position. A C-shaped skin incision is made, beginning in the middle fossa and terminating at the mastoid tip. Two burr holes are placed anterior and two posterior to the transverse and sigmoid sinuses junction. A craniotomy flap exposing the temporal and retromastoid dura is cut. Mastoidectomy with preservation of the labyrinth block and facial nerve canal is the next surgical step. Dura incisions are performed parallel to the middle fossa floor and anterior to the sigmoid sinus. The superior petrosal sinus is

ligated and cut. The inferior temporal lobe and the lateral portion of cerebellum are lightly retracted, preserving the vein of Labbé. The tumor is identified, and cranial nerves VII and VIII are usually displaced inferiorly. A tumor within the cavernous sinus is removed after opening the lateral wall of the cavernous sinus. After total tumor removal, the dura is closed watertight and the skull base is reconstructed with miofascial flaps [28].

### 15.6
### Discussion

TSs are the second most common intracranial schwannoma. There is no "typical clinical syndrome" caused by TSs. The most common symptoms are related to trigeminal nerve dysfunction. Decreased sensation over the involved trigeminal nerve branch or all over the face, and corneal reflex alteration are more frequent than trigeminal pain [21, 30]. Sensory disturbance is described as numbness and paresthesias. Some authors reported that about 10% of patients will not present trigeminal dysfunction as an initial symptom [19,27]. Facial pain may involve either only the affected trigeminal branch or all three divisions. Intensity may vary from light pain to lancinating. It may occur in paroxysms, usually without trigger zones, or may last for hours. According to Day and Fukushima [5], the majority of patients with TS have paroxysmal lancinating facial pain, in episodes that tend to last longer and do not respond to carbamazepine. Only a minority of patients have symptoms of classic trigeminal neuralgia. Some authors [6,20,23,31] reported that trigeminal pain may be absent with tumors originating in the root and is most commonly caused by tumors arising from the ganglion. Other symptoms are headaches, hearing disturbances, hemifacial spasm, hemiparesis, ataxia, diplopia, signs of cerebellar involvement, increased intracranial pressure, and dysfunction of the oculomotor, trochlear, and abducens nerves [2,19,21,23,32]. Malignant tumors are very rare, and anesthesia of all three branches suggests histological malignancy [12,14]. Adequate preoperative neuroradiologic evaluation is fundamental for establishing a correct diagnosis and planning of treatment. Bony changes induced by the tumor, as well as the anatomic bone anatomy of the skull base, are better evaluated with CT scan and plain x-ray examinations. Sharp amputation of the petrous apex, anteromedial erosion of the petrous bone and enlargement of the foramen ovale are usual radiological findings [13,22,25]. On CT scan, TSs appear iso- to hyperdense compared to the surrounding brain, with sharply defined margins, and enhance strongly and uniformly after intravenous contrast administration [10,24]. Cystic changes may be observed. MRI gives the best information concerning the location and extension of the tumor as well as displacement of the neighboring structures and involvement of the cavernous sinus and vessels. On MRI, TSs appear hyperintense on T1-weighted images and hyperintense on T2-weighted images, with intense and homogeneous enhancement after gadolinium administration [29]. Differential diagnoses include meningiomas, epidermoids, metastases, chondrosarcomas, chordomas, chondromas, acoustic schwannomas, and maxillary sinus tumors.

The management strategy for TS includes clinical observation followed by MRI controls for incidental tumors, surgical removal, and radiotherapy (radiosurgery) [1,9,11,16,17,26,34]. Complete or near-total surgical removal can be achieved in over 70% of the patients with skull-base approaches and microsurgical dissection. Involvement of the cavernous sinus is one cause of subtotal resection. In most cases, a clear cleavage plane between the tumor capsule and the cavernous sinus structures can be found and completely dissected, thus achieving total resection. With modern neurosurgical techniques, recurrence is rare. Surgical outcomes are usually favorable; the most frequent symptom after surgery is trigeminal hypoesthesia, and this is transient in many cases. Facial pain may persist after surgery, but most patients experience improvement or total relief. Diplopia, CSF leak, meningi-

tis and hydrocephalus are other described complications. Most new cranial nerves deficits present resolution within 4–6 months. Contemporary series present no mortality or major surgical complications [5,7,9,30]. Good results have been reported with radiosurgery. This treatment is usually indicated as primary therapy for small tumors or for tumor remnants within the cavernous sinus [11]. Long-term follow-up of patients treated with this method is needed in order to evaluate the exact role of radiosurgery. No patient will be cured from this benign tumor with radiotherapy or radiosurgery.

## References

1. Al-Mefty O, Ayoubi S, Gaber E (2002) Trigeminal schwannomas: removal of dumbbell-shaped tumors through the expanded Meckel cave and outcomes of cranial nerve function. J Neurosurg 96:453–463

2. Arseni C, Dumitrescu L, Constantinescu A (1975) Neurinomas of the trigeminal nerve. Surg Neurol 4:497–503

3. Bordi L, Compton J, Symon L (1989) Trigeminal Neuroma. Surg Neurol 31:272–276

4. Burt AM (1993) Textbook of Neuroanatomy – Synopsis of the Cranial Nerves. Saunders, Philadelphia, pp 403–430

5. Day JD, Fukushima T (1998) The surgical management of trigeminal neuromas. Neurosurgery 42:233–241

6. De Benedittis G, Bernasconi V, Ettorre G (1977) Tumors of the fifth cranial nerve. Acta Neurochir 38:37–64

7. Dolenc VV (1994) Frontotemporal epidural approach to trigeminal neurinomas. Acta Neurochir (Wien) 130:55–65

8. Frazier CH (1918) An operable tumor involving the gasserian ganglion. Am J Med Sci 156:483–490

9. Goel A, Muzumdar D, Raman C (2003) Trigeminal neuroma: analysis of surgical experience with 73 cases. Neurosurgery 52:783–790

10. Goldberg R, Byrd S, Winter J (1980) Varied appearance of trigeminal neuromas on CT. Am J Radiol 134:57–60

11. Hasegawa T, Kida Y, Yoshimoto M, Koike J (2007) Trigeminal schwannomas: results of gamma knife surgery in 37 cases. J Neurosurg 106:18–23

12. Hedeman LS, Lewinsky BS, Lochridge GK, Trevor R (1978) Primary malignant schwannoma of the gasserian ganglion: report of two cases. J Neurosurg 48:279–283

13. Holman CB, Olive I, Svien HJ (1961) Roentgenologic features of neurofibromas involving the gasserian ganglion. Am J Radiol 86:148–153

14. Jefferson G (1955) The trigeminal neurinomas with some remarks on malignant invasion of the gasserian ganglion. Clin Neurosurg 1:11–54

15. Knudsen V, Kolze V (1972) Neurinoma of the gasserian ganglion and the trigeminal root. Report of four cases. Acta Neurochir 26:159–164

16. Konovalov AN, Spallone A, Mukhamedjanov DJ, Tcherekajev VA, Makhmudov UB (1996) Trigeminal neurinomas. A series of 111 surgical cases from a single institution. Acta Neurochir (Wien) 138:1027–1035

17. Kuo JS, Chen JCT, Yu C, Zelman V, Giannotta SL, Petrovich Z, MacPherson D, Apuzzo ML (2004) Gamma knife radiosurgery for benign cavernous sinus tumors: quantitative analysis of treatment outcomes. Neurosurgery 54:1385–1394

18. Lang J (1993) Anatomy of the posterior cranial fossa. In: Sekhar LN, Janecka IP (eds) Surgery of the Cranial Tumors. Raven, New York, pp 131–146

19. Lesoin F, Rousseaux M, Villette L, Autricque A, Dhellemmes P, Pellerin P, Vaneecloo JM, Leys D, Jomin M (1986) Neurinomas of the trigeminal nerve. Acta Neurochir (Wien) 82:118–122

20. Levinthal R, Bentson JR (1976) Detection of small trigeminal neurinomas. J Neurosurg 45:568–575

21. McCormick PC, Bello JA, Post KD (1988) Trigeminal schwannoma. Surgical series of 14 cases with review of the literature. J Neurosurg 69:850–860

22. Mello LR, Tänzer A (1972) Some aspects of trigeminal neurinomas. Neuroradiology 4:215–221

23. Nager GT (1984) Neurinomas of the trigeminal nerve. Am J Otolaryngol 5:301–331

24. Naidich TP, Lin JP, Leeds NE, Kricheff II, George AE, Chase NE, Pudlowski RM, Passalagua A (1976) Computed tomography in the diagnosis of extra-axial posterior fossa masses. Radiology 120 :333–339

25. Palacios E, MacGee EE (1972) The radiographic diagnosis of trigeminal neurinomas. J Neurosurg 36:153–156

26. Pan L, Wang EM, Zhang N, Zhou LF, Wang BJ, Dong YF, Dai JZ, Cai PW (2005) Long-term results of Leksell gamma knife surgery for trigeminal schwannomas. J Neurosurg 102:220–224

27. Pollack IF, Sekhar LN, Jannetta PJ, Janecka IP (1989) Neurilemmomas of the trigeminal nerve. J Neurosurg 70:737–745

28. Ramina R, Maniglia JJ, Paschoal JR, Fernandes YB, Neto MC, Honorato DC (2005) Reconstruction of the cranial base in surgery for jugular foramen tumors. Neurosurgery 56:337–343

29. Rigamonti D, Spetzler RF, Shetter A, Drayer BP (1987) Magnetic resonance imaging and trigeminal schwannomas. Surg Neurol 28:67–70

30. Samii M, Migliori MM, Tatagiba M, Babu R (1995) Surgical treatment of trigeminal schwannomas. J Neurosurg 82:711–718

31. Schisano G, Olivecrona H (1960) Neurinomas of the gasserian ganglion and trigeminal root. J Neurosurg 17:306–322

32. Shrivastava RK, Sem C, Post KD (2004) Trigeminal schwannomas. In: Winn HR (ed) Youmans Neurological Surgery. Saunders, Philadelphia, pp 1343–1350

33. Yasui T, Hakuba A, Kim SH, Nishimura S (1989) Trigeminal neurinomas: operative approach in eight cases. J Neurosurg 71:506–511

34. Yoshida K, Kawase T (1999) Trigeminal neurinomas extending into multiple fossae: surgical methods and review of the literature. J Neurosurg 91:202–211

# Facial Nerve Schwannomas

# 16

Ricardo Ramina, Maurício Coelho
Neto, Erasmo Barros da Silva Junior,
Ronaldo Vosgerau, André Giacomelli
Leal, and Yvens Barbosa Fernandes

## Contents

## 16.1
## Introduction

Facial nerve schwannomas (FNSs) are uncommon; extremely slow growing, benign tumors that frequently present without facial dysfunction. Malignant FNSs are extremely rare. They can arise at the cerebellopontine angle (CPA), internal meatus, geniculate ganglion, peripheral nerves in the mastoid bone, or in muscle (Fig. 1). The tumor arises from Schwann cells in a focal manner as a solitary and well-encapsulated mass. The most common sites are the geniculate ganglion and internal auditory canal. This study reviews the surgical anatomy, clinical presentations, radiological diagnosis, appropriate planning for the management, surgical approaches, and the predictive outcomes of surgical management. Surgery is clearly indicated when the patient already presents with facial nerve palsy. If the facial function is normal and the tumor is not compressing the brainstem, conservative management is considered.

## 16.2
## Surgical Anatomy

The relationship between the facial nerve, petrous apex, and temporal bone must be understood in order

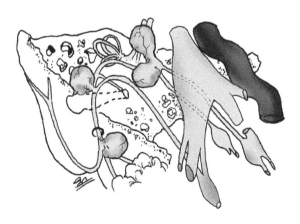

Fig. 1 Sites of origin of facial nerve schwannomas

to choose the best approach with minimal morbidity (Fig. 2). Since it exits from the brainstem, the facial nerve goes into the internal acoustic meatus (meatal segment) to enter the facial canal within the petrous portion of the temporal bone. This portion of the facial nerve, known as the labyrinthic portion, is 3–5 mm in length [16] and contains the geniculate ganglion. The geniculate ganglion is anterior and medial to the arcuate eminence and gives the greater petrosal nerve as its main branch, which runs anteriorly to the pterigopalatyne fossa. In about 15% of cases, the temporal bone is dehiscent over the geniculate ganglion [18]. The facial nerve continues its course inside the temporal bone through its tympanic portion and has a close lateral relationship with the tympanic membrane. The facial nerve exits the skull through the stylomastoid foramen and traverses to the parotid gland, running anteriorly to the digastric muscle. At the stylomastoid foramen, the facial nerve is identified using as landmarks such as the mastoid tip, posterior belly of the digastric muscle, and the cartilaginous portion of the external acoustic meatus. The superior trunk provides innervations to the orbital muscles (temporal and zygomatic branches). Other branches from the superior trunk are the buccal and mandibular nerves. The posterior auricular nerve, the digastric nerve, and cervical nerve branch arise from the inferior trunk.

## 16.3
## Diagnosis

### 16.3.1
### Clinical Symptoms

Establishing a correct preoperative diagnosis of FNS is important for treatment planning and to advise the patient. Preoperative differentiation of a small intracranial FNS from an intracanalicular vestibular schwannoma may be difficult, especially if the patient has no facial nerve palsy. The correct diagnosis is achieved only during

surgery and the surgeon is faced with a difficult decision: remove the tumor, causing an unexpected facial palsy, or abort the procedure.

Facial schwannomas usually manifest with insidious symptoms and different clinical features; the symptoms depend on the site of tumor origin. Facial palsy and hearing disturbances are the predominant presenting symptoms, but it depends on the location and extent of the lesion. Facial paresis is often slowly progressive and preceded by facial twitching [14]. It occurs more frequently in patients with intratemporal tumors. Facial paresis in Bell's palsy has a sudden onset often accompanied by periauricular pain and hyperacusis. FNS is the cause of paresis in about 5% of patients with diagnosis of Bell's palsy. Saito and Baxter [19] found an 84% incidence of facial palsy in intratemporal tumors and 34% in extratemporal tumors. O'Donoghue et al. [12] found facial palsy in only 45% of 48 reported cases. Extratemporal parotid tumors present as parotid masses. Facial palsy is rare in these cases [6]. Hearing loss is observed in patients with intratemporal tumors. According to its location, this loss may be sensorineural or conductive. Tumors in the labyrinthine segment, near to the geniculate ganglion, can present with sensorineural hearing loss. Conductive hearing loss is observed in tumors arising in the horizontal segment. Some patients can be totally asymptomatic [12,17]

According to Chung et al. [3], patients with intratemporal tumors showed more severe symptoms such as hearing loss, tinnitus, dizziness, and facial weakness or pain, than patients with extratemporal schwannomas.

### 16.3.2
### Radiological Findings

There is a universally acceptable imaging description of these lesions as enhancing tubular masses (magnetic resonance imaging, MRI) in a smoothly enlarged facial canal (computed tomography, CT). However, the term "jack of all trades" seems to be applicable for this classic

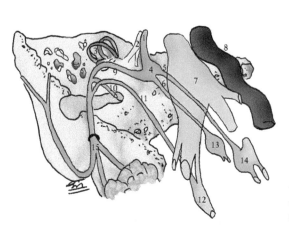

Fig. 2 Drawing of facial nerve anatomy. *1* Intracanalicular portion, *2* cochlear nerve, *3* semicircular canals, *4* geniculate ganglion, *7* Gasserian ganglion, *8* internal carotid artery, *9* labyrinthic and mastoid portions, *15* extratemporal portion

description, since it has been described in the recent literature, in an almost definitive research on such the subject by Wiggins et al. [23], with at least five other possible imaging appearances for these entities. Stasolla et al. [22] have described a FNS with cisternal and intracanalicular components extending to the geniculate ganglion through an enlarged labyrinthine segment of the fallopian canal, configuring an important sign: "the labyrinthine tail." On coronal plane, this tumor featured a short but clear "dural tail," emphasizing the lack of specificity of this sign, which is most often related to meningiomas.

### 16.3.2.1
### Imaging Aspects

On MRI, the classic description of this tumor is a well-circumscribed, fusiform, enhancing mass along the course of the intratemporal facial nerve on T1-enhanced studies. On CT with bone algorithm, a sharp canal enlargement is observed. These statements are not enough to encompass all possible imaging appearances regarding these tumors. Modern imaging techniques are capable of better depicting the effects on the surrounding anatomic landmarks related to these lesions and offer not only the correct diagnosis, but better surgical planning. Regardless of the anatomic location, schwannomas present as heterogeneously or homogenously enhancing soft-tissue attenuation isoattenuated to gray matter on enhancing CT, and may present cystic foci. In the temporal bone, FNS will appear as a benign-appearing scalloping and remodeling of surrounding bony structures. It is not true erosion, but

rather a more benign osseous expansion. MRI can show heterogeneity within a large FNS and predominant hyperintensity on T2-weighted sequences, and iso- to hypointensity on T1-weighted series. Homogenous enhancement is the rule on post-contrast-enhanced MRI (better demonstrated with fat-suppression techniques, especially intracanalicular and intratemporal lesions). Larger lesions may undergo cystic degeneration. Special attention should be paid to the increasing use of three-dimensional contrast interference with steady state sequences. These sequences are submillimetric, T2-weighted acquisitions that better depict structures immersed in cerebrospinal fluid (CSF), mostly cranial nerves and anatomic landscapes in the vicinity of (or interfaced with) CSF. There is a good conspicuity of cysternal, meatal segments of the cranial nerves VII and VIII, the internal auditory canal and its fundus, and the cochlea and vestibule when using this type of sequence. Its usefulness has been proven and now makes up part of the standard imaging protocol at our institution when facing patients with vertigo, facial palsy, or hearing loss, among several other indications.

### 16.3.2.2
### Radiological Findings Relative to the Site of Origin

A dumbbell-shaped tumor may be present if there is an extension from the internal auditory canal through the labyrinthic segment of the facial canal into the geniculate fossa (Fig. 3). This aspect, when associated with a T1-weighted MRI appearance as a sharply enhanced,

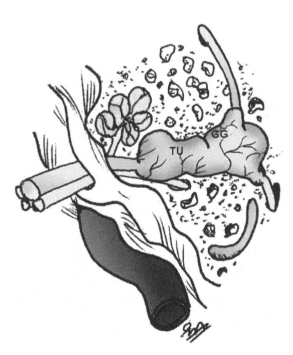

Fig. 3 Facial nerve schwannoma (*TU*) with extension to the geniculate ganglion (*GG*)

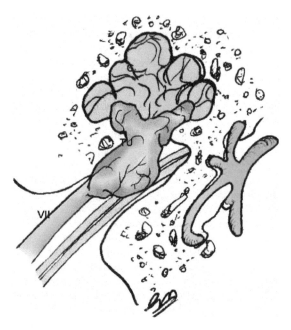

Fig. 4 Drawing showing facial nerve schwannoma with extension into the cochlea (*C*)

scalloped or fusiform enlargement of the facial nerve canal, is diagnostic of FNS. However, it should be differentiated from a transmodiolar acoustic schwannoma when there is extension into the cochlea through the modiolus in a cochlear nerve schwannoma (Fig. 4). When the geniculate fossa is involved primarily, or there is involvement of the greater superficial petrosal nerve, the appearance is distinct. It seems like an extra-axial middle cranial fossa mass. This situation requires inspection of the geniculate ganglion or the grater superficial petrosal nerve to search for possible sites of origin. When the geniculate ganglion is affected, there is a "bulbous" appearance of the middle cranial fossa. FNSs originating in the greater superficial petrosal nerve scallop the anterior margin ganglion and adjacent bony petrous apex. The FNS involving the tympanic segment of the facial nerve has a different morphology and is usually multilobular instead of the classic fusiform appearance, since in this segment the bony structure is more fragile. A fistula to the semicircular canal may develop if there is medial or superior extension. Inferior and lateral extension can cause lateral displacement of the ossicular chain and lead to conductive hearing loss.

The appearance of an FNS involving the mastoid segment is quite distinctive. In this segment, the facial nerve canal is surrounded by delicate, thin-walled bony septations separating air cells, and expansion of the tumor can result in an aggressive aspect due to a breakthrough into these aerated cells. Without bearing this context in mind, misdiagnosis is possible and should raise a possibility of facial nerve hemangioma or other locally invasive entity.

### 16.3.3
### Differential Diagnosis

Differential diagnostic considerations regarding FNS include: cholesteatoma, facial nerve hemangioma, and perineural parotid malignancy. Intratemporal facial nerve enlargement is present in these entities. Congenital or acquired cholesteatoma involving the facial nerve canal does not enhance on T1-enhanced MRI. Facial nerve hemangioma of the facial nerve canal and adjacent bone presents a more aggressive aspect with irregular margins and may even have a "mouth-eaten" appearance.

Ossifying fibroma can present as a calcified honeycomb matrix. A parotid mass may spread its malignancy from distal to proximal along an enlarged facial nerve canal. Idiopathic Bell's palsy is another differential diagnostic consideration that should be paid attention. Indeed, some patients with mild facial nerve palsy can receive this diagnosis. The typical Bell's palsy patient usually presents an enhancing "tuft" in the internal auditory canal fundus plus enhancement of all or part of the facial nerve. Bell's palsy patients, however, do not present an enlarged facial nerve canal on CT and this feature can, indeed, separate these two entities. When involving the CPA-internal auditory canal, FNS can be indistinguishable from acoustic schwannomas if there is no extension through the labyrinthine segment of the facial nerve. Hence, recently diagnosed acoustic schwannomas should be inspected for a "labyrinthine tail," since the presenting symptoms will not always suggest the site of origin of the tumor.

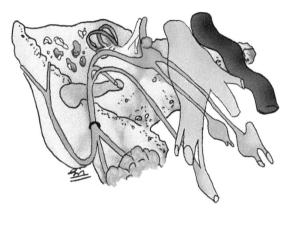

Fig. 5 Drawing of an intracanalicular facial nerve schwannoma.

## 16.4
## Surgical Indication and Planning

The decision on how to treat these patients, the timing of intervention, and the surgical approach should be individualized, depending on the extent of the tumor, grade of facial palsy, hearing function, surgical experience, and informed patient consent. When moderate-to-total facial palsy is already present and for large tumors in the CPA compressing the brainstem, complete resection is indicated [1]. When the patient has no symptoms or only mild facial dysfunction, conservative management (clinical and radiological observation) should be considered [8, 11]. The best postoperative facial function obtained after tumor resection and nerve reconstruction is following treatment for a House-Brackmann (H-B) grade III palsy. These tumors have a slow growth rate. Liu and Fagan [8] treated ten patients conservatively. Eight patients maintained normal facial function for up to 10 years after presentation and no significant tumor growth was observed on serial radiological imaging control. Planning surgery should include detailed explanation to patients, presenting the rationale behind the timing of intervention, and the alternative management (conservative and radiosurgery). Complete tumor removal should include proximal and distal nerve margin, verified by histology of frozen sections. The nerve graft donor site (greater auricular or sural nerve) is prepared. Hypoglossal/facial anastomosis is indicated only if a proximal stump cannot be found. Tumor removal preserving the nerve has been described for cases of small FNS, but in the majority of cases the nerve must be transected. Postoperative eye protection measures (tharsorrhaphy or implant of gold weight) are anticipated. Pure-tone audiogram, electroneuronography, facial-nerve action potential, and photography of a patient's face are measures for assessing facial and cochlear nerves preoperative function, making postoperative comparison possible.

## 16.5
## Surgical Approaches

The choice of surgical approach is based on the anatomic location and extension of the tumor, and the hearing status in both ears. Intracanalicular FNS in patients with good preoperative hearing may be approached through the extradural middle fossa route if the extension into the CPA is small, or through the retrosigmoid/transmeatal approach if the tumor is large in the posterior fossa, compressing the brainstem (Figs. 5–7). If the tumor fills the entire internal auditory canal, identification of the proximal facial nerve stump may be difficult. In some cases, the correct diagnosis of FNS is made only during surgery of a supposed vestibular schwannoma. Facial nerve reconstruction is not possible with the retrosigmoid approach alone because there is no access to the distal stump of the facial nerve (labyrinthine segment). In these cases, the facial nerve is grafted through an additional surgical access (Samii and Draf or Dott's technique). The presigmoid approach with opening of the internal auditory canal may be an alternative. Most of these patients with large tumors are already deaf preoperatively and a translabyrinthine approach is used. Intratemporal tumors are removed via transmastoid, transtemporal approaches (Fig. 8). After tumor removal in small cases, mobilization and rerouting of the facial nerve is performed and an end-to-end anastomosis is possible (Fig. 9). If the gap after tumor removal is too large, a nerve graft is used. Extratemporal FNSs are removed through parotidectomy, and the facial nerve is reconstructed with sural grafts (Fig. 10). In a large case in our series the tumor extended from the parotid region until the middle fossa, causing erosion of the mastoid. This case was removed via parotidectomy combined with a transmastoid approach.

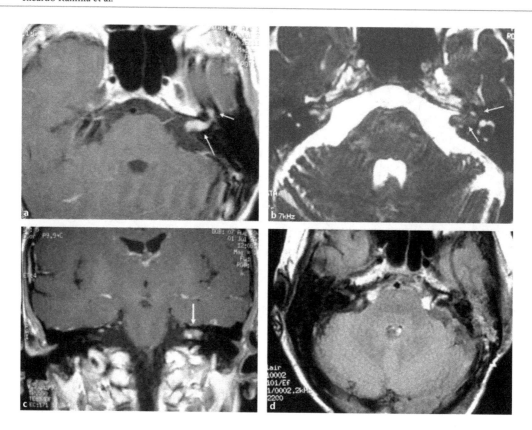

Fig. 6 **a,b** Magnetic resonance imaging (MRI) scan axial view showing a facial nerve schwannoma with extension to the geniculate ganglion (*arrows*). **c** Coronal view showing the tumor within the internal auditory canal (*arrow*). **d** Postoperative MRI

## 16.6
## Postoperative Care and Complications

Postoperative management is similar to other posterior fossa craniotomies, temporal bone surgery, or parotidectomy. Preventing complications of facial nerve palsy is mandatory. Protection of the eye (lid occlusion, tharsorrhaphy, gold-weight insertion) and assistance with speech and swallowing are very important measures. Complications of surgery are related to the surgical approach. These complications include: CSF leak, meningitis, hearing loss, infection, hematoma, and seizures.

## 16.7
## Clinical Material

From 1987 to 2006, eight patients with FNS (six males and two females) were treated in our clinic. Six patients underwent tumor resection. Two patients presented with otologic symptoms without facial nerve palsy and small

FNSs on MRI. These patients were treated conservatively (clinical observation and MRI controls). Four patients presented with intratemporal FNS, facial paresis (H-B grades III–V) and had their tumors removed through a transmastoid approach. One presented conductive hearing loss. The facial nerve was grafted with great auricular nerve graft in three and in one an end-to-end anastomosis was performed. Facial nerve function returned after surgery to grade III (H-B) palsy in all cases. One patient presented with hearing loss, no facial palsy, and an enhancing tumor within the internal auditory canal. With a diagnosis of intracanalicular vestibular schwannoma, the lesion was exposed through a retrosigmoid/transmeatal approach. The surgical finding was a small tumor anterior to the vestibular nerves and superior to the cochlear nerve. The lesion extended into the facial nerve canal, and the intracanalicular portion was totally removed. A sural nerve graft was sutured to the facial nerve stump at the brainstem. The mastoid portion of the facial nerve was exposed via a transmastoid approach and the distal portion of the sural nerve graft sutured

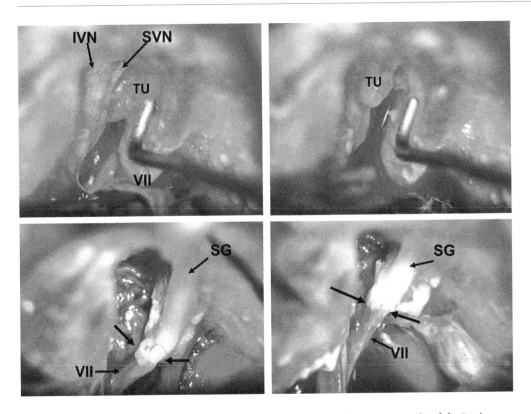

Fig. 7  Surgical pictures. *SVN* Superior vestibular nerve, *IVN* inferior vestibular nerve, *SG* sural graft for Dott's procedure, *VII* facial nerve

to it. At the clinical control 6 months after surgery, the patient presented facial nerve palsy grade IV (H-B). The last patient complained of hearing loss, progressive facial nerve palsy, and presence of a mass in the parotid. CT scan disclosed a large tumor from the parotid region to the middle fossa. Total resection via parotidectomy and a transmastoid approach was performed. A sural nerve graft was used to reconstruct the nerve. A grade IV palsy (H-B) was achieved. There were no surgical complications in this series.

## 16.8
## Radiotherapy

Radiosurgery and conformational radiotherapy have been used to treat small vestibular schwannomas with very good tumor growth control rates [9]. FNSs should respond similarly and recent studies showed good results related to tumor growth control and preservation of facial nerve function [15, 24]. With this treatment, no patient

will actually be cured from its benign tumor and late deleterious effects of radiation may occur.

## 16.9
## Discussion

FNSs are uncommon, slow-growing benign tumors. Most studies report only single or few cases. Lipkin et al. [7] presented a literature review of 239 cases. Sherman et al. [21] reviewed the literature and found 427 cases. The larger series collected 20–30 patients [4, 8, 17]. FNSs may arise along the entire course of the facial nerve, but the majority arise from the intratemporal portion of the facial nerve [4]. The clinical presentation tends to be insidious, depending on the site of tumor origin along the nerve. Facial paresis, otologic symptoms, and a tumor mass in the parotid region are the main clinical manifestations. Normal facial nerve function can be normal in many cases [13, 20]. Differential diagnosis from vestibular schwannomas at the CPA is usually very difficult. Clinical

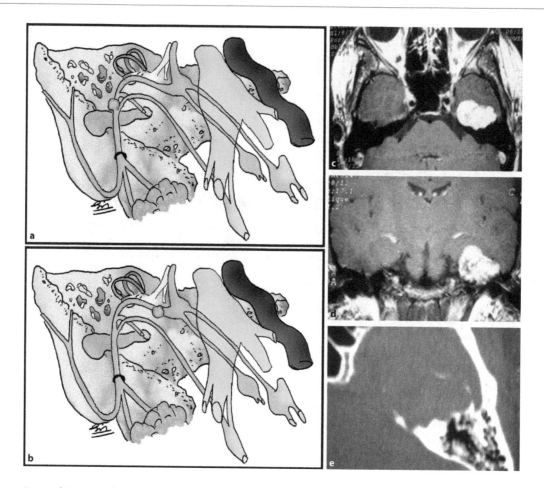

Fig. 8 **a,b** Drawings depicting the tumor site within the temporal bone. **c,d** MRI with gadolinium enhancement showing the intratemporal tumor. **e** Computed tomography (CT) scan demonstrating petrous bone erosion and calcification

presentation of facial palsy and tinnitus with a tumor at the CPA is strongly suspected for FNS. Tumors arising from the chorda tympani are rare and the patients presents with a mass obstructing the external auditory canal, causing conductive hearing loss [2, 10]. This subgroup of FNS is difficult to differentiate from other tumors in the external auditory canal.

Extratemporal FNSs are usually diagnosed as a parotid mass and a fine-needle biopsy will confirm it. Radiological diagnosis of tumors within the internal auditory canal is difficult. High-resolution CT is performed to study the bone structures and the facial canal. High-resolution MRI may give some clues to a correct diagnosis if erosion of the labyrinthine facial nerve canal is observed and there is gadolinium enhancement.

Treatment of FNS varies from radical resection to clinical observation. Timing of surgery is controversial in patients with mild symptoms. In patients without facial dysfunction, a conservative strategy consisting of clinical

and radiological observation should be considered as a treatment option [11]. Liu and Fagan [8] reported that delaying surgical resection of FNS may allow patients to retain normal facial function indefinitely. A variety of surgical accesses is used to resect these tumors. Choice of surgical approach is related to the location, extension of the lesion, and preoperative hearing status. Facial nerve grafting should be planned in every case, including preparation of the nerve graft donor site. There are some reports of removing the tumor with preservation of the facial nerve [5, 12, 17], but this has been more an exception than the rule. The facial nerve should be repaired immediately by end-to-end anastomosis or grafting. These patients will not obtain a better recovery than H-B grade III palsy [8]. Intracanalicular FNSs may be removed via middle fossa, retrosigmoid/transmeatal, or presigmoid approaches when the patient has preoperative hearing. The retrosigmoid/transmeatal access is usually used when there is a tumor mass in the CPA. In these cases,

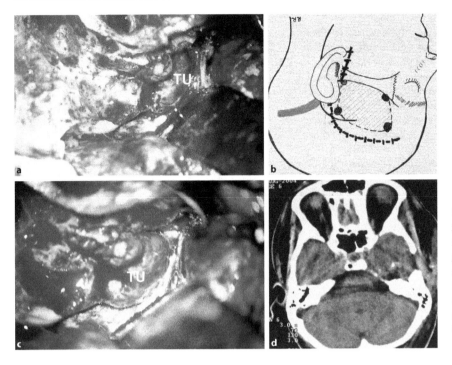

Fig. 9  **a,b** Surgical view of facial nerve schwannoma involving the geniculate ganglion (middle fossa approach). **c** Drawing showing the approach. **d** Postoperative CT scan after total removal of the tumor

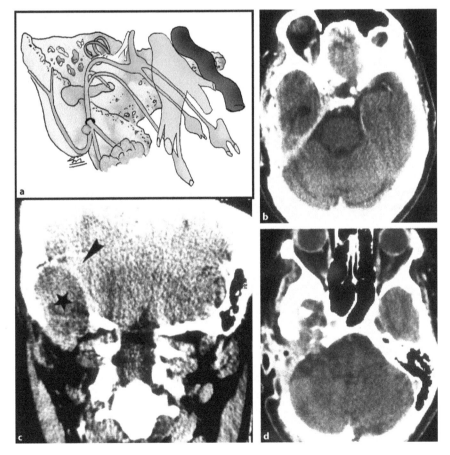

Fig. 10  **a** Drawing showing extratemporal origin of the tumor. **b** CT scan of a large facial nerve schwannoma of extratemporal origin and extension into the temporal bone (*arrow* and *star*). **c,d** Postoperative CT scans

facial nerve reconstruction needs additional dissection of the nerve in the temporal bone. If the patient is already deaf, the translabyrinthine approach is used. Intratemporal tumors are removed via transmastoid approaches. The labyrinth block should not be removed or violated if hearing is preserved. Extratemporal tumors are resected via parotidectomy. Radiosurgery may be an alternative, especially for patients with no facial nerve deficits and tumor progression in radiological examinations. Excellent tumor growth control and facial nerve function may be obtained. The patient should, however, be aware that with this treatment there will be no cure of this benign slow-growing lesion, long-term follow-up is needed, further tumor growth will require surgery, and late complications of irradiation may occur.

## References

1. Angeli S, Brackmann DE (1997) Is surgical excision of facial nerve schwannomas always indicated? Otolaryngol Head Neck Surg 117:144–147

2. Biggs ND, Fagan PA (2001) Schwannomas of the chorda tympani. J Laryngol Otol 115:50–52

3. Chung JW, Ahn JH, Kim JH (2004) Facial nerve schwannomas: different manifestations and outcomes. Surg Neurol 62:245–252

4. Dort JC, Fisch U (1991) Facial nerve schwannomas. Skull Base Surg 1:51–56

5. Fenton JE, Morrin MM, Smail M, Sterkers O, Sterkers JM (1999) Bilateral facial nerve schwannomas. Eur Arch Otorhinolaryngol 256:133–135

6. Janecka IP, Sekhar LN. Facial Nerve Neurilemomas. In: Sekhar LN and Janecka IP (Editors) Surgery of Cranial Base Tumors, Raven Press, New York, 1993, 725–730)

7. Lipkin AF, Coker NJ, Jenkins HA, Alford BR (1987) Intracranial and intratemporal facial neuroma. Otolaryngol Head Neck Surg 96:71–79

8. Liu R, Fagan P (2001) Facial nerve schwannoma: surgical excision versus conservative management. Ann Otol Rhinol Laryngol 110:1025–1029

9. Lunsford LD, Niranjan A, Flickinger JC, Maitz A, Kondziolka D (2005) Radiosurgery of vestibular schwannomas: summary of experience in 829 cases. J Neurosurg 102:195–199

10. Magliulo G, Dámico R, Vacaralli S, Ciniglio-Appiani G (2000) Chorda tympani neuroma: diagnosis and management. Am J Otolaryngol 21:65–68

11. Minovi A, Vosschulte R, Hofmann E, Draf W, Bockmühl U (2004) Facial nerve neuroma: surgical concept and functional results. Skull Base 14:195–200

12. O'Donoghue GM, Brackmann DE, House JW, Jackler RK (1989) Neuromas of the facial nerve. Am J Otol 10:49–54

13. Okabe Y, Nagayama I, Takiguchi T, Furukawa M (1992) Intratemporal facial nerve neurinoma without facial nerve paralysis. Auris Nasus Larynx 19:223–227

14. Pillsbury HC, Price HC, Gardiner LJ (1983) Primary tumors of facial nerve. Laryngoscope 93:1045–1048

15. Pollock BE, Kondziolka D, Flickinger JC, Maitz A, Lunsford LD (1993) Preservation of cranial nerve function after radiosurgery for nonacoustic schwannomas. Neurosurgery 33:597–601

16. Proctor B (1989) Canals of the temporal bone. In: Anson BJ, Donaldson JA (eds) Surgical Anatomy of the Ear and Temporal Bone. Thieme Stratton, New York, pp 89–128

17. Pulec JL (1994) Facial nerve neuroma. Ear Nose Throat J 73:721–752

18. Rhoton AL Jr, Hall GM (1968) Absence of bone over the geniculate ganglion. J Neurosurg 28:48–53

19. Saito H, Baxter A (1972) Undiagnosed intratemporal facial nerve neurilemmomas. Arch Otolaryngol 95:415–419

20. Sataloff RT, Frattali MA, Myers DL (1995) Intracranial facial neuromas: total tumor removal with facial nerve preservation: a new surgical technique. Ear Nose Throat J 74:244–256

21. Sherman JD, Dagnew E, Pensak ML, van Loveren HR, Tew JM Jr (2002) Facial nerve neuromas: report of 10 cases and review of the literature. Neurosurgery 50:450–456

22. Stasolla A, Bellussi A, Bibbolino C (2006) Dural tail: another face of facial nerve schwannoma? AJNR Am J Neuroradiol 27:1804

23. Wiggins RH 3rd, Harnsberger HR, Salzman KL, Shelton C, Kertesz TR, Glastonbury CM (2006) The many faces of facial nerve schwannoma. AJNR Am J Neuroradiol 27:694–699

24. Yoshihisa KJ, Yoshimoto M, Hasegawa T (2007) Radiosurgery for facial schwannoma. Neurosurg 106:24–29

# Vestibular Schwannoma: Current State of the Art

# 17

Marcos Tatagiba
and Marcus André Acioly

## Contents

## 17.1
## Introduction

"If any neurologic surgeon were asked to name the most difficult tumor to extirpate, his answer would doubtless be the acoustic tumor." Dandy (1941) [10]

Approximately seven decades separate this comment from current days. In this interim, several developments regarding imaging modalities and microsurgical techniques, as well as intraoperative neuromonitoring have been responsible for significant reductions in the morbidity of patients suffering from cerebellopontine angle (CPA) pathologies [25, 37, 55, 67, 70]. The progress of neurosurgery as a specialty is intrinsically related to the history of treatment for acoustic neuroma (vestibular schwannoma) [70]. Dealing with vestibular schwannomas (VSs) has developed from almost a death sentence at the beginning of the century [29, 55, 67] to the current concept of "functional microsurgery" [68].

"A few surgeons have thought that the attempt to preserve hearing is useful in every case, because each func-

tionally preserved cochlear nerve might be useful now or later in a patient's life, in view of further technological development, and because of the tremendous educational benefit of collecting experiences and gaining microsurgical skills. If all microsurgeons could agree on this, the last decade of the century would be the era not only of microsurgery, but also of functional microsurgery." Samii and Matthies [68].

Herein, we provide an overview of VSs, focusing on current aspects of intraoperative monitoring, treatment modalities, and decision-making.

## 17.2
## Histopathological Remarks

VSs are benign neoplasms that are caused by an overproliferation of Schwann cells on the vestibular branches of the vestibulocochlear nerve [34, 43, 58, 70]. The vestibular nerves are enclosed by proximal neuroglial and distal neurilemmal or Schwann cell sheaths [48]. The VS arises from the distal sheath at or close to the neuroglial–neurilemmal junction [75]. The transition zone is encountered 1 cm away from the pons, commonly occurring at or close to the internal auditory canal (IAC) [70]. However, the position of the central–peripheral interface, as well as the site of origin of these tumors may vary [43], contributing to different clinical and audiological presentations of medially and laterally arising tumors [3, 44].

Macroscopically, VSs appear as lobular, well-encapsulated, solid tumors [70]. The cystic formation is well recognized, although uncommon [70]. The nerves are stretched over the tumor surface by tumor growth [70]. In addition, surrounding blood vessels, such as the anterior inferior and posterior inferior cerebellar arteries, may also be adherent to the tumor capsule [70]. Tumor consistency varies from very soft to firm and adherent [70].

Microscopically, VSs consists of two types of tissue, Antoni A and Antoni B fibers [70]. Antoni B fibers are loose, semipalisading arrangements of Schwann cells, whereas the Antoni A fibers are denser, presenting more nuclei and a firmer cytoplasm [70].

Histologically, the differential diagnosis is limited to meningiomas due to the occurrence in both tumors of xanthomatous cells and lipofucsin, as well as palisading of cells [70]. However, the presence of whorls and psammoma bodies may be useful for the diagnosis of meningioma [70]. VSs containing islets of meningioma are usually described related to neurofibromatosis type 2 (NF2), although it may also be reported in sporadic VS [33]. NF2 is a severe autosomal dominant disease predisposing to multiple tumors of the peripheral and central nervous systems [24, 42]. The hallmark of the disease is the occurrence of bilateral VSs [42].

## 17.3
## Clinical Remarks

The clinical presentation of VSs may vary broadly [3, 5, 35, 37, 43, 53, 70]. In part, the wide variety of symptoms is due to different stages of tumor growth. The evolution comprises four different stages [43]. Initially, the tumor produces otological symptoms such as high-frequency sensorineural hearing loss, tinnitus, vertigo, and disequilibrium [43, 73]. This stage is also known as the otological [43] or intracanalicular stage [73]. As the tumor grows out from the porus acusticus, worsening of the auditory symptoms is observed together with the onset of headache and facial hypoesthesia due to trigeminal compression, when the tumor reaches 2 cm in size [43, 73]. The third stage is characterized by filling of the cerebellopontine cistern, compressing the brainstem, ultimately involving the facial nerve, the cerebellum, and the lower cranial nerves [43, 73]. Finally, the tumor causes a shift of the fourth ventricle and obstructive hydrocephalus [43]. Fortunately, nowadays even the largest tumors seldom reach this stage [70].

As already mentioned, the site of origin of these tumors may vary [43], contributing to different clinical and

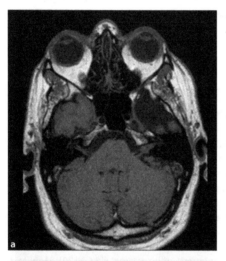
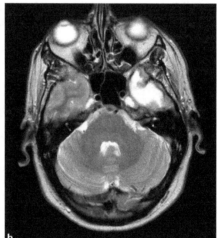
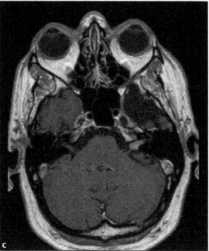

Fig. 1a–c Axial magnetic resonance imaging (MRI) scan showing a small left vestibular schwannoma extending to the cerebellopontine angle cistern. On T1- (**a**) and T2-weighted (**b**) images, the tumor appears isointense. Note the cerebrospinal fluid (CSF) collection between the tumor and the fundus of the internal auditory canal (IAC) (**b**). After gadolinium injection (**c**), homogeneous enhancement is typically observed

audiological presentations [3, 44]. VSs may arise laterally, intermediate (nearby), or medially to IAC [3, 43]. In patients affected by medially arising tumors, hearing is significantly better preserved in comparison to those with intermediate or laterally arising tumors [3, 43]. On the other hand, these patients present with larger tumors that develop without significant auditory symptoms [3, 43]. Smaller tumors along with early hearing complaints are observed frequently in patients affected by laterally arising tumors [3, 43]. The relationship between tumor clinical presentation and tumor morphology may explain some of the differences regarding signs and symptoms, tumor size, and time of disease. Nevertheless, this association has not been corroborated by other authors [35].

Hearing loss is the most frequent clinical symptom of VS [2, 3, 5, 35, 37, 43, 50, 70]. Cochlear nerve disturbances affect 91% of patients suffering from VSs [37]. Normal audiological presentations are rarely observed, comprising 2.7–12% of patients with detected VS [35]. Preoperative deafness occurs chronically in 23% [37] or acutely in 3–13% of patients [5, 35, 37, 44, 50]. The vestibular system is subjectively affected in 61% of patients, followed by the trigeminal nerve in 9%, the facial nerve in 6%, the caudal nerves in 2.7%, and the abducens nerve in 1.8% of patients [37]. The cranial nerves are objectively more involved than noted by the patients [37]. Trigeminal neuralgia and facial hemispasm are rarely reported as presenting symptom of VS [37, 66]. Trigeminal neuralgia is considered to be a sign of large tumors; however, it may also be associated with small tumors as a part of typical vascular compression pathology [66].

## 17.4
## Diagnosis and Classification

A high degree of clinical suspicion is the best key for prompt diagnosis [5, 37, 70]. The clinician should be aware of VS diagnosis in patients complaining of unilateral hearing loss, tinnitus, and vertigo in any combination [70].

Magnetic resonance imaging (MRI) has evolved to become the "gold standard" for VS diagnosis [5, 35, 43, 50]. Tumors as small as 2–3 mm may be diagnosed using MRI [50]. The tumors appear isointense on T1-weighted images, enhancing uniformly after contrast injection [70]. Fortuitously, the tumors exhibit heterogeneous contrast enhancement or cystic degeneration. Hemorrhage is rarely observed [70]. T2-weighted gradient-echo image (three-dimensional Fourier transformation-constructive interference in steady state) is particular useful because of its high contrast and spatial resolution, showing with precision tumor extension to the fundus of the IAC and the signal intensity of the intralabyrinthine fluids [77] (Fig. 1). Hearing is less preserved in tumors that obliterate the fundus in comparison to tumors that do not reach it [77]. In addition, a low intralabyrinthine signal is followed by preserved hearing in solely 20% of cases [77]. Somers et al. [77] believe that the hypointense intralabyrinthine signal is related to vascular compromise of the labyrinth structures caused by mechanical compression. Computed tomography (CT) is still helpful for identifying bone destruction or expansion of the IAC [36, 70]. In addition, preoperative CT is important for surgical planning, for which the position of the labyrinth structures, their relationship to the fundus, and the position of the sigmoid sinus and the emissary vein should be evaluated [36, 70]. Differential diagnoses include meningiomas, hemangiomas, and glomus tumors [70].

With regard to NF2, VSs are encountered in 96% of patients, most of them being bilateral, although unilateral VS is also reported [42]. Tumors that appear multilobulated are suspicious of a lesion of multiple nerve tumors arising from different nerves (i.e., the vestibular, cochlear, and facial nerves; Fig. 2) [65]. Spinal tumors are more common than previously reported, being found in 90% of NF2 patients [42]. Meningiomas (found in 58% of NF2 patients) and trigeminal schwannomas (found in 29% of NF2 patients) are also part of the clinical spectrum of the disease [42].

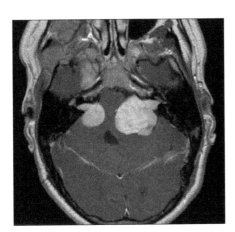

Fig. 2 Axial T1-weighted gadolinium-enhanced MRI of a neurofibromatosis type 2 (NF2) patient revealing bilateral vestibular schwannomas, which is the hallmark of the disease. The tumor on the left side shows a rather lobulated aspect, which may represent tumors arising from different cranial nerves

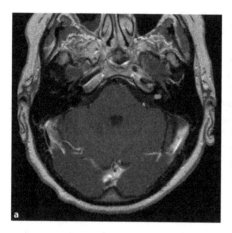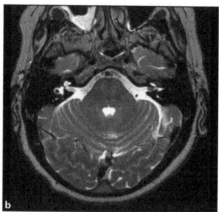

**Fig. 3a,b** Vestibular schwannoma, Hannover class T1. Axial T1-weighted, gadolinium-enhanced (**a**) and T2-weighted MRI (**b**) demonstrating a purely intracanalicular vestibular schwannoma on the left side. Note the rim of CSF between the tumor and the end of the IAC (**b**)

Patients are classified regarding tumor extension as follows: T1, purely intrameatal; T2, intra- and extrameatal; T3a, filling the cerebellopontine cistern; T3b, reaching the brainstem; T4a, compressing the brainstem; and T4b, severely dislocating the brainstem and compressing the fourth ventricle (Figs. 3–7, Table 1) [36–38, 67, 68]. A complete audiological evaluation is performed based on patient's pure-tone audiogram (PTA), speech discrimination scores (SDS), and brainstem auditory evoked potentials (BAEPs). VS may cause hearing loss of any frequency; however, hearing loss affecting high frequencies is the most common audiometric finding [3, 46, 50]. Flat loss, trough-shaped loss, and low-tone loss have been also reported in evaluating the PTA of patients suffering from VS [3, 46, 50]. High-frequency hearing loss together

with a marked reduction in SDS is a landmark sign of an eighth-nerve lesion, such as VS [46]. The auditory function is analyzed by using the New Hannover classification, as follows: H1 (normal hearing), 0–20 dB and 95–100% SDS; H2 (useful hearing), 21–40 dB and 70–94% SDS; H3 (moderate hearing), 41–60 dB and 40–69% SDS; H4 (poor hearing), 61–80 dB and 10–39% SDS; H5 (no functional hearing), >80 dB and 0–9% SDS (Table 2) [68].

BAEP recording is considered to be the most sensitive audiologic test for the diagnosis of VS [3, 38]. Nevertheless, a lower sensitivity is expected in patients with normal audiological findings [35] showing additionally a significant variation with tumor size [5]. In tumors smaller than 1 cm, the BAEP wave morphology was abnormal solely in 76.5% of patients, whereas in tumors larger than

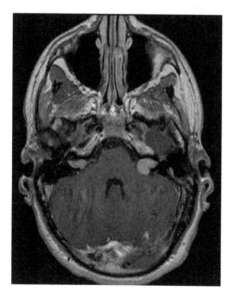

**Fig. 4** Vestibular schwannoma Hannover classes T2 and T3a. Axial T1-weighted, gadolinium-enhanced MRI in a patient suffering from NF2, revealing an intra- and extrameatal tumor on the right side and a tumor that fills the cerebellopontine cistern on the left side

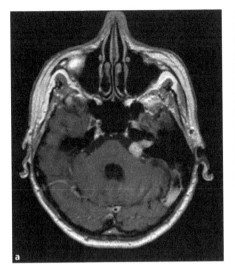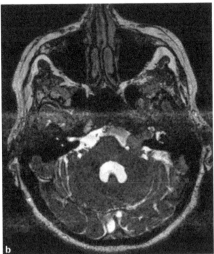

Fig. 5a,b Vestibular schwannoma Hannover class T3b. Axial T1-weighted, gadolinium-enhanced (**a**) and T2-weighted (**b**) MRI showing a vestibular schwannoma on the left side that reaches the brainstem

2 cm, it was abnormal in 100% [5]. Given the relevance of early diagnosis of VS along with the aforementioned lower sensitivity, MRI is recommended whenever there is clinical suspicion of VS [5].

The patients are further classified according to Nordstadt's BAEP typing system, consisting of types B1–B5 (Table 3) [38]. Preoperative prediction of hearing preservation may be more accurately evaluated when combin-

ing clinical data from the patient's audiometry, the radiological data of tumor extension, and neurophysiological parameters [38]. These data are currently used for patient counseling regarding the timing of surgery [38]. Patients suffering from small tumors, together with good-to-fair hearing and BAEP types B1 and B2 attain the best hearing preservation rates [38]. The House-Brackmann scale is used to assess facial function [20].

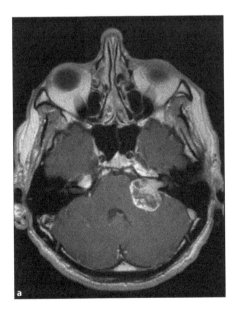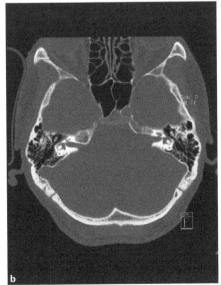

Fig. 6a,b Vestibular schwannoma Hannover class T4a. Axial T1-weighted, gadolinium-enhanced MRI (**a**) demonstrating a large tumor that compresses the brainstem. Thin-slice, bone-window, computed tomography (**b**) showing the typical bony expansion of the IAC

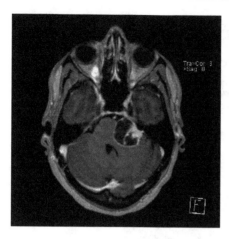

Fig. 7 Vestibular schwannoma Hannover class T4b. Axial T1-enhanced MRI revealing a large tumor that compresses and displaces the brainstem together with compression of the fourth ventricle. Note the hypointense areas of cystic degeneration

Table 1 Hannover classification of tumor extension (adapted from references [36–38, 67, 68])

| Class | Extension |
| --- | --- |
| T1 | Purely intrameatal |
| T2 | Intra- and extrameatal |
| T3a | Filling the cerebellopontine cistern |
| T3b | Reaching the brainstem |
| T4a | Compressing the brainstem |
| T4b | Dislocating the brainstem and compressing the fourth ventricle |

Table 2 New Hannover classification of hearing function (adapted from reference [68]). *SDS* Speech discrimination scores

| Hearing class | Audiological evaluation |
| --- | --- |
| H1 (normal hearing) | 0–20 dB and 95–100% SDS |
| H2 (useful hearing) | 21–40 dB and 70–94% SDS |
| H3 (moderate hearing) | 41–60 dB and 40–69% SDS |
| H4 (poor hearing) | 61–80 dB and 10–39% SDS |
| H5 (no functional hearing) | >80 dB and 0–9% SDS |

## 17.5
## Treatment Options

The treatment comprises clinical and radiological observation, surgery, and radiotherapy. Patients are advised of all treatment modalities and the choice is made together with the medical team.

Conservative management is a viable treatment alternative for VS, being advocated by some authors in selected cases such as those with advanced age, poor general health, small tumors with minimal or no symptoms (especially intracanalicular), tumors in the only or better-hearing ear, NF2, patient preference, and any combination of these [4, 19, 61, 74, 76, 80, 82]. Nevertheless, conservative management carries a significant risk of hearing loss [4, 19, 61, 74, 76, 80, 82] even in nongrowing tumors [16]. Therefore, when hearing preservation is considered, earlier intervention should be taken into account [4, 61]. In addition, the chances of hearing preservation are better in cases of short symptom duration [35, 68]. In addition to hearing deterioration, loss of patient compliance should be considered in choosing conservative management [4, 19, 76].

## 17.5.1
## Surgery

The surgical indications include:
1. Large tumors (brainstem compression).
2. Cystic tumors.
3. Young patients (<50 years).
4. Vestibular-related main symptoms.
5. Bilateral tumors in NF2 patients.
6. Patient's individual decision.

Table 3 Nordstadt's brainstem auditory evoked potential (BAEP) classification system (adapted from reference [38])

| BAEP type | BAEP waves |
| --- | --- |
| B1 | Waves I, III and V are present<br>Latency I-III is normal or slightly increased (within two standard deviations, 2.1±0.28 ms) |
| B2 | Waves I, III and V are present<br>Latency I–III is severely increased (>2.66 ms) |
| B3 | Wave III is lost |
| B4 | Solely wave I or wave V is present |
| B5 | All waves are lost |

Concerning NF2 patients, the first surgery is recommended as soon as possible. If hearing preservation is not a goal, the surgeon may adopt a wait-and-see attitude for the second tumor while the patients are scheduled for lip-reading learning. On the other hand, if hearing preservation is a goal, the second surgery is planned for the next 2 or 3 months, at which time total or deliberate subtotal resection may be performed with the assumption of function preservation, particularly in the last hearing ear.

VSs may be operated on using the retrosigmoid approach, the middle fossa approach, and the translabyrinthine approach.

"The risk implied for patients is minimized if the surgeon and the team use the approach with which they are most familiar." Samii and Matthies [68]

We perform solely the retrosigmoid approach at our department for VS because it provides a wide exposure of the CPA allowing superior and inferior extensions of the approach for treating multiple tumors within a single procedure (as often occur in NF2 patients), as well as preservation or reconstruction of the cranial nerves [68].

The operative nuances of the retrosigmoid approach for VS resection and auditory brainstem implant (ABI), as well as the preoperative and postoperative precautions are detailed in Chapter 14.

### 17.5.1.1
### Intraoperative Monitoring

### Cochlear Nerve Monitoring

The introduction of intraoperative neurophysiological monitoring techniques for auditory function emerged in the 1970s and the beginning of the 1980s together with the first attempts at hearing preservation in CPA surgery [38, 45]. The goal of intraoperative auditory function monitoring is to provide information about the status of the auditory pathways during surgery in order to prevent damage to auditory function [9] and consequent hearing loss. Early detection of the damage through a near-real-time electrophysiological recording technique is required to alert the surgical team, resulting in immediate interruption or change of the microsurgical maneuvers, with the aim of reversing the damaging process. This may enable wave recovery and thus spare hearing loss [9, 39].

The brainstem auditory evoked potencial (BAEP) is the most widely used intraoperative electrophysiological method for auditory function monitoring because it has a high sensitivity [9] and reliability to detect cochlear nerve damage [60]. However, BAEP recording requires from 30 s to 4 min to detect reliably changes to response waves [39, 46], which is a disadvantage of the method. In this time, permanent damage to the cochlear nerve could occur before the surgical team is able to detect and avoid it [9]. Direct auditory nerve manipulation [17, 39, 81],

cerebellar retraction [17, 39, 81], and drilling of the internal auditory canal [39] are identified events that lead to intraoperative BAEP changes and, ultimately, could interfere with the postoperative hearing outcome.

During intraoperative BAEP monitoring, three changes can happen: latency increase, amplitude decrease, and wave loss [39]. Latency increase and amplitude decrease are usually observed as precursors to wave loss [39].

When to warn the surgeon still is a matter of debate between authors. Empirical and divergent warning criteria have been used for different electrophysiological teams to warn the surgeon about the deteriorating BAEP: (1) a latency increase of 0.3 ms or amplitude decrease of 50% [39]; (2) a wave V latency increase of 0.5 ms [9]; (3) a wave V latency increase of 0.07 ms/min or more than 1.5 ms (absolute value) [17]; or (4) a wave V latency increase of 1.0 ms and amplitude decrease of 50% [9, 23, 32].

A wave V latency increase of 1.0 ms and amplitude decrease of 50% are the most widely used criteria [9, 23, 32]. However, the observation of hearing impairment in CPA tumor surgeries following an increased wave V latency of less than 1 ms together or not with an amplitude decrease smaller than 50% shows that these criteria may be not sensitive as "warning signs" for hearing preservation in this group of patients [23]. Conversely, in patients affected by non-neoplastic CPA diseases, such as neurovascular compression (e.g., trigeminal neuralgia, facial hemispasm), these criteria seemed to be too sensitive since a wave V latency increase of 1.0 ms and amplitude decrease of 50%, or even wave V loss did not predict hearing loss in this group of patients [23].

The reasonable answer to this dilemma is thus: "It depends on the disease that you are dealing with" [23, 32]. For CPA tumor, a stricter criteria should be used and, therefore, we use latency increase of more than 0.3 ms or amplitude decrease greater than 50% as our reference in such surgeries [39].

As reported previously by Matthies and Samii [39], each temporary or permanent wave I, III, or V loss carries a risk of deafness, as follows: for wave I loss, the risk is 65%; for wave III loss, the risk is 65 %; for wave V loss, the risk is 78%. Whether or not these losses are concomitant, that is permanent waves I, III, and V loss or type B5, they is associated with 96% of deafness postoperatively [39]. The loss of wave III is the most precocious and sensitive sign for predicting postoperative deafness, whereas loss of wave V is the most definitive sign of postoperative deafness [39]. Other authors also emphasize the relevance of loss of waves I and V for hearing preservation, alone or in combination [17, 81].

BAEP stability during CPA tumor surgery indicates a high hearing preservation rate [49, 81]. Patients with preoperative types B1 and B2 have a higher rate of hearing preservation (up to 80%), whereas those with types B4 and B5 have reduced chances of hearing preservation (12% and 17%, respectively) [38].

BAEP monitoring is performed throughout the procedure at our department in all patients that have types B1–B4 BAEPs; the microsurgical maneuvers are modified if BAEP changes occur that are known to have impact on postoperative hearing.

## Facial Nerve Monitoring

Even though there is an increasing rate of reported facial nerve preservation following VS surgery [69], facial nerve paresis or paralysis remains a significant risk to patients [1]; it is a frequent postoperative sequela of major concern [69]. Indeed, the increasing rates of facial nerve preservation are supported by the introduction of routine intraoperative facial nerve monitoring [1, 51, 59, 69]. Conversely, some authors believe that monitoring serves only to speed up the dissection, thereby reducing the operating time substantially [70].

Various monitoring techniques have become routine in dealing with complex cranial base lesions [1]. Direct electrical stimulation, continuous electromyography (EMG), and monitoring of facial nerve motor evoked potentials (fMEPs) are useful adjuncts to CPA surgery [1, 51, 59].

Direct electrical stimulation is performed by using a monopolar stimulation probe; the responses are recorded by needle electrodes placed subdermally into the ipsilateral orbicularis oculi and orbicularis oris. The stimuli allow direct identification of the facial nerve fibers over the tumor surface [59]. Hence, dissection can be performed without risking the integrity of the flattened nerve bundle [59]. In addition, the stimuli may be applied intermittently, assuring the surgeon that the nerve is preserved distal to the stimulation point [59]. Compound muscle action potentials comparing the response from stimulation at the brainstem to the response at the internal auditory canal may be predictive of the functional integrity of the facial nerve [1]. A minimal stimulus intensity of 0.05 mA or less together with a response amplitude of 240 μV or greater are used to predict House-Brackmann grades I and II outcome in 85% of patients at 1-year follow-up [51]. Disadvantages of the method include its intermittent use and difficulty in locating the facial nerve at the brainstem in large tumors [1, 59].

Continuous EMG is better than direct electrical stimulation alone, improving the rate of facial nerve preservation during cranial base surgery [1, 59]. The spontaneous facial activity registered by EMG shows five typical waveforms that can be classified into spikes, bursts, A, B, and C trains [59]. "A" trains are sustained periodic EMG activities presenting a sinusoidal pattern that produce a high-frequency sound from the loudspeaker [59]. They occur following tumor dissection in the vicinity of the facial nerve, as well as during dissection of the nearby brainstem, and intrameatal decompression [59]. The appearance of A trains has a sensitivity of 86% and a specificity of 89% in demonstrating postoperative deterioration of facial function [59].

To assess the functional integrity of the facial nerve, Akagami et al. [1] utilized fMEP monitoring during cranial base surgery. The stimulus is applied transcranially, contralateral to the operating side being recorded by the same electrodes used for EMG [1]. They found that satisfactory facial function was obtained in 88% of surgeries for VS. fMEP monitoring can be performed throughout the procedure at the demand of the surgeon, as well as following neurotonic discharges recorded by EMG or after extensive dissection on the facial nerve [1].

We routinely accomplish direct electrical stimulation and continuous EMG in all of our patients. Currently, fMEP has been performed increasingly at our department as part of an ongoing study to provide further evidence of the usefulness of the method in skull-base surgery. Just as for cochlear nerve monitoring, the surgical steps are modified or even interrupted if facial nerve changes happen that are known to be significant with regard to the postoperative deterioration of facial function.

17.5.1.2
## Surgical Outcomes

Samii and Matthies evaluated a large series of 1000 VSs [67–69] and found that complete resection was achieved in 97.9% of patients, whereas deliberate subtotal resection was performed in 2.1%. The recurrence rate was 0.8% in patients not affected by NF2 [68]. The mortality rate of the series was 1.1% [67]. Hemiparesis was observed in ten patients (1%), tetraparesis was found in 1 (0.1%), and caudal cranial nerves palsies were documented in 5.5% of the patients [67]. In addition, permanent ataxia was observed in two patients (0.2% of the series) [67].

The cochlear nerve was anatomically preserved in 68% of patients and functionally preserved in 39.5% [67, 68]. With regard to only small tumors (T1 and T2) and patients with good or normal hearing function, hearing was preserved in up to 88% of patients [68]. The overall anatomical facial nerve preservation rate was 93% [69]. Normal facial nerve function was documented in 51% of the patients [67]. Forty-five percent of the patients showed some reduction in facial nerve function (House-Brackmann grade 2 in 13%, grade 3 in 15%, grade 4 in 6%, and grade 5 in 11%); however, they accomplished good recovery within 1 year postoperatively [67]. Facial paralysis was experienced by 4% of the patients, although only 1.7% did not show any recovery following hypoglossal–facial nerve anastomosis [67].

In 2002, this series was updated to 1800 VSs considering only hearing function [40]. Again, there were significant differences in the rates of hearing preservation according to tumor extension and preoperative hearing. This work is worth mentioning because it showed that hearing preservation should be considered in patients affected by large VSs, such as classes T3 and T4. In patients with normal or good preoperative hearing, the chance of preserving hearing function was 58% for those with T3 tumors and 29% for those with T4 tumors [40]. In summary, this work showed that "the summit of hearing preservation has not been reached as improvements are still achieved even in most difficult conditions." This sentence has been somewhat prophetic since better results were then presented in evaluating the last 200 VSs [64]. Anatomical facial nerve preservation was achieved in 98.5% of patients, together with an overall functional hearing preservation rate of 51% [64]. There was no permanent surgery-related morbidity and mortality in this current series [64]. Undoubtedly, the expertise gained from over 3200 patients operated on by Professor Samii [15] may be one reason for these sound results.

## Neurofibromatosis Type 2

The surgical outcomes for patients affected by NF2 are worse than those achieved in patients not affected by it. Complete resection was achieved in 87.5% of the patients [65]. The facial nerve was anatomically preserved in 85%, whereas the cochlear nerve was preserved in 59% [65]. The overall hearing preservation rate was 36% [65]. Just as for individuals not affected by NF2, the chances of achieving hearing preservation are greater with early surgery and good preoperative hearing function [65].

Deliberate subtotal resection was performed for brainstem decompression and principally for hearing preservation in the last hearing ear, and was successful in 8 of 11 patients [65]. Therefore, subtotal resection with functional preservation for the last hearing ear is recommended [65].

## Trigeminocardiac Reflex and Vasoactive Treatment

Trigeminocardiac reflex (TCR) is a phenomenon that occurs during intraoperative manipulations or traction of the fifth cranial nerve during its intra- or extracranial course [13, 14, 26, 71]. For neurosurgical procedures, TCR is defined as a decrease in the main arterial blood pressure (MABP) of 20% or more associated with bradycardia lower than 60 beats/min after direct or indirect traction of the trigeminal nerve [14, 26, 71]. TCR occurs in 11% of patients undergoing VS surgery [14]. The hypotension caused by this reflex has a negative prognostic impact for hearing preservation in patients harboring large tumors, such as classes T3 and T4 [14].

In patients affected by VS, there is an increased internal auditory canal pressure and thereby a compromised vascular supply to the auditory apparatus [2, 14, 30]. The acute hypotension that follows TCR occurs in this ischemic environment and may lead to a further decrease in the vascular supply and ultimately to cochlear nerve damage [14]. This is the most likely mechanism to explain the negative impact on the auditory function following TCR [14].

Since 2001, there has been increasing interest in the study of the vasoactive treatment for hearing preservation following VS surgery [78]. The rationale for such research was that surgical manipulation elicits nerve edema, vasospasm, and somehow triggers a chain mechanism of microcirculation disturbances, nerve ischemia, and consequently delayed hearing loss [78, 79]. This process begins during surgery and remains thereafter [52]. According to BAEP at the end of tumor resection, the patients were subjected to medical therapy with hemodilution, attempting to improve the microcirculation, and a calcium-channel blocker schema with the assumption that it would serve as a neuronal protective agent [52, 78]. By using hydroxyethyl starch and nimodipine, Strauss et al. [78] were able to achieve 66.6% of hearing preservation in the treated group, whereas in the nontreated group, the hearing preservation rate was 30%.

Several authors studied the hemorheological and hemodynamic effects of hypervolemic hemodilution [47] and isovolemic hemodilution [11]. During hypervolemic hemodilution, the systolic blood pressure increases by up to 20% in these patients. Induced hypertension, hemodilution, and calcium-channel blockers are also widely used for treating cerebral arterial vasospasm following subarachnoid hemorrhage, in order to avoid neurological deficits [11]. The induced hypertension that occurs in conjunction with the hemodilution might also play a role in the so-called "vasoactive treatment" for hearing preservation, not only postoperatively, but also intraoperatively. At the moment, we are conducting a prospective study to evaluate the effects of the increased MABP in the TCR that occurs during CPA tumor surgery and, ultimately, in hearing function, as a part of the "vasoactive treatment".

17.5.1.3
## Auditory Brainstem Implants and Future Perspectives

Despite the reports of hearing preservation among NF2 patients [8, 68], they have typically became deaf as a result of tumor progression or surgical removal of bilateral VSs [8, 31, 54, 63, 68]. These patients develop neural deafness because of the loss of continuity along the cochlear nerve and are therefore unable to profit from cochlear implants [31, 54, 63]. A central auditory prosthesis that stimulates proximally to the damaged cochlear nerve is the only available treatment modality for hearing restoration among NF2 patients [63]. The current option for these patients is ABI, which directly stimulates the cochlear nucleus [8, 31, 54, 63].

The electrode is placed at the end of the first- or second-side VS removal surgery into the lateral recess of the fourth ventricle, particularly over the cochlear nuclear complex, which bulges into the floor of the lateral recess [8, 54]. Then, the correct position of the electrode is achieved by using electrically stimulated BAEPs, thereby detecting the auditory pathway response and avoiding false stimulation of the cranial nerve nuclei or long sensory or motor tracts [8, 41]. Facial and glossopharyngeal nerves monitoring by EMG confirms that these nerves are not activated by ABI stimulation [8].

Six weeks postoperatively, the patient is subjected to initial stimulations [8, 54]. Channels that induce unpleasant sounds or nonauditory effects are excluded [8]. ABI provides useful auditory sensations that improve the patient's ability to recognize environmental sounds and lip-reading capacities [8, 31, 54, 63]. However, only a few patients are able to detect auditory-only word recognition [8, 31, 54, 63].

The irregular tonotopic arrangement of the cochlear nucleus complex is believed to be the reason for these results [8, 31, 63]. Nevertheless, a special device, namely a penetrating ABI that was designed for better alignment of the tonotopic gradient of the cochlear nucleus, did not improve hearing performance significantly [31, 63]. This observation, together with the fact that some of ABI recipients not affected by NF2 achieved higher levels of speech perception, gives rise to the possibility that these limitations observed in NF2 patients may be associated with damage to the cochlear nucleus caused by the tumor or tumor resection [63].

So, a new device that bypasses the damaged cochlear nucleus was developed in order to overcome these limitations, called the auditory midbrain implant (AMI) [31, 63]. The inferior colliculus, more specifically the central nucleus of the inferior colliculus, is a useful site for a central auditory prosthesis because it collects almost every kind of preprocessed auditory information that comes from the brainstem and because it has a well-defined tonotopic organization [31, 63]. Animal studies suggest that behavioral responses produced by stimulation of the central nucleus of the inferior colliculus are due to detected auditory sensations [31]. Of course, further studies are necessary to establish the usefulness of this auditory device.

Additional indications for ABI include VS in the last hearing ear, total deafness in patients with head trauma, or cochlear nerve aplasia [8]. At the moment, however, only NF2 patients are enrolled for ABI at our department.

## 17.5.2
### Stereotactic Radiotherapy

Alternative treatment options for VS include fractionated stereotactic radiotherapy [27], and stereotactic radiosurgery by using both linear accelerator (LINAC)- [62] and gamma-knife-based approaches [7, 18, 28, 56], or even with Cyberknife fractionated radiosurgery [6, 21]. Initially, the indications for VS radiosurgery included elderly patients, patients with high surgical risk, and patients with residual or recurrent tumors following surgical resection [56, 57]. Thereafter, some authors extended these concepts, recommending radiosurgery as the first line treatment for VS [28].

Undoubtedly, there have been many advances regarding radiosurgery so that better results are currently achieved [6, 7, 18, 21, 28]. The reduction of treatment doses to 12–13 Gy show that tumor growth was similarly controlled but side effects were reduced in terms of hearing loss and function of the trigeminal and facial nerves [12]. Staging the dose as performed in the Cyberknife radiosurgery regimen may reduce injury to adjacent normal cranial nerves, thereby improving hearing preservation in VS patients undergoing radiosurgery [6, 21].

The rates of 5-year tumor control following radiosurgery are approximately 95% [18, 28, 62]. Hearing preservation rates range from 51 to 93% [6, 7, 18, 21, 28, 62] and worsening of facial nerve function varies from 0 to 21% [6, 7, 18, 21, 28, 62]. Trigeminal dysfunction is also broadly described, varying from 0 to 27% [6, 7, 18, 21, 28, 62].

It is worth mentioning that up to 5% of patients may fail radiosurgery so that tumors keep growing beyond expected swelling [22, 57, 72]. For these patients, the surgery is more difficult to perform due to destruction of the arachnoid plane [68, 72]. Conversely, other authors believe that there is no relationship between ease or difficulty in surgery following radiosurgery [57]. Despite this controversy, the fact is that microsurgical treatment after failed radiosurgery is somewhat disastrous, with less favorable results [22, 57, 68].

Proponents of radiosurgery continue to compare results of the earlier surgical series with more recent radiosurgery clinical studies. Interestingly, they did not realize that microsurgical treatment is also under continuous development toward the concept of functional microsurgery. Stricter neurophysiological criteria have been developed to improve the rates of hearing and facial nerve preservation. As mentioned earlier, a recent surgical study showed complete tumor resection in 98% of patients, together with 100% anatomical facial nerve preservation following surgery for only Hannover classes T1–T3 tumors. At the last follow-up examination, excellent or good facial nerve function was obtained in 81% of the patients, with no total facial palsy [64]. Moreover, in patients affected by small tumors along with normal-to-moderate preoperative hearing, the hearing preservation rates reached up to 88% [68]. So, the indications for radiosurgery remain elderly patients, patients in a poor general clinical conditions, patients with residual or recurrent tumors following surgery, and the patient's decision.

## References

1. Akagami R, Dong CC, Westerberg BD (2005) Localized transcranial electrical motor evoked potentials for monitoring cranial nerves in cranial base surgery. Neurosurgery 57:ONS78–85

2. Badie B, Pyle GM, Nguyen PH, Hadar EJ (2001) Elevation of internal auditory canal pressure by vestibular schwannomas. Otol Neurotol 22:696–700

3. Berrettini S, Ravecca F, Sellari-Franceschini S, Bruschini P, Casani A, Padolecchia R (1996) Acoustic neuroma: correlations between morphology and otoneurological manifestations. J Neurol Sci 144:24–33

4. Bozorg Grayeli A, Kalamarides M, Ferrary E, Bouccara D, El Gharem H, Rey A, Sterkers O (2005) Conservative management versus surgery for small vestibular schwannomas. Acta Otolaryngol 125:1063–1068

5. Chandrasekhar SS, Brackmann DE, Devgan KK (1995) Utility of auditory brainstem response audiometry in diagnosis of acoustic neuromas. Am J Otol 16:63–67

6. Chang SD, Gibbs IC, Sakamoto GT, Lee E, Oyelese A, Adler JR Jr (2005) Staged stereotactic irradiation for acoustic neuroma. Neurosurgery 56:1254–1263

8. Colletti V, Fiorino FG, Carner M, Giarbini N, Sacchetto L, Cumer G (2000) The retrosigmoid approach for auditory brainstem implantation. Am J Otol 21:826–836

7. Chung WY, Liu KD, Shiau CY, Wu HM, Wang LW, Guo WY, Ho DM, Pan DH (2005) Gamma knife surgery for vestibular schwannoma: 10-year experience of 195 cases. J Neurosurg 102:S87–96

9. Colletti V, Fiorino FG, Mocella S, Policante Z (1998) ECochG, CNAP and ABR monitoring during vestibular Schwannoma surgery. Audiology 37:27–37

10. Dandy WE (1941) Results of removal of acoustic tumours by the unilateral approach. Arch Surg 42:1026–1033

11. Ekelund A, Reinstrup P, Ryding E, Andersson AM, Molund T, Kristiansson KA, Romner B, Brandt L, Saveland H (2002) Effects of iso- and hypervolemic hemodilution on regional cerebral blood flow and oxygen delivery for patients with vasospasm after aneurysmal subarachnoid hemorrhage. Acta Neurochir (Wien) 144:703–713

12. Flickinger JC, Kondziolka D, Niranjan A, Lunsford LD (2001) Results of acoustic neuroma radiosurgery: an analysis of 5 year's experience using current methods. J Neurosurg 94:1–6 14. Gharabaghi A, Koerbel A, Samii A, Kaminsky J, von Goesseln H, Tatagiba M, Samii M (2006) The impact of hypotension due to the trigeminocardiac reflex on auditory function in vestibular schwannoma surgery. J Neurosurg 104:369–375

13. Gharabaghi A, Acioly de Sousa MA, Tatagiba M (2006) Detection and prevention of the trigeminocardiac reflex during cerebellopontine angle surgery. Acta Neurochir (Wien) 148:1223

15. Gharabaghi A, Samii A, Koerbel A, Rosahl SK, Tatagiba M, Samii M (2007) Preservation of function in vestibular schwannoma surgery. Neurosurgery 60:ONS124–128

16. Graamans K, Van Dijk JE, Janssen LW (2003) Hearing deterioration in patients with a non-growing vestibular schwannoma. Acta Otolaryngol 123:51–54

17. Grundy BL, Jannetta PJ, Procopio PT, Lina A, Boston JR, Doyle E (1982) Intraoperative monitoring of brain-stem auditory evoked potentials. J Neurosurg 57:674–681

19. Hoistad DL, Melnik G, Mamikoglu B, Battista R, O'Connor CA, Wiet RJ (2001) Update on conservative management of acoustic neuroma. Otol Neurotol 22:682–685

20. House JW, Brackmann DE (1985) Facial nerve grading system. Otolaryngol Head Neck Surg 93:146–147 18. Hasegawa T, Fujitani S, Katsumata S, Kida Y, Yoshimoto M, Koike J (2005) Stereotactic radiosurgery for vestibular schwannomas: analysis of 317 patients followed more than 5 years. Neurosurgery 57:257–265

21. Ishihara H, Saito K, Nishizaki T, Kajiwara K, Nomura S, Yoshikawa K, Harada K, Suzuki M (2004) CyberKnife radiosurgery for vestibular schwannoma. Minim Invasive Neurosurg 47:290–293

22. Iwai Y, Yamanaka K, Yamagata K, Yasui T (2007) Surgery after radiosurgery for acoustic neuromas: surgical strategy and histological findings. Neurosurgery 60:ONS75–82

23. James ML, Husain AM (2005) Brainstem auditory evoked potential monitoring. when is change in wave V significant? Neurology 65:1551–1555

24. Kluwe L, Mautner V, Heinrich B, Dezube R, Jacoby LB, Friedrich RE, MacCollin M (2003) Molecular study of frequency of mosaicism in neurofibromatosis 2 patients with bilateral vestibular schwannomas. J Med Genet 40:109–114

25. Koerbel A, Gharabaghi A, Safavi-Abbasi S, Tatagiba M, Samii M (2005) Evolution of vestibular schwannoma surgery: the long journey to current success. Neurosurg Focus 18:e10

26. Koerbel A, Gharabaghi A, Samii A, Gerganov V, von Gosseln H, Tatagiba M, Samii M (2005) Trigeminocardiac reflex during skull base surgery: mechanism and management. Acta Neurochir (Wien) 147:727–733

27. Koh ES, Millar BA, Menard C, Michaels H, Heydarian M, Ladak S, McKinnon S, Rutka JA, Guha A, Pond GR, Laperriere NJ (2007) Fractionated stereotactic radiotherapy for acoustic neuroma: single-institution experience at The Princess Margaret Hospital. Cancer 109:1203–1210

28. Kondziolka D, Lunsford LD, McLaughlin MR, Flickinger JC (1998) Long-term outcomes after radiosurgery for acoustic neuromas. N Engl J Med 339:1426–1433

29. Krause F (1911) Surgery of the Brain and Spinal Cord, vol. II. Rebmann, New York, pp 3–32

30. Lapsiwala SB, Pyle GM, Kaemmerle AW, Sasse FJ, Badie B (2002) Correlation between auditory function and internal auditory canal pressure in patients with vestibular schwannomas. J Neurosurg 96:872–876

31. Lenarz T, Lim HH, Reuter G, Patrick JF, Lenarz M (2006) The auditory midbrain implant: a new auditory prosthesis for neural deafness-concept and device description. Otol Neurotol 27:838–843

32. Loiselle DL, Nuwer MR (2005) When should we warn the surgeon? Diagnosis-based warning criteria for BAEP monitoring. Neurology 65:1522–1523

33. Ludemann W, Stan AC, Tatagiba M, Samii M (2000) Sporadic unilateral vestibular schwannoma with islets of meningioma: case report. Neurosurgery 47:451–454

34. Luse SA (1960) Electron microscopic studies of brain tumors. Neurology 10:881–905

35. Magdziarz DD, Wiet RJ, Dinces EA, Adamiec LC (2000) Normal audiologic presentations in patients with acoustic neuroma: an evaluation using strict audiologic parameters. Otolaryngol Head Neck Surg 122:157–162

36. Matthies C, Samii M, Krebs S (1997) Management of vestibular schwannomas (acoustic neuromas): radiological features in 202 cases – their value for diagnosis and their predictive importance. Neurosurgery 40:469–482

37. Matthies C, Samii M (1997) Management of 1000 vestibular schwannomas (acoustic neuromas): clinical presentation. Neurosurgery 40:1–10

38. Matthies C, Samii M (1997) Management of vestibular schwannomas (acoustic neuromas): the value of neurophysiology for evaluation and prediction of auditory function in 420 cases. Neurosurgery 40:919–930

39. Matthies C, Samii M (1997) Management of vestibular schwannomas (acoustic neuromas): the value of neurophysiology for intraoperative monitoring of auditory function in 200 cases. Neurosurgery 40:459–466

40. Matthies C, Samii M (2002) Vestibular schwannomas and auditory function: options in large T3 and T4 tumors? Neurochirurgie 48:461–470

41. Matthies C, Thomas S, Moshrefi M, Lesinski-Schiedat A, Frohne C, Battmer RD, Lenarz T, Samii M (2000) Auditory brainstem implants: current neurosurgical experiences and perspective. J Laryngol Otol Suppl 27:32–36

42. Mautner VF, Lindenau M, Baser ME, Hazim W, Tatagiba M, Haase W, Samii M, Wais R, Pulst SM (1996) The neuroimaging and clinical spectrum of neurofibromatosis 2. Neurosurgery 38:880–886

43. Moffat DA, Golledge J, Baguley DM, Hardy DG (1993) Clinical correlates of acoustic neuroma morphology. J Laryngol Otol 107:290–294

44. Moffat DA, Hardy DG, Baguley DM (1989) Strategy and benefits of acoustic neuroma searching. J Laryngol Otol 103:51–59

45. Moller AR, Jannetta PJ (1983) Monitoring auditory functions during cranial nerve microvascular decompression operations by direct recording from the eighth nerve. J Neurosurg 59:493–499

46. Moller MB (1994) Audiological evaluation. J Clin Neurophysiol 11:309–318

47. Mori K, Arai H, Nakajima K, Tajima A, Maeda M (1995) Hemorheological and hemodynamic analysis of hypervolemic hemodilution therapy for cerebral vasospasm after aneurysmal subarachnoid hemorrhage. Stroke 26:1620–1626

48. Nager GT, Baltimore MD (1969) Acoustic neuromas. Arch Otolaryngol 89:68–95

49. Nakamura M, Roser F, Domiani M, Samii M, Matthies C (2005) Intraoperative auditory brainstem responses in patients with cerebellopontine angle meningiomas involving the inner auditory canal: analysis of the predictive value of the responses. J Neurosurg 102:637–642

50. Neary WJ, Newton VE, Laoide-Kemp SN, Ramsden RT, Hillier VF, Kan SW (1996) A clinical, genetic and audiological study of patients and families with unilateral vestibular schwannomas. II. Audiological findings in 93 patients with unilateral vestibular schwannomas. J Laryngol Otol 110:1120–1128

51. Neff BA, Ting J, Dickinson SL, Welling DB (2005) Facial nerve monitoring parameters as a predictor of postoperative facial nerve outcomes after vestibular schwannoma resection. Otol Neurotol 26:728–732

52. Neu M, Strauss C, Romstock J, Bischoff B, Fahlbusch R (1999) The prognostic value of intraoperative BAEP patterns in acoustic neurinoma surgery. Clin Neurophysiol 110:1935–1941

53. Olivecrona H (1967) Acoustic tumors. J Neurosurg 26:6–13

54. Otto SR, Brackmann DE, Hitselberger WE, Shannon RV, Kuchta J (2002) Multichannel auditory brainstem implant: update on performance in 61 patients. J Neurosurg 96:1063–1071

55. Penzholz H (1984) Development and present state of cerebellopontine angle surgery from the neuro- and otosurgical point of view. Arch Otorhinolaryngol 240:167–174

56. Pollock BE, Lunsford LD, Flickinger JC, Clyde BL, Kondziolka D (1998) Vestibular schwannoma management. Part I. Failed microsurgery and the role of delayed stereotactic radiosurgery. J Neurosurg 89:944–948

57. Pollock BE, Lunsford LD, Kondziolka D, Sekula R, Subach BR, Foote RL, Flickinger JC (1998) Vestibular schwannoma management. Part II. Failed radiosurgery and the role of delayed microsurgery. J Neurosurg 89:949–955

58. Rand RW, Kurze T (1968) Preservation of vestibular, cochlear, and facial nerves during microsurgical removal of acoustic tumors. Report of two cases. J Neurosurg 28:158–161

59. Romstock J, Strauss C, Fahlbusch R (2000) Continuous electromyography monitoring of motor cranial nerves during cerebellopontine angle surgery. J Neurosurg 93:586–593

60. Rosahl SK, Tatagiba M, Gharabaghi A, Matthies C, Samii M (2000) Acoustic evoked response following transection of the eighth nerve in the rat. Acta Neurochir (Wien) 142:1037–1045

61. Rosenberg SI (2000) Natural history of acoustic neuromas. Laryngoscope 110:497–508

62. Rutten I, Baumert BG, Seidel L, Kotolenko S, Collignon J, Kaschten B, Albert A, Martin D, Deneufbourg JM, Demanez JP, Stevenaert A (2007) Long-term follow-up reveals low toxicity of radiosurgery for vestibular schwannoma. Radiother Oncol 82:83–89

63. Samii A, Lenarz M, Majdani O, Lim HH, Samii M, Lenarz T (2007) Auditory midbrain implant: a combined approach for vestibular schwannoma surgery and device implantation. Otol Neurotol 28:31–38

64. Samii M, Gerganov V, Samii A (2006) Improved preservation of hearing and facial nerve function in vestibular schwannoma surgery via the retrosigmoid approach in a series of 200 patients. J Neurosurg 105:527–535

65. Samii M, Matthies C, Tatagiba M (1997) Management of vestibular schwannomas (acoustic neuromas): auditory and facial nerve function after resection of 120 vestibular schwannomas in patients with neurofibromatosis 2. Neurosurgery 40:696–706

66. Samii M, Matthies C (1995) Acoustic neurinomas associated with vascular compression syndromes. Acta Neurochir (Wien) 134:148–154

67. Samii M, Matthies C (1997) Management of 1000 vestibular schwannomas (acoustic neuromas): surgical management and results with an emphasis on complications and how to avoid them. Neurosurgery 40:11–23

68. Samii M, Matthies C (1997) Management of 1000 vestibular schwannomas (acoustic neuromas): hearing function in 1000 tumor resections. Neurosurgery 40:248–262

69. Samii M, Matthies C (1997) Management of 1000 vestibular schwannomas (acoustic neuromas): the facial nerve-preservation and restitution of function. Neurosurgery 40:684–695

70. Sampath P, Long DM (2004) Acoustic Neuroma. In: Winn HR (ed) Youmans Neurological Surgery. Saunders, Philadelphia, pp 1147–1168

71. Schaller B, Probst R, Strebel S, Gratzl O (1999) Trigemino-cardiac reflex during surgery in the cerebellopontine angle. J Neurosurg 90:215–220

72. Sekhar LN (2007) Surgery after radiosurgery for acoustic neuromas: surgical strategy and histological findings. Neurosurgery 60:ONS82

73. Selesnick SH, Jackler RK (1992) Clinical manifestations and audiologic diagnosis of acoustic neuromas. Otolaryngol Clin North Am 25:521–551

74. Shin YJ, Lapeyre-Mestre M, Gafsi I, Cognard C, Deguine O, Tremoulet M, Fraysse B (2003) Neurotological complications after radiosurgery versus conservative management in acoustic neuromas: a systematic review-based study. Acta Otolaryngol 123:59–64

75. Skinner HA (1929) The origin of acoustic nerve tumours. Br J Surg 16:440–463

76. Smouha EE, Yoo M, Mohr K, Davis RP (2005) Conservative management of acoustic neuroma: a meta-analysis and proposed treatment algorithm. Laryngoscope 115:450–454

77. Somers T, Casselman J, de Ceulaer G, Govaerts P, Offeciers E (2001) Prognostic value of magnetic resonance imaging findings in hearing preservation surgery for vestibular schwannoma. Otol Neurotol 22:87–94

78. Strauss C, Bischoff B, Neu M, Berg M, Fahlbusch R, Romstock J (2001) Vasoactive treatment for hearing preservation in acoustic neuroma surgery. J Neurosurg 95:771–777

79. Strauss C, Fahlbusch R, Romstock J, Schramm J, Watanabe E, Taniguchi M, Berg M (1991) Delayed hearing loss after surgery for acoustic neurinomas: clinical and electrophysiological observations. Neurosurgery 28:559–565

80. Walsh RM, Bath AP, Bance ML, Keller A, Rutka JA (2000) Consequences to hearing during the conservative management of vestibular schwannomas. Laryngoscope 110:250–255

81. Watanabe E, Schramm J, Strauss C, Fahlbusch R (1989) Neurophysiologic monitoring in posterior fossa surgery. II. BAEP-waves I and V and preservation of hearing. Acta Neurochir (Wien) 98:118–128

82. Yamakami I, Uchino Y, Kobayashi E, Yamaura A (2003) Conservative management, gamma-knife radiosurgery, and microsurgery for acoustic neurinomas: a systematic review of outcome and risk of three therapeutic options. Neurol Res 25:682–690

# Functional Microsurgery of Vestibular Schwannomas

Cordula Matthies

**18**

Contents

## 18.1
## Background

The introduction of the operating microscope into oto-rhinolaryngology in the 1960s and into neurosurgery in 1968 [21] meant a breakthrough for these disciplines and brought about a fundamental change in a patient's chances of survival in general, and specifically in skull base surgery. Rates of morbidity were significantly improved by microsurgery [2, 27], but a functional technique for performing neurosurgery of skull base lesions was only developed 10–20 years later by implementing neuromonitoring [4, 20].

Vestibular schwannomas (VSs) constitute the most frequent pathology of the cerebellopontine angle (CPA), affecting mostly patients of middle age, but becoming symptomatic in virtually all age classes. Under ideal conditions, VSs can be cured, that is removed completely with a risk of recurrence of below 0.1% [25](Samii & Matthies 1997), with completely intact neurological function and no subjective complaints. Due to the nature and location of VSs, however, the majority of patients are threatened by facial palsy and vestibular and auditory dysfunction.

## 18.2
## Objective

Over a period of 25 years, from 1977 to 2002, 2300 patients with VSs were treated according to principles set up by Madjid Samii at Nordstadt Hospital, the teaching hospital of Hannover Medical School, in Germany. From

1985 onwards, neuromonitoring was started in selected cases until it was implemented as a routine tool and sufficient experience had evolved to the development of functional microsurgery of the CPA.

Numerous new experiences and insights have been gathered along the way, initiating changes in the concept of the treatment protocol, and have been adopted by other colleagues and centres. The goal of this chapter is to outline the principles of functional microsurgery and some of the most important experiences and related clinical results.

## 18.3
## Methods

### 18.3.1
### Technique of Functional Microsurgery

Insights into neurological function and adequate handling of the patient are the basic principles of functional neurosurgery, which begin with preoperative preparations.

#### 18.3.1.1
#### Preoperative Testing and Decision Regarding Operative Positioning

As outlined previously [23–25], the suboccipital route with the patient in the semisitting position offers fundamental advantages with regard to functional nerve preservation. As an alternative, the supine position with the head slightly elevated and rotated to the contralateral side may be a sensible option.

Preoperative conventional radiography of the cervical spine and craniocervical junction are carried out in order to detect advanced degenerative disease, hypermobile spine, hypermobility, or instability. The patient is subjected to positioning testing, whereby the surgeon stands behind the sitting patient and rotates and bends his/her head to the tumour side for 5 min to detect radiating paresthesias or cervical or brachial pain. In the latter case, additional imaging to detect a spinal lesion is indicated. In some patients, primary cervical disk surgery might become necessary before the cranial approach. If a space-occupying lesion has been excluded, but the position test remains positive, neuromonitoring of the positioning must be recommended.

#### 18.3.1.2
#### General Anaesthesia

Total intravenous anaesthesia is the internationally accepted standard for posterior fossa surgery; cardiovascular strain is thus minimised and the registration of any kind of electrophysiological potentials is enabled. In the case of large brainstem compressive schwannomas and/or cervical lesions, fibre-optic endoscopic intubation is the mode of choice. Only short-acting muscle relaxants are administered at the induction of anaesthesia, while no further relaxants are applied later on. For anaesthesiological monitoring, transoesophageal ultrasound and precordial ultrasound are combined for highest safety in detecting any air embolism, with the option of fast air removal and control of its success. One precondition to this is a further catheter placement in the right atrium beforehand.

#### 18.3.1.3
#### Patient Positioning for Surgery

After induction of anaesthesia, with the patient in the supine position, electrodes are set up for multimodality monitoring. At first, bilateral median nerve somatosensory evoked potentials (MSEPs) are set up in an alternating left/right mode and documented as baselines. Under continuous stimulation and recording, the patient is placed in a semisitting position, the patient's neck is extended, anteflexed and rotated by 20–30° to the tumour side. Attention is paid to avoiding any narrow angle between the neck and chin and to use only moderate neck extension. In the case of unilateral MSEP deterioration, some correction of the position should be undertaken by reducing rotation and increasing the extension; the latter in particular will bring about fast recovery. In critical cases, where no immediate recovery on correction is reported or where bilateral deterioration develops, the rotation should be stopped for some seconds or minutes until recovery, and then repositioning should be attempted with limited flexion and rotation. It may be necessary to spend some time on good positioning, as it is a prerequisite to good surgery.

#### 18.3.1.4
#### Preparation for Multimodality Neuromonitoring

The neurophysiological set-up includes monitoring of the auditory pathway and motor cranial nerve monitoring.

#### 18.3.1.5
#### Preparation for Motor Cranial Nerve Monitoring

For recording of motor nerve activation, continuous free-run electromyography (EMG) is indicated; motor evoked potentials (MEPs) may also be recommended.

#### EMG Recording

For EMG recording, pairs of monopolar electrodes are set subcutaneously above, rather than into the muscle of interest; free-run activity is recorded as well as activity on indirect and direct mechanic nerve manipulation and on electrical stimulation. During and at the end of surgery, the comparison of responses elicited by proximal stimulation close to the brainstem and distal within the internal auditory canal (IAC) are tested and compared to each other.

## MEP Recording

For MEP recording, the same recording electrodes are used while stimulation is performed by contralateral, multipulse, sequential motor cortex activation, enabling a uniform activation of the motor pathway proximal to the lesion [1, 7].

Motor cranial nerves that are routinely recorded are the trigeminal and the facial nerves. In the case of far-caudal tumour extension to the level of the jugular foramen, or specifically in the case of suspected schwannoma origin of the caudal cranial nerves, additional recording from the levator veli palatini muscle (cranial nerve IX), the vocalis muscle (cranial nerve X), the trapezius muscle (cranial nerve XI) the tongue (cranial nerve XII) is indicated and achieved using the same principles. This is especially sensible in case of suspected neurofibromatosis enlargement of the jugular foramen.

### 18.3.1.6
#### Preparation for Auditory Pathway Monitoring

Conventional auditory brain response (ABR) recording is recommended simultaneously for both sides in order to detect activity of crossing parts of the pathway. Separate right- and left-sided acoustic stimulation is performed with bilateral recording. Hereby, side comparison is enabled, which allows simple peak analysis and the detection of false positive ipsilateral responses and of brainstem disturbances in very large brainstem-compressive lesions. In general, multimodality monitoring of the eighth nerve is to be recommended for all retrocochlear lesions, and especially in schwannomas. This includes conventional recording ipsilateral and contralateral to the lesion side, and nearfield potentials such as electrocochleography (ECoch) and direct nerve recording or brainstem recording [11, 12, 15, 16, 30, 31].

### 18.3.1.7
#### Surgical Approach

After surgical disinfection and draping of the whole electrophysiological set-up needs to be controlled in order to identify any electrode dislocation, slipping or disconnection before the start of surgery, and to allow refixation.

The suboccipital approach is performed by lateral suboccipital craniotomy within the sinus angle of transverse and sigmoid sinuses [25]. The borders of both have to be exposed as this will allow pulling the dura in an outward direction. The 1 or 2 mm thus gained will give about 5° more of inspection angle (see below).

After craniotomy and haemostatic measures under jugular venous compression, control electrophysiological potentials are recorded. Continuous auditory and motor cranial nerve monitoring is started and the microscope is placed. The microscopic view is transferred to a screen for the neurophysiology team, or integrated into the monitoring screen.

## Auditory Nerve Function

### Right Vestibular Schwannoma T.P. 54y – Operative Steps (1)

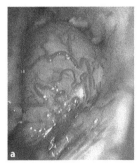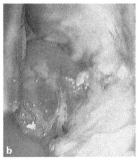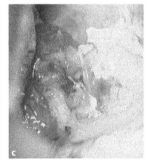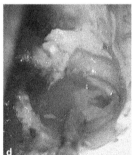

Fig. 1  **a** Right vestibular schwannoma exposed via the lateral suboccipital approach. **b** The dura of the petrous bone is resected. **c** The posterior wall of the internal auditory canal (IAC) is opened with the aid of a diamond drill. **d** The content of the IAC is exposed. **e–p** *see next page*

## Auditory Nerve Function
### Right Vestibular Schwannoma T.P. 54y – Operative Steps (2)

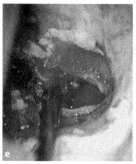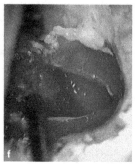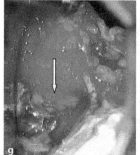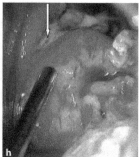

## Auditory Nerve Function
### Right Vestibular Schwannoma T.P. 54y – Operative Steps (3)

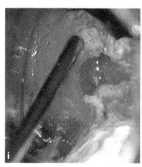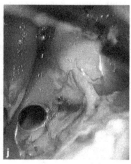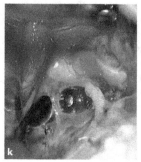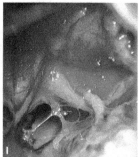

## Cranial Nerve Function
### Right Vestibular Schwannoma T.P. 54y – Operative Steps (4)

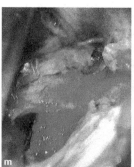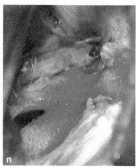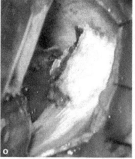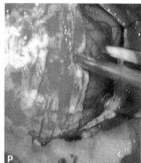

**Fig. 1** *(continued)* **e** The intrameatal tumour part is mobilised out of the fundus. **f** The intrameatal tumour is enucleated and removed stepwise up to the porus. **g** The tumour is lifted and pulled upwards to expose the arachnoid at the border between tumour and cochlear nerve (*arrow*) **h** The tumour is pulled down and backwards, and a hint of the facial nerve appears at the upper border (*arrow*). **i** The tumour is pulled lateral for further enucleation and decompression of the brainstem. **j** The tumour capsule is lifted up exposing the caudal cranial nerves and cochlear nerve. **k** The tumour is pulled upwards and the cochlear nerve can be loosened in the arachnoid layer. **l** Most of the cochlear nerve is prepared free from the tumour and a part of the facial nerve becomes visible. **m** The tumour is completely removed with preservation of the facial and cochlear nerves. A moist fibrin sponge is positioned under the nerve bundle. **n** The exposed nerves are covered by a moist piece of fibrin sponge at the intrameatal portion. The petrous vein is observed under jugular venous compression. **o** The IAC is closed by layers of dura, muscle and fibrin plaster. **p** The cerebellum and dura are in an optimal state. **q** *see next page*

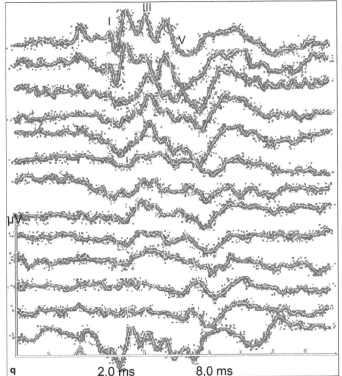

1. Baseline after Positioning
2. After craniotomy, CSF drainage, retractor
3. Drilling, I flat, latency increase, Stop! Break.

4. Stop! Amplitude decrease, break.
5. Slow recovery, still delayed

6. Drilling finished, amplitudes
7. Dissection in IAC, II and III flat

8. Traction lateralwards, I smaller

9. Enucleation, V smaller, stop!

10. Traction backwards, all amplitudes flat, stop!
11. Muscle on IAC → ABR smaller

12. Change to smaller muscle, V recovery
13. Normal ABR class A1, normal hearing at 11dB, stable hearing at 6 years follow-up

Fig. 1 *(continued)* **q** Intraoperative auditory brainstem response (ABR) monitoring with functional preservation of the cochlear (VIIIth) nerve. *CSF* Cerebrospinal fluid

## Microsurgical Steps

The subsequent microsurgical steps (Fig. 2) are to be undertaken and closely correlated with changes of EMG and ABR:
1. Baseline (after patient positioning).
2. Second baseline after craniotomy/craniectomy.
3. Cerebrospinal fluid release.
4. Retraction of cerebellum.
5. Arachnoid dissection and exposure of the nerves and tumour.
6. Bone removal of the posterior wall of the IAC (conservation of labyrinthine structures).
7. Intrameatal tumour dissection.
8. Tumour mobilisation at the fundus of the IAC.
9. Volume reduction (by 50%) of space-occupying lesion in the CPA.
10. Stretching of the tumour–nerve bundle.
11. Direct dissection at the tumour–nerve plane.
12. Complete resection of the space-occupying lesion.
13. Measures for haemostasis.
14. Sealing of the IAC.
15. Retractor removal.
16. Dura closure.

### 18.3.1.8
### Microscopic Approach

The dura is opened in a laterally convex mode within the sinus angle and pulled outward by two to three sutures. The cerebellum is lifted up with a retractor blade and the arachnoid over the caudal cranial nerves and the cisterna magna is opened for release of cerebrospinal fluid. If evoked potentials are stable, a definite retractor blade is positioned, otherwise retraction must be loosened, until evoked potential recovery occurs. In large tumours, considerable deterioration is observed already at this early step. Tension exerted by retraction is minimised by dissection of any arachnoid cover (Figs. 2a and 2b).

In tumour extension classes 1, 2 and 3, the next step is the opening of the IAC. In extension class 4 and in all other cases with critical evoked potentials, some tumour enucleation is performed first in order to reduce nerve traction.

For opening of the IAC, the vascularisation of the dura of the petrous bone is coagulated (Fig. 2c) and the dura is excised (Fig. 2d) and is kept in most tissue for closure later on. The posterior wall of the IAC is opened with diamond drills. Respecting the labyrinthine system is facilitated, the posterior wall of the IAC is preserved for at 3.5 mm; the

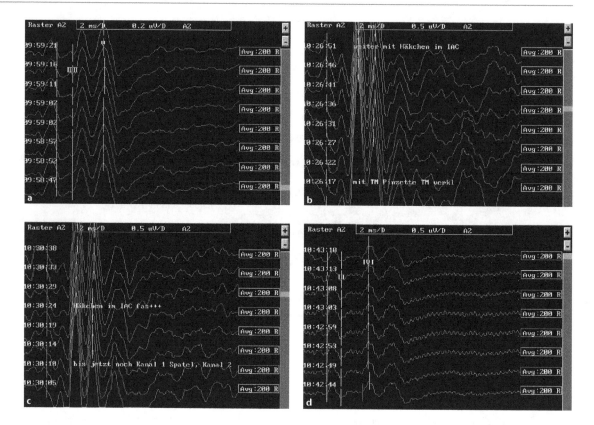

Fig. 2 **a** Conventional ABR **b** Nearfield ABR: tumour enucleation **c** Nearfield ABR: intrameatal dissection **d** Preserved conventional ABR

latter may be measured easily with the aid of an angulated hook [12]. During drilling, repeated breaks are necessary, as no reliable ABR responses can be obtained simultaneous to any drilling. In addition to ABR, ECoch should be performed, providing fast information regarding any deterioration of inner ear function. Opening or destruction of the labyrinthine system is indicated by a steep amplitude loss of wave I or of the ECoch potential. This will be followed by a general decline of all ABR components. If a considerable decline of wave I and of the ECoch is observed, a fenestration of the bone layer of a semicircular canal must be presumed. Immediate sealing of the semicircular canal with microsurgical fibrin plaster can be tried. In this case one can expect a significant drop of post-operative quality of hearing.

#### 18.3.1.9
### Intrameatal Dissection

After IAC opening, intrameatal tumour reduction and nerve mobilisation at the lateral end in the fundus are the next and risky steps. The identification of the facial nerve at the upper anterior part of the IAC is performed by slight mobilisation of the upper tumour part. The tumour movement causes some facial nerve activation in

the EMG recordings. At the dorsal surface, the superior and inferior vestibular nerves are identified and inspected for tumour infiltration; in most cases both nerves are tumorous and are transected. The intrameatal tumour portion is reduced in size by stepwise enucleation. Hereafter, the lateral tumour end may be luxated out of the fundus. During these steps, special attention must be paid to ABR components I and II. If the ABR amplitude decreases repeatedly by 50%, even with intermittent recovery, this is regarded as critical and some longer period for recovery to the original state is indicated. If this does not develop, the implantation of a small fibrin sponge soaked with nimodipine or papaverine solution under or on the nerve bundle may be helpful. If recovery of the cochlear and nerve potentials I and II remains poor, a change to a different site of action may be wise.

#### 18.3.1.10
### Tumour Dissection in the CPA Cistern

The tumour portion in the CPA is enucleated by use of the Cavitron Ultrasonic Surgical Aspirator, the platelet-shaped knife and microforceps as far as possible in order to reduce the compression to the brainstem and the tension on the nerves. The inner tumour parts are dissected while the tumour capsule is maintained as long as possible. During the period of reduction, intermittent ABR deterioration may occur, especially if the tumour sinks down onto the eighth nerve. The facial and trigeminal nerves might show intermittent activity; as long as this occurs only on surgical activity, this is acceptable. If, however, post-manipulation activity occurs, then the traction on the nerves must be reduced and irrigation with Ringer solution containing some vasodilating (nimodipine, papaverine) solution is indicated.

### 18.3.1.11
### Tumour Dissection at the Tumour–Nerve Border

After extensive debulking of the tumour, its capsule is gripped and lifted upwards. This may cause EMG responses and usually a rather improved ABR. Then the arachnoid layer is taken by a very fine forceps and pulled away from the tumour towards the course of the nerves. In large tumours, the caudal cranial nerves are released from the tumour first; then the eighth nerve is loosened along its course from the brainstem to the porus. If the connection with the tumour is still too tight and ABR responses become critical, then there are three possibilities to safe nerve handling: (1) the inferior tumour part needs further enucleation, (2) sharp dissection is performed leaving some tumour remnants along the course of the nerve or (3) dissection of this site is left for later.

The next working direction is the dissection at the border between brainstem and tumour towards the origin of the facial and trigeminal nerves. The tumour traction is now in a lateral and slightly upward direction where the facial nerve will become visible at its brainstem origin. For easier identification direct electric stimulation at 0.5 mA is performed with a bipolar microforceps. The same mode of microsurgical action with soft, short movements is performed for dissection of the arachnoid layer towards the nerve. If this leads again to serious traction and electrophysiological deterioration, then further tumour enucleation is necessary.

Thereafter, the tumour may be pulled backwards and downwards to expose the superior and anterior part of the tumour where the facial nerve is usually adherent and spread apart in diverted fascicle groups. Dissection of its arachnoid, lifting the nerve slowly away from the tumour provokes EMG responses and allows the identification of the whole nerve up to the porus. While this is the moment of facial nerve identification and conservation, these actions may be most dangerous to the cochlear nerve. Traction downwards and backwards is critical to the cochlear nerve and leads to deterioration of ABR components III–V. This may be counteracted by repeated breaks during which the tumour is lifted up to temporarily reduce the tension on the eighth nerve.

Both the cochlear and facial nerves are most adherent to the tumour medial to the porus of the IAC. Dissection at this site is usually not possible in a soft mode, but sharp dissection may be necessary. Beforehand, it is essential to identify and secure both nerves at either side of this difficult region. After maximal tumour removal within the cistern, the IAC is approached again to remove the final intrameatal tumour parts and to identify the courses of the facial and cochlear nerves. The tumour remnant is then lifted up and dissected off the cochlear nerve. Thereafter, the tumour remnant at the facial nerve is removed stepwise with intermittent use of electrical stimulation to differentiate between facial nerve fascicle groups and tumorous parts, until complete tumour resection. Direct nerve stimulation at the brainstem origin and within the IAC is performed and responses are compared to each other. The nerves in the IAC are covered by a moist fibrin sponge.

After control of all electrophysiological parameters, careful inspection of the operating field is performed, then repeated under jugular venous compression; unapparent opening of cerebellar and tentorial veins is thus identified and will be sealed by bipolar coagulation or by fibrin plaster (Fig. 1).

### 18.3.1.12
### Closure

The IAC is reconstructed in part by implantation of the dura piece previously taken from the petrous bone. Sealing of any mastoid cells of that area is accomplished by implantation of a piece of muscle combined with fascia taken during the surgical approach; fixation is done with some fibrin glue or plaster. During muscle placement, ABRs must be controlled carefully, as compression by the muscle may lead to deterioration of auditory potentials (Fig. 1). If deterioration of wave III or waves I–III occurs, immediate removal of the muscle must be performed; after wave recovery, reimplantation may be attempted, possibly with a smaller piece of muscle.

Finally, the tumour capsule may be set under traction away from the nerves and the tumour is dissected off the nerves within the arachnoid plane by traction or by sharp dissection. Closure of the approach consists of dural closure in a watertight mode, covering the dura with a layer of muscle fascia and covering the external mastoid cells with muscle fascia. The bone flap is fixed or substituted by methylmethacrylate.

### 18.3.2
### Special Aspects for Selected Cases

Some patients pose a greater challenge to the neurosurgical team due to individual conditions, such as very large schwannoma, schwannoma recurrence with some facial palsy, schwannoma with only hearing ear and a poor conventional ABR

### 18.3.2.1

## Special Considerations for Facial Nerve and Multimodality Control in Large Schwannomas

In large schwannomas, the conventional free-run EMG for motor cranial nerve control is of limited use. For a long period of this surgical procedure, the facial and other nerves are not visible and cannot be tested by direct stimulation. While debulking the tumour, the surgeon does not know whether the motor nerves are still in continuity. If a part of a motor nerve is finally exposed, this may still be at a rather distal portion of the nerve course. Furthermore, only parts of the nerve may be identified and amenable to stimulation and testing. MEPs can be of great help for these conditions. By contralateral anodal activation of the motor pathway using a transcranial electrical multipulse stimulation technique, a reproducible activation of the motor cranial nuclei and nerves is initiated and motor evoked EMG responses can be recorded. MEP monitoring can be performed throughout surgery and long before direct nerve exposure. Due to artefact contamination, performance and analysis are by no means simple (Fig. 4a, 4b). The usefulness of MEP is threefold: (1) MEP recording can be performed independent of nerve exposure, (2) MEPs indicate a pre-existing lesion and (3) MEPs are a helpful tool for prognostic measures.

Figure 4.c demonstrates an intraoperative facial MEP record in a patient with a long-standing facial paresis. Due to the paresis, the MEP latency is severely increased from an average of 14 ms to 18 ms; furthermore during surgery a great variability in latency and amplitude is observed; preservation of the MEP up to the end of surgery correlated well with preserved facial function at House-Brackmann grade 4 and subsequent recovery to grade 3 within 6 weeks.

Regarding motor cranial nerve EMG, all actions with some traction should cause some EMG activity. If this is diminished or absent and if the course of the facial nerve is difficult to identify, then electrical stimulation is useful in order to differentiate tumour nerve fibres and different motor nerves (Fig. 3). Stimulation should be kept at a limited intensity of 0.5–1 mA and rather at a low stimulation frequency in order to prevent any nerve block.

### 18.3.2.2

## Special Considerations for the Auditory Pathway and Multimodality Control in Critical Hearing Function

In some patients, despite normal-to-good hearing, conventional ABR may be severely deformed or not routinely reproducible. However, preservation of auditory function

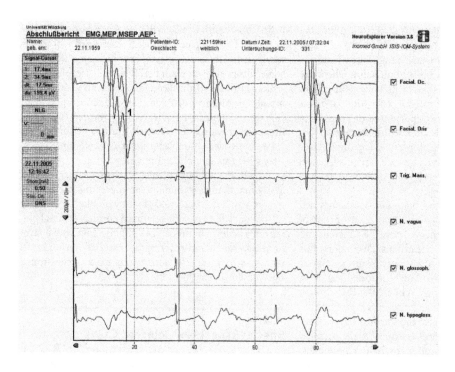

Fig. 3 Electromyography motor cranial nerves in the cerebellopontine angle (CPA): muscle action potentials evoked by direct nerve stimulation at 0.5 mA. A stimulus artefact is visible in all recordings. *EMG* Electromyography, *MEP* motor evoked potential, *MSEP* median nerve somatosensory evoked potential, *AEP* auditory evoked potential

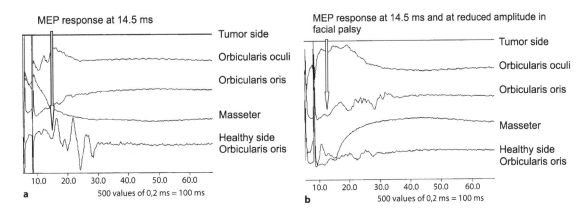

MEP response at 14.5 ms

———— Tumor side

———— Orbicularis oculi

———— Orbicularis oris

———— Masseter

———— Healthy side
Orbicularis oris

10.0  20.0  30.0  40.0  50.0  60.0
**a**          500 values of 0,2 ms = 100 ms

MEP response at 14.5 ms and at reduced amplitude in facial palsy

———— Tumor side

———— Orbicularis oculi

———— Orbicularis oris

———— Masseter

———— Healthy side
Orbicularis oris

10.0  20.0  30.0  40.0  50.0  60.0
**b**          500 values of 0,2 ms = 100 ms

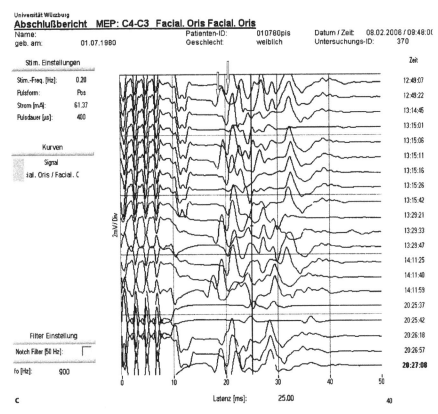

**c**

Fig. 4  **a** Stimulation M4/M3 on the healthy side: MEP response at 14.5 ms. **b** Stimulation M4/M3 on the tumour side: MEP response at 14.5 ms and at reduced amplitude in a case of facial palsy. **c** Stimulation M4/M3 on the tumour side: MEP response at 17.5 and 20 ms (*white arrows*) in a case of facial palsy

may be essential for their further life course, as in the case of the last hearing ear or in professionals with a special need for bilateral hearing. Advanced techniques of functional microsurgery then become necessary, namely, the support by nearfield monitoring. By principle, in contrast to conventional farfield electrophysiolgical monitoring, nearfield monitoring requires special electrode positioning as close to the site of the potential generators as pos-

sible in order to register larger-amplitude potentials and avoid the process of averaging potentials over 15 s or longer. Nearfield recording offers the unique option of so-called online information without delay of averaging and processing. Furthermore, thanks to the close position, potentials may be obtained in patients for whom conventional recording fails, and thus in whom only with the nearfield technique is some monitoring is enabled.

### 18.3.3
## Electrocochleography

ECoch may be performed by a transtympanal penetrating needle electrode or by a non-invasive tympanal surface electrode on the involved side. The non-invasive technique of electrocochleography is carried out under visual control by otoscopy: a small ball electrode with some electrode contact jelly is placed on the tympanum. It is important to restrict the size of the electrode and the amount of surface jelly in order to contain the flexibility of the tympanum and to allow the simultaneous insertion of the earphone. Using this nearfield technique, a cochlear microphonic and a large peak I are registered; in addition, due to the increasing distance of the generating anatomic structures, components II, III, IV and V of the ABR are also visible.

### 18.3.4
## Brainstem Recording

A small ball electrode is placed at the lateral recess and covered with some cotton or one or two ball electrodes are mounted to the cerebellar retractor (Fig. 2). The latter technique may be performed in a bipolar fashion or with the Cz reference used generally for ABR. The same nearfield electrode may be changed in position in order to be set closer to or directly on the auditory nerve during the microsurgical process. Recording produces a nearfield ABR containing components III, IV and V. It may also show components I and II in an inverted mode.

The obtained potentials are at minimum ten-fold larger, and ten recordings form a well discernible response within two seconds, but even if 60 averaged recordings are used this process will take at maximum 5 s.

### 18.3.5
## Principles of Neurophysiological Cooperation

During microsurgery, continuous exchange must take place between the neurosurgeon and the neurophysiologist. The neurophysiologist will report any deterioration with an atmosphere of reassurance as long as it is not critical. Once any deterioration proceeds towards a critical direction, he or she will indicate this in order to give the surgeon a chance to prevent harmful changes by performing an early break in time. This might mean a true break with waiting for a recovery, some irrigation with Ringer solution or a vasoactive substance, or the change of the site of action to another less sensitive area for some time. Similarly, the experienced surgeon will predict and announce to the neurophysiologist those actions he or she is planning and regard as potentially critical for the

monitoring. Within an experienced team, the microsurgical process is therefore not slower, but in general rather faster than without monitoring because those periods with stable recording are used in an optimal way by the surgeon – if he or she has gained some positive experience.

The criteria to follow during monitoring are manyfold. Conservation of ABR waves I and V are the first-line goals. In order to achieve this, all of the changes occurring beforehand must be detected and counteracted, namely critical changes of components II and III. Those components are endangered under special microsurgical conditions, at most on traction backwards and downwards, but a special risk also exists during dissection within the IAC or at the tumour–nerve border. In addition, traction away from the brainstem and away from the cochlea are to be judged as critical and require close observation.

In multiple studies performed in the Hannover series, the reversibility of the ABR changes has been demonstrated, forming the basis for fruitful monitoring.

### 18.4
## Results

### 18.4.1
## Hannover Series of Vestibular Schwannomas

Between 1977 and 2003, 2289 patients were operated via the suboccipital approach and were registered for detailed analysis. Data exist for 1927 patients operated by M. Samii and for 362 patients operated by his associates C. Matthies, S. Mirzai, G. Penkert, A. Sepehrnia, M. Tatagiba and P. Vorkapic. All of the patients were registered in a special database containing clinical and surgical information.

### 18.4.2
## Surgical Aspects and Mortality

Out of the series of 2289 patients, all were operated by the lateral suboccipital approach. In the first 1000 patients, the mortality rate was 1.1%. In the second part of the series, including 1289 patients, mortality was 0.15% (two patients operated by Samii's associates; Table 1).

Postoperative haemorrhage was reduced from 2.2% to 1.2% in the second part of the series; the necessity for surgical revision was also reduced from 1.5% to 0.7%. The occurrence of cerebrospinal fistulas was considerably reduced from an incidence of 9.2% to 5.2% in the second part of the series, but the need for surgical revision increased from 1.6% to 2.8%. Other problems such as wound healing disturbances were further substantially reduced.

Table 1 Complications in vestibular schwannoma (VS) surgery. *CSF* Cerebrospinal fluid

| Surgical sequelae | Group I Patients 1–1000 | Group II Patients 1001–2289 |
|---|---|---|
| Haemorrhage | 2.2% | 1.2% |
| Revision for haemorrhage | 1.5% | 0.7% |
| Hydrocephalus | 2.3% | 2.2% |
| CSF fistula | 9.2% | 5.2% |
| Revision for fistula | 1.6% | 2.8% |
| Bacterial meningitis | 1.3% | - |
| Wound revision | 0.8% | 0.7% |
| Mortality | 1.1% | 0.15% |

## 18.4.3
## Facial Nerve

Facial nerve preservation was increased throughout the series from 90% to 96% of patients. In the case of preserved facial nerve continuity, 70% showed good facial nerve function (House-Brackmann grades 1–3) within the first 2 weeks. In the case of any facial palsy, patients were regularly controlled at 3-month intervals to control adequate recovery or set the indication for secondary nerve repair by hypoglossal–facial anastomosis.

## 18.4.4
## Auditory Function

Auditory function could be preserved in 45.5% of cases in Samii's personal series and in 40% of his associates' series.

These data contain a learning curve with an initial preservation rate of 28% to nearly 50% in the most recent 600 patients. Some details are presented in four tables on pre- and postoperative hearing function (Tables 2–5). Auditory function is classified according to the Hannover Hearing Classification in classes of 20 dB and related speech discrimination scores [26].

Table 2 Auditory function in 362 patients operated by the associates of Madjid Samii (C. Matthies, S. Mirzai, G. Penkert, A. Sepehrnia, M. Tatagiba and P. Vorkapic): overall preservation rate 40%

| Preoperative class | | Postoperative hearing class | | | | | Total | Preservation rate |
|---|---|---|---|---|---|---|---|---|
| | | H1 | H2 | H3 | H4 | H5 | | |
| H1 | n | 12 | 28 | 12 | 2 | 50 | 104 | |
| | % | 11.5% | 27% | 11.5% | 2% | 48% | | 52% |
| H2 | n | 5 | 18 | 20 | 9 | 79 | 131 | |
| | % | 4% | 14% | 15% | 7% | 60% | | 40% |
| H3 | n | – | 3 | 7 | 6 | 51 | 67 | |
| | % | | 4.5% | 10.5% | 9% | 76% | | 24% |
| H4 | n | – | – | – | 1 | 8 | 9 | |
| | % | | | | 11% | 89% | | 11% |
| H5 | n | – | 1 | – | – | 50 | 51 | |
| | % | | 2% | | | 98% | | 2% |
| Total | | 17 | 50 | 39 | 18 | 238 | 362 | |

Table 3  Auditory function in 1927 patients operated by Madjid Samii: overall preservation rate 45.5%

| Preoperative class | | Postoperative hearing class | | | | | Total | Preservation rate |
|---|---|---|---|---|---|---|---|---|
| | | H1 | H2 | H3 | H4 | H5 | | |
| H1 | n | 107 | 140 | 69 | 19 | 215 | 550 | |
| | % | 19.5% | 25.5% | 12.5% | 3.5% | 39% | | 61% |
| H2 | n | 8 | 113 | 95 | 26 | 318 | 560 | |
| | % | 1% | 20% | 17% | 5% | 57% | | 43% |
| H3 | n | 1 | 10 | 72 | 31 | 277 | 391 | |
| | % | 0.3% | 2.7% | 18% | 8% | 71% | | 29% |
| H4 | n | – | – | 4 | 9 | 50 | 63 | |
| | % | | | 6% | 14% | 80% | | 20% |
| H5 | n | – | – | 5 | 2 | 356 | 363 | |
| | % | | – | 1.4% | 0.6% | 98% | | 2% |
| Total | | 116 | 263 | 245 | 87 | 1216 | 1927 | |

Table 4  Auditory function in 1025 small VSs operated by Madjid Samii: overall preservation rate 57%

| Preoperative class | | Postoperative hearing class | | | | | Total | Preservation rate |
|---|---|---|---|---|---|---|---|---|
| | | H1 | H2 | H3 | H4 | H5 | | |
| H1 | n | 90 | 108 | 41 | 11 | 111 | 361 | |
| | % | 25% | 30% | 11% | 3% | 31% | | 69% |
| H2 | n | 6 | 90 | 72 | 14 | 139 | 321 | |
| | % | 2% | 28% | 22% | 4% | 43% | | 57% |
| H3 | n | 1 | 6 | 51 | 21 | 135 | 214 | |
| | % | 0.5% | 3% | 24% | 10% | 63% | | 37% |
| H4 | n | – | – | 3 | 4 | 18 | 25 | |
| | % | | | 3% | 4% | 18% | | 28% |
| H5 | n | – | – | 4 | 2 | 98 | 104 | |
| | % | | | 4% | 2% | 94% | | 6% |
| Total | | 97 | 204 | 171 | 52 | 501 | 1025 | |

Table 5  Auditory function in 859 large VSs operated by Madjid Samii: overall preservation rate 28%

| Preoperative class | | Postoperative hearing class | | | | | Total | Preservation rate |
|---|---|---|---|---|---|---|---|---|
| | | H1 | H2 | H3 | H4 | H5 | | |
| H1 | n | 13 | 27 | 27 | 7 | 100 | 174 | |
| | % | 7.5% | 15.5% | 15.5% | 4% | 57.5% | | 42.5% |
| H2 | n | 1 | 22 | 21 | 10 | 171 | 225 | |
| | % | 0.5% | 10% | 9% | 4.5% | 76% | | 24% |
| H3 | n | – | 4 | 18 | 10 | 139 | 171 | |
| | % | | 2% | 10.5% | 6.5% | 81% | | 19% |
| H4 | n | – | – | 1 | 5 | 29 | 35 | |
| | % | | | 3% | 14% | 83% | | 17% |
| H5 | n | – | – | 1 | – | 253 | 254 | |
| | % | | | 0.4% | | 99.6% | | 0.4% |
| Total | | 14 | 53 | 68 | 32 | 692 | 859 | |

The chances of hearing preservation are better in smaller tumours up to 30 mm diameter, correlating to tumour extension classes T1, T2 and T3a, with an average preservation rate of 57%. Furthermore, it is important to notice that the chances of preserving hearing at the preoperative level are 25–30%. In addition, attention should be paid to the finding that in some patients, improvement of hearing function by one or two classes may be obtained by surgery, especially in cases of very poor preoperative hearing.

## 18.5
## Discussion

In the discussion on techniques and chances of improving functional outcome in vestibular schwannoma surgery, a fundamental change has developed over the past 20 years. At the end of the 1980s (about 10 years after introduction of monitoring techniques to some unique operating teams and units [4]), the focus of discussion was still whether any trial of hearing preservation was worthwhile at all. It took about a further decade to adapt and refine neurophysiological monitoring to the operating conditions and to demonstrate that rates and quality of preserved nerve functions (facial and cochlear) increased, while the next decade was spent introducing and standardising those techniques to all major clinics and to make more handy machinery available. Numerous studies now show the advancements thus achieved for the pa-

tients and prove the long-term stability of the preserved nerve functions [3].

Despite all enthusiasm, it has to be conceded that there were repeated periods of a certain drawback from regular neuromonitoring because of frequent difficulties with artefacts and often no chance of continuous monitoring. Even those centres with successful routine monitoring application, ABRs posed a problem with artefacts, deformation and limited reliability. It has to be stressed that the most refined technique in electrode placement, cable guidance and powerful hardware application are essential.

Moreover, the interpretation of the intraoperative neurophysiological findings had to be developed on completely different grounds than in the neurological laboratory. It took considerable time to prove that first of all each evoked potential component is of considerable importance and that it should always be related to the ongoing microsurgical action [9, 10, 12, 18]. In the beginning, investigators focused their interest solely on the presence of ABR component V. To date, this still holds true as the important factor with regard to the reliability on postoperative hearing or deafness: If wave V is lost, there is about a 90% probability of complete hearing loss [12]. Exceptions may be identified; for example, in the case of immense fluid effusion of the mastoid and middle ear during surgery. On the other hand, it could be shown that a short-term, temporary loss of ABR wave V, with final presence of wave V at the end of surgery was followed by deafness in only 14% of cases. Both aspects, however, are the major causes for the concept of focussing on other aspects in the goal of hearing preservation. Relevant aspects are those changes with a higher chance of reversibility: waves II and III are particularly sensitive to manipulation along the nerve up to the brainstem entry, but they have a good chance of recovery if the surgeon reacts fast to critical changes, such as a 30% or 50% amplitude reduction or 0.5 ms latency increase. These changes occur long before a critical change or loss of wave V, except for in extreme microsurgical manoeuvres with severe brainstem compression or cerebellar retraction. In conclusion, wave V may be used to predict postoperative function; components I, II and III should be focussed on during the monitoring process.

Regarding the type of ABR changes, the primary focus must be amplitude changes. Experimental studies correlating ABR changes, recovery and immunohistochemical investigations demonstrate a very reduced reliability of normalised ABR latencies [28].

In order to improve the recording options and the identification of all ABR components, nearfield recording techniques are recommended by several investigators. Several centres have tried out nearfield and direct recording techniques with various types of electrodes in an attempt to increase the speed and sensitivity of ABR recording [11, 15–17]. Furthermore, direct nerve recording provides the opportunity to differentiate between the cochlear and other nerve fibres [19, 22]. To date, it is a minority that applies such techniques regularly, while most would like to try them and clearly list all of the advantages involved [28]. Moller and Jannetta [15, 16] were among the very first to apply and report direct recording techniques of the auditory nerve and to underline the advantage of online information. Colletti et al. [5] also advocate the use of immediate feedback monitoring: "The fundamental prerequisite for obtaining optimal benefits from monitoring is the use of techniques of direct and continuous electrophysiologic recording with instantaneous feedback to the surgeon, such as compound nerve action potentials...".

With regard to the anatomical topography, nearfield, recording in the vicinity of the cochlea, cochlear nerve and cochlear nucleus must be most useful for the control of the microsurgical effects on those structures. Direct recording techniques give larger and faster responses and may allow faster and more helpful microsurgical manoeuvres [11, 14, 30, 31].

Today, all centres performing regular CPA surgery and aiming for functional nerve preservation apply monitoring of the auditory pathway. The overall preservation rate, independent of tumour size and hearing quality, varies between 40 and 50% for schwannomas and is higher for all the other pathologies. Recent data show that there are impressive phenomena of learning curves. In the material presented here, the initial hearing preservation rate, in the premonitoring era, was 28%, and augmented in M.

Samii's personal series continuously. In his recent report on 200 cases, a further improvement in preservation rate to 51% was documented. Furthermore, Samii's personal pupils and associates altogether achieved a preservation rate of 40%. This result may reflect the importance of longstanding surgical assistance, the value of the developed treatment guidelines and the essential influence and support of neurophysiological monitoring.

In addition to the preservation rate, the quality of the preserved hearing is of increasing interest. If refined neuromonitoring is performed successfully, not only are rates of hearing preservation improved, but there is a chance of improving the quality of functional outcome [14]. Regarding the quality of the preserved hearing, up to one-third of cases of small schwannomas retain their preoperative hearing level, and around 20% in cases of medium-sized schwannomas that are filling out the CPA cistern. The perspective for the patients has changed completely. The challenge and the options to the surgeons have also undergone tremendous change where neuromonitoring should be used with the same ease and expertise as the microinstruments, the microscope and navigation tools.

## References

1.  Akagami R, Dong CCJ, Westerberg BD (2005) Localized transcranial electrical motor evoked potentials for monitoring cranial nerves in cranial base surgery. Neurosurgery 57 (ONS Suppl 1):ONS78–ONS85

2.  Bentivoglio P, Cheesman AD, Symon L (1988) Surgical treatment of acoustic neuromas during the last five years: part II – Results for facial and cochlear nerve function. Surg Neurol 29:205–209

3.  Betchen SA, Walsh J, Post KD (2005) Long-term hearing preservation after surgery for vestibular schwannoma. J Neurosurg 102:6–9

4.  Cohen NL (1979) Acoustic neuroma surgery with emphasis on preservation of hearing. Laryngoscope 89:886–896

5.  Colletti V, Fiorino FG (1998) Advances in monitoring of seventh and eighth cranial nerve function during posterior fossa surgery. Am J Otol 19:503–512

6.  Colletti V, Fiorino FG, Carner M, Giarbini N, Sacchetto L, Cumer G (2000) The retrosigmoid approach for auditory brainstem implantation. Am J Otol 21:826–836

7.  Dong CCJ, MacDonald DB, Akagami R, Westerberg B, Al Khani A, Kanaan I, Hassounah M (2005) Intraoperative facial motor evoked potential monitoring with transcranial electrical stimulation during skull base surgery. Clin Neurophysiol 116:588–596

8.  Frohne C, Matthies C, Lesinski-Schiedat A, Frohne C; Illg A, Rost U, Matthies C, Battmer RD, Samii M, Lenarz Th (2000) Auditory brainstem implant in the rehabilitation of patients with Neurofibromatosis II. J Laryngol Otology 114:11–14

9. James ML, Husain AM (2005) Brainstem auditory evoked potential monitoring: when is change in wave V significant? Neurology 65:1551–1555

10. Legatt AD (2002) Mechanisms of intraoperative brainstem auditory evoked potential changes. J Clin Neurophysiol 19:396–408

11. Matthies C, Samii M (1997) Direct brainstem recording of auditory evoked potentials during vestibular schwannoma resection: nuclear BAEP recording. Technical note and preliminary results. J Neurosurg 86:1057–1062

12. Matthies C, Samii M (1997) Management of vestibular schwannomas: the value of neurophysiology for intraoperative monitoring of auditory function in 200 cases. Neurosurgery 40:459–468

13. Matthies C, Samii M (2002) Vestibular schwannomas and auditory function: options in large T3 and T4 tumors? Neurochirurgie 48:461–70

14. Moller AR, Jannetta PJ (1983) Monitoring auditory functions during cranial nerve microvascular decompression operations by direct recording from the eighth nerve. J Neurosurg 59:493–499

15. Moller AR, Jannetta PJ (1984) Monitoring auditory nerve potentials during operations in the cerebellopontine angle. Otolaryngol Head Neck Surg 92:434–439

16. Moller AR, Colletti V, Fiorino FG (1994) Click-evoked responses from the exposed intracranial portion of the eighth nerve during vestibular nerve section: bipolar and monopolar recordings. Electroencephalogr Clin Neurophysiol 92:17–29

17. Nakamura M, Roser F, Dormiani M, Samii M, Matthies C (2005) Intraoperative auditory brainstem responses in patients with cerebellopontine angle meningiomas involving the inner auditory canal: analysis of the predictive value of the responses. J Neurosurg 102:637–642

18. Nguyen BH, Javel E, Levine SC (1999) Physiologic identification of eighth nerve subdivisions: direct recordings with bipolar and monopolar electrodes. Am J Otol 20:522–534

19. Ojemann RG, Levine RA, Montgomery WM, MacGaffigan P (1984) Use of intraoperative auditory evoked potentials to preserve hearing in unilateral acoustic neuroma removal. J Neurosurg 61:938–948

20. Rand R, Kurze T (1968) Case reports and technical notes: preservation of vestibular, cochlear and facial nerves during microsurgical removal of acoustic tumours. J Neurosurg 28:158

21. Robertson J, Senne A, Brackmann D, Hitselberger WE, Saunders J (1996) Direct cochlear nerve action potentials as an aid to hearing preservation in middle fossa acoustic neuroma resection. Am J Otol 17:653–657

22. Samii M, Matthies C (1995) Preservation of hearing in acoustic tumor surgery. Adv Tech Stand Neurosurg 22:343–373

23. Samii M, Matthies C (1997) Management of 1,000 vestibular schwannomas (acoustic neuromas): surgical management and results with an emphasis on complications and how to avoid them. Neurosurgery 40:12–23

24. Samii M, Matthies C (1997) Management of 1000 vestibular schwannomas (acoustic neuromas): hearing function in 1000 tumor resections. Neurosurgery 40:248–262

25. Samii M, Gerganov V, Samii A (2006) Improved preservation of hearing and facial nerve function in vestibular schwannoma surgery via the retrosigmoid approach in a series of 200 patients. J Neurosurg 105:527–535

26. Samii M, Turel KE, Penkert G (1985) Management of seventh and eighth nerve involvement by cerebellopontine angle tumors. Clin Neurosurg 32:242–272

27. Sekiya T, Shimamura N, Yagihashi A, Suzuki S (2002) Axonal injury in auditory nerve observed in reversible latency changes of brainstem auditory evoked potentials (BAEP) during cerebellopontine angle manipulations in rats. Hear Res 173:91–99

28. Schmerber S, Lavieille JP, Dumas G, Herve T (2004) Intraoperative auditory monitoring in vestibular schwannoma surgery: new trends. Acta Otolaryngol 124:53–61

29. Yingling CD, Gardi JN (1992) Intraoperative monitoring of facial and cochlear nerves during acoustic neuroma surgery. Otolaryngol Clin North Am 25:413–448

30. Wazen JJ (1994) Intraoperative monitoring of auditory function: experimental observations and new applications. Laryngoscope 104:446–455

# Surgery of Large and Giant Residual/ Recurrent Vestibular Schwannomas

**19**

Ricardo Ramina, Mauricio Coelho Neto, Tobias Alecio Mattei, Rogerio Santos Clemente, and Yvens Barbosa Fernandes

## Contents

## 19.1

## Introduction

Surgical removal of vestibular schwannomas (VSs) has been performed routinely in most neurosurgical centers in the world. The goals of surgery are: no mortality, complete removal to achieve cure of this benign lesion, and preservation of the facial nerve and, in selected cases, functionally the cochlear nerve. However, in some occasions, total resection may be not possible even when the surgery is performed by the most experienced surgeon. If the tumor remnant is small the patients are followed with magnetic resonance imaging (MRI). When the remnant of tumor presents progressive growth they are usually treated by surgery or stereotactic radiosurgery with good results [1, 8, 14, 17]. Patients presenting on recurrence large tumors are rare because in most cases where the original tumor was subtotally removed, they are closely controlled with follow-up radiological examinations. Many series of small and medium-sized residual/recurrent VSs have been reported in the literature [1, 14, 17, 18]. Series dealing with large recurrent tumors cannot be found. The only treatment of these large lesions is surgical removal. These procedures are usually difficult

due to the presence of scar tissue and adherences to the cranial nerves, vessels, and brainstem.

## 19.2

## Material and Methods

From 1987 to 2006, 280 patients with VS were operated by the senior author (RR). In this series, 21 patients presented with residual/recurrent tumors. Nineteen cases were operated on elsewhere and 15 of these patients presented with large or giant tumors. Two patients operated on in our clinic presented with recurrence of the tumor. In these patients, the tumors were small, intracanalicular, residual tumors. The VSs were totally removed, as evidenced by postoperative MRI examination. One patient presented a large cystic schwannoma and the other one a 2-cm tumor. These tumors recurred 2 and 3.5 years, respectively, after surgery. Giant VSs are those with a diameter exceeding 4.5 cm, and large VSs are those with a diameter larger than 3.5 cm. These tumors caused compression of the brainstem. There were ten giant and five large VSs in this series (Table 1). Most patients were young, with a mean age of 37.8 years (range 21–58 years). Clinical symptoms were: deafness (all patients), ataxia (ten patients), complete facial nerve palsy (eight patients), facial numbness (six cases), and hoarse voice and swallowing difficulties (five patients). Tracheotomy and gastrostomy was performed in one patient after two surgeries and conformational stereotactic radiotherapy. Gamma-knife radiosurgery was carried out in two cases and conformational radiotherapy in one. One previous surgery had been performed in six cases, two in seven cases, and three in two cases. Tumor size at first surgery varied from 3.5 to 5.0 cm, and four were cystic (Table 1). Subtotal removal by previous surgery(ies) was performed in all cases. The mean time that had elapsed between the last surgery and the definitive surgery in our department was 2.8 years (range 1.5–5 years). Causes for subtotal removal were: extensive bleeding, adherences to the brainstem and facial nerve, and cerebellar edema. The internal

Table 1  Patients with large and giant residual/recurrent vestibular schwannoma (VS). *GKS* Gamma knife surgery, *CSR* conformational stereotactic radiotherapy

| Patient | Age (years) | No. of previous surgeries | Size of first operation (cm) | Tumor types | Grade resection last surgery | Radiation therapy after previous surgery(ies) | Size before definitive surgery (cm) | Time between last surgery and definitive surgery (years) |
|---|---|---|---|---|---|---|---|---|
| MEVB | 23 | 1 | 4.0 | Solid | 40% | No | 4.5 | 3 |
| IC | 27 | 2 | 4.0 | Cystic | 30% | No | 5.0 | 2 |
| JL | 58 | 1 | 4.0 | Solid | 40% | No | 3.5 | 5 |
| FRB | 21 | 1 | 4.5 | Solid | 30% | No | 4.5 | 1.5 |
| HHS | 29 | 3 | 5.0 | Cystic | 60% | No | 5.0 | 3 |
| IA | 52 | 2 | 4.5 | Solid | 40% | No | 4.0 | 4 |
| AV | 38 | 1 | 4.0 | Solid | 30% | No | 4.0 | 3 |
| PL | 42 | 3 | 4.0 | Solid | 40% | No | 4.5 | 2.5 |
| JB | 47 | 1 | 4,0 | Solid | 40% | No | 4.0 | 2 |
| LAB | 40 | 2 | 4,5 | Solid | 30% | CSR | $,5 | 2 |
| MMM | 35 | 2 | 5,0 | Solid | 50% | No | 5.0 | 4 |
| JML | 47 | 2 | 4.0 | Cystic | 50% | GKS | 5.0 | 3.5 |
| LF | 28 | 2 | 4.5 | Cystic | 30% | No | 4.5 | 1.5 |
| CSY | 39 | 2 | 4.0 | Solid | 50% | No | 4.5 | 4 |
| VRS | 42 | 1 | 3.5 | Solid | 30% | GKS | 4.0 | 2.5 |

auditory canal (IAC) had been opened in five cases. All patients were reoperated in our department through the retrosigmoid/transmeatal approach in the dorsal position (Fig. 1) and with facial nerve monitoring in cases of preserved facial nerve. Twelve patients needed a shunt insertion for hydrocephalus. The mean postoperative follow-up was 5.6 years (range 1–11 years).

## 19.3
## Results and Surgical Complications

Surgery was indicated to completely remove these large/giant recurrent tumors so as to decompress the brainstem and save the patient's life. This was achieved in all patients (Table 2). The surgical procedure was more difficult than in nonoperated cases. Fibrosis caused by the previous surgery made dissection of the dura mater and

identification of the sigmoid sinus difficult. After opening of the dura mater there was no clear arachnoid plane. Those cases that had submitted to radiotherapy presented more adherences. Dissection of the cranial nerves, vessels, and brainstem with preservation of these structures was the main task of the surgery. Facial nerve monitoring helped to preserve the nerve. When the previous surgeon had not opened the IAC, identification and dissection of the facial nerve within the IAC was easier. Anatomical preservation of the facial nerve was possible in six out of seven patients with preoperative facial nerve function. Hypoglossal-facial anastomosis was performed 2 or 3 weeks after surgery in seven of the remaining eight cases. House and Brackmann (H-B) facial palsy grades III–IV were obtained in these patients.

Transient trigeminal nerve deficits occurred in three patients. The major complications in this series were meningitis in one case and transient palsy of the caudal

Table 2 Patients with large and giant residual/recurrent VS. *VII CN* cranial nerve VII, *V CN* cranial nerve V, *CSF* cerebrospinal fluid

| Patient | Preoperative VII CN grade[a] | Other preoperative neurological deficits | Postoperative VII CN grade[a] | Hydrocephalus | Extent of Removal | Follow-up | Complications |
|---|---|---|---|---|---|---|---|
| MEVB | II | Ataxia | IV | Yes | Total | 10 years | No |
| IC | VI | Ataxia, V CN, dysphasia | VI | Yes | Total | 9 years | CSF leak/ meningitis |
| JL | I | No | III | No | Total | 9 years | CSF leak |
| FRB | IV | Ataxia | VI | No | Total | 8 years | None |
| HHS | VI | Ataxia, V CN, dysphasia | VI | Yes | Total | 8 years | Facial numbness |
| IA | VI | Ataxia, V CN | VI | Yes | Total | 8 years | None |
| AV | I | No | I | Yes | Total | 5 years | None |
| PL | VI | Ataxia | VI | Yes | Total | 4 years | IX, X (transient) |
| JB | III | No | IV | No | Total | 3 years | None |
| LAB | VI | Ataxia, V CN, dysphasia. Tracheotomy, gastrostomy | VI | Yes | Total | 3 years | Facial numbness |
| MMM | VI | Ataxia, V CN | VI | Yes | Total | 3 years | CSF leak |
| JML | VI | Ataxia, dysphasia | VI | Yes | Total | 2 years | None |
| LF | VI | Ataxia, dysphasia, V CN | VI | Yes | Total | 1.5 years | IX, X (transient), facial numbness |
| CSY | III | No | III | Yes | Total | 4 months | None |
| VRS | I | No | III | Yes | Total | 4 months | None |

[a] House and Brackmann [6]

cranial nerves in two. One of these patients needed transient tracheotomy and gastrostomy. There was no permanent morbidity. One patient was admitted to our clinic after two surgical procedures and conformational radiotherapy with tracheostomy and gastrostomy. After radical resection the facial nerve was rehabilitated with a VII/XII anastomosis and the tracheotomy and gastrostomy were removed 3 months thereafter. This patient recovered well, and 1 year after the definitive surgery returned to her previous job as an elementary school teacher. The histological findings in all cases revealed benign schwannomas.

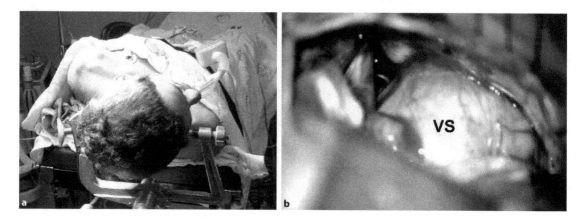

Fig. 1a,b  Patient's position (**a**) and exposition of the vestibular schwannomas (*VS*; **b**)

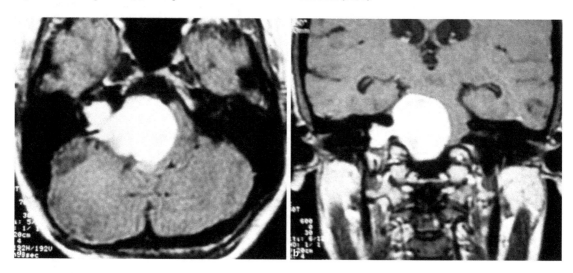

Fig. 2a,b  Magnetic resonance imaging (MRI) – 2 years after surgery for a giant residual/recurrent VS (case 1)

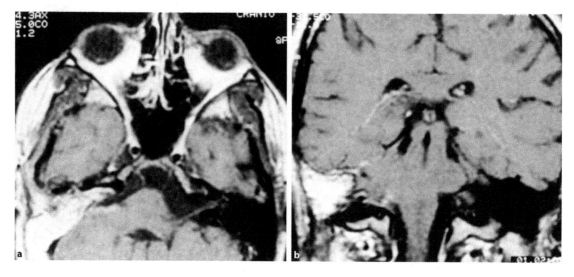

Fig. 3a,b  Postoperative MRI after total removal (case 1)

### 19.3.1
### Case 1

This 23-year-old woman underwent surgical resection of a large VS 2 years before admission. The retrosigmoid approach had been used and only subtotal removal could be achieved. She developed facial paralysis H-B grade IV and hydrocephalus. The hydrocephalus was treated with shunt insertion. At admission to our clinic, MRI revealed a giant residual/recurrent VS (Fig. 2). The tumor was removed totally using the retrosigmoid-transmeatal approach. The facial nerve could be preserved and the patient presented no additional deficit (Fig. 3).

### 19.3.2
### Case 2

This 38-year-old woman was admitted to our clinic with a history of previous surgery for removal of a 3.5-cm VS 4 years before in another clinic. Partial removal had been performed and at admission to our clinic she presented a facial paresis H-B grade II. A shunt had been inserted for hydrocephalus. MRI revealed a giant residual/recurrent VS (Fig. 4). Total removal of the tumor and preservation of the facial nerve was achieved (Fig. 5); the postoperative course was uneventful.

### 19.3.3
### Case 3

This 40-year-old woman presented with a giant VS and hydrocephalus. The hydrocephalus was treated initially by shunt and with two surgical approaches for the VS.

Only partial resection of the tumor was achieved. After the second surgery the patient developed brain edema and remained in a coma for 1 week in the intensive care unit. She developed complete facial nerve paralysis and swallowing disturbance, requiring tracheotomy. She was admitted to our clinic with tracheotomy and gastrostomy, was unable to walk due severe ataxia, and presented with complete facial nerve paralysis. Conformational radiotherapy had been performed after the second surgical procedure. The tumor showed further growth in the control MRIs and the residual lesion had received no treatment (Fig. 6). This giant recurrent/residual tumor was totally resected using the retrosigmoid/transmeatal approach (Fig. 7). There was no postoperative complication and the facial nerve was rehabilitated with a VII/XII anastomosis. The tracheotomy and gastrostomy were removed 3 months thereafter. The patient was able to return to her previous function as elementary school teacher 1 year after surgery.

### 19.4
### Discussion

With the development of new radiological procedure, especially high-definition MRI, VSs are easily diagnosed. Most tumors are small- or medium-sized when diagnosis is established and surgical removal with preservation of the facial nerve, no mortality, and no additional morbidity can be accomplished in the majority of cases. Surgical difficulties to achieve total removal with preservation of the facial nerve, no mortality, and no further morbidity are encountered with large and giant VSs. These tumors, may be partially removed, either intentionally or unintentionally, for various reasons [11, 17]. After subtotal re-

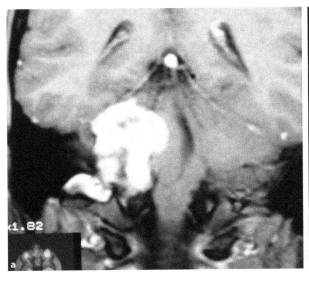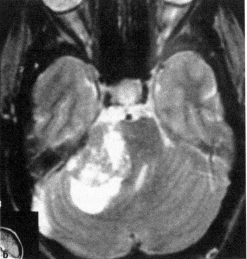

Fig. 4a,b Preoperative MRI of giant residual recurrent VS (case 2)

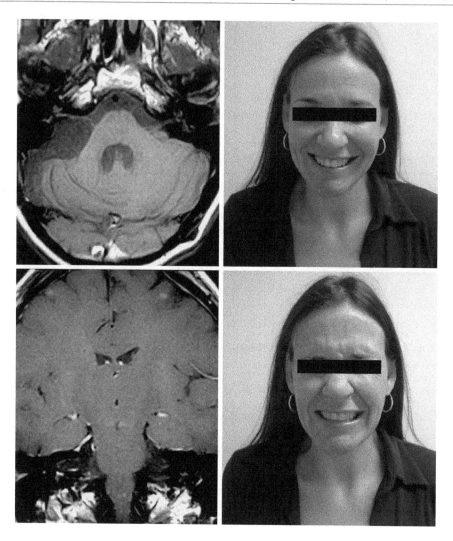

Fig. 5 Postoperative MRI and patient with preservation of facial nerve (case 2)

section, tumor remnants present an unpredictable growth rate [1, 3, 4, 12].

Recurrent tumors are those that present a new growth after total removal and residual tumors are those subtotally removed [19]. After incomplete excision, the recurrence rate is usually high. Sakaki et al. [15] reported recurrence rates of 29% (5 out of 17 patients) after subtotal resection. Other series [2] reported 52 patients with subtotal removal, 33 with near-total resections (remnant ≤25 mm and ≤2 mm thick), and 19 with subtotal resections (any larger remnant). Recurrences occurred in 1 (3%) of 33 patients who had a near-total resection and in 6 (32%) of 19 patients who had a subtotal resection. All recurrences were observed in the mid-cerebellopontine angle following the translabyrinthine approach. It is, however, not easy to differentiate subtotal from near-total resection. We prefer to classify the grade of resection as

either complete or incomplete. A very low recurrence rate is observed after complete tumor removal [5, 10, 13, 16], but higher recurrence rates after total excision have also been reported [20]. As the growth of the remnant tumor has no clear pattern, the patients in this series were classified as residual/recurrent.

There are few reports on the treatment and outcome of residual VSs [1, 14, 17]. Published studies on the surgical management of large and giant residual/recurrent vestibular schwannomas (acoustic neurinoma) were not found using a keyword search through Pub-Med. In the majority of cases, patients who underwent subtotal resection of a VS are followed carefully with MRI and if the tumor remnant grows, further treatment is indicated. Therefore, recurrent tumors are usually treated when they are small. Samii and Matties [16] published the largest series on VS operated by one surgeon. Sixty-two patients of

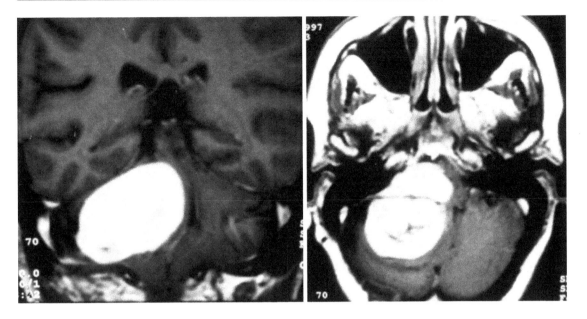

Fig. 6 MRI after two previous surgeries and radiotherapy. Giant residual/recurrent VS (case 3)

his series had residual/recurrent tumors (56 underwent surgery in other hospitals). The sizes and outcomes of these cases were not presented. Two patients died after surgery for recurrent tumors. In other reported series of 179 cases, 11 patients (6%) had undergone previous surgery [5]. Tumor sizes and outcomes of these cases were also not described. A series of 23 residual VS was reported [17], four patients presented large lesions (up to 4.0 cm in

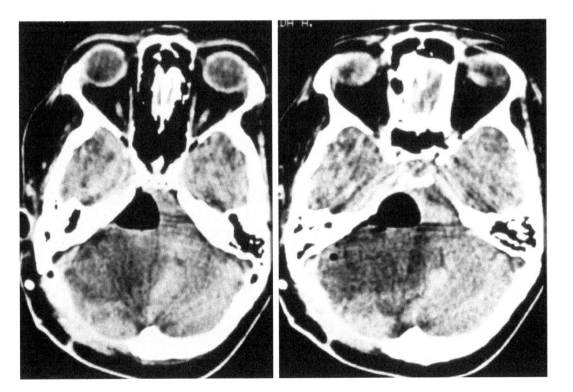

Fig. 7 Postoperative computed tomography scan after total removal of the giant residual/recurrent VS

diameter) and one a giant VS (5.0 cm in diameter). Total resection was achieved in four of these patients and the facial nerve was not preserved in any case. The lesions were removed through the transcochlear approach (three patients) and translabyrinthine (two patients).

Our series presents 15 patients with large and giant residual/recurrent VSs. All patients had been operated on elsewhere and the majority presented complications after the previous surgeries. Nine patients underwent at least two previous surgical procedures. Tumor growth of the residual tumors was observed in control MRI examinations, but patients and surgeons were afraid of new surgical procedures or treatment with radiotherapy.

Resection of residual VSs is usually difficult due to scar tissue and absence of a clear arachnoid plane between the tumor and brainstem, vessels and nerves. When the recurrent tumor is large or giant, surgical removal is even more difficult because the structures around the tumor capsule are adherent and displaced. Total excision could be achieved in all our patients through the retrosigmoid-transmeatal approach. Seven patients presented facial nerve function preoperatively. Facial nerve preservation was possible in six. Transient trigeminal nerve and caudal cranial nerve deficits developed in three and two patients, respectively. There was no mortality. Facial nerve rehabilitation is performed with XII/VII anastomosis. This procedure should be avoided, however, in patients with complete caudal cranial nerve paralysis. In these cases, rehabilitation of the face is performed through plastic surgery procedures or/and cross-face anastomosis.

Radiotherapy and radiosurgery have been recommended to treat subtotally resected VSs. Good outcomes in 50 patients treated with gamma-knife radiosurgery after previous microsurgical subtotal resection or recurrence after total resection of VS was reported [21]. The median treatment volume was 3.4 ml, and with a median follow-up of 75 months (range 42–114 months), the control rate of tumor growth was 96%. Radiosurgery is not recommended for large lesions with significant brainstem compression. These tumors usually require surgical resection [9]. Radiosurgical doses and tumor dimensions were considered the two most important risk factors for injury to cranial nerves VII and V [7]. In our series, three patients were treated after previous surgery with radiosurgery or conformational radiotherapy. These tumors presented further growth. For large and giant VSs, surgical excision is the only definitive treatment.

## 19.5
## Conclusion

Large and giant recurrent/residual VSs are rare. Most recurrent VSs are small and have an unpredictable growth rate. Surgical removal is the only curative treatment for these large and giant lesions. Total resection with low morbidity and mortality can be achieved through the retrosigmoid/transmeatal approach. Absence of scar tissue, adherence to the brainstem, cranial nerves, and vessels are the main surgical difficulties.

## References

1. Beatty CW, Ebersold MJ, Harner SG (1987) Residual and recurrent acoustic neuromas. Laryngoscope 97:1168–1171
2. Bloch DC, Oghalai JS, Jackler RK (2004) The fate of the tumor remnant after less-than-complete acoustic neuroma resection. Otolaryngol Head Neck Surg 130:104–112
3. El-Kashlan HK, Zeitoun H, Arts HA (2000) Recurrence of acoustic neuroma after incomplete resection. Am J Otol 21:389–392
4. Gamache F, Patterson R (1992) Growth rates for residual and recurrent acoustic neuroma. In: Tos M, Thomsen J (eds) Acoustic Neuroma. Kugler, Amsterdam, pp 705–707
5. Gormley WB, Sekhar LN, Wright DC, et al (1997) Acoustic neuromas: results of current surgical management. Neurosurgery 41:50–60
6. House JW, Brackmann DE (1985) Facial nerve grading system. Otolaryngol Head Neck Surg 93:146–147
7. Ito K, Shin M, Matsuzaki M, et al (2000) Risk factors for neurological complications after acoustic neurinoma radiosurgery: refinement from further experiences. Int J Radiat Oncol Biol Phys 48:75–80
8. Iwai Y, Yamanaka K, Ishiguro T (2003) Surgery combined with radiosurgery of large acoustic neuromas. Surg Neurol 59:283–291
9. Kondziolka D, Lunsford LD, Flickinger JC (2003) Acoustic tumors: operation versus radiation – making sense of opposing viewpoints. Part II. Acoustic neuromas: sorting out management options. Clin Neurosurg 50:313–328
10. Lanman TH, Brackmann DE, Hitselberger WE, et al (1999) Report of 190 consecutive cases of large acoustic tumors (vestibular schwannoma) removed via the translabyrinthine approach. J Neurosurg 90:617–623
11. Matthies C, Samii M (2002) Vestibular schwannomas and auditory function: options in large T3 and T4 tumors? Neurochirurgie 48:461–470
12. Pace-Balzan A, Lye RH, Ramsden RT, et al (1992) Growth characteristics of acoustic neuromas with particular reference to the fate of capsule fragments remaining after tumor removal: implications for patient management. In: Tos M, Thomsen J (eds) Acoustic Neuroma. Kugler, Amsterdam, pp 701–703
13. Ramina R, Maniglia JJ, Meneses MS, et al (1997) Acoustic neurinomas. Diagnosis and treatment. Arq Neuropsiquiatr 55:393–402
14. Roberson JB Jr, Brackmann DE, Hitselberger WE (1996) Acoustic neuroma recurrence after suboccipital resection: management with translabyrinthine resection. Am J Otol 17:307–311

15. Sakaki S, Nakagawa K, Hatakeyama T, et al (1991) Recurrence after incompletely resected acousticus neurinomas. Med J Osaka Univ 40:59–66
16. Samii M, Matthies C (1997) Management of 1000 vestibular schwannomas (acoustic neuromas): surgical management and results with an emphasis on complications and how to avoid them. Neurosurgery 40:11–23
17. Sanna M, Falcioni M, Taibah A, et al (2002) Treatment of residual schwannoma. Otol Neurotol 23:980–987
18. Shea JJ 3rd, Hitselberger WE, Benecke JE Jr, et al (1985) Recurrence rate of partially resected acoustic tumors. Am J Otol Suppl:107–109
19. Shelton C (1995) Unilateral acoustic tumors: how often do they recur after translabyrinthine removal? Laryngoscope 105:958–966
20. Thomassin JM, Pellet W, Epron JP, et al (2001) Recurrent acoustic neurinoma after complete surgical resection [in French]. Ann Otolaryngol Chir Cervicofac 118:3–10
21. Unger F, Walch C, Papaefthymiou G (2002) Radiosurgery of residual and recurrent vestibular schwannomas. Acta Neurochir (Wien) 144:671–677

# Arachnoid Cysts of the Posterior Fossa

# 20

Gustavo Adolpho de Carvalho
and Michael Hinojosa

Contents

## 20.1
## Introduction

Intracranial arachnoid cysts (ACs) are presumably congenital malformations that are thought to be formed by the splitting of the arachnoid membrane due to an increased pulsation of the cerebrospinal fluid (CSF) [4, 12, 13]. They represent only 1% of all intracranial lesions and are most commonly found in the middle fossa [2,4,20,40]. ACs involving the posterior fossa, especially the cerebellopontine angle (CPA), represent the second most common location and are found in 10–11% of all cases [17, 31, 39].

Despite modern diagnostic imaging (magnetic resonance imaging, MRI), a definitive preoperative diagnosis is sometimes still controversial [17, 38]. ACs involving the posterior fossa may be asymptomatic or may produce a wide variety of posterior fossa symptoms with little specificity like headache, ataxia, dizziness, tinnitus and hearing loss. Patients affected are usually between the fourth and fifth decade of life.

Different methods of surgical treatment have been proposed for the management of intracranial ACs [10]. Stereotactic punction, cystoperitoneal shunting, cyst fenestration or marsupialisation into the subarachnoid space, and radical resection of the cyst are the most common procedures [2, 10, 24].

## 20.2
## Formation and Growth of ACs

Regarding the formation of ACs, two major steps are of interest: (1) the development and (2) the possible growth. The aetiology of ACs has been discussed extensively in the past [4, 13, 15]. Infection, trauma and/or alteration of the CSF flow and/or pressure were the common hypotheses to explain their origin [9, 20, 25]. Sporadic findings of inflammatory and ependymal cells have been reported, but in the majority of cases, histological studies with electron and light microscopy found a duplication of the arachnoid membrane [26, 36]. ACs are probably congenital malformations that are formed during development due to a local alteration in the CSF pressure and flow, resulting in a splitting of the arachnoid membrane [24, 26].

A progressive increase in cyst volume may occur in many cases [1,2]. Several mechanisms can be responsible for a gradual enlargement of an AC. Intracystic haemorrhage, an osmotic gradient allowing a passive fluid-diffusion into the cyst, a ball-valve mechanism or an active secretion from the cyst wall are the main theories to explain cyst growth [27, 39]. Fluid secretion of the cyst wall is controversial, but may be responsible for the growth of cysts that consist mainly of ependymal cells [5, 26]. Haemorrhage may happen not only into the cyst, but also into the subdural or extradural space [19, 22]. However, it is usually of acute onset and unlikely to cause continuous slow growth [23, 35]. Nevertheless, the presence of a ball-valve mechanism and therefore intermittent entrapment of CSF is usually responsible for gradual cyst enlargement in most of the lesions [5, 20].

## 20.3
## Relationship Between ACs and CSF Flow

A computed tomography (CT) cisternogram and new MRI with CSF dynamic studies have clarified the relationship between the AC and CSF pathways [14]. There are cysts that communicate with the CSF pathways (communicating cysts) and those that do not (non-communicating cysts) [1, 13].

Based on CT cisternography findings, Galassi et al. [11] and Crisi et al. [8] further divided the communicating cysts into two main categories: slowly communicating cysts and rapidly communicating cysts. The dynamic MRI technique shows fluid movements such as the eventual communication of the cyst with the CSF pathways and the CSF pulsation inside the AC in cases of communicating cysts.

## 20.4
## Radiological Diagnosis of ACs

Pneumoencephalography was the main diagnostic tool to detect AC in the past. Only with the advent of modern radiological techniques (high-resolution CT scans and MRI) has a significant improvement in the preoperative diagnosis of ACs been achieved [18]. CT and MRI scans usually show a non-calcified homogeneous extra-axial lesion, without contrast enhancement, with the same characterises as the CSF. Elevated signal intensity on T1-weighted images is described in cases of high protein content due to previous intracystic haemorrhage or secondary to infection. In the past, accurate diagnosis was sometimes difficult, especially in non-communicating ACs, and therefore they could be confused preoperatively with epidermoid cysts and other cystic lesions [29, 33, 34, 39]. Nowadays, however, the diffusion MRI technique can usually readily differentiate ACs from epidermoid tumours.

## 20.5
## Classification of ACs According to their Location in the Posterior Fossa

In our opinion, three different main groups of AC can be identified depending on their major location and extension: Group I: AC of the CPA (Fig. 1); group II: AC of the CPA with extension dorsal to the brainstem (Fig. 2); group III: AC located at the CPA extending into the internal auditory canal (IAC; Fig. 3). Mass effect with compression of the surrounding structures can be evident in all different groups.

## 20.6
## Surgical Treatment of ACs

The indication for surgery and the mode of surgical treatment are still a matter of debate [7, 12, 13, 16, 39]. In many cases, ACs are asymptomatic and do not grow progressively. Conservative management with regular radiological control will identify those cases with gradual cyst enlargement who need surgical treatment. Surgical indication and technique should be based on the following criteria: (1) type of AC (communicating or non-communicating), (2) growth of the cyst, (3) compression or displacement of the surrounding neurovascular structures, and most important (4) the patient's symptoms and signs, and especially on-going clinical worsening.

Different types of surgical approaches can be performed [3, 7, 13]. Cyst fenestration, stereotactic punction, endoscopic cyst fenestration, cystoperitoneal shunt, cyst marsupialisation into the subarachnoid space and com-

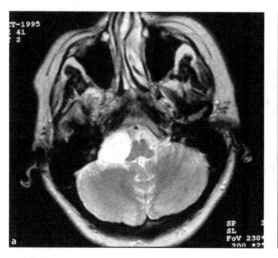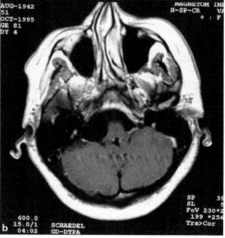

Fig. 1a,b  T1- (a) and T2-weighted (b) axial magnetic resonance imaging (MRI) scans revealing a big arachnoid cyst located at the cerebellopontine angle (CPA)

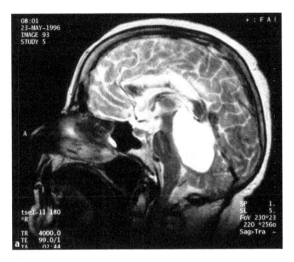
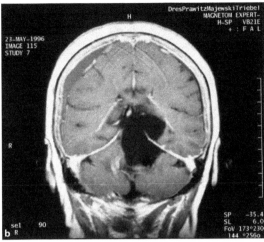

Fig. 2a,b T1- and T2-weighted gadolinium-enhanced MRI scans displaying a huge arachnoid cyst located dorsal to the brainstem, mainly at the posterior fossa and partially extending into the middle fossa. The sagittal (**a**) and coronal images (**b**) show the important dorsal compression of the brainstem and supratentorial extension of the lesion through the tentorial notch

plete or partial resection of the cyst wall are the main options [7, 10, 17, 40]. The advantages and disadvantages of each surgical treatment have been discussed extensively [7, 32]. Among the most frequently used techniques are aspiration techniques like stereotactic punction or endoscopic punction. Reclosure of the cyst wall or insufficient fenestration and therefore inadequate drainage into the subarachnoid space are the main reasons for recurrence and regrowth. Cystoperitoneal shunting also carries a considerable rate of obstruction and/or recurrence. Nevertheless, cyst shunting presents good results with a small likelihood of recurrence for ACs located in the middle fossa associated with hydrocephalus [6, 7, 30, 32].

In our experience, the most likely prevention of cyst recurrence is open surgery with resection of the entire cyst wall, especially for ACs located at the posterior fossa. Because of the close relationship between the cyst and many important neurovascular structures in this area (e.g.

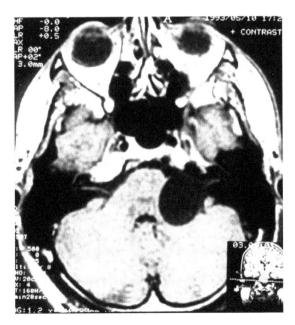

Fig. 3 Axial T1-weighted MRI scan showing an arachnoid cyst located in the CPA, extending into the internal auditory canal, with the same signal intensity as the cerebrospinal fluid, compressing the brainstem. T1-weighted, gadolinium-enhanced MRI scan displaying the mass effect caused from the cystic lesion on to the brainstem. Note that there is no contrast-enhancement of the cyst wall

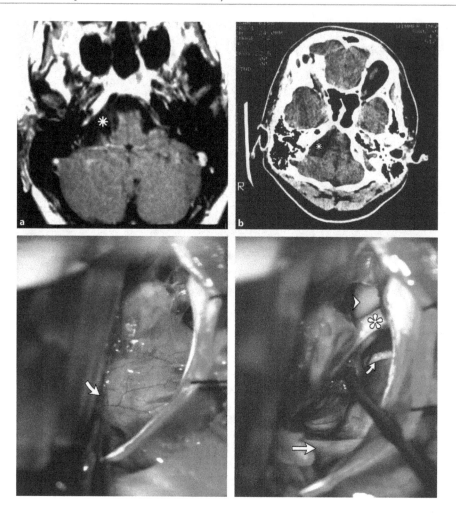

Fig. 4 **a,b** Axial T1-weighted MRI picture after gadolinium and axial computed tomography scan displaying the AC at the CPA, compressing the brainstem **c** After a lateral suboccipital retrosigmoid approach and retraction of the cerebellum, the AC (*arrow*) at the CPA can be displayed covering and surrounding the cranial nerves **d** After careful radical removal of the AC, the trigeminal nerve (*arrowhead*), abducens nerve (*upwards arrow*), facial-cochlear nerve complex and the caudal cranial nerves (*arrow*) can be well recognised

the brainstem and cranial nerves IV–XII), cyst shunting, punction or endoscopic procedures may be hazardous in these cases.

Patients with posterior fossa ACs with compression of the brainstem or surrounding neurovascular structures and correlating symptoms will usually profit from surgical treatment. Suboccipital craniotomy permits a good and safe exposure of the cyst and surrounding neurovascular structures. Radical resection of the cyst and careful resection of the cyst parts adherent to vessels and cranial nerves minimise the chance of recurrence. Furthermore, patients with additional vascular compression syndromes, as in one of our cases, will more likely improve following open surgery, wide cyst resection and, if necessary, microsurgical vascular decompression.

In some particular cases, strong adhesion between the cyst wall and the neurovascular structures may be found. A trial of radical removal of the cyst wall in such cases may result in post-operative cranial nerve deficits (e.g. facial palsy, hearing loss and swallowing disturbance). Extensive resection and wide opening of the cyst without direct manipulation of the surrounding cranial nerves will provide considerable connection of the AC to the cisterns and will avoid such post-operative morbidity. Regular follow-up on such cases is especially indicated in order to detect a possible recurrence.

In cases of posterior fossa communicating ACs with associated hydrocephalus, ventriculoperitoneal shunting should be attempted first. If no relief of the preoperative symptoms is achieved and serial post-operative scans demonstrate no shrinking of the cyst, open surgery should be performed.

Around 50 cases of posterior fossa AC with CPA involvement have been reported in the literature. All of these cases were treated according to different treatment protocols. Therefore, the rate of recurrence, regrowth and clear decision-making concerning the best surgical technique are still unclear.

Samii et al. [28] published a report of 12 patients who underwent surgery of ACs involving the posterior fossa. In seven cases the AC was located within the CPA, in three cases in the CPA with major extension dorsal to the brainstem and in two cases at the CPA extending into the IAC. A suboccipital retrosigmoid approach was performed in all patients. Radical resection of the cyst could be accomplished in all but one case. There was no mortality. Major post-operative morbidity was present in one case due to intraoperative air embolism in the semisitting position and strong adherence of the cyst wall with the surrounding neurovascular structures. Short- and long-term follow-up (over 3.3 years) displayed improvement of most preoperative symptoms. The suboccipital approach provided a good and safe exposure of vascular structures and cranial nerves in the CPA. Complete resection with few exceptions is obviously tolerated very well, as demonstrated by our series. This emphasises the chances and advantages of this concept.

## 20.7
## Conclusion

Microsurgical treatment of ACs located in the posterior fossa is usually beneficial. Good exposure of the vascular and cranial nerve structures in the CPA is essential for a safe removal of these cysts. The suboccipital approach allows a radical resection of most cysts without endangering the surrounding structures and reducing the chances of cyst recurrence.

Complete cyst resection is the most reliable option for prevention of recurrence. The fact that it is so well tolerated provides the best reason for application of this mode of treatment. Long-term follow-up has demonstrated the improvement of the majority of the preoperative symptoms.

## References

1. Becker T, Wagner M, Hofmann E, et al (1991) Do arachnoid cysts grow? A retrospective CT volumetric study. Neuroradiology 33:341–345
2. Berens P, Ostertag CB (1992) Zystische Fehlbildungen des Gehins: Stereotaktische Diagnostik und Therapie. Nervenarzt 63:725–730
3. Bourekas EC, Raji MR, Dastur KJ, et al (1992) Retroclival arachnoid cyst. AJNR Am J Neuroradiol 13:353–354
4. Brooks ML, Mayer DP, Sataloff RT, et al (1992) Intracanalicular arachnoid cyst mimicking acoustic neuroma: CT and MRI. Comp Med Imag Graph 16:283–285
5. Cao GX (1989) Intracranial arachnoid cyst: report of 23 cases. Chung Hua Wai Ko Tsa Chih 27:426–427
6. Caruso R, Salvati M, Cervoni L (1994) Primary intracranial arachnoid cyst in the elderly. Neurosurg Rev 17:195–198
7. Ciricillo SF, Cogen PH, Harsh GR, et al (1991) Intracranial arachnoid cyst in children. A comparison of the effects of fenestration and shunting. J Neurosurg 74:230–235
8. Crisi G, Calo M, De Santis M, et al (1984) Metrizamide-enhanced computed tomography of intracranial arachnoid cysts. J Comput Assist Tomogr 8:928–935
9. di Rocco C, Caldarelli M, di Trapani G (1981) Infratentorial arachnoid cysts in children. Childs Brain 8:119–133
10. Eiras Ajuria J, Alberdi Vinas J (1991) Endoscopic treatment of intracranial lesions. Apropos of 8 cases. Neurochirurgie 37:278–283
11. Galassi E, Tognetti F, Pozzati E, et al (1986) Extradural hematoma complicating middle fossa arachnoid cyst. Childs Nerv Syst 2:306–308
12. Haberkamp TJ, Monsell EM, House WF, et al (1990) Diagnosis and treatment of arachnoid cysts of the posterior fossa. Otolaryngol Head Neck Surg 103:610–614
13. Handley MN, Grahm TW, Daspit CP, et al (1985) Otolaryngologic manifestations of posterior fossa arachnoid cysts. Laryngoscope 95:678–681
14. Higashi S, Yamashita J, Yamamoto Y, et al (1992) Hemifacial spasm associated with a cerebellopontine angle arachnoid cyst in a young adult. Surg Neurol 37:289–292
15. Inoue T, Matsushima T, Fukui M, et al (1988): Immunohistochemical study of intracranial cysts. Neurosurgery 23:576–581
16. Jallo GL, Woo HH, Meshki C, et al (1997) Arachnoid cysts of the cerebellopontine angle: diagnosis and surgery. Neurosurgery 40:31–38
17. Lange M, Oeckler R (1987) Results of surgical treatment in patients with arachnoid cysts. Acta Neurochir 87:99–104
18. Leo JS, Pinto RS, Hulvat GF, et al (1979) Computed tomography of arachnoid cysts. Radiology 130:675–680
19. Lisovoski F, Danziger N, Helias A, et al (1992) Arachnoid cyst of the temporal fossa. Subdural hematoma. Contribution of MRI. Rev Neurol Paris 148:150–151
20. Little JR, Gomez MR, MacCarty CS (1973) Infratentorial arachnoid cyst. J Neurosurg 39:380–386
21. McAndrew PT, Land N, Sellar RJ (1995) Case report: a case of intracranial septated arachnoid cyst. Clin Radiol 50:502–503
22. Olsen NK, Madsen HH (1990) Arachnoid cyst with complicating intracystic and subdural haemorrhage. Rontgenblatter 43:166–168
23. Pasquini U, Bevilacqua F, Salvolini U, et al (1993) An intracranial arachnoid cyst with a repeated intracystic hemorrhagic complication. Radiol Med Torino 86:145–148
24. Punzo A, Conforti R, Martiniello D, et al (1992) Surgical indications for intracranial arachnoid cysts. Neurochirurgia 35:35–42

25. Rakier A, Feinsod M (1995) Gradual resolution of an arachnoid cyst after spontaneous rupture into the subdural space. Case report. J Neurosurg 83:1085–1086

26. Rengachary SS, Watanabe I (1981) Ultrastructure and pathogenesis of intracranial arachnoid cysts. J Neuropathol Exp Neurol 40:61–83

27. Ruscalleda J, Guardia E, dos Santos FM, et al (1980) Dynamic study of arachnoid cysts with metrizamide. Neuroradiology 20:185–189

28. Samii M, Carvalho GA, Schuhmann MU, et al (1999) Arachnoid cysts of the posterior fossa. Surg Neurol 51: 376–383

29. Samii M, Tatagiba M, Piquer JP (1996) Surgical treatment of epidermoid cysts of the cerebellopontine angle. J Neurosurg 84:14–19

30. Sato H, Sato N, Katayama S, et al (1991) Effective shunt-independent treatment for primary middle fossa arachnoid cyst. Childs Nerv Syst 7:375–381

31. Schuknecht HF, Gao YZ (1983) Arachnoid cyst in the internal auditory canal. Ann Otol Rhinol Laryngol 92:535–541

32. Serlo W, von Wendt L, Heikkinen E, et al (1985) Shunting procedures in the management of intracranial cerebrospinal fluid cysts in infancy and childhood. Acta Neurochir Wien 76:111–116

33. Summer TE, Benton C, Marshak G (1975) Arachnoid cyst of the internal auditory canal producing facial paralysis in a three-year-old child. Radiology 114:425–426

34. Tamas LB, Wyler AR (1985) Intracranial mucocele mimicking arachnoid cyst: case report. Neurosurgery 16:85–86

35. Tortelly Costa AC, de Freitas MR, de Sa RM, et al (1985) Intracranial arachnoid cyst associated with subdural hygroma: report of a case. Arq Neuropsiquiatr 43:91–97

36. Vaquero J, Carrilo R, Cabezudo JM, et al (1981) Arachnoid cyst of the posterior fossa. Surg Neurol 16:117–121

37. Wakisaka S, Yoneda K, Kitano I, et al (1986) Arachnoid cyst in the quadrigeminal cistern. Surg Neurol 26:52–58

38. Wiener SN, Pearlstein AE, Eiber A (1987) MR imaging of intracranial arachnoid cysts. J Comput Assist Tomogr 11:236–241

39. Yamakawa H, Ohkuma A, Hattori T, et al (1991) Primary intracranial arachnoid cyst in the elderly: a survey on 39 cases. Acta Neurochir Wien 113:42–47

40. Yokota JI, Imai H, Okuda O, et al (1993) Inverted Bruns' nystagmus in arachnoid cysts of the cerebellopontine angle. Eur Neurol 33:62–64

# Facial and Cochlear Nerve Function After Surgery for Cerebellopontine Angle Meningiomas

# 21

Makoto Nakamura

## Contents

## 21.1
## Introduction

Meningiomas are the second most common tumors of the cerebellopontine angle (CPA) after vestibular schwannomas, comprising 6–15% of cases [3, 19, 34]. They share a common location, the area of the CPA, but their site of dural origin and their relationship to surrounding neurovascular structures of the CPA are variable. Therefore, the clinical presentation and outcome after surgery may be different.

Rokitansky in 1856 [23] was the first to report a tumor, which is classified as a CPA meningioma, and Virchow later described a psamomma originating from the posterior lip of the meatus acusticus [36]. In 1928, Cushing and Eisenhardt reported a series of seven patients with meningiomas "simulating acoustic neuromas," emphasizing the high surgical risk in dealing with these tumors [5].

Posterior fossa meningiomas involving the CPA have been recognized as a particular entity since then [8, 13, 15, 22, 24, 31]. With the advent of microsurgical techniques, Yasargil et al. [38], Sekhar and Janetta [32], Ojemann [21], Al-Mefty et al. [1, 11, 12], and Samii et al. [17, 25, 26, 28] reported results after resection of these tumors. The term CPA meningioma has been used to include meningiomas, which share a common location, that is, occupancy of the CPA. Despite this common location, these tumors may have diverse origins with regard to the site of dural attachment, which can be outside the CPA. Accordingly, the relationship of the tumor to the surrounding neurovascular structures, especially the facial and cochlear nerve, can be quite variable [17, 25, 28, 30, 37].

Previous reports have indicated that the clinical presentation and outcome differs between CPA meningiomas lying anterior or posterior to the IAC [25, 30]. The surgical series of CPA meningiomas at the Nordstadt Hospital, Hannover, Germany, allowed further detailed investigation of the tumor location related to the inner auditory canal (IAC), with special consideration of the pre- and postoperative facial and cochlear nerve function. A subclassificaiton of CPA meningiomas into five groups was enabled based on the large number of patients treated at our institution.

## 21.2
## Patients and Methods

Between 1978 and 2002, a total of 1800 cases of meningiomas were operated at the Nordstadt Hospital. Among them, there were 421 CPA meningiomas. Evaluation of pre- and postoperative clinical data, with special emphasis on audiologic and facial nerve findings, and neuroradiological imaging studies was based on 347 patients with complete data material.

Our clinical data analysis included 270 females (77.8%) and 77 males (22.2%). The mean age of the patients was 53.4 years (range 17.6–84 years). The pre- and postoperative facial nerve function was examined according to the House and Brackmann (H&B) grading system [14]. Data was available in 334 patients. Pre- and postoperative hearing function was graded according to the Hannover Audiological Classification in steps of 20-dB hearing loss, calculated as the mean of air conduction data at 1, 1.5, 2, and 3 kHz in the pure tone average (PTA, class H1: good, 0–20 dB; H2: useful, 21–40 dB; H3: moderate, 41–60 dB; H4: poor, 61–80 dB; H5: functional deafness, >81 dB) [16]. The best speech discrimination score for each patient was classified as normal (100–95%), useful (90–70%), moderate (65–40%), poor (35–5%), or nonexistent (<5%). Complete audiologic data was available in 333 patients. The patients were evaluated immediately before surgery and 10–14 days postoperatively. The mean follow-up time was 62.3 months (range 2–214 months).

The pre- and postoperative status of the facial and cochlear nerve function was compared among groups using the chi$^2$-test with one degree of freedom. A $p$-value was calculated for each comparison, with significance assumed at the 0.05 level.

## 21.3
## Results

### 21.3.1
### Tumor Location

Tumor location of CPA meningiomas was classified according to their topographical location to the IAC. Meningiomas originating at the petrous ridge anterior to

the IAC ($n$=114, 32.9%) were declared as group 1 tumors (Fig. 1). Tumors revealing involvement of the IAC itself were classified as group 2 tumors (22.2%, Fig. 2). Tumors originating superior to the IAC were defined as group 3 tumors (70 tumors, 20.2%, Fig. 3); those having their origin inferior to the IAC as group 4 tumors (41 tumors, 11.8%, Fig. 4), and tumors with their matrix located posterior to the IAC as group 5 tumors (45 tumors, 12.9%, Fig. 5).

### 21.3.2
### Nerve–Tumor Relationship

In any case of CPA meningioma, the facial and cochlear nerves are displaced in characteristic directions, due to their intimate anatomic relationship in the CPA. The direction of nerve displacement was dependent on the site of tumor origin at the CPA.

In CPA meningiomas with their origin anterior to the IAC (group 1), the facial and cochlear nerves were most commonly displaced posteriorly (45.2%, Fig. 1b). Inferior displacement was observed in 42.9% and superior displacement in 9.5%.

The trigeminal nerve was mostly displaced superiorly (59.5%); anterior displacement was observed in 26.2% and inferior displacement in 14.3%. Cranial nerves IX–XI were inferiorly displaced in only 16.7% of cases.

The nerve–tumor relationship in CPA meningiomas involving the IAC is much less predictable. Most commonly, the facial and cochlear nerves were surrounded by the tumor (29.2%, Fig. 2b). Displacement to the superior and inferior direction was observed in 25%

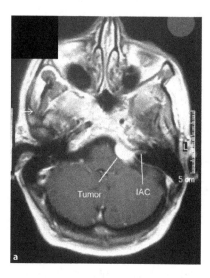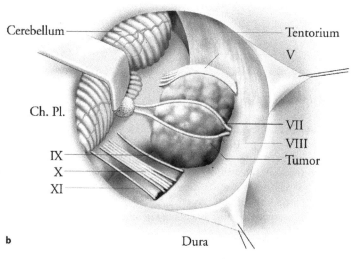

Fig. 1  **a** Example of a group 1 tumor. A 58-year-old female with a left-sided cerebellopontine angle (CPA) meningioma located anterior to the inner auditory canal (*IAC*). **b** Illustration of a group 1 tumor displacing the facial (*VII*) and cochlear (*VIII*) nerves posteriorly (45.2%) and compressing the trigeminal nerve (*V*) superiorly (59.5%). An inferior displacement of the facial and cochlear nerves was observed in 42.9% (not shown in illustration). *Ch. Pl.* Choroid plexus, *IX* glossopharyngeal nerve, *X* vagus nerve, *XI* accessory nerve

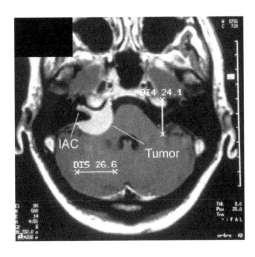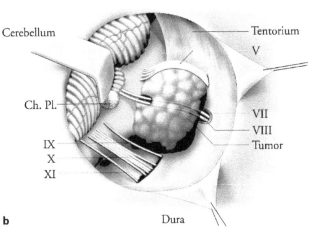

Fig. 2   **a** Example of a group 2 tumor. A 44-year-old female with a right-sided CPA meningioma involving the IAC. **b** Illustration of a group 2 tumor involving the IAC. The posterior wall of the IAC is removed. The tumor may either originate in the IAC or involve the IAC secondarily. The facial and cochlear nerves lie within the tumor in 29.2% of cases. Superior or inferior displacement was observed each in 25% (not shown). The majority of tumors (70.8%) did not displace the trigeminal nerve, but in larger tumors, the displacement was observed mainly to the superior (16.7%) and anterior (8.3%) direction

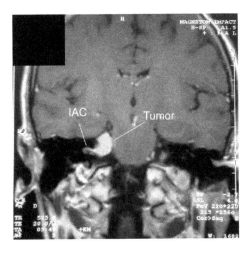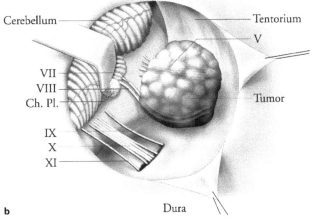

Fig. 3   **a** Example of a group 3 tumor. A 58-year-old female with a right-sided CPA meningioma located superior to the IAC. **b** Illustration of a group 3 tumor displacing the facial and cochlear nerves inferiorly and compressing the trigeminal nerve inferiorly. Inferior displacement of the facial and cochlear nerves was observed in 77.8%; the trigeminal nerve was most commonly displaced inferiorly in large tumors (33.3%)

each. Posterior (12.5%) and anterior (8.3%) displacement was less common. In large tumors, the trigeminal nerve was displaced superiorly in 16.7% of cases. Cranial nerves IX–XI were inferiorly displaced in 29.2% of cases.

As it may be anticipated, tumors originating superior to the IAC (group 3) most commonly displaced the facial and cochlear nerves inferiorly (77.8%, Fig. 3b). An anterior displacement was observed in only 16.7%. The trigeminal nerve was displaced inferiorly in large tumors in 33.3% of cases (Fig. 3b). Similarly, in group 4 tumors, the facial and cochlear nerves were displaced superiorly in 68.75% (Fig. 4b) and anteriorly in 18.75%. In 68.75% of

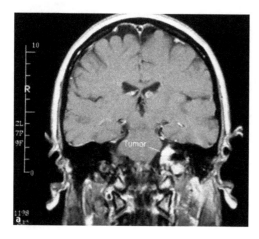
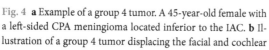
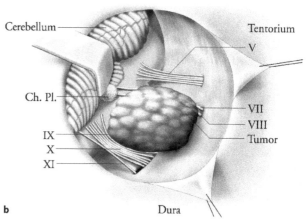

Fig. 4 **a** Example of a group 4 tumor. A 45-year-old female with a left-sided CPA meningioma located inferior to the IAC. **b** Illustration of a group 4 tumor displacing the facial and cochlear nerves anterosuperiorly (68.75%) and compressing the glossopharyngeal and vagus nerves inferiorly (56.25%)

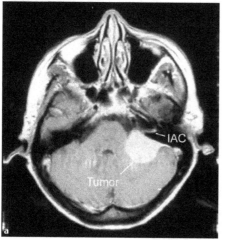
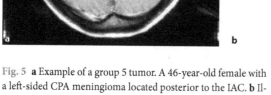
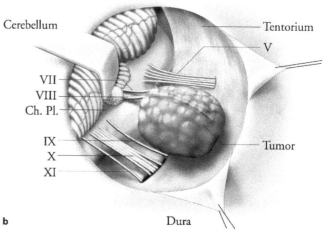

Fig. 5 **a** Example of a group 5 tumor. A 46-year-old female with a left-sided CPA meningioma located posterior to the IAC. **b** Illustration of a group 5 tumor displacing the facial and cochlear nerves anteriorly (62.5%). Inferior displacement of these nerves was observed in 25% (not shown). The glossopharyngeal and vagus nerves were displaced inferiorly in 50% (not shown)

cases, the trigeminal nerve was not involved, but in large tumors, displacement was observed in the superior direction in 25%. Cranial nerves IX–XI were displaced inferiorly in 56.25% of cases (Fig. 4b).

Finally, group 5 tumors showed displacement of the facial and cochlear nerves to the anterior direction in 62.5% (Fig. 5b). Inferior displacement was observed in 25%. There was no relationship to the trigeminal nerve in 87.5% of cases, and anterior displacement was only observed in large tumors in 12.5% of cases. Cranial nerves IX–XI were most commonly displaced to the inferior direction (50%); they were equally displaced anteriorly or were surrounded by the tumor in 12.5%.

### 21.3.3
### Tumor Resection

Patients were most commonly operated through a lateral suboccipital retrosigmoid approach (330 patients) in the semisitting position. In tumors with significant extension to the petroclival region, a combined supra-infratentorial presigmoidal approach was performed (17 patients). In all procedures, the intracranial part of surgery was carried out with the aid of an operating microscope. Intraoperative neuromonitoring of the facial and the cochlear nerves has been utilized since 1986 and standardized protocols were routinely used since 1990 (Medelec, Surrey, UK).

Total tumor resection, including Simpson grades 1 and 2 [33], could be achieved in 95 tumors (83.3%) in group 1, 68 tumors (88.3%) in group 2, 63 tumors (90%) in group 3, 32 tumors (78%) in group 4, and 40 tumors (88.9%) in group 5. Altogether, 85.9% of patients underwent complete tumor resection and 14.1% a subtotal removal of the tumor.

The rate of total tumor resection in the subgroup of patients who underwent surgery through the combined supra-infratentorial presigmoidal approach was lower (70.58%) due to tumor involvement of the cavernous sinus in five patients.

## 21.3.4
## Complications

The most common complication that was encountered after surgery of CPA meningiomas was cerebrospinal fluid (CSF) fistula and postoperative hydrocephalus (4.6% of cases each). Few patients with CSF fistula required a temporary lumbar drainage (2.8%) or a surgical revision (0.8%). Patients with hydrocephalus were treated with temporary external ventricular drainage (3.2%) or a ventriculoperitoneal shunt (1.4%).

Postoperative hemorrhage occurred in 3.5% of patients, requiring surgical evacuation in 2.6%.

The rate of postoperative sigmoid sinus thrombosis was rare following a lateral suboccipital approach (0.3%), but had a higher incidence after the combined supra-infratentorial presigmoid approach (5.8%).

In this clinical series, two patients (0.6%) died perioperatively, one due to aspiration on the third postoperative day (following a combined supra-infratentorial presigmoid approach) and the other due to a hematoma on the 2nd day after surgery following tumor removal via the lateral suboccipital approach.

## 21.3.5
## Facial Nerve Function

The pre- and postoperative facial nerve function was evaluated on the basis of clinical data of 334 patients. In group 1, tumors ($n$=109) most of the patients ($n$=93,

85.3%) presented initially with no facial paresis (H&B grade 1). Preoperative H&B grades 2, 3, 4, and 5/6 paresis were observed in 8.3%, 2.8%, 1.8%, and 1.8% of patients, respectively. Both patients with preoperative complete facial palsy were already operated in an outside hospital and presented with a recurrent tumor.

In group 2 tumors involving the IAC ($n$=76), 81.6% of the patients presented with no facial nerve paresis preoperatively; 6.6% presented with a facial nerve paresis of H&B grade 2, 3.9% with H&B grade 3, 3.9% with H&B grade 4, 2.6% with H&B grade 5, and 1.3% with complete facial nerve paresis.

Of the patients with a group 3 tumor, 87.9% ($n$=66) had no preoperative facial nerve deficit; 10.6% of patients presented with a facial nerve paresis of H&B grade 2 and 1.5% with a complete facial nerve palsy (after previous surgery).

Of the patients with a group 4 tumor, 79.5% ($n$=39) presented without any facial nerve deficit; 12.8% had a mild facial nerve paresis of H&B grade 2, 5.1% presented with H&B grade 3, and 2.6% with H&B grade 4.

In group 5 tumors ($n$=44), 90.9% of patients presented without a facial nerve deficit; 9.1% had a mild facial nerve paresis before surgery (H&B grade 2).

Comparison among groups showed that preoperative facial nerve paresis was less common among group 5 tumors (9.1%) compared to group 4 (20.5%) and group 2 (18.4%), although the difference was not statistically significant (group 5 vs group 4, $p$=0.1397; group 5 vs group 2, $p$=0.1678). The immediate postoperative result of facial nerve function in patients with preoperative good function was best in group 5 (preservation of H&B grade 1 score in 90%) followed by group 4 (preservation of H&B grade 1 score in 87%) and group 3 (preservation of H&B grade 1 in 84.5%). Preservation of preoperative good facial nerve function was less common in group 1 (76.3% H&B grade 1) and in group 2 tumors (79% H&B grade 1), although it was still achieved in the majority of cases (Table 1). The difference between group 5 and group 1 was statistically significant at $p$=0.0414; the difference between group 5 and group 2 did not reach statistical significance ($p$=0.1467).

Improvement of facial nerve function in the immediate postoperative period was observed in all four patients with group 5 tumors presenting with a mild paresis (H&B

Table 1 Rate of functional facial nerve preservation at the same preoperative level after surgery (including improvements). *H&B* House and Brackmann grade

| Grade | Group 1 | Group 2 | Group 3 | Group 4 | Group 5 |
|---|---|---|---|---|---|
| H&B 1 | 71/93 (76.3%) | 49/62 (79%) | 49/58 (84.5%) | 27/31 (87%) | 36/40 (90%) |
| H&B 2 | 6/9 (66.6%) | 2/5 (40%) | 7/7 (100%) | 5/5 (100%) | 4/4 (100%) |
| H&B 3 | 2/3 (66.6%) | 0/3 (0%) | | 1/2 (50%) | |

grade 2). Recovery from mild facial paresis was also observed in other groups. There was no improvement of facial nerve function in the immediate postoperative period in patients with tumors involving the IAC (group 2).

The outcome of facial nerve function depending on the surgical approach did not reveal any significant difference.

The influence of tumor size as a possible relevant factor for facial nerve outcome was examined separately. There were 149 tumors (44.6%) with a diameter <3 cm, and 129 patients among them had a normal preoperative facial nerve function (H&B grade 1, 86.6%). In 82.9% of these patients, normal facial nerve function was preserved postoperatively. Tumors of >3 cm were observed in 185 patients (55.4%); among them, 155 patients had normal preoperative facial nerve function (H&B grade 1, 83.8%). Normal facial nerve function after surgery could be achieved in 80.6%.

Statistical comparison did not reveal any significant difference concerning facial nerve outcome between both groups ($p=0.6177$). The relationship between the extent of tumor resection and facial nerve function was also investigated, but did not show any significant difference between the patient group with total compared to subtotal tumor resection.

### 21.3.6
## Auditory Function

Results of pre- and postoperative auditory function based on PTA and speech discrimination tests were obtained in 333 patients. Among 109 patients with group 1 tumors, 45% had normal preoperative hearing (class 1), 15.6% presented with class H2, 17.4% with class H3, 11.9% with class H4 hearing, and 10.1% were already deaf (class H5).

Due to intrameatal tumor infiltration, normal preoperative hearing (class H1) was less frequently encountered in patients harboring group 2 tumors (only 28.9%, 22 of 76 patients); 22.4% patients had class H2, 18.4% had class H3, 7.9% had class 4, and 22.4% of patients were already functionally deaf at time of surgery (class H5).

In group 3 tumors ($n=65$), 49.2% had normal hearing (class H1) before surgery; 18.5% had class H2, 15.4% had class 3, 4.6% presented with class 4, hearing and 12.3% were already deaf before surgery.

In group 4 tumors ($n=39$), 28.2% of patients presented with normal hearing (class H1) before surgery; 25.6% had class H2, 10.3% presented each with class H3 and H4 hearing, and 25.6% were already deaf on the affected side before surgery.

In group 5 tumors ($n=44$), 47.7% of patients presented with normal hearing (class H1) before surgery; 22.7% had class H2 hearing, 15.9% presented with class H3, 6.8% with class H4 hearing, and 6.8% patients were already deaf on the affected side before surgery.

The comparison among groups showed that normal preoperative hearing was more common in group 3 (49.2%) and group 5 (47.7%) compared to group 2 (28.9%) and group 4 (28.2%) tumors. The immediate postoperative results of auditory function in patients with preoperative normal hearing was best in group 3 and 5 (preservation of normal hearing in 81.3% and 81%, respectively) followed by group 1 (preservation of normal hearing in 63.3%) and group 4 (preservation of normal hearing in 54.5%). Preservation of preoperative normal hearing was less common in group 2 (22.7%; Table 2). The differences between group 2 versus groups 3, 5, and 1 were highly significant ($p<0.0001$, $p=0.0001$, and $p=0.0016$, respectively).

Recovery of auditory function from preoperative functional deafness (class H5) in the immediate postoperative course was most commonly observed in group 5 (66.6%) followed by group 4 (20%) and group 3 (12.5%; Table 2). Recovery from preoperative deafness occurred in only 1 of 17 patients (5.9%) in group 2.

The outcome of auditory function depending on the surgical approach did not reveal any significant difference.

Tumor size as a possible relevant factor concerning outcome of postoperative hearing function was examined. There were 149 tumors (44.6%) with a diameter <3 cm; 67 patients among them had normal preoperative hearing function (class H1, 45%). Of these 67, normal hearing function was preserved postoperatively in 61.2%. A tumor size of >3 cm was observed in 185 patients (55.4%). Among them, 68 patients had normal preoperative hearing function (class H1, 36.8%). Preservation of normal hearing after surgery was achieved in 64.7%. Statistical comparison did not reveal any significant difference concerning outcome of hearing function between both groups ($p=0.6727$).

The relationship between the extent of tumor resection and hearing function was also investigated and did not reveal any difference between tumors with total or subtotal resection.

### 21.3.7
## Long-term Follow Up

The long-term follow up of facial nerve function was available in 324 patients. The mean clinical follow-up time was 62.3 months (2–214 months). Further improvement of facial nerve function could be observed during clinical follow up. In 38.4% of patients with postoperative H&B grade 3 ($n=13$) or grade 4 ($n=13$) paresis, facial nerve paresis improved to H&B grade 1–2 during long-term follow up. One of six patients with postoperative H&B grade 5 improved to good facial nerve function (H&B grade 1–2), and five patients to H&B grade 3.

Of patients with postoperative H&B grade 6, 11.1% ($n=18$) improved to H&B grade 1–2 and 55.6% showed

Table 2 Preservation rate of auditory function on the same level after surgery (including improvements). Hearing function was graded according to the Hannover Audiological Classification

|  | Group 1 | Group 2 | Group 3 | Group 4 | Group 5 |
| --- | --- | --- | --- | --- | --- |
| Class H1 | 31/49 (63.3%) | 5/22 (22.7%) | 26/32 (81.3%) | 6/11 (54.5%) | 17/21 (81%) |
| Class H2 | 12/17 (70.6%) | 7/17 (41.2%) | 6/12 (50%) | 3/10 (30%) | 8/10 (80%) |
| Class H3 | 13/19 (68.4%) | 6/14 (42.9%) | 7/10 (70%) | 4/4 (100%) | 7/7 (100%) |
| Class H4 | 7/13 (53.8%) | 3/6 (50%) | 3/3 (100%) | 3/4 (75%) | 2/3 (66.6%) |
| Class H5[a] | 1/11 (9%) | 1/17 (5.9%) | 1/8 (12.5%) | 2/10 (20%) | 2/3 (66.6%) |

[a] Improvements

improvement to H&B grade 3, including five cases of facial nerve reconstruction. Altogether, 297 of 334 patients (88.9%) had good facial nerve function (H&B grade 1–2) on long-term follow up.

Data concerning auditory function was available from 313 of 333 patients on long-term follow up. Hearing improved to normal level during follow up in 58.1% of patients with postoperative class H2 hearing, 40% of patients with class H3, 17.6% of patients with class H4, and even 7% of patients with postoperative functional deafness.

In summary, 169 of 333 patients (50.8%) had normal hearing (class H1) on long-term follow up. Hearing preservation (postoperative hearing function of class H1–4) was possible on long-term follow up in 258 of 284 patients (90.8%) presenting with hearing function of class H1–4 preoperatively.

## 21.4
## Discussion

Due to their intimate anatomical relationship, the facial and cochlear nerves are often involved in CPA meningiomas. The degree of facial and cochlear nerve involvement is influenced not only by the tumor size, but also by the tumor location in relation to the IAC. Also, the outcome of facial nerve function or auditory function after surgical removal of these tumors may depend on the type of nerve displacement encountered during surgery.

The literature reveals only few reports that have analyzed the outcome of facial nerve function and audiometric data after surgery for CPA meningiomas. In recent microsurgical series, normal facial nerve function could be preserved in 60 and 70% of patients harboring CPA meningiomas [29, 37] after surgery through different approaches. Although, when facial weakness was already present before surgery, the risk of further deterioration increased [29]. In our series, patients presenting with H&B grade 2–3 preoperatively showed worsening of facial nerve function in 28.9% on average in all tumor

groups. The frequency of preoperative facial nerve paresis was different depending on the location and origin of the tumor at the CPA. As it may be presumed, preoperative facial weakness was more common in tumors involving the IAC (group 2). Compression of the facial nerve from the anterior direction (group 1) revealed higher rates of preoperative facial weakness compared to compression from above (group 3) or from the posterior direction (group 5). Improvement of facial nerve paresis was also more frequently observed in the latter groups.

The clinical outcome of surgery for CPA meningiomas appears to be dependent on their premeatal or retromeatal location [2, 25, 30, 37]. Several series indicated that the postoperative outcome of facial nerve function was substantially worse in premeatal than in retromeatal tumors [2, 29, 37]. Consistent with these previous findings, we have observed substantial differences in facial nerve outcome depending on the tumor location. Normal preoperative facial nerve function could be preserved in the majority of cases, but ranged from 76.3% in group 1 tumors (lying anterior to the IAC) to 90% in group 5 tumors (lying posterior to the IAC). In tumors involving the IAC (group 2), normal facial nerve function could be maintained in 79% of cases. The more intimate relationship between intrameatal tumors and the facial nerve may account for the slightly lower likelihood of preservation of normal facial nerve function postoperatively. In tumors located anterior to the IAC with frequent posterior displacement of the facial nerve, the facial nerve represents a continuous obstacle during surgery through the lateral suboccipital approach, and therefore the risk of damage to the facial nerve during surgery is increased with less favorable outcome of facial nerve function.

In any case, it is mandatory to attempt facial nerve preservation during surgery as the clinical course on long-term follow up showed further improvement of postoperative facial paresis, finally resulting in 88.9% of all cases with good facial nerve function (H&B grade 1–2).

The audiometric data after surgery of CPA meningiomas has been analyzed in only a few previous reports. The surgical management of CPA meningiomas with regard to attempts to preserve hearing also differed depending on the preference of different approaches used for tumor removal. The rate of hearing preservation ranged from 65 to 75% [9, 20, 30] and showed that in the majority of cases hearing preservation was possible; however, it has to be pointed out that hearing preservation was attempted in only selected cases in whom preoperative hearing was either normal or only mildly impaired [10,20]. In other cases, hearing-destructive approaches were often considered for surgery.

Similar to the facial nerve findings, tumor location affected strongly the outcome of auditory function after retrosigmoid tumor removal in our series. Preservation of normal hearing could be achieved most frequently in group 3 and 5 tumors (81.3% and 81%, respectively), followed by group 1 (63.3%) and group 4 (54.5%). Normal hearing was preserved in only 22.7% of group 2 tumors. Although tumors with premeatal location (group 1) or intrameatal involvement (group 2) present more commonly with hearing deficits preoperatively (class H2-4), preservation of hearing at least at the same level or improved hearing could be achieved in 55.8% (average of both groups). In tumors involving the IAC, the cochlear and facial nerves have an intimate relation to the tumor, especially during their intrameatal course. This subgroup of meningioma requires more frequent preparation at the nerve–tumor border, and this may be the reason for the less likely preservation of normal hearing in this subtype of tumor.

Interestingly, patients harboring tumors that were located inferior to the IAC (group 4) had a less favorable preservation rate of normal hearing compared to other tumor subgroups (group 2 excluded). It is unclear whether this is due to the more frequently encountered superior displacement of the cochlear nerve in this type of tumor. It is also worth mentioning that patients with group 4 tumors were less likely to present with normal preoperative hearing (class H1, only 28.2%), similar to patients with group 2 tumors. These findings would favor a hypothesis that the cochlear nerve is generally more impaired when displaced superiorly and even more susceptible to surgical manipulation during tumor removal in this unusual position.

Retromeatal tumors (group 5) revealed the highest rate of hearing preservation, at 85% (class H2–4 preoperatively), compared to tumors in other locations.

One remarkable finding regarding CPA meningiomas is recovery of hearing from preoperative deafness, which was observed in seven cases in our series. In one deaf patient with a retromeatal tumor (group 5), even dramatic hearing recovery to normal hearing was observed. Few case reports have demonstrated previously that hearing restoration can occur with CPA meningiomas, even in the face of profound preoperative deficit [4, 7, 18, 35]. In our view, these cases show that it is worth attempting to preserve hearing in as many patients as possible, even in case of bad or no clinical preoperative hearing.

Compared to surgery for vestibular schwannomas, the rate of hearing preservation is more favorable for CPA meningioma surgery [6, 27]. Analysis of 2000 vestibular schwannomas operated at our department showed that the rate of hearing preservation depended on the preoperative hearing quality and the tumor size. Good chances of hearing preservation were encountered in cases with normal or good preoperative hearing, with 70% for intrameatal tumors (T1), 65% for tumors with intra-extrameatal extension (T2), 56% for medium-sized tumors (T3), and 25% for tumors with brainstem compression or even dislocation (T4).

In our series of CPA meningiomas, hearing preservation among patients presenting with functional hearing (class H1-4), was achieved in 90.8%, including those cases with improvement on long-term follow up. The results were dependent on tumor extension and location, but not on the tumor size. Reviewing these data, the overall possibility of hearing preservation is superior for CPA meningiomas compared to vestibular schwannomas. The observed difference in results may be due to the more intimate involvement of vestibular schwannomas with the cochlear nerve or its blood supply. Direct trauma to the cochlear nerve or deterioration of the blood supply during manipulation for tumor removal in vestibular schwannomas may result in lower success rate in hearing preservation. Although the pathophysiological changes at the tumor–nerve border in schwannomas and meningiomas and the differences in either group are not well understood, every attempt has to be made to preserve hearing in as many cases as possible. In particular for CPA meningiomas, ours and previous results have shown that restoration of auditory function is possible even in cases with preoperatively profound hearing deficit or functional deafness. Hearing preservation should not be limited to retromeatal meningiomas (group 5 in our series) with good or serviceable preoperative hearing. These tumors had also the best success rate in our series, but hearing conservation or improvement is also possible in tumors in a more challenging location.

The presented data with continuous improvement of functional outcome along with a high rate of surgical radicality were also accomplished thanks to the support of intraoperative neurophysiological monitoring. The significance of neuromonitoring has been demonstrated in a recent study on large vestibular schwannomas with brainstem involvement, where not only the rates of functional nerve preservation were improved, but also the quality of preserved hearing [16]. Multimodality functional control during each microsurgical step has increased the knowledge on ongoing changes due to microsurgical maneuvers as well as their safety. By recording the electromyography of motor cranial nerves, early nerve identification and delicate handling of the nerve during tumor resection are enabled. Thus the rate of anatomical facial nerve preservation will increase along with surgical radicality. Intraoperative monitoring of auditory brainstem responses intensifies the surgeons' awareness as well as the rate of functional preservation of the cochlear nerve. It may be summarized that neurophysiological monitoring also increases surgical radicality and the quality of functional outcome of surgery for CPA tumors.

## 21.5
## Conclusion

The outcome of facial and cochlear nerve function is different for CPA meningiomas depending on the topographic classification of these tumors. Better results are achieved for tumors located posterior (group 5) or superior (group 3) to the IAC, compared to tumors with premeatal location (group 1) or intrameatal involvement (group 2). Hearing preservation or even improvement is also possible in less favorable tumors with premeatal or intrameatal extension, using the lateral suboccipital retrosigmoid approach; we therefore do not recommend the use of hearing-destructive skull-base approaches in any case of CPA meningioma. Preservation of the cochlear nerve should be attempted in every patient, bearing in mind that recovery of hearing has also been observed in preoperatively deaf patients.

## References

1. Al-Mefty O, Fox JL, Smith RR (1988) Petrosal approach for petroclival meningiomas. Neurosurgery 22:510–517
2. Batra PS, Dutra JC, Wiet RJ (2002) Auditory and facial nerve function following surgery for cerebellopontine angle meningiomas. Arch Otolaryngol Head Neck Surg 128:369–374
3. Brackmann DE, Bartels LJ (1980) Rare tumours of the cerebellopontine angle. Otolaryngol Head Neck Surg 88:555–559
4. Christiansen CB, Greisen O (1975) Reversible hearing loss in tumours of the cerebello-pontine angle. J Laryngol Otol 89:1161–1164
5. Cushing H, Eisenhardt L (1962) Meningiomas: Their Classification, Regional Behaviour, Life History and Surgical End Results. Hafner, New York, pp 199–207
6. Gardner G, Robertson JH (1988) Hearing preservation in unilateral acoustic neuroma surgery. Ann Otol Rhinol Laryngol 97:55–66
7. Goebel JA, Vollmer DG (1993) Hearing improvement after conservative approach for large posterior fossa meningioma. Otolaryngol Head Neck Surg 109:1025–1029
8. Grand W, Bakay L (1975) Posterior fossa meningiomas. A report of 30 cases. Acta Neurochir (Wien) 32:219–233
9. Grey PL, Baguley DM, Moffat DA, et al (1996) Audiovestibular results after surgery for cerebellopontine angle meningiomas. Am J Otol 17:634–638
10. Grey PL, Moffat DA, Hardy DG (1996) Surgical results in unusual cerebellopontine angle tumours. Clin Otolaryngol 21:237–243
11. Haddad GF, Al-Mefty O (1994) The road less traveled: transtemporal access to the CPA. Clin Neurosurg 41:150–167
12. Harrison MJ, Al-Mefty O (1997) Tentorial meningiomas. Clin Neurosurg 44:451–466
13. Hoffman GR, De Busscher J, De Haene A (1957) Le meningiome de l'angle pontocerebelleux. Neurochirurgie 3:123–137
14. House JW, Brackmann DE (1985) Facial nerve grading system. Otolaryngol Head Neck Surg 93:146–147
15. Markham JW, Fager CA, Horrax G, et al (1955) Meningiomas of the posterior fossa: their diagnosis, clinical features, and surgical treatment. Arch Neurol Psychiatry 74:163–170
16. Matthies C, Samii M (2002): Vestibular schwannomas and auditory function: options in large T3 and T4 tumours? Neurochirurgie 48:461–470
17. Matthies C, Carvalho G, Tatagiba M, et al (1996) Meningiomas of the cerebellopontine angle. Acta Neurochir Suppl (Wien) 65:86–91
18. Maurer PK, Okawara SH (1988) Restoration of hearing after removal of cerebellopontine angle meningioma: diagnostic and therapeutic implications. Neurosurgery 22:573–575
19. Moffat DA, Saunders JE, McElveen JT, et al (1993) Unusual cerebello-pontine angle tumours. J Laryngol Otol 107:1087–1098
20. Nassif PS, Shelton C, Arriaga M (1992) Hearing preservation following surgical removal of meningiomas affecting the temporal bone. Laryngoscope 102:1357–1362
21. Ojemann RG (1985) Meningiomas: clinical features and surgical management. In: Wilkins RH, Rengachary SS (eds) Neurosurgery. McGraw-Hill, New York, pp 648–651
22. Petit-Dutaillis D, Daum S (1949) Les meningiomes de la fosse posterieure. Rev Neurol 81:557–572
23. Rokitansky C (1856) Lehrbuch der pathologischen Anatomie. Wilhelm Braumüller, Wien
24. Russell JR, Bucy PC (1953) Meningiomas of the posterior fossa. Surg Gynecol Obstet 96:183–192
25. Samii M, Ammirati M (1991) Cerebellopontine angle meningioma. In: Al-Mefty O (ed): Meningiomas. Raven, New York, pp 503–515
26. Samii M, Ammirati M (1992) Posterior pyramid meningiomas (cerebellopontine angle meningioma). In: Samii M, Ammirati M (eds) Surgery of Skull-Base Meningioma. Springer, Berlin, Heidelberg, New York, pp 73–85
27. Samii M, Matthies C (1997) Management of 1000 vestibular schwannomas (acoustic neuromas): hearing function in 1000 tumour resections. Neurosurgery 40:248–260
28. Samii M, Turel KE, Penkert G (1985): Management of seventh and eighth nerve involvement by cerebellopontine angle tumours. Clin Neurosurg 32:242–272
29. Schaller B, Heilbronner R, Pfaltz CR, et al (1995) Preoperative and postoperative auditory and facial nerve function in cerebellopontine angle meningiomas. Otolaryngol Head Neck Surg 112:228–234

30. Schaller B, Merlo A, Gratzl O, et al (1999) Premeatal and retromeatal cerebellopontine angle meningioma. Two distinct clinical entities. Acta Neurochir (Wien) 141:465–471

31. Scott M (1972) The surgical management of the meningiomas of the cerebellar fossa. Surg Gynecol Obstet 135:545–550

32. Sekhar LN, Jannetta PJ (1984) Cerebellopontine angle meningiomas. Microsurgical excision and follow-up results. J Neurosurg 60:500–505

33. Simpson D (1957) The recurrence of intracranial meningiomas after surgical treatment. J Neurol Neurosurg Psychiatry 20:22–39

34. Thomsen J (1976) Cerebellopontine angle tumours, other than acoustic neuromas. A report on 34 cases. A presentation of 7 bilateral acoustic neuromas. Acta Otolaryngol 82:106–111

35. Vellutini EA, Cruz OL, Velasco OP, et al (1991) Reversible hearing loss from cerebellopontine angle tumours. Neurosurgery 28:310–312

36. Virchow RLK (1863) Die krankhaften Geschwülste, Dreissig Vorlesungen gehalten während des Wintersemesters 1862–1863 an der Universität zu Berlin. A. Hirschwald, Berlin

37. Voss NF, Vrionis FD, Heilman CB, et al (2000) Meningiomas of the cerebellopontine angle. Surg Neurol 53:439–446

38. Yasargil MG, Mortara RW, Curcic M (1980) Meningiomas of the basal posterior cranial fossa. In: Krayenbhul H (ed) Advances and Technical Standards in Neurosurgery. Springer, Vienna, pp 3–115

# Jugular Foramen Tumors – Diagnosis and Management

**22**

Ricardo Ramina, Joao Jarney Maniglia,
Yvens Barbosa Fernandes, Jorge Rizzato
Paschoal, and Maurício Coelho Neto

## Contents

## 22.1
## Introduction

Jugular foramen (JF) tumors are rare, deeply located skull-base lesions that may involve important neurovascular structures and present diagnostic and management difficulties. Precise knowledge of the anatomy of the JF and related regions (temporal bone, posterior fossa, and high cervical region) is necessary to approach these lesions. Several anatomical studies have been performed, but the surgical anatomy of this region remains poorly understood [23, 28]. Total removal of the tumor with preservation of cranial nerves and vessels is the aim of treatment, but it remains a challenge in spite of all developments in skull-base surgery and interventional neuroradiology. The main surgical difficulties with these tumors are related to the deep location of the lesion, hypervascularization, involvement of cranial nerves (VII, VII, IX, X, and XI) and vessels like the internal carotid artery (ICA) and the vertebral artery (VA) and its branches. The multidisciplinary management of these tumors by neurosurgeons, ear, nose, and throat (ENT) surgeons, and interventional neuroradiologists has led to a better understanding of diagnosis, preoperative evaluation, and treatment of these patients. Paragangliomas are the most frequent JF tumors. They have been called chemodectomas, nonchromaffin tumors, and glomus tumors. These neoplasms are histologically benign in most cases, highly vascularized, and may invade bone, blood vessels, the dura mater, and cranial nerves. The initial symptoms of JF paragangliomas are pulsatile tinnitus and hearing loss. Other common JF tumors are schwannomas and meningiomas. Malignant and invasive tumors usually present pain in the ear and temporal region associated with paralysis of cranial nerves as initial symptoms. Several surgical approaches have been used [13, 15, 20, 21, 37, 47]. Most approaches are often not adequate for large tumors with extension into the posterior fossa and retropharyngeal space, making tumor removal incomplete. The development of multidisciplinary skull-base teams (neurosurgeons, ENT surgeons, interventional neuroradiologists, and neurointensivists) gives the patient the best chance of radical surgical removal with preservation of the involved structures. Postoperative cerebrospinal fluid (CSF) leak is one of the most common complications in surgery for JF tumors [20, 21, 24], but surgical damage to functioning caudal cranial nerves is the most dangerous complication due to the risk of aspiration pneumonia.

## 22.2
## Clinical Material and Methods

### 22.2.1
### Patient Population

Between 1987 and 2006, 111 patients with JF tumors were treated surgically. The most frequent lesion was paraganglioma (62 cases) followed by schwannoma (19 cases) and meningioma (11 cases; Table 1). In the group with paragangliomas, there was a 4:1 female:male ratio), and the mean age was 42.5±12 years (range 18–72 years). Pulsatile tinnitus and hearing loss were the most common initial clinical symptom of paragangliomas. Three patients related a family history of JF or carotid body tumors, and two of these patients presented with bilateral JF paragangliomas. Tumor-secreting catecholamines (norepinephrine) were observed in two cases. These tumors require careful perioperative treatment with ß-blockers to avoid complications of catecholamine overload. Four paragangliomas were malignant. These patients presented lower cranial nerve deficits as initial complaints. There were 11 JF meningiomas. All patients with JF meningiomas presented initially with low cranial nerves palsy, and six cases were malignant lesions or tumors with malignant behavior. In this group, two were histologically malignant and four presented with malignant behavior. Nineteen patients presented with JF schwannoma (lower cranial nerve schwannomas). Chordomas and chondrosarcomas (seven cases), malignant tumors (carcinomas; four cases), aneurysmatic bone cyst (two cases), cholesteatomas (two cases), chondroma (one case), lymphangioma (one case), and inflammatory granuloma (one case) were other lesions in this series (Table 1). Patients with malignant tumors complained of pain in the ear and mastoid region. Eleven patients (10%) had undergone surgery previously at other institutions.

### 22.2.2
### Radiological Examination

High-definition computed tomography (CT) scan examination is useful for analysis of bone structures of the cranial base, tumor calcification, hyperostosis, and bone erosion in cases of meningiomas, aneurysmatic bone cysts, and chondrosarcomas (Fig. 1). Preoperative magnetic resonance imaging (MRI) with gadolinium (Gd) enhancement is very useful to demonstrate the characteristics of the tumor, its vascularization, extension, and relationship with neighboring structures. Magnetic resonance angiography is performed to study tumor vascular-

ization, venous circulation, and occlusion of the sigmoid sinus. Paragangliomas are well-vascularized lesions with heterogeneous Gd enhancement (Fig. 2). Schwannomas enhance homogenously with Gd, present a regular contour, may be cystic, and some cases present an extension into the high cervical region (Fig. 2). Meningiomas present Gd enhancement that may extend into the cervical region and present a "dura tail" (Fig. 3). Chordomas and chondrosarcomas are heterogeneous, presenting some areas with contrast enhancement. Digital subtraction angiography (DSA) is performed for diagnosis and to guide preoperative embolization in cases of highly vascularized lesions. DSA is performed routinely when the lesion is well vascularized. Branches of the external carotid artery (ascending pharyngeal artery) are usually feeders of JF paragangliomas. Invasion of the walls of the ICA may become visible in angiography. Patients harboring lesions surrounding or invading the ICA are submitted to balloon test occlusion. In these cases, sacrifice of the ICA may be necessary. When the tumor is hypervascularized, feeders from the external carotid artery (ascending

Table 1 Histology and grade of tumor resection

| Histology | No. of cases | Grade of resection | |
|---|---|---|---|
| | | Total | Sub-total |
| Paragangliomas | 62 | 48[a] | 12[b] |
| Schwannomas | 19 | 19 | 0 |
| Meningiomas | 11 | 6 | 5 |
| Aneurysmatic bone cyst | 02 | 2 | 0 |
| Chondrosarcoma | 06 | 1 | 5 |
| Chordoma | 02 | 0 | 2 |
| Malignant Tumor | 04 | 0 | 4 |
| Cholesteatoma | 02 | 1 | 1 |
| Chondroma | 01 | 1 | 0 |
| Lymphangioma | 01 | 1 | 0 |
| Inflammatory granuloma | 01 | 1 | 0 |
| **TOTAL** | **111** | **80 (72%)** | **31 (28%)** |

[a] Three present recurrence of tumor
[b] Four malignant, three reoperation

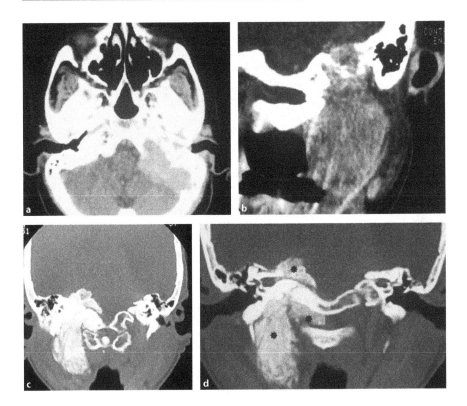

Fig. 1a–d Computed tomography (CT) scan showing large paragangliomas with skull-base bone erosion (**a,b**) and a large calcified jugular foramen (JF) meningioma (**c,d**)

pharyngeal, internal maxillary, and occipital arteries), the ICA (carotid tympanic branches), and the VA (posterior inferior cerebellar artery) are embolized with Gelfoam® and Ivalon® particles through superselective catheterization, 3–5 days prior to surgery. The venous circulation, position, and patency of the jugular bulb are better evaluated with the venous phase of DSA. A highly located and hypertrophic jugular bulb may cause symptoms of tinnitus and hearing loss. It is easily demonstrated by the venous phase of DSA.

## 22.3
## Surgical Technique

### 22.3.1
### Surgical Anatomy

The JF is described as having two portions, the nervous and the venous portions. The nervous portion contains the glossopharyngeal nerve, the inferior petrosal sinus, and the meningeal branches of the ascending pharyngeal artery, and the venous portion contains the sigmoid sinus, and the vagus and accessory nerves. Other authors describe three portions [23]: two venous and one nervous

(intrajugular). The nervous portion is localized between the two venous portions and contains cranial nerves IX, X, and XI. The cranial nerves lie anteromedial to the jugular bulb and maintain a multifascicular histoarchitecture (particularly the Xth cranial nerve) [48]. The vagus nerve is formed by multiple fascicles, and the glossopharyngeal and accessory nerves by one and two fascicles, respectively. The tympanic branch of the glossopharyngeal nerve (Jacobson's nerve) and the auricular branch of vagus nerve (Arnold's nerve) cross the JF. Intradurally, the JF is related to the caudal cranial nerves IX, X, and XI (with its spinal portion), nerves VII and VIII, the vertebral, posterior inferior, and anterior inferior cerebellar arteries, the lower brainstem, and the upper cervical cord. The anatomical parameters required to expose the facial nerve at the stylomastoid foramen region are: the mastoid tip posteriorly, the "pointer" superiorly, and the posterior belly of the digastric muscle inferiorly. The structures of the temporal bone related to the surgical approach to the JF are: the sigmoid, transverse, superior, and inferior petrosal sinuses, the mastoid cells and its antrum, the semicircular canals, the ossicles, the facial nerve canal, and the tympanic bone. The ICA runs medial to the tympanic bone and gives off the carotid-tympanicum branches. Structures related to neck dissection are:

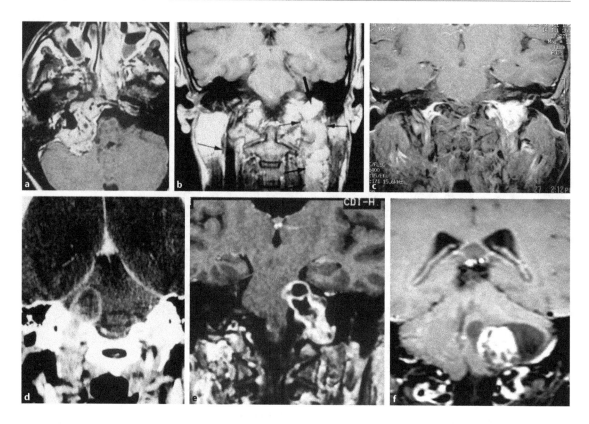

Fig. 2a–f Magnetic resonance imaging (MRI) with gadolinium enhancement showing JF paragangliomas (**a–c**) and cystic JF schwannomas (**d–f**)

1. Muscles: anterior border of the sternocleidomastoid muscle (SCM), the digastric, splenius capitis, obliquus capitis superior and inferior, and splenius cervicis muscles.
2. Vessels: common carotid, external carotid artery with its branches and internal carotid arteries, VA at the cranial cervical junction, common facial vein, and external and internal jugular veins.
3. Nerves: greater auricular nerve, cranial nerves X, XI, and XII, and the sympathetic trunk.

### 22.3.2
### Position of Patient and Skin Incision

All patients are placed in the dorsal position with the head held in a Mayfield clamp and turned 45° to the opposite side (Fig. 4). The contralateral internal jugular vein must be free. The facial, cochlear, and caudal cranial nerves are monitored. All contact areas are protected for the long duration of the procedure. A nasogastric tube is inserted. The skin incision is C-shaped, starting in the temporal region, and circumscribing the ear as far as the anterior border of the SCM (Fig. 4). After folding the

scalp skin anteriorly, the great auricular nerve is identified. This nerve may be used as a graft to reconstruct the facial nerve. The external auditory canal is exposed. If the patient has no hearing and there is tumor invasion with destruction of the ossicular chain, it is cut at the osteocartilaginous junction. The external auditory canal is closed in two layers to avoid CSF fistula.

### 22.3.3
### Reconstruction of the Cranial Base

The large surgical defect is closed in three layers. This technique of skull-base reconstruction using vascularized tissues fascia muscle flaps was developed by our group to avoid postoperative CSF leaks and obtain good cosmetic results (Fig. 5) [40]. The first layer is watertight dura closure or resection of the infiltrated dura and use of a temporalis fascia graft with fibrin glue. Use of an abdominal fat graft is avoided. The second layer is a vascularized temporalis muscle flap. The posterior half of the temporalis muscle is incised, dissected, turned down, and sutured in the cervical and parotid fasciae to cover the dura mater at the end of surgery to fill the surgical defect in the mastoid cavity. The third layer is a myofascial flap

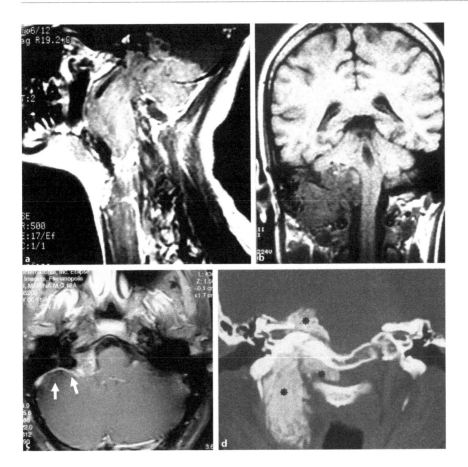

Fig. 3  **a–c** MRI images of JF meningiomas showing the dural "tail" (*arrows* in **c**). **d** CT scan showing large JF meningioma

formed by the temporalis muscle fascia, cervical fascia and SCM. The temporalis muscle fascia is incised in the middle portion of the temporal region and dissected inferiorly as far as the temporal line. The cervical fascia is cut posterior to the external auditory canal, mastoid tip, and over the SCM. The insertion of the SCM is removed from the mastoid and a vascularized myofascial flap formed by the temporalis muscle fascia; the cervical fascia and the SCM are turned posterior and inferiorly. This flap is secured with sutures in the temporalis fascia, and in the parotid and cervical fascia. It is turned back to cover the temporalis muscle flap and the entire surgical field.

### 22.3.3.1
### Neck Dissection

The next surgical step is neck dissection (Fig. 6). The anterior border of the SCM is identified and the major vessels of the neck (common carotid artery, ICA, external carotid artery and its branches, and the internal jugular vein) are dissected. The external jugular vein is ligated

with suture/ligature and cut. A key muscle for neck dissection is the digastric muscle. The digastric muscle is used as a guide for dissection of cranial nerves VII and XII. Cranial nerve XII crosses the external carotid artery inferior to the digastric muscle. In the majority of cases the accessory nerve is located laterally to the internal jugular. Cranial nerve X and the sympathetic trunk run lateroinferior to the common carotid artery. The VA is dissected at the lateral process of C1 (Fig. 6). Proximal control of this vessel is important in infiltrative tumors of the posterior fossa.

### 22.3.3.2
### Facial Nerve Management

The facial nerve exits the stylomastoid foramen superiorly to the digastric muscle. This nerve is identified at the stylomastoid foramen using the following parameters: the mastoid tip, the posterior belly of the digastric muscle, the "pointer" and the tympanomastoid suture (Fig. 7). If this nerve is not infiltrated by the tumor, it is not necessary

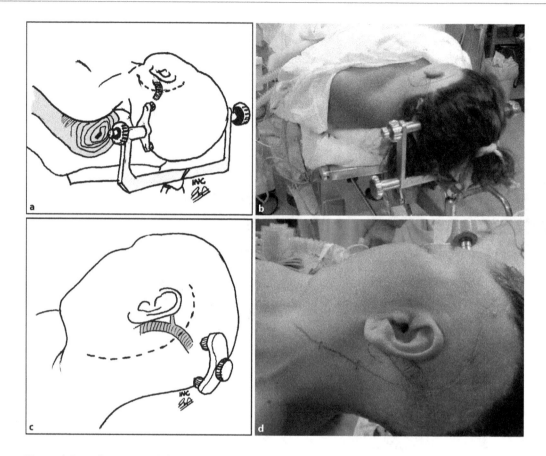

Fig. 4 **a,b** Patient's position. **c,d** Skin incision

to remove it from its bony canal. Tumor is resected anteriorly and posteriorly to the facial canal. This technique avoids postoperative facial paralysis by rerouting cranial nerve VII. When necessary facial nerve reconstruction is accomplished with grafts from the great auricular or sural nerves.

### 22.3.3.3
### Temporal Bone Dissection

Temporal bone dissection and radical mastoidectomy is performed with identification of the facial nerve canal, the labyrinth, mastoid antrum, ossicles, and the sinodural angle (Fig. 7). The sigmoid sinus and the jugular bulb are completely skeletonized. The retrofacial mastoid cells are removed. The posterior and anterior walls of the external auditory meatus are drilled to better expose the tumor in the ear. Any tumor within the ear, Eustachian tube, and mastoid cells is resected after removal of the tympanic membrane. Removal of the tympanic bone exposes the ICA (distal control) allowing bipolar coagulation of the carotid–tympanic branches (branches of ICA) that very often are tumor feeders.

### 22.3.4
### Craniectomy and Opening of the JF

A small craniectomy (3 cm in diameter) exposing the posterior fossa dura and the posterior portion of the JF is the next surgical step (Fig. 8). The emissary mastoid vein is coagulated and cut. The sigmoid sinus is totally dissected. Any tumor within the cervical region and jugular bulb is exposed by widely opening of the JF, communicating the cervical with the cranial portion of the JF. The lateral process of C1 and the posterior border of the JF are removed with a drill and a small Kerrison punch.

### 22.3.4.1
### Extradural Tumor Removal

Small dura incisions are performed in front and behind the sigmoid sinus, below the superior petrosal sinus. The sigmoid sinus is ligated with two sutures (Fig. 8). The internal jugular vein is double-ligated (suture/ligature). The posterior wall of the sigmoid sinus is incised and the intraluminal portion of the lesion is dissected with microsurgical techniques from the anterior wall of the

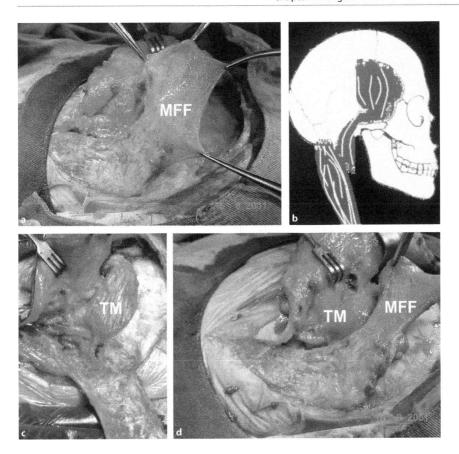

Fig. 5a–d Reconstruction technique. **a** Myofascial flap (*MFF*). **b,c** Temporal muscle (*TM*) rotation. **d** Final aspect

sigmoid sinus and jugular bulb. Bleeding from the inferior petrosal sinus may occur. This sinus is packed with Gelfoam® or Surgicel® after complete tumor removal from the JF. After all of this surgical dissection, removal of the extradural tumor is accomplished (Fig. 9). Tumor extensions anteriorly compressing the ICA and infiltrating the tympanic bone is dissected and removed. In case of tumors not invading the sigmoid sinus like schwannomas, tumor removal may be accomplished without ligation of the sigmoid sinus.

### 22.3.4.2
### Intradural Tumor Removal

The medial wall of the sigmoid sinus is incised to expose the posterior fossa. Minimal cerebellar retraction is needed to open the cerebellomedularis cistern, exposing the intradural JF region (Fig. 10). Cranial nerves VII and VIII are identified. In small tumors, the lower cranial

nerves are easily identified at the brainstem. An intra and extradural dissection of these nerves from the tumor capsule permits total resection with preservation of these structures if the nerves are not infiltrated (Fig. 10). Large intradural tumors are initially coagulated and debulked. Identification of cranial nerves is difficult in large lesions compressing the brainstem. In these cases, especially in paragangliomas, step-by-step shrinkage of the tumor mass with bipolar coagulation and intracapsular tumor removal permits identification of the cranial nerves at the brainstem. Intraoperative monitoring of the caudal cranial nerves is helpful for preservation of these structures. Fascicles of cranial nerves IX, X, and XI may be infiltrated and total removal is possible only if the patient presents preoperatively with deficits of these nerves. Radical tumor removal requires resection of all infiltrated bone and dura mater. It should be performed in all cases of benign noninvasive lesions. Aggressive and malignant tumors show infiltrated the surrounding structures and there is no clear cleavage plane. Total removal is usually not pos-

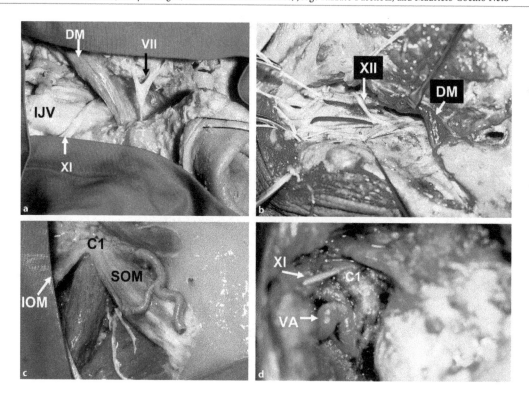

Fig. 6 **a–c** Anatomical specimen showing neck dissection. Digastric muscle (*DM*), cranial nerves VII, XI, and XII, internal jugular vein (*IJV*), superior and inferior oblique muscles (*SOM* and *IOM*, respectively). **d** Surgical picture. *VA* Vertebral artery

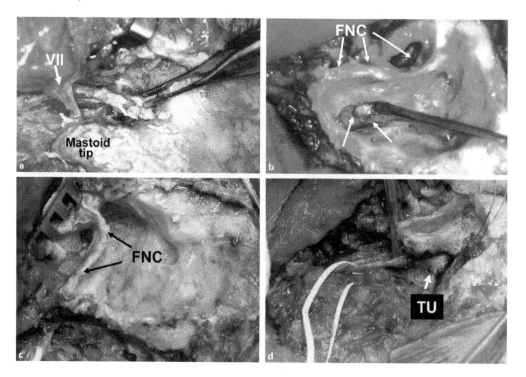

Fig. 7 **a** Facial nerve (VII) dissection. **b,c** Mastoidectomy, facial nerve canal (*FNC*), retrofacial mastoid cells (*arrows*). **d** Jugular bulb with tumor (*TU*)

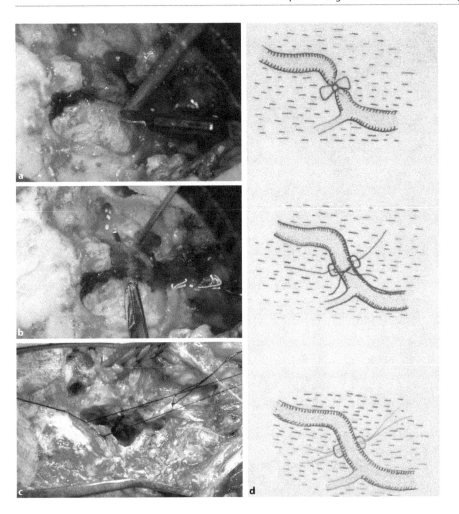

Fig. 8 **a** Craniectomy, dura incision posterior to the sigmoid sinus. **b** "Mosquito" clamp under the sigmoid sinus. **c** Sigmoid sinus ligature. **d** Drawing showing sigmoid sinus ligature technique

sible in these cases. The skull-base defect is closed with the reconstruction technique described earlier. Postoperative lumbar drainage is avoided it is used only if the dural defect could not be closed in a watertight fashion.

## 22.3.5
### Postoperative Care

Postoperative measures are the same as for a major intracranial surgery. The patient is taken intubated to the intensive care unit. To avoid aspiration, extubation is carried out only after the patient is completely awake and the function of the lower cranial nerves can be carefully examined. If the patient presents swallowing difficulty with recurrent aspiration, tracheostomy should be performed as early as possible.

## 22.4
### Results of this Series

Paragangliomas (62 cases) were the most common tumors, followed by schwannomas (19 cases), meningiomas (11 cases), chordomas and chondrosarcomas (7 cases), malignant tumors (4 cases), aneurismal bone cysts (2 cases), cholesteatomas (2 cases), and chondroma, lymphangioma, and inflammatory granuloma (one case each).

## 22.4.1
### Resectability

Radical tumor resection could be obtained in 79 cases (72%) and in 86% of benign tumors (Table 1). Total resection of benign paragangliomas was possible in 48

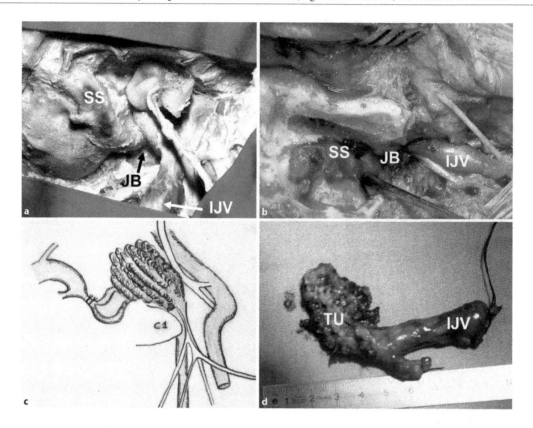

Fig. 9  **a** Anatomical specimen showing the internal jugular vein, jugular bulb (*JB*), and sigmoid sinus (*SS*). **b** Surgical picture. **c** Drawing showing SS ligation and extradural tumor removal. **d** Surgical specimen: paraganglioma

patients. Three of these patients with paragangliomas presented with recurrence of the lesion, with a mean postoperative follow-up of 3 years. These cases were reoperated. Total resection was not possible in 12 patients with paragangliomas. Four of these tumors were malignant and received postoperative radiotherapy. Three had been operated on previously elsewhere. Invasion of the lower cranial nerves or brainstem was the reason for subtotal removal of benign paragangliomas. These patients were followed with MRI examination and radiotherapy was carried out if the tumor remnant showed further growth. Involvement of the ICA was a frequent finding in cases of paragangliomas. This vessel could be dissected from the tumor in the majority of cases (Fig. 11). Two patients with benign paragangliomas showed infiltration of the walls of the ICA and reconstruction of the vessel was performed with a high-flow saphenous bypass (Fig. 12). Radical removal was possible in all cases of schwannomas and in six patients with benign meningiomas. Invasive and malignant meningiomas, chondrosarcomas, chordomas and other malignant tumors could not be totally resected due to infiltration of the brainstem, cranial nerves, dura, and bone. Postoperative radiotherapy was performed in these cases.

### 22.4.2
### Postoperative Complications

Damage to the lower cranial nerves was the most frequent complication. New deficits of lower cranial nerves were the more dangerous complication, and were the cause of postoperative death in two cases. Ten patients developed lower cranial nerves palsy, which was permanent in six cases. Facial nerve and cochlear nerve paralysis occurred in eight cases.; facial nerve function returned spontaneously in three. In five patients, the facial nerve was resected due to tumor infiltration and the facial nerve was reconstructed with nerve grafts (great auricular nerve) or cranial nerve XII/VII anastomosis (one case). All of these patients attained good functional recovery. CSF leakage occurred in four patients (3.6%). These CSF fistulas were treated with repeated surgery (one case) or conservatively with lumbar drainage (three cases). Three of these patients developed meningitis. Four patients (3.6%) died after surgery. The main cause of death was surgical damage to the lower cranial nerves, which was complicated by aspiration pneumonia and septicemia (two patients). Other causes of death were: pulmonary embolism (one patient) and large cervical hematoma causing tracheal

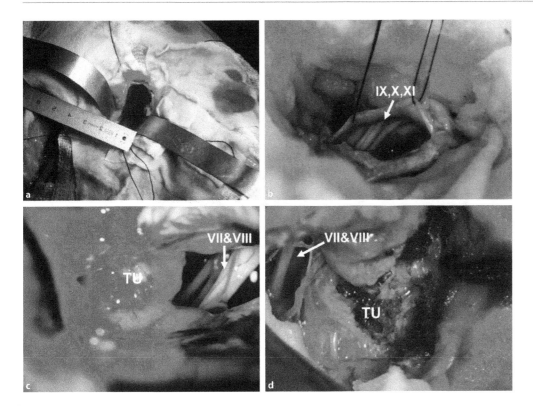

Fig. 10  **a** Dura opening. **b** Intradural identification of the caudal cranial nerves. **c,d** Intradural paragangliomas (TU), cranial nerves VII and VIII

deviation and hypoxia (one patient). This patient died due to secondary complications of brain hypoxemia in spite of hematoma removal and intubation. The hematoma was caused by bleeding from the internal jugular vein. This vessel was ligated during surgery, but the suture opened postoperative after the patient experienced a coughing crisis. Since this episode we performed double suture/ligature of the internal jugular vein in all cases. The complications are listed in Table 2.

## 22.5
## Discussion

The most frequent tumor arising in the JF region is paraganglioma. Multiple terms have been used to describe paragangliomas: glomus tumor, chemodectoma, glomerocytoma, nonchromaffin tumor, tympanic body tumor, and receptoma are the most common [18]. The term "glomus jugulare body" was first used by Guild in 1941 [17] to describe carotid-body-like structures in the temporal bone. In April 1942, Rosenwasser [45, 46] operated on a patient with a bleeding mass that arose in the middle ear and protruded from the ear canal. Histologically, this tumor was identical to benign carotid body tumors. In 1945, Rosen-

wasser [45] published the first description of a middle-ear paraganglioma and associated these tumors with the glomus jugulare bodies. In 1962, Alford and Guilford [1] classified these lesions as glomus tympanicum and glomus jugulare tumors. Chemoreceptor cells are non-chromaffin-staining paraganglion cells developed from the neural crest region during embryogenesis[51, 56]. In 1941, Guild [17] observed the normal occurrence of these structures

Table 2  Surgical complications. *CSF* Cerebrospinal fluid

| Complication | Number |
| --- | --- |
| New cranial nerve deficits | |
| VI | 1 |
| VII | 8 (3 transient) |
| VIII | 8 |
| IX, X, XI | 10 (4 transient) |
| CSF leak | 04 (3.6%) |
| Hemiparesis | 1 |
| Mortality | 4 (3.6%) |

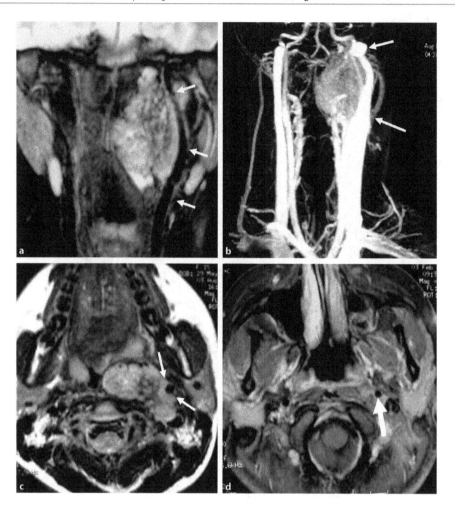

Fig. 11a–d  MRI (**a,c**) and magnetic resonance angiography (**b**) showing involvement of the internal carotid artery (*arrows*). **d** MRI after total removal and preservation of the ICA (*arrow*)

in the temporal bone and called them glomus jugulare bodies. Accumulations of chemoreceptor cells are found in the head and neck region. They are found in the adventitia of the jugular bulb beneath the floor of the middle ear, in the bony walls of the tympanic canals related to the tympanic branches of the glossopharyngeal and vagus nerves, and in the bone of the promontory, close to the mucosal lining of the middle ear in the ciliary ganglion, the ganglion nodosum of the vagus nerve, and in the walls of large arteries [8, 30]. The ascending pharyngeal artery, through its inferior tympanic branch, provides these bodies with an arterial blood supply. Glomus caroticum and glomus aorticum have same histological features, and paragangliomas are similar in all locations. Familial cases present with a much higher incidence of multicentricity [53]; in these cases the paternal allele is the determining factor [54]. There is a 50% incidence of male carrier offspring and 0% female carrier offspring with paraganglioma. This genetic abnormality is created by mutations

located on chromosome 11 at 11q13 and q2.7 [5]. Most frequent location of paragangliomas are: the jugular bulb region (glomus jugulare), the middle ear (glomus tympanicum), and along the course of the vagus nerve (glomus vagale). Other frequent tumors originating in the JF are schwannomas of lower cranial nerves, meningiomas, and chondrosarcomas [42]. The most frequent complains of patients with JF lesions are related to hearing and swallowing symptoms. Patients with paragangliomas usually present as initial symptoms pulsatile tinnitus, hearing loss, and cranial nerve involvement. Growing of the lesion will cause facial paralysis, polypoid mass in the external auditory canal, vertigo, hoarseness, paralysis of the tongue, and in more advanced cases cerebellar symptoms and hemiparesis hypertension, headache, arrhythmias, nausea, and palpitations occur when the tumor secretes norepinephrine. These patients should receive perioperative treatment with ß-blockers. Benign tumors may be very large at diagnosis, and clinical signs and symptoms

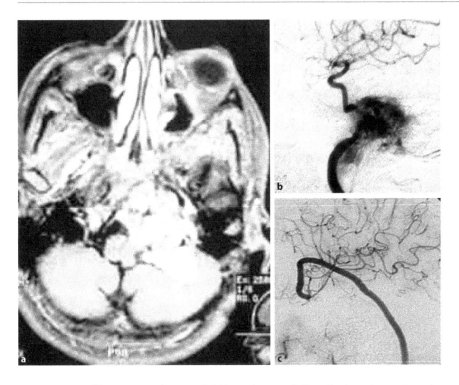

Fig. 12 **a** MRI of large paraganglioma with ICA involvement. **b** Digital subtraction angiography shows ICA infiltration. **c** High-flow bypass between the middle cerebral artery and the external carotid artery with saphenous graft

may not accurately indicate the extension of the lesion. Schwannomas of the JF are usually benign, noninfiltrative lesions [9]. Meningiomas arise from arachnoid cells in the jugular bulb and infiltrate surrounding bone and nerve tissue [32]. Complete tumor removal with preservation of the cranial nerves and vessels is the goal to be achieved. Benign JF tumors can be totally removed and cured [13, 16, 20, 31, 38, 39, 44, 47]. Resection of large benign paragangliomas with extensive intracranial extension and skull-base infiltration may, however, be controversial [8, 13]. The main surgical difficulties with these lesions are: deep location, hypervascularization, involvement of cranial nerves and vessels, infiltration of the brainstem, bone infiltration at the cranial base, and large extension within the posterior fossa [36, 41]. Preoperative evaluation includes complete otological and neurological examination, CT, magnetic resonance imaging (MRI), MRA, and DSA. DSA is performed in cases of highly vascularized lesions. If the ICA is involved or encased, balloon test occlusion is performed. A high-flow shunt (saphenous vein or radial artery graft) is used to reconstruct this vessel in selected cases. New endovascular techniques with placement of stents have been developed and may be helpful when the ICA is involved. Preoperative embolization of highly vascularized lesions, as large paragangliomas and some meningiomas, is performed to reduce bleeding and surgical time [33]. The multidisciplinary approach associating the expertise of neurosurgeons and ENT surgeons gives the best chance of radical removal with preservation of the cranial nerves, vessels, and brainstem. Surgical morbidity and mortality are usually associated with damage to the lower cranial nerves [6]. The surgical strategy to preserve cranial nerves is to first dissect them in a "healthy" plane in the neck, follow them to the JF, and, after dura opening, identify the nerves at the brainstem. If the nerves are infiltrated yet still functioning, subtotal resection leaving a small piece of tumor around the nerves and postoperative radiotherapy (if there is proven postoperative residual tumor growth) seems to be the best treatment. CSF leakage is common and may be a serious complication after resection of JF lesions [2, 21, 24, 55]. Several techniques for reconstruction of a surgical defect have been described. The cranial base is usually reconstructed with: abdominal fat graft, rotation of local and distant pedicled muscle flaps, and free muscle flaps vascularized with microsurgical vessel anastomosis [3, 13, 22, 35]. These procedures have disadvantages: an additional skin incision is required, the fat tissue is not vascularized, a foreign body reaction may occur, and compression of the brainstem [11] and cases of lipoid meningitis are described in the literature [19, 43]. Regional muscle flap rotation increases surgical time, necessitates additional incisions, and may produce poor cosmetic results [4, 14, 34]. Free muscle flaps vascularized with microsurgical techniques have the following disadvantages: increased surgical time and risk of infection, an additional surgical team is required, and there is a higher morbidity rate in elderly patients [3, 4, 10]. Postoperative lumbar drainage is used by many authors [13, 49]. This procedure may have serious morbidity [50]. The cranial-base reconstruction technique we have developed has several advantages when compared with the other approaches. This technique is easy to perform, uses two vascularized flaps, can be employed for small and large defects, causes no additional deficits, is effective in CSF leakage prevention, reduces the need of postoperative lumbar drainage, and produces very good cosmetic results [40].

Radiation therapy is recommended by some authors as the initial treatment for paragangliomas, because resection of these tumors is associated with damage to the lower cranial nerves [29, 52]. The beneficial effects of radiation therapy for paragangliomas of the temporal bone remains, however, uncertain [16]. The effect of irradiation appears to be on the blood vessels and fibrous elements of the lesion [7, 26, 52]. Over 80% tumor control after radiation therapy is reported [12, 25, 26]. The development of radiation-induced neoplasms has been described after radiotherapy for benign glomus jugulare tumors [27]. Malignant tumors should be treated with radio- and chemotherapy.

## 22.6
## Conclusion

Surgical removal remains the treatment of choice and may be curative in cases of schwannomas, benign meningiomas, noninfiltrative paragangliomas, and other benign JF tumors. Radical resection of malignant and invasive tumors with preservation of the cranial nerves is not possible. Large paragangliomas of the JF with intracranial extension may be excised radically through a multidisciplinary approach, with preservation of the lower cranial nerves if they present no infiltrative behavior. Postoperative morbidity and mortality were related to the size and histological features of the lesions. Paralysis of the lower cranial nerves with dysphasia remains the most serious complication related to surgery. Preoperative embolization is very useful in most cases of paragangliomas and highly vascularized tumors, reducing surgical time and blood loss. Adequate reconstruction of the skull base is necessary to avoid postoperative CSF leak.

## References

1. Alford BR, Guilford FR (1962) A comprehensive study of tumors of the glomus jugulare. Laryngoscope 72:765–805
2. Al-Mefty O, Teixeira A (2002) Complex tumors of the glomus jugulare: criteria, treatment, and outcome. J Neurosurg 97:1356–1366
3. Anand V (1989) Reconstruction in cranial base surgery. In: Al-Mefty O (ed) Surgery of the Cranial Base. Kluwer Academic, Boston, pp 297–314
4. Ariyan S (1990) Pectoralis major muscle and musculocutaneous flaps. In: Strauch B, Vasconez LO, Hall-Findlay EJ (eds) Grabb's Encyclopedia of Flaps. Little, Brown, Boston, pp 512–522
5. Bikhazi PH, Roeder E, Attaie A, et al (1999) Familial paragangliomas: the emerging impact of molecular genetics on evaluation and management. Am J Otol 20:639–643
6. Bowdino B, Farrell P, Moore G, et al (2004) Long-term surgical results for glomus temporale tumors. Neurosurg Q 14:19–26
7. Brackmann DE, House WF, Terry R, et al (1972) Glomus jugulare tumors: effect of irradiation. Trans Am Acad Ophthalmol Otolaryngol 76:1423–1431
8. Brown JS (1985) Glomus jugulare tumors revisited: a ten-year statistical follow-up of 231 cases. Laryngoscope 95:284–288
9. Carvalho GA, Tatagiba M, Samii M (2000) Cystic schwannomas of the jugular foramen: clinical and surgical remarks. Neurosurgery 46:560–566
10. Chang DW, Langstein HN, Gupta A, et al (2001) Reconstructive management of cranial base defects after tumor ablation. Plast Reconstr Surg 107:1346–1357
11. Chen TC, Maceri DR, Levy ML, et al (1994) Brain stem compression secondary to adipose graft prolapse after translabyrinthine craniotomy: case report. Neurosurgery 35:521–524
12. Cummings BJ, Beale FA, Garrett PG, et al (1984) The treatment of glomus tumors in the temporal bone by mega voltage radiation. Cancer 53:2635–2640
13. Fisch U (1982) Infratemporal fossa approach for glomus tumors of the temporal bone. Ann Otol Rhinol Laryngol 91:474–479
14. Gal TJ, Kerschner JE, Futran ND, et al (1998) Reconstruction after temporal bone resection. Laryngoscope 108:476–481
15. Glasscock ME, Harris PF, Newsome G (1974) Glomus tumors: diagnosis and treatment. Laryngoscope 84:2006–2032
16. Green JD, Brackmann DE, Nguyen CD, et al (1994) Surgical management of previously untreated glomus jugular tumors. Laryngoscope 104:917–921
17. Guild SR (1941) A hitherto unrecognized structure: the glomus jugularis in man. Anat Rec 79:28 (abstract)
18. Gulya AJ (1993) The glomus tumor and its biology. Laryngoscope 103:7–15
19. Hwang PH, Jackler RK (1996) Lipoid meningitis due to aseptic necrosis of a free fat graft placed during neurotologic surgery. Laryngoscope 106:1482–1486
20. Jackson CG, Glasscock ME, Nissen AJ, et al (1982) Glomus tumor surgery: the approach, results and problems. Otolaryngol Clin North Am 15:897–916
21. Jackson CG, Woods CI, Chironis PN (1993) Glomus jugulare tumors. In: Sekhar LN, Janecka IP (eds) Surgery of Cranial Base Tumors. Raven, New York, pp 747–768

22. Jones NF, Schramm VL, Sekhar LN (1987) Reconstruction of the cranial base following tumour resection. Br J Plast Surg 40:155–162

23. Katsuta T, Rhoton AL Jr, Matsushima T (1997) The jugular foramen: microsurgical anatomy and operative approaches. Neurosurgery 41:149–202

24. Kempe LG (1982) Glomus jugulare tumor. In: Youmans JR (ed) Neurological Surgery, 2nd edn. Saunders, Philadelphia, pp 3285–3298

25. Kim JA, Elkon D, Lim ML, et al (1980) Optimum dose of radiotherapy for chemodectomas of the middle ear. Int J Radiol Oncol Biol Phys 6:815–819

26. Konefal JB, Pilepich MV, Spector GJ, et al (1987) Radiation therapy in the treatment of chemodectomas. Laryngoscope 97:1331–1335

27. Lalwani AK, Jackler RK, Gutin PH (1993) Lethal fibrosarcoma complicating radiation therapy for benign glomus jugulare tumor. Am J Otol 14:398–402

28. Lang J (1989) Anatomy of the jugular foramen. In: Samii M, Draf W (eds) Surgery of the Skull Base. Springer, Berlin, pp 59–64

29. Larner JM, Hahn SS, Spaulding CA, et al (1992) Glomus jugulare tumors: long-term control by radiation therapy. Cancer 69:1813–1817

30. Lattes R, Waltner JG (1949) Nonchromaffin paraganglioma of the middle ear. Cancer 2:447–468

31. Mattos JP, Ramina R, Borges W, et al (2004) Intradural jugular foramen tumors. Arq Neuropsiquiatr 62:997–1003

32. Molony TB, Brackmann DE, Lo WW (1992) Meningiomas of the jugular foramen. Otolaryngol Head Neck Surg 106:128–136

33. Murphy TP, Brackmann DE (1989) Effects of preoperative embolization on glomus jugular tumors. Laryngoscope 99:1244–1247

34. Neligan PC, Mulholland S, Irish J, et al (1996) Flap selection in cranial base reconstruction. Plast Reconstr Surg 98:1159–1168

35. Netterville JL, Civantos EJ (1993) Defect reconstruction following neurologic skull base surgery. Laryngoscope 103:55–63

36. Ramina R, Maniglia JJ, Barrionuevo CE (1988) Glomus jugulare tumors: classification and treatment. Presented at the International Symposium on Cranial Base Surgery, September 13–17, Pittsburgh, USA

37. Ramina R, Maniglia JJ, Barrionuevo CE (1993) Surgical excision of petrous apex lesions. In: Sekhar LN, Janecka IP (eds) Surgery of Cranial Base Tumors. Raven, New York, pp 291–306

38. Ramina R, Maniglia JJ, Fernandes YB, et al (2004) Jugular foramen tumors: diagnosis and treatment. Neurosurg Focus 17:E5

39. Ramina R, Maniglia JJ, Fernandes YB, et al (2005) Tumors of the jugular foramen: diagnosis and management. Neurosurgery 57:59–68

40. Ramina R, Maniglia JJ, Paschoal JR, et al (2005) Reconstruction of the cranial base in surgery for jugular foramen tumors. Neurosurgery 56:337–343; discussion 337–343

41. Ramina R, Maniglia JJ, Pedrozo AA, et al (1996) Surgical treatment of jugular foramen tumors. Zentralbl Neurochir 57:47 (in German)

42. Ramina R, Neto MC, Fernandes YB, et al (2006) Meningiomas of the jugular foramen. Neurosurg Rev 29:55–60

43. Ricaurte JC, Murali R, Mandell W (2000) Uncomplicated postoperative lipoid meningitis secondary to autologous fat graft necrosis. Clin Infect Dis 30:613–615

44. Robertson JT, Clark WC, Robertson JH, et al (1990) Glomus jugulare tumors. In: Youmans JR (ed) Neurological Surgery, 3rd edn. Saunders, Philadelphia, pp 3654–3666

45. Rosenwasser H (1945) Carotid body like tumor involving the middle ear and mastoid Bone. Arch Otolaryngol 41:64–67

46. Rosenwasser H (1952) Glomus jugulare tumors. Laryngoscope 62:623–633

47. Samii M, Tatagiba M (1996) Tumors of the jugular foramen. Neurosurg Q 6:176–193

48. Sen C, Hague K, Kacchara R, et al (2001) Jugular foramen: microscopic anatomic features and implications for neural preservation with reference to glomus tumors involving the temporal bone. Neurosurgery 48:838–848

49. Shapiro AS, Scully T (1992) Closed continuous drainage of cerebrospinal fluid via a lumbar subarachnoid catheter for treatment or prevention of cranial/spinal cerebrospinal fluid fistula. Neurosurgery 30:241–245

50. Snow RB, Kuhel W, Martin SB (1991) Prolonged lumbar spinal drainage after the resection of tumors of the skull base: a cautionary note. Neurosurgery 28:880–882

51. Spector GJ, Ciralsky R, Maisel RH, et al (1975) IV. Multiple glomus tumors in the head and neck. Laryngoscope 85:1066–1075

52. Springate SC, Weichselbaum RR (1990) Radiation or surgery for chemodectoma of the temporal bone: a review of local control and complications. Head Neck 12:303–307

53. van Baars F, van den Broek P, Cremers C, et al (1981) Familial nonchromaffinic paragangliomas (glomus tumors): clinical aspects. Laryngoscope 91:988–996

54. van der Mey AG, Maaswinkel-Mooy PD, Cornelisse CJ, et al (1989) Genomic imprinting in hereditary glomus tumors: evidence of a new genetic theory. Lancet 2:1291–1294

55. Watkins LD, Mendoza N, Cheesman AD, et al (1994) Glomus jugulare tumours: a review of 61 cases. Acta Neurochir 130:66–70

56. Zak FG (1954) An expanded concept of tumors of glomic tissue. N Y State J Med 54:1153–1165

# IV Specific Surgical Management

# Diagnosis and Treatment of Adult Hydrocephalus

Petra M. Klinge

## Contents

## 23.1
## Introduction

Despite a long history, adult-type hydrocephalus is still challenging when it comes to the decision of when and whether shunt treatment should be performed in the individual case. Modern technical achievements in the design of shunt valves, which allow a noninvasive pressure and flow adjustment, have not substantially improved the overall outcome and treatment-related risks over the past decades.

In adult-type hydrocephalus, we are fronting a chronic illness where symptoms occur insidiously, at first glance appearing mild and fluctuating, hard to capture or to measure. Also, the origin and pathology is often not clearly understood, like in idiopathic normal-pressure hydrocephalus (NPH), or assigned an unknown period of pathology, such as long-standing overt ventriculomegaly (LOVA) and idiopathic aqueductal stenosis, both of which have a possible relationship to childhood or being preterm. In those hydrocephalic patients who survive infancy and childhood, the majority of cases with spina bifida and its associated problems, when becoming an adult, are almost a forgotten population, lost in the space between pediatric and adult neurosurgeons.

In NPH, we have finally learned that comorbidity represents an important factor that alters the diagnosis and the pathology (e.g., aging, cerebrovascular and Alzheimer's comorbidity in idiopathic NPH) as well the antecedent event (e.g., traumatic brain injury, hemorrhage or tumor surgery), confounding with the clinical symptoms in secondary NPH. As a result, data on the incidences and prevalences of adult-type hydrocephalus are sparse.

Both the more traditional methods (e.g., measurement of resistance to cerebrospinal fluid, CSF, outflow – $R_{out}$) and/or the intracranial pressure–volume index, analysis of intracranial pressure oscillations ("B-waves"), and the nontraditional methods, cerebral blood flow and metabolic imaging, have failed improve diagnostic accuracy or to identify the best candidates for shunt surgery.

The recently published guidelines on idiopathic NPH [30] concluded that no standard criteria for the diagnosis and treatment of adult hydrocephalus presently exist. This has been attributed to a lack of well-designed prospective multicenter trials in the various fields regarding the etiology, pathophysiology, diagnosis, treatment, and outcome.

Scientists are presently paying more attention to the fact that chronic hydrocephalus couldn't be simply a matter of intracranial pressure and "disturbed CSF-dynamics." It is understood that we need to establish the metabolic consequences of hydrocephalus. One has to consider both the brain CSF dynamics and biomechanics for a better understanding of the underlying disease. This has recently opened the field for studies on brain function and metabolism both in the clinical and experimental field. A consensus statement from a National Institutes of Health funded meeting held in Bethesda (USA), 29–30 September 2005: "Hydrocephalus: Myths, New Facts, and Clear Directions" indicated that it would be an important step to promote hydrocephalus research, creating networks among scientists with evidence from clinical and basic research covering the various aspects of pathophysiology, diagnosis, and treatment. It is hoped, that such a cooperative effort will finally allow a more comprehensive knowledge of "the locus of dysfunction" in a brain that at first glance is affected by ventriculomegaly. Finally, finding the "point of no return," the stage at which irreversible damage occurs during that chronic illness, and to avoid it in our patients.

## 23.2
### Diagnosis and Symptoms Related to Chronic Hydrocephalus

An association between chronic ventricular enlargement and clinical symptoms related to gait, cognitive, and urinary disturbances has been observed in many clinical study over the past decades [15]. This clinical triad is found in both the communicating as well as the noncommunicating types of adult hydrocephalus (e.g., LOVA [34] and idiopathic aqueductal stenosis, or other forms of chronic hydrocephalus [34, 44]).

Dizziness, gait instability, and slowing of thoughts and action are often the first symptoms to be reported [15], when patients start experiencing problems. Headaches and vision problems are more frequently reported in noncommunicating hydrocephalus, and are thought to be attributable to episodes of elevated pressure, which are rarely found in NPH [38]. Generally, investigators most readily look at gait difficulties (e.g., using computer-aided video analysis) [40]; however, with regard to the motor disturbances, the importance of problems of posture and balance in hydrocephalus in determining the gait disorder has been established [4]. In addition, a more general involvement of the motor system including disturbances of the upper limb kinetics has been demonstrated [32], which certainly explains the difficulties in writing sometimes observed in patients showing a narrowed and reduced scripture.

Electromyography and motor-evoked potentials have contributed to an understanding of the potential origin of motor disturbances in hydrocephalus, suggesting that the walking and motor dysfunction are more likely to be of extrapyramidal origin than a result of a major pyramidal tract involvement [48]. Based on the findings, the gait disorder in chronic hydrocephalus is suggested to reflect a subcortical motor control disorder affecting the substantia nigra and the basal ganglia output connection pathways to structures in the frontal lobes. However, not all gait and motor disturbances in hydrocephalus can be narrowed down to an extrapyramidal problem. A detailed analysis of postural function in patients with NPH has recently revealed an involvement of sensorimotor integration and a misinterpretation of afferent visual stimuli in the brainstem postural center [46].

The cognitive profile of NPH patients has been described as a deficit in attention, a slowing of thought processes, apathy, inertness, and loss of motivation associated with memory disorders [13]. As such, it was designated as "subcortical dementia" [10]. However, compared to gait, there seems to be the highest variability in cognitive disturbances before shunting, and in changes in this parameter after shunting [43]. Furthermore, psychiatric problems such as hostility, aggressiveness, and depression were frequently reported [25]. The appearance of depression in patients with hydrocephalus could not only be a consequence of the underlying brain disease, but it could also arise in response to the associated physical and mental disabilities and to the psychomotor retardation [38]. Giving the impression of a variable improvement, cognitive symptoms can be subtle and changes after shunting may go undetected, and so may not have been reliably assessed without the aid of psychometric measures [13]. A certain "profile" of cognitive symptoms has also been detected using various neuropsychological tests: overall, verbal performance was better than nonverbal performance, showing an impairment of attention, executive function, visuospatial function, object perception, object memory, and visuoconstructive function [13, 14].

With regard to urinary incontinence, patients mostly present a clinical picture of "urge incontinence," with an increased frequency of urination during the day and night. In later stages of the disease, it is certainly affected by gait and mental incapabilities. In elderly patients, incontinence is affected by comorbidities, which is why it is argued to be the least specific syndrome of the triad [38].

It has been confirmed in the Hydrocephalus Guidelines [30], that identification of ventriculomegaly by neuroimaging and clinical findings (e.g., related to the clinical triad) is a mainstay of establishing the diagnosis. Patients with ventriculomegaly in the absence of any of the symptoms are generally not considered as candidate for shunting, and vice versa. The differential diagnosis of adult hydrocephalus, however, includes the wide spectrum of the classic forms of neurodegenerative diseases, among the most important being vascular dementia (Alzheimer's and Parkinson's) [38]. In NPH, for example, 75% of the patients had additional akinetic, tremulous, hypertonic, and/or hyperkinetic movement disorders [23]. Their prevalence was highest in patients with idiopathic NPH (56/65 patients, 86%). The most frequent movement disorder was upper extremity bradykinesia, which responded favorably to CSF diversion in 80% of a subset of this group.

With regard to cerebrovascular disease, there is high prevalence (83%) of systemic hypertension in idiopathic NPH patients [6, 24]. The various problems of the elderly, such as orthopedic problems, spinal lumbar stenosis, neuropathies, and prostatism, for example, play an important role in idiopathic NPH [38].

## 23.3
### Diagnostic Tests in the Evaluation of Hydrocephalus

The so-called "diagnostic-tests" may be more helped with the term "prognostic tests," as they have been implemented in the prediction of the result of shunting, particularly in those patients with a questionable diagnosis in the presence of unexpected findings. Traditionally, invasive testing is required in order to identify a defective CSF flow and a CSF circulatory disorder, or probatory drainage: cisternography, long-term intracranial pressure measurement and B-wave analysis (Fig. 1), measurement of resistance to CSF outflow (Rou) or compliance [5, 41], high-volume spinal tap test (50 cm³), and controlled continuous lumbar drainage [31]. As they all reflect the traditional idea about hydrocephalus pathophysiology being a primary disorder of CSF absorption, invasive tests have somehow become considered a standard investigation in numerous services over the past decades. As a matter of fact, only a few tests have been studied prospectively so as to allow a reliable determination of their accuracy in predicting the results of shunting [29]. As a general observation, the positive predictive value (PPV) of that test parameter is relatively high, ranging from 70 to 90%, while the negative predictive value (NPV) is disappointingly low (less than 30%). Also, patients show a wide range of physiological values, in part a matter of center-specific methods and thresholds; however, a patient should never be excluded from shunt treatment based on negative tests results, as long as the clinical impression is supportive [30].

Recently, a single-center study on external lumbar drainage (ELD), done in a larger series of 151 patients with idiopathic NPH, provided comparably high figures for both PPV (90.5%) and NPV (77.7%) [31]. In that study, 76 of the 84 patients with a positive drainage response improved with a shunt, and 14 of the 18 patients in whom drainage gave no improvement did not benefit from the shunt, suggesting that a drainage protocol might be most favorable in mimicking a shunt response. Although the risks associated with ELD (e.g., nerve root irritation, infection, and headache) are reported to be low, the true disadvantages (e.g., hospitalization and compliance) remain to be calculated.

In summary, the diagnostic tests reveal evidence of a heterogeneous patient population in adult chronic hydro-cephalus, where no constant morphological and physiological element exists. As a consequence, more than one test is routinely applied in the hope of improving the prognostic accuracy; however, the result is a "diagnostic puzzle." Regardless of the rationale underlying the use of a combination of test procedures in the individual patient, such a concept is questioned by many clinicians, stating that there is clearly a need for a single standardized, as well a practicable diagnostic protocol.

## 23.4
## Neuroimaging and Brain/CSF Metabolism

Basically, ventriculomegaly is indicated by Evan's index or the frontal horn index, defined as the largest diameter of the frontal horns divided by the largest diameter of the brain at the level of the anterior commissure or at the level of the frontal horns: a value of this parameter above 0.3 or 0.4 is indicative of hydrocephalus. These indices are possibly the only findings obligatory for establishing the diagnosis of hydrocephalus, while all other imaging findings are optional [38], for example large temporal horns, dilated third ventricle, enlarged perisylvian fissures or both focal dilatation and obliteration of the cortical sulci (so-called periventricular edema, Fig. 2a), increased callosal angle, and aqueductal flow void (Fig. 2b).

Attention should be drawn to periventricular white matter lesions (PWMLs) and deep white matter lesions (DWMLs), as observed in T2-weighted MRI or in fluid-attenuated inversion-recovery sequences (Fig. 3). These have been clearly associated with cerebrovascular co-morbidity and have been observed in a subgroup of patients with idiopathic NPH [45]. A negative correlation of DWMLs and PWMLs with the outcome in patients was found, although exclusion of an individual patient based on the finding of white-matter lesions is not justified, as before shunting, there was no difference in either PWMLs or DWMLs between outcome groups in that study.

In a comparison of NPH and Binswanger's disease, it was found that they share, for the major part, MRI

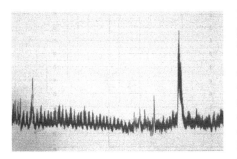

Fig. 1 Photograph of a paper record made while monitoring intracranial pressure epidurally in a patient with normal pressure hydrocephalus (NPH). Sequences of symmetrical B-waves, initially described by Lundberg in the 1960s, displaying an amplitude ranging from 10 to 50 mmHg with a frequency of 0.5–3/min have been associated with chronic hydrocephalus. If those waves are recorded for more than 50% of the time, when assessed during overnight monitoring (48 h), they have been reported to be a good predictor of outcome in a subset of patients. So-called "plateau waves" with amplitudes of up to 100 mmHg over a period of 5–20 min are rarely observed in chronic hydrocephalus. B-wave activity, however, has been associated with rapid-eye-movement sleep activity, thereby questioning the validity for hydrocephalus diagnosis. It is assumed that B-waves are of vascular nature (i.e. related to changes and oscillations in the systemic blood pressure)

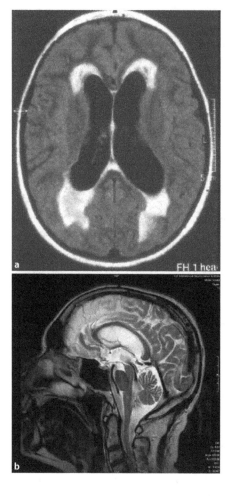

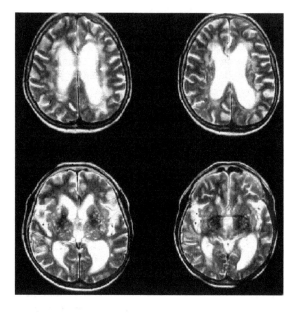

Fig. 3 T2-weighted magnetic resonance imaging (MRI) in NPH showing abundant and variable white matter lesions in the periventricular region. They are located in the vicinity of the ventricles, however, distinct from the subependymal zone (**upper images**). Located in the subcortical regions (**lower images**), the basal ganglia, they are assigned as deep white matter lesions. These lesions have been attributed to vascular pathology (e.g. chronic subcortical infarctions, normally seen in patients with subcortical arteriosclerotic encephalopathy), systemic hypertension being the most important risk factor

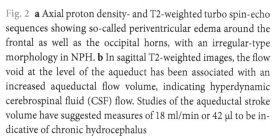

Fig. 2 **a** Axial proton density- and T2-weighted turbo spin-echo sequences showing so-called periventricular edema around the frontal as well as the occipital horns, with an irregular-type morphology in NPH. **b** In sagittal T2-weighted images, the flow void at the level of the aqueduct has been associated with an increased aqueductal flow volume, indicating hyperdynamic cerebrospinal fluid (CSF) flow. Studies of the aqueductal stroke volume have suggested measures of 18 ml/min or 42 µl to be indicative of chronic hydrocephalus

changes with regard to white matter lesions, which the authors suggested indicates a common pathophysiological pattern [45]. Mechanisms are explained by an increased pulse pressure in periventricular and subcortical arteriosclerotic vessels, which may cause enlargement of ventricles in the absence of raised intracranial pressure in that subgroup of patients.

Although blood flow and metabolic studies have so far shown a variable correlation with the clinical outcome

[35], those methods, have been suggested to allow access to the brain disease in hydrocephalus, and studies are promising in this regard.

Using [$^{15}$O]H$_2$O-positron emission tomography (PET), global cerebral blood flow and cerebrovascular reserve capacity before and after application of 1 g Diamox were quantified before, 1 week, and 7 months after surgery in 70 patients with idiopathic NPH (Fig. 4) [17, 18]. Global blood flow was significantly lower in the "shunt-

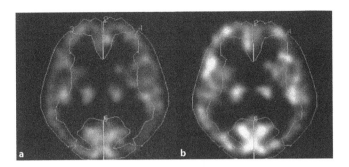

Fig. 4a,b [$^{15}$O]H$_2$O-positron emission tomography (PET) before (**a**) and after (**b**) after intravenous application of 1 g Diamox in a patient with NPH. Diamox (acetazolamide) increases cerebral blood flow through cerebral vessel dilatation. If blood flow increases by more than 30%, the so-called cerebrovascular reserve capacity is considered intact. [$^{15}$O]H$_2$O-PET is considered a routine tool in the diagnosis of cerebrovascular diseases. Both blood flow and cerebrovascular reserve capacity in hydrocephalic patients were measured, averaging the measures in the regions of interests according to the vascular territories of the anterior, middle, and posterior cerebral arteries

responder." The predictive accuracy increased to 88% with the finding of a decreased blood flow, when compared to the accuracy score of 76% obtained by a combination of dynamic CSF tests. Furthermore, the cerebrovascular reserve capacity was correlated with clinical changes after shunt placement: after 1 week, shunt responders showed considerable improvement (>30%) in reserve capacity and nonresponders did not, suggesting that neurological improvement after shunting is related to early restoration of the hemodynamic reserve and to improved conditions in the chronic hypoxic environment of the hydrocephalic brain [17].

Using statistical parametric mapping (SPM 99, Welcome Department of Cognitive Neurology, London, UK) in a series of idiopathic NPH, significant regional decreases in frontal, frontomedial, and temporomedial cortical areas were found, which positively correlated with the clinical impairment using a score based on a formal assessment of both gait and mental function (Fig. 5). These areas could have been attributed to the frontal association cortex, the frontomesial and the supplementary motor cortex, and to the inner and outer limbic cortex after transformation into a standard stereotaxic space (Montreal Neurological Institute default template of SPM 99 for $^{15}$O regional cerebral blood flow studies). In addition, after shunting, clinical responders exhibited increases in regional blood flow in supplemental motor areas, while nonresponder did not.

Other PET studies using an anatomic region-of-interest analysis on coregistered magnetic resonance done in both secondary and idiopathic NPH, demonstrated a reduction in cerebral blood flow in the basal ganglia and the thalamus. This was correlated with the level of function in patients, related to the motor disorder [36].

Disturbances in brain and neuronal metabolism have also been evidenced by $^1$H- and $^{31}$P-MRI spectroscopy investigations in NPH patients [8]: lactate peaks in the periventricular areas and reduced N-acetylaspartate/total creatine ratios in the cortex differed from those in controls and in other forms of dementia. Very recent studies in microdialysis have indicated a situation of postischemic recovery in patients with chronic hydrocephalus [1].

In the light of these observations, the CSF contents of neuronal metabolites and peptides, neurotransmitters, and of products reflecting neuronal degeneration (Tau, A-beta, neurofilament and sulfatide) have emphasized the potential advantage of investigating neuronal and brain metabolism, and have shown to be effective diagnostic and prognostic markers in adult hydrocephalus [42].

23.5

## Pathophysiology of Chronic Hydrocephalus

Whether an increased $R_{out}$ and/or B-waves is linked to the pathophysiology of chronic hydrocephalus has been discussed. Early investigations have shown an association between an elevated $R_{out}$ and a reduced compliance with CSF malabsorption [41]. These parameters have since been associated with chronic hydrocephalus and, it has been suggested, are important diagnostic tools [7].

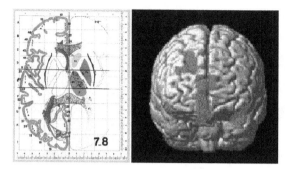

Fig. 5 Using statistical parametric mapping (SPM 99, Wellcome Department of Cognitive Neurology, London, UK), regional blood flow was correlated with clinical impairment in 70 patients with idiopathic NPH. On the voxel level, statistical correlations were attributed to Broadman areas (**right**) after transformation into anatomic standard (Montreal Neurological Institute): thresholds for statistical inferences: $Z > 3.09$, uncorrected $p$-value on voxel level $p < 0.001$, extend threshold at least 6 voxel. The more the patient was clinically impaired, areas with diminished blood flow were found in the frontal association cortex, the frontomesial and the supplementary motor cortex, and to the inner and outer limbic cortex, as plotted in the three-dimensional MRI surface image (**right**)

Biopsy specimens taken at the time of shunt surgery in patients diagnosed with NPH did not show any correlation between an increased $R_{out}$ and arachnoids fibrosis, although arachnoid fibrosis was previously supposed to be the morphological correlate causing CSF malabsorption [2]. There is no normative data on any of these physiological parameters, regardless of the methodology used

to estimate $R_{out}$ and/or intracranial compliance; this questions the significance of $R_{out}$ for diagnosing chronic hydrocephalus. It is meanwhile acknowledged that $R_{out}$ naturally increases with age in otherwise healthy individuals [11]. As such, in the subgroup of chronic hydrocephalus of the elderly, much higher cut-off values are likely to be indicative of the disease [5].

In the aforementioned cortical biopsy studies, a high incidence of amyloid plaques and neurofibrillary tangles has been observed in patients with idiopathic NPH [2]; 30–50% of patients have Alzheimer's disease on cortical biopsy [16]. It has therefore been suggested that the two diseases may have some common pathophysiology (e.g., diminished clearance of extracellular amyloid-beta peptides, Aβ, and hyperphosphorylated tau proteins, hpTau, from the brain interstitial fluid) [39]. Altered CSF dynamics and decreased expression of Aβ transport proteins at the capillary endothelium may be causal.

These findings were corroborated by an experimental study of kaolin-induced hydrocephalus in aged rats: Aß[1–42] and Aß[1–40] accumulation was evident at 6 and 10 weeks post-hydrocephalus induction [22]. Kaolin-induced blockage of CSF circulation in the basal subarachnoidal space results in hydrocephalus (Fig. 6a) and increased resistance to CSF absorption. In the later stages, intracranial pressure normalizes; however, resistance remains above normal values [9]. Increasing amyloid burden at CSF absorption sites, in vessel walls and perivascular spaces, and within the parenchyma was observed (Fig. 6b). Low-density lipoprotein-receptor-related protein 1 (LRP-1), the primary capillary endothelial receptor for transport of Aβ out of the brain interstitial fluid, also showed reduced expression [22]. The findings suggest that the age-related impairment of the CSF circulation decreases the clearance or washout of potentially toxic

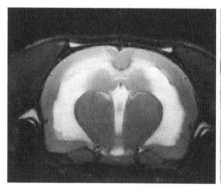

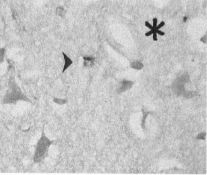

Fig. 6 **a** Coronal MRI (4.7 Tesla, Bruker-Spect, Magdeburg, Germany) of kaolin-induced hydrocephalus in a rat. Note the periventricular hyperintensities, obvious at a stage where intracranial pressure normalizes, and resistance to CSF outflow remains above normal levels, indicating a disturbed CSF circulation and turnover. **b** At that stage, using specific immunostaining of anti-A-beta-40 and anti-A-beta-42 proteins in the aged rats with kaolin-induced hydrocephalus, larger "plaque-like" accumulations (*arrowhead*) in the cortical as well as hippocampal parenchyma were observed; ×1000 microscopic magnification; *cerebral microvessel

products of brain metabolism from the brain interstitial fluid (e.g., beta amyloid), leading to Alzheimer's disease pathology in chronic hydrocephalus of the elderly.

Other experimental studies have furthermore supported the role for chronic ischemia causing neuronal injury in vulnerable brain regions, and adaptive vascular and neuronal processes [21, 27], playing a more important role in the disease than ventricular enlargement and CSF dynamic parameters.

Experimental studies have contributed to many of the clinical-pathological aspects of chronic hydrocephalus. They allow, however, a more structured insight into the biomechanical as well as the biochemical mechanisms. As a consequence, they have opened the field for adjunct neuroprotective strategies [12].

Since very recently, a proportion of patients in a large idiopathic NPH cohort with large head circumference (HC) has been identified, who presumably have congenital hydrocephalus that has not become clinically apparent until late in life. It is clear that our traditional classification scheme in adult-type hydrocephalus is no longer valid [47].

## 23.6
## Treatment and Outcome

Practically speaking, decision making for shunt surgery results in a variety of different strategies: a strict investigator considers shunting only in patients presenting with the complete triad, marked ventriculomegaly and other supportive clinical and imaging findings. A liberal investigator shunts nearly everybody, even in the presence of an incomplete triad, comorbid conditions, and/or unexpected clinical and radiological findings. The first investigator may miss an occasionally treatable patient and the second may perform many useless and risky surgical interventions. Neither of the strategies will eventually help to improve the quality of our treatment of NPH, but rather, may increase the risk of an upcoming "therapeutic nihilism."

Across studies, overall improvement rates to shunt treatment range between 30 and 96% [18]. Adjustable valves allow noninvasive treatment of problems related to over- and underdrainage, which are the most frequent complications related to shunt treatment [3]. In a larger study of 218 NPH patients, nontraumatic subdural effusion occurred in 15 patients; however, 8 were treated by adjustment alone [49]. The 5-year shunt survival rate was 80.2%. Outcomes were excellent or good in 71 of 90 patients (78.9%) with idiopathic NPH and in 30 (69.8%) of 43 patients with secondary NPH. Via magnetic force, pressure changes can easily be administered transcutaneously in an outpatient setting (Fig. 7).

Ventriculostomy is the first option in the cases of noncommunicating hydrocephalus [33]. It has also been implicated in the treatment of NPH in order to overcome the shunt-related problems. So far, studies report contradictory results, and there are still few long-term data [3]. There is evidence that patients have later failed to improve and were treated with a shunt [26].

In this regard, one issue that has not been very well addressed in the past is the fact that postoperative management still lacks protocols for patient follow up and the assessment of clinical outcome and clinical improvement [18]. As long as there are no clear criteria for assessing shunt success, the definite value of shunting NPH may never be clarified. In the literature, long-term and short-term outcome are lumped together [18]. It is known from studies of long-term outcome of idiopathic NPH, however, that particularly in that elderly age group, a lot of comorbid factors (e.g., ischemic brain or heart diseases) do affect the long-term outcome, and clinical deterioration occurs unrelated to the shunt [28]. Overall improvement decreased from 64% to 26% when comparing outcomes at 3 months with those at 3 years.

Some authors introduced scales either by rating the degree of cognitive impairment, gait, and urinary disturbances before shunting, or by grading the magnitude of improvement in each symptom after surgery. None of these scales has gained a wide acceptance and or have been shown to be advantageous for the clinical assessment. Some authors have used scales from the rehabilitation field (e.g., the Rankin scale, the Barthel index, and the Katz index), or other neurological scales (e.g., the Mini Mental State Examination, or the Glasgow Coma Outcome Scale); however, these have not been validated for the assessment of hydrocephalus.

Neuropsychological methods have been used to assess the clinical improvement more reliably and to mea-

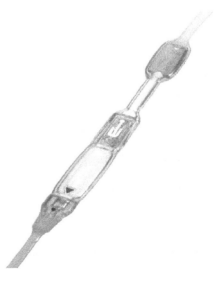

Fig. 7 The Codman programmable differential pressure valve allows pressure changes of 10 mm $H_2O$ within a range of 30–200 mm $H_2O$ (photograph of the internal parts of the valve)

PRE OP

POST OP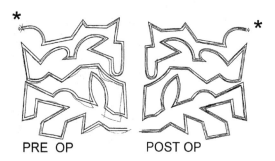

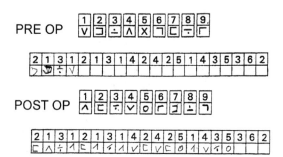

PRE OP POST OP

Fig. 8 The pencil-paper-test "digit-symbol": an example of considerable improvement in visual attention at 1 week after shunt treatment in a patient with good clinical outcome. The pencil-paper-test "line-tracing": parallel to a marked improvement in gait-profiles at 1 week after shunt treatment, the patient made considerably less errors and took less time to complete the line-tracing, a measure of motor precision. Both tests were originally a part of the adult Wechsler's test battery. *PRE OP* Preoperative, *POST OP* postoperative

sure improvement of function after shunt treatment. It has been shown by various investigators that there is considerable improvement in neuropsychological function, which is correlated with improvement in the daily activities. Raftopoulos et al. have shown a 66% improvement in psychometric function, which contributed to an improvement in the Black-outcome scale of 96% [37]. Thereby, neuropsychological measures may provide early and reliable measures of functional outcome in hydrocephalus. In follow-up examination, these tests may offer a practical and standardized tool to monitor patient status, since assessment of gait function alone might not contribute sufficiently to monitoring of the patient's functional outcome after shunt placement. More simple tests are needed, for example tests that are assessable in a larger cohort of patients (e.g., pencil paper tests; Fig. 8), simple, can be applied as bedside tests, and that can define the degree of dementia pre- and postoperatively [20]. Prospective randomized studies incorporating standardized measures for clinical improvement and outcome instruments with attention to inter-rater reliability and construct validity will be key in the development or selection of a useful outcome measure.

Finally, the management of nonresponders has virtually not been addressed in the literature. It remains unclear in these cases whether this is attributable to an ineffective shunt (blockage or underdrainage), selection of a poor candidate, or irreversible damage. Presently, these questions cannot be answered properly as long as follow-up studies have not been systematically performed in a prospective design [19].

## 23.7
## Future Concepts and Conclusion

Hydrocephalus needs basic research on the basis of experimental studies looking at the brain injury and its reversibility in chronic hydrocephalus, narrowing down the potential mechanisms related to a disturbed blood flow, blood–brain barrier breakdown, and altered CSF clearance function, all balancing the homeostasis of the brain interstitial fluid.

The natural course of chronic hydrocephalus remains to be established. It is not clear whether and how the disease progresses, and what is the determining factor for irreversible brain damage.

To address the various unsolved clinical issues, multicenter cooperations, providing larger number of patients, and assessed in a standardized and prospective manner, must be the future hallmarks for clinical hydrocephalus research.

The currently ongoing prospective European multicenter study on the prediction of outcome in patients with idiopathic NPH, which started in October 2005, joined by 15 European neurosurgical and neurological centers, will report 1 year postoperative results from 200 prospectively evaluated patients. Patients will be included on the basis of clinical and imaging findings, and a battery of clinical tests will be applied before shunt surgery. As a new approach, data will be registered electronically in a Web-based database located at the International Neuroscience Institute, Hannover. Quantitative measures of gait and balance and of cognitive function will provide objective and standardized measures of improvement and outcome. It is hoped that this cooperation will evolve into a growing network of scientists and researches, aiming to create a "loop of evidence" based on prospective clinical trials, patient registries, and ongoing basic, experimental, and clinical studies, improving the outcome for hydrocephalus.

## References

1. Agren-Wilsson A, Roslin M, Eklund A, et al (2003) Intracerebral microdialysis and CSF hydrodynamics in idiopathic adult hydrocephalus syndrome. J Neurol Neurosurg Psychiatry 74:217–221

2. Bech RA, Waldemar G, Gjerris F, et al (1999) Shunting effects in patients with idiopathic normal pressure hydrocephalus; correlation with cerebral and leptomeningeal biopsy findings. Acta Neurochir (Wien) 141:633–639

3. Bergsneider M, Black PM, Klinge P, et al (2005) Surgical management of idiopathic normal-pressure hydrocephalus. Neurosurgery 57:S29–S39

4. Blomsterwall E, Svantesson U, Carlsson U, et al (2000) Postural disturbance in patients with normal pressure hydrocephalus. Acta Neurol Scand 102:284–291

5. Boon AJ, Tans JT, Delwel EJ, et al (1997) Dutch normal-pressure hydrocephalus study: prediction of outcome after shunting by resistance to outflow of cerebrospinal fluid. J Neurosurg 87:687–693

6. Boon AJ, Tans JT, Delwel EJ, et al (1999) Dutch normal-pressure hydrocephalus study: the role of cerebrovascular disease. J Neurosurg 90:221–226

7. Borgesen SE, Gjerris F, Sorensen SC (1979) Intracranial pressure and conductance to outflow of cerebrospinal fluid in normal-pressure hydrocephalus. J Neurosurg 50:489–493

8. Braun KP, Vandertop WP, Gooskens RH (2000) NMR spectroscopic evaluation of cerebral metabolism in hydrocephalus: a review. Neurol Res 22:51–64

9. Brinker T, Beck H, Klinge P, et al (1998) Sinusoidal intrathecal infusion for assessment of CSF dynamics in kaolin-induced hydrocephalus. Acta Neurochir (Wien) 140:1069–1075

10. Caltagirone C, Gainotti G, Masullo C, et al (1982) Neurophysiological study of normal pressure hydrocephalus. Acta Psychiatr Scand 65:93–100

11. Czosnyka M, Czosnyka ZH, Whitfield PC, et al (2001) Age dependence of cerebrospinal pressure–volume compensation in patients with hydrocephalus. J Neurosurg 94:482–486

12. Del Bigio MR, Massicotte EM (2001) Protective effect of nimodipine on behavior and white matter of rats with hydrocephalus. J Neurosurg 94:788–794

13. De Mol J (1977) [Neuropsychological study of mental troubles in normal pressure hydrocephaly and their short term evolution after spinal fluid derivation] Etude neuropsychologique des troubles mentaux dans l'hydrocephalie normotensive et de leur evolution a court terme apres derivation du liquide cephalo-rachidien. Acta Psychiatr Belg 77:228–253

14. Devito EE, Pickard JD, Salmond CH, et al (2005) The neuropsychology of normal pressure hydrocephalus (NPH). Br J Neurosurg 19:217–224

15. Fisher CM (1977) The clinical picture in occult hydrocephalus. Clin Neurosurg 24:270–284

16. Golomb J, Wisoff J, Miller DC, et al (2000) Alzheimer's disease comorbidity in normal pressure hydrocephalus: prevalence and shunt response. J Neurol Neurosurg Psychiatry 68:778–781

17. Klinge P, Berding G, Brinker T, et al (2002) The role of cerebral blood flow and cerebrovascular reserve capacity in the diagnosis of chronic hydrocephalus – a PET-study on 60 patients. Acta Neurochir Suppl 81:39–41

18. Klinge PM, Berding G, Brinker T, et al (1999) A positron emission tomography study of cerebrovascular reserve before and after shunt surgery in patients with idiopathic chronic hydrocephalus. J Neurosurg 91:605–609

19. Klinge P, Marmarou A, Bergsneider M, et al (2005) Outcome of shunting in idiopathic normal-pressure hydrocephalus and the value of outcome assessment in shunted patients. Neurosurgery 57:S40–S52

20. Klinge P, Ruckert N, Schuhmann M, et al (2002) Neuropsychological testing to improve surgical management of patients with chronic hydrocephalus after shunt treatment. Acta Neurochir Suppl 81:51–53

21. Klinge PM, Samii A, Mühlendyck A, et al (2003) Cerebral hypoperfusion and delayed hippocampal response after induction of adult kaolin hydrocephalus. Stroke 34:193–199

22. Klinge PM, Samii A, Niescken S, et al (2006) Brain amyloid accumulates in aged rats with kaolin-induced hydrocephalus. Neuroreport 17:657–660

23. Krauss JK, Regel JP, Droste DW, et al (1997) Movement disorders in adult hydrocephalus. Mov Disord 12:53–60

24. Krauss JK, Regel JP, Vach W, et al (1996) Vascular risk factors and arteriosclerotic disease in idiopathic normal-pressure hydrocephalus of the elderly. Stroke 27:24–29

25. Lindqvist G, Andersson H, Bilting M, et al (1993) Normal pressure hydrocephalus: psychiatric findings before and after shunt operation classified in a new diagnostic system for organic psychiatry. Acta Psychiatr Scand Suppl 373:18–32

26. Longatti PL, Fiorindi A, Martinuzzi A (2004) Failure of endoscopic third ventriculostomy in the treatment of idiopathic normal pressure hydrocephalus. Minim Invasive Neurosurg 47:342–345

27. Luciano MG, Skarupa DJ, Booth AM, et al (2001) Cerebrovascular adaptation in chronic hydrocephalus. J Cereb Blood Flow Metab 21:285–294

28. Malm J, Kristensen B, Stegmayr B, et al (2000) Three-year survival and functional outcome of patients with idiopathic adult hydrocephalus syndrome. Neurology 55:576–578

29. Marmarou A, Bergsneider M, Klinge P, et al (2005) The value of supplemental prognostic tests for the preoperative assessment of idiopathic normal-pressure hydrocephalus. Neurosurgery 57:S17–S28

30. Marmarou A, Bergsneider M, Relkin N, et al (2005) Development of guidelines for idiopathic normal-pressure hydrocephalus: introduction. Neurosurgery 57:S1–S3

31. Marmarou A, Young HF, Aygoc GA, et al (2005) Diagnosis and management of idiopathic normal-pressure hydrocephalus: a prospective study in 151 patients. J Neurosurg 102:987–997

32. Matousek M, Wikkelso C, Blomsterwall E, et al (1995) Motor performance in normal pressure hydrocephalus assessed with an optoelectronic measurement technique. Acta Neurol Scand 91:500–505

33. Oi S, Hidaka M, Honda Y, et al (1999) Neuroendoscopic surgery for specific forms of hydrocephalus. Childs Nerv Syst 15:56–68

34. Oi S, Shimoda M, Shibata M, et al (2000) Pathophysiology of long-standing overt ventriculomegaly in adults. J Neurosurg 92:933–940

35. Owler BK, Pickard JD (2001) Normal pressure hydrocephalus and cerebral blood flow: a review. Acta Neurol Scand 104:325–342

36. Owler BK, Momjian S, Czosnyka Z, et al (2004) Normal pressure hydrocephalus and cerebral blood flow: a PET study of baseline values. J Cereb Blood Flow Metabol 24:17–23

37. Raftopoulos C, Deleval J, Chaskis C, et al (1994) Cognitive recovery in idiopathic normal pressure hydrocephalus: a prospective study. Neurosurgery 35:397–404

38. Relkin N, Marmarou A, Klinge P, et al (2005) Diagnosing idiopathic normal-pressure hydrocephalus. Neurosurgery 57:S4–16

39. Silverberg GD (2004) Normal pressure hydrocephalus (NPH): ischaemia, CSF stagnation or both. Brain 127:947–948

40. Stolze H, Kuhtz-Buschbeck JP, Drucke H, et al (2001) Comparative analysis of the gait disorder of normal pressure hydrocephalus and Parkinson's disease. J Neurol Neurosurg Psychiatry 70:289–297

41. Tans JT, Poortvliet DC (1989) Relationship between compliance and resistance to outflow of CSF in adult hydrocephalus. J Neurosurg 71:59–62

42. Tarnaris A, Watkins LD, Kitchen ND (2006) Biomarkers in chronic adult hydrocephalus. Cerebrospinal Fluid Res 3:11

43. Thomsen AM, Borgesen SE, Bruhn P, et al (1986) Prognosis of dementia in normal-pressure hydrocephalus after a shunt operation. Ann Neurol 20:304–310

44. Tisell M, Tullberg M, Hellstrom P (2003) Neurological symptoms and signs in adult aqueductal stenosis. Acta Neurol Scand 107:311–317

45. Tullberg M, Jensen C, Ekholm S, et al (2001) Normal pressure hydrocephalus: vascular white matter changes on MR images must not exclude patients from shunt surgery. AJNR Am J Neuroradiol 22:1665–1673

46. Wikkelso C, Blomsterwall E, Frisen L (2003) Subjective visual vertical and Romberg's test correlations in hydrocephalus. J Neurol 250:741–745

47. Wilson RK, Williams MA (2007) Evidence that congenital hydrocephalus is a precursor to idiopathic normal pressure hydrocephalus (INPH) in only a subset of patients. J Neurol Neurosurg Psychiatry 78:508–511

48. Zaaroor M, Bleich N, Chistyakov A, et al (1997) Motor evoked potentials in the preoperative and postoperative assessment of normal pressure hydrocephalus. J Neurol Neurosurg Psychiatry 62:517–521

49. Zemack G, Romner B (2002) Adjustable valves in normal-pressure hydrocephalus: a retrospective study of 218 patients. Neurosurgery 51:1392–1400

# Primary Tethered Cord Syndrome

## 24

Steffen K. Rosahl

## Contents

## 24.1
## Introduction

While tethered cord syndrome (TCS) has often been referred to as a single entity in the past, this view is beginning to change. Secondary forms like those associated with myelomeningocele, lipoma, or trauma may be entirely different from primary ones. Criteria that had been thought to be important, like low conus medullare, thick filum terminale, and permanent cord traction, are also now being questioned with respect to their contribution to the pathophysiology and to the clinical picture. Primary TCS may be entirely different from secondary forms related to trauma, myelomeningocele repair, or dysraphism in general. The disorder remains a challenge for both diagnostic and therapeutic measures. Today there is no question, however, that neurosurgery plays an important role in its treatment, and indications for surgery have recently widened rather than narrowed. Early diagnosis to prevent neurological deterioration is an urgent requirement, and even prophylactic surgery is now

being advocated [2, 20, 59, 67]. On the other hand, there is evidence that a low conus and/or a thick filum do not necessarily lead to clinical symptoms typical for TCS [47, 56].

## 24.2
## History and Definitions

Although there was an early report by Jones in 1891 with the illustrative title "Spina bifida occulta: no paralytic symptoms until 17 years of age; spine trephined to relieve pressure on the cauda equina; recovery" that describes a patient with neonatal history of spina bifida in whom a "fibrous band" crossing the spinal canal had been transected and removed [29], the specific term "tethered cord syndrome" itself was first applied by Garceau in 1953 [15]. The initial definition included a conus medullare situated below the level of L1/2 and a thickened filum as "hard criteria." Recently, an entity of an occult tight filum terminale syndrome, characterized by clinical findings consistent with a TCS, but with the conus ending in a normal position, has been recognized [77].

It is because of this controversy, that one is hesitating to come up with strong criteria to define the condition. In 1993, Warder and Oaks, in a larger series of patients, demonstrated that a low conus is not a necessary condition for TCS [75, 76]. At that time they stated that the disorder is diagnosed by progressive symptoms and a thickened filum terminale. By 2001 the thick filum was no longer a primary issue anymore, and Warder then defined TCS rather along clinical observations as being a progressive form of neurological deterioration that results from spinal cord tethering by various dysraphic spinal abnormalities [74]. Yet 2 years later, tethered spinal cord is still defined by other authors as "...a condition in which the conus medullaris ends at a level below the L1–2 intervertebral space" [67].

It has been indicated that TCS may rather be a functional disorder of the lumbosacral spinal cord, and the only morphological abnormality at the macro level is a firm attachment of the spinal cord to the spinal canal. Otherwise, gross anatomical information is not adequate to diagnose the disorder. In a significant number of patients who present with the typical clinical picture of TCS, the diameter of the filum terminale is found to be within normal limits and the caudal end of the spinal cord is located in the normal position [79]. The combination of an elongated cord and a thick filum terminale, demonstrated by magnetic resonance imaging (MRI) or at operation, is not an essential feature for the diagnosis of TCS [80].

Excessive tension in the lumbosacral cord appears to be the most crucial factor in the pathogenesis of the disorder. Tension in the lower cord is related to impairment of oxidative metabolism in this region [78].

Posterior displacement of the conus and filum on MRI, lack of viscoelasticity by the stretch test of the filum during surgery, and fibrous displacement of glial tissue within the filum by histological studies, according to Yamada et al. (2004) would be the prevailing criteria to establish the diagnosis [79]. This would mean, however, that the exact diagnosis is only established after surgery. However, the same author has suggested that for TCS diagnosis, emphasis should rather be on its characteristic clinical picture [80].

For this review, we may therefore elaborate on a definition of TCS given by Yamada et al. as early as 1981 [84]. Keeping in mind that spinal cord adhesion is the basic relevant pathogenetic factor, TCS is a clinical entity that is manifested by back and leg pain, progressive motor and sensory changes in the legs, urinary and sphincter control deficiencies, and spinal deformities like kyphoscoliosis. Research has added that it represents a functional disorder caused by lumbosacral neuronal dysfunction due to traction and tension in the lower spinal cord [32, 79].

This overview focuses on TCS without dysraphism. Clinical signs in this group of patients may develop later in childhood or even in adulthood. The symptoms and findings are often distinct and point to the diagnosis [59]. The tight filum terminale is one major pathogenetic factor in this group of patients.

On imaging, posterior displacement of the conus and filum that attach the posterior arachnoid membrane are often the only radiological criteria [83]. This type of primary TCS may be considered a role model for the pathophysiology of the disorder, and release of the filum is less controversial than in other forms of occult spinal dysraphism or tethering due to tumors. Secondary causes such as arachnoiditis, trauma, and retethering after previous operations will not be discussed here, although they often also deserve the attention of the neurosurgeon.

## 24.3
## Epidemiology and Prevalence

Data regarding the prevalence of primary TCS are rare. A recent survey in 5499 Turkish primary school children including all primary causes ranging from tight filum terminale over myelomeningocele to intraspinal tumors, suggested a prevalence of 0.1% overall and of 1.4% in 422 enuretic children [2]. Although the first symptoms usu-

ally occur between the ages of 5 and 15 years, adult onset of the syndrome is well documented in the literature [1, 16, 20, 33, 34, 40, 42, 44, 49, 57, 83].

Associated developmental disorders, such as cavovarous foot, length differences between the lower limbs, scoliosis, and cutaneous alteration in the lumbar and sacral regions (lipomas, hypertrichosis, hemangiomas, and dimples), may occur with varying frequencies [52, 59].

## 24.4
## Etiology

### 24.4.1
### Normal Anatomy of the Filum and the Conus

The filum terminale is a fibrovascular band that is composed mainly of 5- to 20-μm-thick longitudinal bundles of type 1 collagen separated by 3- to 10-μm intervals. A delicate (0.05–1.5 μm) meshwork of predominantly type 3 collagen transverse fibers connects these bundles. Abundant longitudinally oriented elastic and elaunin fibers are found inside collagen bundles, which along with vascular structures add up to a complex three-dimensional structure [12].

It is commonly believed that in healthy humans, the filum fuses with the dura of the lower spinal canal at the level of the second sacral segment. While this is true in the majority, there is a wide range of fusion sites. In a more recent study by Hansasuta et al. (1999), the fusion was found to be located from L5 to S3 [24]. Moreover, the dural sac itself mostly ends at S2, with a range from S1 to S3. Interestingly, in 4 of 27 cases, the fila fused above the S1 level, and off-the-midline fusion was found in 3 cases. At birth, the conus medullare rests at L2/3 and, because of the growth of the spine relative to the spinal cord within the first 2 months, it comes to rest at its adult location of L1/L2 [59].

Yundt et al. (1997) measured the diameters of the filum terminale in vivo in the operating room on 31 children aged between 2 and 14 years who underwent selective dorsal rhizotomy for spastic cerebral palsy. None of the children had clinical evidence of TCS. The authors found the diameter of the filum at 10 and 15 mm caudal to the conus to be around 1.2 mm, with a standard deviation of little over 0.2 mm [85].

In another study with fresh adult cadavers, the mean diameter at the origin of the filum was slightly greater (1.38 mm), and more variable, with a range of 0.4–2.5 mm [56]. With a filum thickness of more than 2 mm and with two fila originating below the L2 level, 6 of 41 cadavers fulfilled one of the original anatomic diagnostic criteria for TCS, although there was no medical history of the respective symptoms.

In 104 TCS patients without spinal dysraphism, Yamada et al. (2004) found the conus at the L2–3 intervertebral space or above in 37, and below the L2–3 level in 67 patients. The diameter of the filum was <2 mm in 60, and ≥2 mm in 44 patients [83]. The authors concluded that combination of an elongated cord and a thick filum terminale, demonstrated by MRI or at operation, is no longer an essential feature for the diagnosis of TCS [82].

## 24.4.2
## Pathophysiology

Genetically, TCS has recently been linked to modifications on chromosomes 21 and 22 [48]. The embryopathy underlying tethering of the filum terminale is not yet satisfactorily understood. George et al. (2003) have immunostained 34 fila from patients with TCS [17]. The caudal neural tube developmental markers H4C4 (CD44) and NOT1 exhibited significant alterations in tethered fila compared to controls. The authors suggested that the change in expression of these markers may be indicative of altered cell identity in the filum and constitute the predisposition to tethering [17].

Embryologically, the disorder is apparently different from overt myelomeningocele and associated Arnold-Chiari type II malformation. Clinically, however, the association of TCS with spinal dysraphic disorders is so striking and obvious [3, 21, 26, 40, 47, 52, 59, 86] that a clear separation into different entities has not yet become well established. It has been postulated that primary TCS is a manifestation of local dysmorphogenesis of all three germ layers at the lumbosacral area, possibly triggered by a hemorrhagic, inflammatory, or some other local lesion occurring in embryogenesis [64].

TCS has also frequently been diagnosed in association with spinal tumors, especially with lipomas [7, 8, 20, 49, 59]. Oi et al. (1990) reported that the presence of lipomyelocele may delay development of neurological deficits [47].

The basic mechanical cause of primary TCS without spinal dysraphism is clearly to be found in an anchoring of the caudal end of the spinal cord by an altered, less elastic filum terminale. Selcuki et al. (2003) on histology found that "more connective tissue with dense collagen fibers, some hyalinization and dilated capillaries" were present in the fila from a group of patients presenting with clinical symptoms of TCS and normal MRI appearance of the fila. They suggested that this may reflect a decreased elasticity within the filum terminale [67].

When the spinal column grows after birth, it usually does so faster than the spinal cord, which is fastened to the base of the brain, the dentate ligaments, and the nerve roots along its course. Stretching of the spinal cord can also occur with flexion and extension movement. During surgery, a rostral-to-caudal decrease in diameter, pallor, and absence of pulsation of the spinal cords all indicate traction [59]. Upon release, there is noticeable retraction of the cone in the rostral direction, and the formerly lin-early oriented and small blood vessels become undulating and widen. Both the lumbosacral spinal cord and the cauda equina fibers have been shown to be most susceptible to stretch and elongation, which may initiate metabolic, vascular, and conduction changes [6]. The tethering effect of the tight filum terminale is transmitted to the spinal cord up to the level of D12. Above this level, the dentate ligaments mostly prevent further propagation of the tethering effect. Consequently, the tethering force is exerted mainly on the conus medullare [49, 63].

Constant or intermittent stretching induces traction and tension in the cord, giving rise to functional changes that in turn are responsible for the development of symptoms. Electrophysiological activity is depressed [13] and shifts in metabolism such as those indicated by an altered reduction/oxidation ratio of cytochrome oxidase in the mitochondria of the lower cord ensue [78, 84]. The latter suggests that there is impairment of oxidative metabolism, and other experimentors have confirmed this view [69]. These putative functional changes in TCS occur mainly within the lumbosacral portion of the spinal cord [82]. It is not yet clear to what extent they are a direct consequence of micromechanical injury to neurovascular structures or secondary to ischemia due to decreased blood supply. With the application of laser Doppler flowmetry before and after surgical release it was shown, however, that there is a threefold increase in blood flow 2–3 cm rostral to the site of tethering [65]. Prolonged or accentuated neuronal dysfunction may lead to structural damage to the neuronal perikarya, and later, of the axons [84]. In animal experimentation, axonal transport of cholinergic enzymes has been shown to be compromised in spinal cord ischemia [41]. Kocak et al. (1997) found hypoxanthine and lipid peroxidation levels to be significantly elevated in a guinea pig model of TCS [35], consistent with the picture in ischemic injury. Subsequently, the latencies of the somatosensory (SSEP) and motor evoked potentials (MEPs) significantly increased, and the amplitudes decreased, indicating a defective conduction in the motor and sensory nerve fibers. Aside from reversible changes like edema, the group also reported irreversible changes like scarcity of neurofilaments and destruction in axons, and damage in myelin sheaths [35].

Thus, it appears that the pathophysiological mechanisms that give rise to the clinical findings in TCS are both axonal and neuronal, both elements being adversely affected by traction and ischemia.

## 24.5
## Clinical Findings

TCS is diagnosed primarily on the basis of its characteristic symptomatology, accentuated by postural changes, since it is a functional disorder of the lumbosacral spinal cord [80]. The most common presenting symptoms of primary TCS are lumbar pain radiating to the lower limbs and lower limb palsy. Patients may also exhibit urinary, anal sphincter control deficiencies, and kyphoscoliosis due to imbalance of the muscles innervated by the deficient cauda [52, 53, 81].

The appearance and progression of these symptoms are highly variable and may depend upon age, growth, physical activity, and overlap with changes caused by associated lesions. While changes like neurogenic bladder facilitate early recognition, preexisting neurological deficits, slow development, and acceptance of minor deficiencies may mask the disease [59].

Skeletal abnormalities like foot or leg length discrepancies, pes cavus, and varus or valgus deformities are always suspicious of TCS [45], as are cutaneous abnormalities often pointing to the diagnosis of occult dysraphism [20, 22, 34, 76, 77]. Syringomyelia may be associated or even caused by TCS, and the symptoms can overlap with those of primary TCS [11]. In children, recurrent meningitis of unknown cause as well as recurrent urinary tract infection should raise prompt further clinical investigation.

Late presentation of TCS has been suggested to be related to the degree of tethering and the cumulative effect of repeated microtrauma during flexion and extension [20]. In order to establish an early diagnosis, patients with persistent back or leg pain, neurological deficits, or skeletal deformities should be investigated with MRI.

TCS can have far reaching consequences for the patient, potentially causing major disability if it is not diagnosed and treated properly [9]. Even the growth rate of children harboring the disorder may be decreased [62]. For early diagnosis, it is important to notice minor changes. Back pain, enuresis, stress incontinence, and delayed toilet training in children should not be taken casually by the observer. Lower-extremity fatigue requiring frequent rest periods, unsteady gait, and postural changes may be important signs in the early phase of spinal cord tethering. This constellation of symptoms, possibly combined with skeletal abnormality, is not confined to childhood and adolescence [30, 47, 49]. In adults, however, onset of clinical symptoms is often precipitated by traumatic events, presumably causing stretch to the conus and the cauda, and clinical changes usually begin more suddenly.

## 24.6
## Imaging and Other Diagnostic Techniques

MRI is generally the method of choice for investigating primary TCS without spinal dysraphism [1, 7, 23, 47, 52, 59]. Radiological criteria for an abnormal filum terminale in the past include a caliber of more than 2 mm, the conus situated below the L2 vertebral level, and presence of fatty tissue at the level of conus medullaris [43]. These criteria have been rightfully been challenged on the basis of evidence that a significant proportion of TCS patients do not show these features on imaging, as discussed earlier. What can be seen on imaging, however, is poste-

rior displacement of the conus and filum with attachment on the dura of the lower spinal canal [83]. Although in general the filum may be surgically sectioned at any level over its entire length, identification and distinction of the structure from the nerve roots of the cauda equina under the surgical microscope may not always be trivial. Thus, precise information on the site of the tether is desirable in the planning of a neurosurgical intervention. On T2-weighted images, nerve roots are as well visualized as the filum terminale, and it is often hard to tell them apart, even on axial images. Constructive interference of steady-state sequences (CISS) may overcome this dilemma by suppressing the root signal, such that the filum terminale can then be clearly visualized in its entire length (Fig. 1) [61].

The cause of this effect is not yet clearly known. A reduced partial volume effect of the thinner slices in CISS images would seem unlikely, because often there is no significant difference in the diameter of the filum and the surrounding nerve roots. It is possible that the distinction may be caused by the motion of nerve roots as opposed to the relative stillness of the filum.

Scoliosis may present another problem, especially in adults, because it is difficult to capture the entire width of the spinal canal in sagittal images [59]. Plain radiographs and computed tomography should always complement MRI in suspected spinal dysraphism [49, 52, 59, 81]. Apart from signs of spina bifida, kyphosis and scoliosis, vertebral body fusion, fused lamina, increased interpeduncular distance, prominent or absent spinous processes, and midline hypercalcifications may be detected [59].

It has also been hypothesized that a horizontally angulated sacrum may predate the clinically appreciable symptoms of a tethered spinal cord after myelomeningocoele repair [71]. Ultrasonography can be effective in screening for spinal cord location and tethering as well as for associated meningocele, diastematomyelia, teratoma, and lipoma [58].

SSEPs to tibial and peroneal nerve stimulation are valuable in correlation with static neurological deficit, in demonstrating deterioration on serial investigations before a permanent neurological deficit occurs, and during surgery for monitoring purposes [5, 12, 14, 16, 27, 35, 37, 38, 50, 51, 54, 63, 73, 78, 82, 84].

Since a fixed deficit in bladder function is irreversible by surgical untethering in most cases, early recognition of TCS assumes greater importance. This may be accomplished by urocystometry and pelvic electromyography (EMG) [31].

## 24.7
## Indications for and Timing of Surgery

In a recent series of 60 children aged 3–18 years who met typical clinical criteria for TCS, Webby et al. (2004) retrospectively analyzed the outcome over a mean fol-

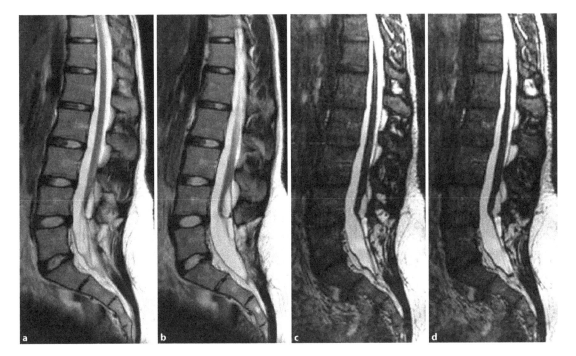

Fig. 1 **a,b** Sagittal magnetic resonance imaging scan of a patient with tethered cord syndrome. An associated lipoma in the lumbar spine had been operated on several years ago. While the nerve roots of the cauda equina and the lipoma give a clear signal in T2-weighted images, the filum and exact site of tethering cannot be identified unequivocally. **c,d** Sagittal constructive interference of steady-state sequences of the lumbar spine of the same patient. The nerve root signal is almost completely suppressed in the median sections of the spinal canal, and the filum terminale is easily recognized

low-up period of 13.9 months after sectioning of a tight filum terminale [77]. All patients in this series had their conus in a normal position on MRI. After surgery, urinary deficiency completely resolved in 52% and markedly improved in 35%. Fecal incontinence resolved in 56% and improved in 41%. Weakness, sensory abnormalities, and pain improved or resolved in all patients. Surgery was indicated only when there were signs of spina bifida occulta, progressive neurogenic bladder instability unresponsive to conservative measures, and two or more of the following: fecal incontinence or chronic constipation, lower-extremity weakness, gait changes, reflex/tone abnormalities, sensory disturbances, back/leg pain, limb length discrepancy, scoliosis/lordosis, recurrent urinary tract infections, abnormal voiding cystourethrogram/ultrasound, syringomyelia, or neurocutaneous stigmata.

This comprehensive list illustrates the complex clinical workup involved in decision making for the surgical indication in TCS patients. The study also demonstrates that significant improvement of neurogenic bladder disturbances may be achieved even in patients in whom the disorder has already caused some urinary deficiency as long as primary symptoms are not ignored or accepted and a diagnosis of TCS is established early by employing the whole range of diagnostic criteria.

When surgery is delayed over a longer period in established disease, results are not as favorable [34, 46, 47, 53, 55, 59, 80]. Since the disease leads to progressive neurological deterioration in most patients with neuroradiologically proven TCS, including a low conus and spina bifida occulta, prophylactic surgery has been suggested and performed in children and adults with good results for several years follow up in asymptomatic patients [60, 72].

Previous surgery (e.g., for myelomeningocele or spinal tumors) does not appear to compromise the results of surgical untethering [33] and therefore should not be a criterion to delay an operation in clinically progressive disease with clear radiological signs of TCS.

Having observed histological changes that reflect decreased elasticity of the filum terminale in urinary incontinent patients with normal results in radiological studies, Selcuki et al. (2003) even suggested sectioning of the filum terminale in all of these patients [67].

While there is no consensus about the timing of surgery in primary TCS today, there is clearly a tendency toward early operation in established disease, especially when there are progressive clinical signs. Conservative wait-and-see management in patients with a clinical manifestation possibly related to primary tethering of the spinal cord and no radiological markers would at least necessitate a search for associated anomalies [46], urodynamic investigation, and close follow up. On the other hand, asymptomatic patients with clear radiological signs of TCS may not become symptomatic for years [10, 28], but should be referred to surgery on appearance of the first symptoms [46, 60].

## 24.8
## Operative Technique and Intraoperative Monitoring

Adherence to some general neurosurgical principles will help to improve operative results. With the patient in prone position, special efforts to ensure that the abdomen is free of pressure should be undertaken in order to reduce abdominal venous pressure and prevent unnecessary blood loss. In the presence of spinal curvature, this may be difficult. A midline incision will usually be carried out, which avoids additional cutaneous manifestations and follows scoliotic deformities. In the presence of associated malformations and in recurrent surgery, as a rule the surgeon will work from normal to abnormal anatomy.

In primary TCS without associated lesions, hemilaminectomy will be sufficient to approach and transect the filum. Laminectomy and laminotomy will be necessary in cases of additional tumors or myelomeningocele; the latter should be carefully considered in the presence multiple arch defects [34, 52, 59].

If primary dural closure cannot be achieved due to a small dural sac or a large surface after tumor resection that would promote retether, dural plasty with either thoracolumbar fascia or artificial material will be required [59]. This may be combined with retention sutures, which may help to maintain a relatively normal position of the spinal cord within the thecal sac, thus decreasing the potential adherence of the dorsally scarred aspect of the dysmorphic cord to an overlying graft [70].

Intraoperative monitoring with anal sphincter EMG has long been introduced in surgery for TCS [27]. A more elaborate setup with continuous EMG recording of leg muscles, continuous recording of tibial nerve SSEPs, recording of MEPs evoked by transcranial electrical stimulation, and recording of compound muscle action potentials or SSEPs from the scalp upon electrical stimulation of the nerve roots (mapping) provides the surgeon with functional information about the state of the motor and sensory pathways and enables the anatomical identification of nerve roots and their distinction from fibrous or neoplastic structures [37, 38, 51, 54].

Because electrical stimulation of the filum will also lead to motor activation due to activation of neighboring nerve roots, and because there is considerable interpatient variability in the electrical thresholds of nerve fibers, von Koch et al. (2002) have proposed a ratio, rather than an absolute number, for establishing the electrical criteria for the distinction of the filum and the roots [73]. In over 70% of their 63 patients, muscle activation via the filum required 100 times the voltage needed to activate a motor root.

## 24.9
## Results and Outcome

Because of the progressive clinical course of the disorder and the good results of untethering, there is general agreement that surgery is the method of choice for the treatment of primary TCS. The condition is easily dealt with surgically, with little risk of additional injury. It is also universally accepted that the likelihood of some improvement in neurologic function and the elimination of pain is high [1, 3, 19, 20, 26, 34, 36, 40, 42, 46, 52, 57, 59, 66, 68, 73, 81]. There are, however, differences in outcome with respect to the extent of tethering and displacement of the conus, the presence of additional lesions like myelomeningocele and tumors, and the age of the patient at onset of symptoms.

Neurogenic bladder may not improve after surgery at all [36, 46], or only in a small percentage of patients [4, 20, 60, 73], most probably depending on the duration and severity of the disease. The main urologic improvement seen is in bladder capacity [18], probably related to normalization of neurogenic detrusor overactivity [19]. Complete restoration of urinary function to a normal level was reported in all patients in a series of infants up to 3 years of age when surgery is performed shortly after occurrence of the first clinical signs, while untethering in children presenting at birth with upper motor neuron symptoms may result in poorer outcome [10]. Johnson and Levy (1995) suggested that children with markedly decreased cord motion on phase MRI would not improve after surgery [28].

In adult patients with primary TCS, neurologic findings and urinary deficits show a favorable long-term surgical outcome after tethered cord release, as most patients report improvement or stabilization of their symptoms. In addition, the overall postoperative complication rate is low [40]. A short duration from onset of symptoms to surgery is also associated with a good prognosis [25].

Albeit rare, possible complications of surgical untethering include: deterioration of motor function [66], postoperative urinary tract infections [73], deterioration of preoperative normal bladder function [18, 19], erectile dysfunction [4], incomplete untethering [33], and cerebrospinal fluid leak [68]. Retethering may also occur [33, 39, 66], and can usually be released surgically with good results.

## 24.10
## Concluding Remarks

In the literature, the term primary TCS apparently stand for at least three different entities – tight filum terminale with and without low conus medullare, as well as TCS associated with myelomeningocele and tumors. These entities are diagnosed at various different stages. It is this variety that mainly accounts for the different outcome reports and the ambiguity with respect to the indication for surgery. Nevertheless, there is common ground: neurological deterioration in a majority of patients with untreated primary TCS is natural and obvious. It is thus important that the diagnosis is established as early as possible. Surgical untethering ultimately remains the method of choice and should be offered to all patients who experience worsening of their condition. In some with clear evidence of TCS, even prophylactic surgery may be indicated.

### References

1. Akay KM, Ersahin Y, Cakir Y (2000) Tethered cord syndrome in adults. Acta Neurochir (Wien) 142:1111–1115
2. Bademci G, Saygun M, Batay F, et al (2006) Prevalence of primary tethered cord syndrome associated with occult spinal dysraphism in primary school children in Turkey. Pediatr Neurosurg 42:4–13
3. Begeer JH, Wiertsema GP, Breukers SM, et al (1989) Tethered cord syndrome: clinical signs and results of operation in 42 patients with spina bifida aperta and occulta. Z Kinderchir 44:5–7
4. Boemers TM, van Gool JD, de Jong TP (1995) Tethered spinal cord: the effect of neurosurgery on the lower urinary tract and male sexual function. Br J Urol 76:747–751
5. Boor R, Schwarz M, Reitter B, Voth D (1993) Tethered cord after spina bifida aperta: a longitudinal study of somatosensory evoked potentials. Childs Nerv Syst 9:328–330
6. Breig A (1970) Overstretching of and circumscribed pathological tension in the spinal cord: a basic cause of symptoms in cord disorders. J Biomechanics 3:7–13
7. Brophy JD, Sutton LN, Zimmerman RA, et al (1989) Magnetic resonance imaging of lipomyelomeningocele and tethered cord. Neurosurgery 25:336–340
8. Byrne RW, Hayes EA, George TM, McLone DG (1995) Operative resection of 100 spinal lipomas in infants less than 1 year of age. Pediatr Neurosurg 23:182–186
9. Cartwright C (2000) Primary tethered cord syndrome: diagnosis and treatment of an insidious defect. J Neurosci Nurs 32:210–215
10. Cornette L, Verpoorten C, Lagae L, et al (1998) Tethered cord syndrome in occult spinal dysraphism: timing and outcome of surgical release. Neurology 50:1761–1765
11. Erkan K, Unal F, Kiris T (1999) Terminal syringomyelia in association with the tethered cord syndrome. Neurosurgery 45:1351–1359
12. Fontes RB, Saad F, Soares MS, et al (2006) Ultrastructural study of the filum terminale and its elastic fibers. Neurosurgery 58:978–984
13. Fujita Y, Yamamoto H (1989) An experimental study on spinal cord traction effect. Spine 14:698–705
14. Fukui J, Kakizaki T (1980) Urodynamic evaluation of tethered cord syndrome including tight filum terminale: prolonged follow-up observation after intraspinal operation. Urology 16:539–552
15. Garceau GJ (1953) The filum terminal syndrome. J Bone Joint Surg Am 35:711–716
16. George TM, Fagan LH (2005) Adult tethered cord syndrome in patients with postrepair myelomeningocele: an evidence-based outcome study. J Neurosurg 102:150–156
17. George TM, Bulsara KR, Cummings TJ (2003) The immunohistochemical profile of the tethered filum terminale. Pediatr Neurosurg 39:227–233
18. Gross AJ, Michael T, Godeman F, et al (1993) Urological findings in patients with neurosurgically treated tethered spinal cord. J Urol 149:1510–1511
19. Guerra LA, Pike J, Milks J, et al (2006) Outcome in patients who underwent tethered cord release for occult spinal dysraphism. J Urol 176:1729–1732
20. Gupta SK, Khosla VK, Sharma BS, et al (1999) Tethered cord syndrome in adults. Surg Neurol 52:362–369
21. Guthkelch AN, Hoffmann GT (1981) Tethered spinal cord in association with diastematomyelia. Surg Neurol 15:352–354
22. Guyotat J, Bret P, Jouanneau E, et al (1998) Tethered cord syndrome in adults. Neurochirurgie 44:75–82
23. Hall WA, Albright AL, Brunberg JA (1988) Diagnosis of tethered cords by magnetic resonance imaging. Surg Neurol 30:60–64
24. Hansasuta A, Tubbs RS, Oakes WJ (1999) Filum terminale fusion and dural sac termination: study in 27 cadavers. Pediatr Neurosurg 30:176–179
25. Haro H, Komori H, Okawa A, et al (2004) Long-term outcomes of surgical treatment for tethered cord syndrome. J Spinal Disord Tech 17:16–20
26. Hoffman HJ, Hendrick EB, Humphreys RP (1976) The tethered spinal cord: its protean manifestations, diagnosis and surgical correction. Childs Brain 2:145–155
27. James HE, Mulcahy JJ, Walsh JW, et al (1979) Use of anal sphincter electromyography during operations on the conus medullaris and sacral nerve roots. Neurosurgery 4:521–523
28. Johnson DL, Levy LM (1995) Predicting outcome in the tethered cord syndrome: a study of cord motion. Pediatr Neurosurg 22:115–119

29. Jones J (1891) "Spina bifida occulta: no paralytic symptoms until seventeen years of age; spine trephined to relieve pressure on the cauda equina; recovery." Reports on the medical and surgical practice in the hospitals and asylums of Great Britain, Ireland and the Colonies. Br Med J 1:173–174

30. Kaplan JO, Quencer RM (1980) The occult tethered conus syndrome in the adult. Radiology 137:387–391

31. Khoury AE, Hendrick EB, McLorie GA, et al (1990) Occult spinal dysraphism: clinical and urodynamic outcome after division of the filum terminale. J Urol 144:426–428

32. Kiechl S, Kronenberg MF, Marosi M, et al (1996) Tethered cord syndrome as cause of spinal cord dysfunction. Lancet 348:342–343

33. Kirollos RW, Van Hille PT (1996) Evaluation of surgery for the tethered cord syndrome using a new grading system. Br J Neurosurg 10:253–260

34. Klekamp J, Raimondi AJ, Samii M (1994) Occult dysraphism in adulthood: clinical course and management. Childs Nerv Syst 10:312–320

35. Kocak A, Kilic A, Nurlu G, et al (1997) A new model for tethered cord syndrome: a biochemical, electrophysiological, and electron microscopic study. Pediatr Neurosurg 26:120–126

36. Kondo A, Kato K, Kanai S, et al (1986) Bladder dysfunction secondary to tethered cord syndrome in adults: is it curable? J Urol 135:313–316

37. Kothbauer K, Schmid UD, Seiler RW, et al (1994) Intraoperative motor and sensory monitoring of the cauda equina. Neurosurgery 34:702–707

38. Kothbauer KF, Novak K (2004) Intraoperative monitoring for tethered cord surgery: an update. Neurosurg Focus 16:E8

39. Lagae L, Verpoorten C, Casaer P, et al (1990) Conservative versus neurosurgical treatment of tethered cord patients. Z Kinderchir 45:16–17

40. Lapsiwala SB, Iskandar BJ (2004) The tethered cord syndrome in adults with spina bifida occulta. Neurol Res 26:735–740

41. Malatova Z, Chavko M, Marsala J (1989) Effect of spinal cord ischemia on axonal transport of cholinergic enzymes in rabbit sciatic nerve. Brain Res 481:31–42

42. Maroun FB, Jacob JC, Murray GP (2000) Tethered cord syndrome in adults. Surg Neurol 54:403

43. McLendon RE, Oakes WJ, Heinz ER, et al (1988) Adipose tissue in the filum terminale: a computed tomographic finding that may indicate tethering of the spinal cord. Neurosurgery 22:873–876

44. McLone DG (1996) The adult with a tethered cord. Clin Neurosurg 43:203–209

45. Michelson DJ, Ashwal S (2004) Tethered cord syndrome in childhood: diagnostic features and relationship to congenital anomalies. Neurol Res 26:745–753

46. Oakes WJ (1996) The borderlands of the primary tethered cord syndrome. Clin Neurosurg 43:188–202

47. Oi S, Yamada H, Matsumoto S (1990) Tethered cord syndrome versus low-placed conus medullaris in an over-distended spinal cord following initial repair for myelodysplasia. Childs Nerv Syst 6:264–269

48. Opitz JM (2005) Genetics of tethered cord "syndrome": The FG syndrome. Am J Med Genet A 132:454–455

49. Pang D, Wilberger JE Jr (1982) Tethered cord syndrome in adults. J Neurosurg 57:32–47

50. Paradiso G, Lee GY, Sarjeant R, et al (2005) Multi-modality neurophysiological monitoring during surgery for adult tethered cord syndrome. J Clin Neurosci 12:934–936

51. Paradiso G, Lee GY, Sarjeant R, et al (2006) Multimodality intraoperative neurophysiologic monitoring findings during surgery for adult tethered cord syndrome: analysis of a series of 44 patients with long-term follow-up. Spine 31:2095–2102

52. Park TS, Kanev PM, Henegar MM, et al (1995) Occult spinal dysraphism. In: Youmans JA (ed) Neurological Surgery, 4th edn. Saunders, Philadelphia, pp 873–898

53. Patterson P (1989) The tethered spinal cord: an overview. Axone 11:38–40

54. Phillips LH, Jane JA (1996) Electrophysiologic monitoring during tethered spinal cord release. Clin Neurosurg 43:163–174

55. Phuong LK, Schoeberl KA, Raffel C (2002) Natural history of tethered cord in patients with meningomyelocele. Neurosurgery 50:989–993

56. Pinto FC, Fontes RB, Leonhardt M de C, et al (2002) Anatomic study of the filum terminale and its correlations with the tethered cord syndrome. Neurosurgery 51:725–729

57. Rafael H (1999) Tethered cord. J Neurosurg 90:175

58. Raghavendra BN, Epstein FJ, Pinto RS, et al (1983) The tethered spinal cord: diagnosis by high-resolution real-time ultrasound. Radiology 149:123–128

59. Reigel DH, McLone DG (1994) Tethered spinal cord. In: Cheek WR (ed) Pediatric Neurosurgery: Surgery of the Developing Nervous System. Saunders, Philadelphia, pp 77–95

60. Rinaldi F, Cioffi FA, Columbano L, et al (2005) Tethered cord syndrome. J Neurosurg Sci 49:131–135

61. Rosahl SK, Kassem O, Piepgras U, et al (2005) High-resolution constructive interference in steady-state imaging in tethered cord syndrome: technical note. Surg Neurol 63:372–374

62. Rotenstein D, Reigel DH, Lucke J (1996) Growth of growth hormone-treated and nontreated children before and after tethered spinal cord release. Pediatr Neurosurg 24:237–241

63. Sarwar M, Crelin ES, Kier EL, et al (1983) Experimental cord stretchability and the tethered cord syndrome. AJNR Am J Neuroradiol 4:641–643

64. Sarwar M, Virapongse C, Bhimani S (1984) Primary tethered cord syndrome: a new hypothesis of its origin. AJNR Am J Neuroradiol 5:235–242

65. Schneider S, Rosenthal A, Greenberg B, et al (1993) A preliminary report on the use of laser Doppler flowmetry during tethered spinal cord release. Neurosurgery 32:214–218

66. Schoenmakers MA, Gooskens RH, Gulmans VA, et al (2003) Long-term outcome of neurosurgical untethering on neurosegmental motor and ambulation levels. Dev Med Child Neurol 45:551–555

67. Selcuki M, Vatansever S, Inan S, et al (2003) Is a filum terminale with a normal appearance really normal? Childs Nerv Syst 19:3–10

68. Sharif S, Allcutt D, Marks C, et al (1997) "Tethered cord syndrome" – recent clinical experience. Br J Neurosurg 11:49–51

69. Tani S, Yamada S, Knighton RS (1987) Extensibility of the lumbar and sacral cord. Pathophysiology of the tethered spinal cord in cats. J Neurosurg 66:116–123

70. Tubbs RS, Oakes WJ (2006) A simple method to deter re-tethering in patients with spinal dysraphism. Childs Nerv Syst 22:715–716

71. Tubbs RS, Wellons JC III, Bartolucci AA, et al (2002) Horizontal sacrum as an indicator of a tethered spinal cord. Pediatr Neurosurg 36:209–213

72. van der Meulen WD, Hoving EW, Staal-Schreinemacher A, et al (2002) Analysis of different treatment modalities of tethered cord syndrome. Childs Nerv Syst 18:513–517

73. von Koch CS, Quinones-Hinojosa A, Gulati M, et al (2002) Clinical outcome in children undergoing tethered cord release utilizing intraoperative neurophysiological monitoring. Pediatr Neurosurg 37:81–86

74. Warder DE (2001) Tethered cord syndrome and occult spinal dysraphism. Neurosurg Focus 10:E1

75. Warder DE, Oakes WJ (1993) Tethered cord syndrome and the conus in a normal position. Neurosurgery 33:374–378

76. Warder DE, Oakes WJ (1994) Tethered cord syndrome: the low-lying and normally positioned conus. Neurosurgery 34:597–600

77. Wehby MC, O'Hollaren PS, Abtin K, et al (2004) Occult tight filum terminale syndrome: results of surgical untethering. Pediatr Neurosurg 40:51–57

78. Yamada S, Iacono RP, Andrade T, et al (1995) Pathophysiology of tethered cord syndrome. Neurosurg Clin N Am 6:311–323

79. Yamada S, Knerium DS, Mandybur GM, et al (2004) Pathophysiology of tethered cord syndrome and other complex factors. Neurol Res 26:722–726

80. Yamada S, Siddiqi J, Won DJ, et al (2004) Symptomatic protocols for adult tethered cord syndrome. Neurol Res 26:741–744

81. Yamada S, Won DJ, Siddiqi J, et al (2004) Tethered cord syndrome: overview of diagnosis and treatment. Neurol Res 26:719–721

82. Yamada S, Won DJ, Yamada SM (2004) Pathophysiology of tethered cord syndrome: correlation with symptomatology. Neurosurg Focus 16:E6

83. Yamada S, Won DJ, Yamada SM, et al (2004) Adult tethered cord syndrome: relative to spinal cord length and filum thickness. Neurol Res 26:732–734

84. Yamada S, Zinke DE, Sanders D (1981) Pathophysiology of "tethered cord syndrome". J Neurosurg 54:494–503

85. Yundt KD, Park TS, Kaufman BA (1997) Normal diameter of filum terminale in children: in vivo measurement. Pediatr Neurosurg 27:257–259

86. Zerche A, Krüger J, Gottschalk E (1997) Tethered cord syndrome after spina bifida: own experiences. Eur J Pediatr Surg 7:54–55

# Dysfunctional Segmental Motion and Discogenic Lumbar Pain. From Fusion to Disc Replacement

**25**

Fernando Schmidt and Robert Schönmayr

## Contents

## 25.1
## Introduction

The most frequent clinical problem of the adult spine is back pain. It is known that 60–80% of people at some time in their lives will have back pain that may affect their general health, activities of daily life, and their working capacity. It is one of the main causes for patients to miss work. There is also a dramatic rise in social benefits for back pain and it is known that 80–90% of healthcare costs associated with back pain are spent by 10% of patients with chronic low back pain (LBP) [26]. LBP is a multifactorial disease with organic, mechanical, and psychosocial aspects. It is assumed that the back pain in only 15% of patients has a defined pathology [27], and among them, dysfunctional segmental motion and discogenic pain are problems that may need to be treated surgically.

According to Professor Edward C. Benzel, there are four categories of instability in the spine: overt acute instability, limited acute instability, glacial instability, and dysfunctional segmental motion-associated instability [3]. The latter describes chronic instability related to the disc or vertebral body degenerative changes associated with abnormal motion that result in the potential for pain. This type of instability has also been called mechanical instability. The patients report characteristic pain usually worsened by activity and improved by rest.

On the other hand, we may have patients with nonmechanical discogenic back pain, probably reflecting the earliest stage of disc degeneration in which obvious mechanical dysfunction of the disc or facets has not yet developed.

The basic structure of a spine functional segment is an anterior column, mechanically supported by a hydraulic cushion and posterior secondary joints, resulting in a strong load-bearing and flexible structure.

The prevalent surgical treatment for chronic LBP is discectomy and fusion, performed with the aim of reducing pain and eliminating neural compression, but not to restore disc or segmental function. Swedish authors have demonstrated the benefits of fusion over nonsurgical treatment in the alleviation of chronic LBP [14]. Studies have shown improvements in the instrumentation techniques, increasing the radiological fusion rate above 94%, but have failed to provide evidence of actual improvements in clinical outcome [21]. Based on retrospective clinical studies, accelerated degeneration of the adjacent motion segment following fusion has come into focus [11]. The quest for a more physiologic surgical solution than fusion has thus initiated the so-called nonfusion technologies. The modern history of disc replacement began in the early 1960s, when Fernström first implanted stainless steel spheres [13]. This history continued with the AcroFlex artificial disc [12] and was followed by the Charité artificial disc [8]. In the meantime, more alternatives have appeared for the treatment of degenerative back pain. These are: disc nucleus replacement, posterior dynamic stabilization systems, interspinous devices, and facet joint arthroplasty.

In this chapter we will provide a brief revision of the anatomy and pathophysiology of lumbar degenerative discs disease, the available surgical treatments, and their development during the last decade.

## 25.2
## Functional Anatomy of the Lumbar Spine

The lumbar spine has a lordotic curve, consists of five vertebrae (L1–L5), and has five intervertebral discs. The vertebral body is a roughly cylindrical mass of cancellous bone enclosed in a cortical shell and has upper and lower endplates. The endplates support the nucleus pulposus and provide points of attachment for the annulus fibrosis. Arising from the posterolateral surfaces of the vertebral bodies there are the pedicles. The lamina, arising from the medial aspect of the posterior extremity of the pedicles, forms the roof of the spinal canal. The laminae unite in the midline, and at this point form the spinous process. The transverse processes project laterally and arise from the lateral surfaces of the pedicle. Situated between each of the vertebral bodies, anteriorly in the spine, are the intervertebral discs, and posteriorly, two typical diarthrodial joints, known as the facets joints.

The discs of the human spine are the largest avascular structures in the body. They are roughly cylindrical and vary in size and shape, becoming a larger, more kidney-shaped structure in the lumbar spine. The intervertebral discs consist of collagen fibers embedded in a highly hydrated extracellular matrix. They comprise a well-hydrated central nucleus pulposus that is surrounded by the firm collagenous lamellae of the annulus fibrosus. Water constitutes about 70–80% of the total nucleus pulposus weight. Aside from water, proteoglycans are the most abundant material in the nucleus. Aggrecan is the major proteoglycan in the intervertebral disc. It has a brush-like structure made up of many glycosaminoglycan molecules attached to a core protein with a swelling propensity. The integrity of the intervertebral disc relies on the proper balance between matrix synthesis and degradation.

The main functional posterior elements of the spine are the facet joints. The disc carries 80% and the facet joints 20% of the axial load. The facets provide 40% of the torsional and shear strength. Their orientation changes from a more sagittal in the upper to a more coronal plane in the lumbar spine. The more sagittal the orientation, the more unable to resist flexion or translation movements they are, whereas they have in common the ability to resist rotation independent from their orientation.

Ligaments connect adjacent vertebrae and extend over several segments, stabilizing the spine and setting limits to the movements. The term "motion segment" is applied to two adjacent vertebrae, the disc, the facet joints, the ligaments, and the muscles between them.

There are nociceptors in the periosteum and accompanying blood vessels in the cancellous bone of the vertebrae, within the dura and nerve root sleeves. The histology of the normal disc suggests that only the most peripheral annulus layers have free nerve endings, and that the facet joint capsules and ligaments and fascia, in contrast, are more richly innervated. The posterior primary rami of the lumbar nerve roots supply all of these structures, overlapping between several adjacent levels.

The lumbar spine is flexible, but at the same time has to carry heavy loads. Movements of the spine produce internal loads on the vertebral body, facet joints, discs, and ligaments. Movement of the spine never occurs as pure flexion or extension in a single plane. There occur always coupled with movements in the other planes. In daily life, we expose our lumbar spine to complex movements and loads.

## 25.3
## Pathophysiology

Back pain that is reproducible during discography has been shown in quite a number of studies [2,15]. The fibrous annulus, consisting of concentric lamellae rich in collagen, harbors in its outer layers free nerve endings, and is therefore capable of signaling pain.

The intervertebral discs undergo changes in metabolism, structure, and mechanical function through the ages. The onset of these changes is influenced by multiple factors like genetics, age, nutrition, lifestyle, and mechanical aspects.

It is thought that the degenerative processes first affect the nucleus pulposus. There is a loss of the normal nucleus matrix, which turns it into a more fibrotic and less cartilaginous structure. The most prominent change with degeneration is progressive loss of proteoglycan, water, and collagen. This may result in a loss of disc height, a decrease in its ability to rehydrate after unloading, and increasing alteration of the intervertebral disc and surrounding tissues. Degeneration also impacts the end plates. The cartilage of the end plates thins and becomes calcified, preventing important nutrients from entering the intervertebral disc and catabolic products such as lactic acid from leaving the disc. Loss of disc height and structure may affect the annulus, resulting in pain, but may – because of altered load and motion pattern – subsequently also expedite wear and degeneration of the facet joints, resulting in arthrogenic pain due to facet arthritis. In addition, bulging of the intervertebral disc may result in nerve root impingement, causing radicular pain. Other painful intervertebral disc-related conditions include spinal stenosis, narrowing of the intervertebral foramina due to loss of disc height, bulging ligaments, and hypertrophic bone and facet joints.

The degenerative process according to Kirkaldy-Willis occurs in three phases [18]: (1) dysfunction, (2) instability, and (3) restabilization. The dysfunctional phase is the least well defined. Activity-related back pain results from dysfunction of the spinal segments, especially in relation to their load-bearing function and mobility. The term used to describe this situation is "instability" or "mechanical" LBP. However, abnormal movements in the dysfunction phase, even if they are present, are not always easy to detect. On the other hand, there are patients who have pain not related to load or motion, which is considered to be chemically generated. This differentiation may be important in the application of new nonfusion techniques.

Investigations for lumbar back pain comprise lateral, anteroposterior, oblique, and flexion–extension radiographs. Radiologically, lumbar segmental instability is defined as sagittal plane translation of more than 4.5 mm, or 15% of vertebral body diameter, or as rotation of more than 15–25°. On computed tomography (CT) scans, the following findings may be associated with instability:

1. Retrolisthesis (on sagittal reformations).
2. Spondylolisthesis.
3. Previous facetectomy.
4. Disc space narrowing and presence of gas.
5. Facet degeneration.
6. Synovial cyst.

On magnetic resonance imaging (MRI), disc degeneration appears with disc space narrowing and a low signal on T2-weighted images. Changes involving the bone marrow adjacent to a degenerated disc are frequent and can be classified into three types according to the description of Modic changes [22].

Although discography is controversial [23], provocative discography with subsequent CT scanning appears to be the most sensitive diagnostic imaging technique for the evaluation of discogenic LBP [28].

## 25.4
## Surgical Treatment

Today, treatment for degenerative disc disease focuses on relieving low back and/or sciatic pain. Treatment begins with conservative care, anti-inflammatory medication, and physiotherapy. Under this regimen, more than 85% of patients are treated successfully. However, the remaining 10–15% of them persist with chronic LBP and require more invasive treatment.

For patients suffering from disabling chronic LBP with or without radiculopathy with any objective findings other than disc degenerative disease, the indication for surgical treatment, and any technique that is going to be used, is controversial up to now. In the 1980s, the spine surgeons believed that abnormal load and/or motion were the primary cause in the generation of chronic LBP in degenerative disc disease. Fusion of the painful segment(s), a procedure performed with the aim of controlling or eliminating spinal segmental instability, would be the appropriate surgical solution. Indication for fusion was seen in patients with radiological evidence of instability and in cases in which removal of the facets or extensive foraminectomy was required for adequate decompression, resulting in secondary instability. Since

then, posterior, intertransverse, posterolateral and anterior/posterior interbody and "360°" fusion techniques have been used to treat chronic LBP. Metallic instrumentation was introduced in order to increase fusion rates and provide reliable anterior support.

The numbers of these procedures increased exponentially in the 1990s. Regardless of these, the results of spine fusion vary extensively. Although successful fusion may be achieved in a high percentage of cases, it fails to provide good clinical results in nearly half of the cases. In spite of partially disappointing results, fusion procedures are still considered as standard technique to be used in the treatment of chronic LBP due to degenerative disc disease. In addition, there are significant undesirable long-term effects associated with spine fusion. For example, lack of motion within the fused segment may lead to accelerated degeneration of the adjacent levels. This is the main reason why during the last two decades a variety of new technologies has been developed with the aim of avoiding fusion and preserving or restoring segmental function.

The currently available nonfusion devices fall into three main categories: total disc replacement (TDR), disc nucleus replacements, and posterior dynamic stabilization including interspinous devices. Other concepts are about to emerge such as facet replacement or total posterior element replacements. Nonfusion surgical approaches aim at removal of the damaged tissue and replacement by a synthetic implant. This approach has been successful for many decades in total knee and hip replacement.

The indication for fusion surgery is, however, not the same as for nonfusion techniques. Patients with mechanical or dysfunctional segmental pain associated with significant instability or advanced structural segmental damage are predominantly candidates for efficient fusion techniques. On the other hand, patients with chronic nonmechanical discogenic LBP or minor instability in the earlier stages of degeneration may qualify for nonfusion techniques.

The task of identifying patients who will benefit more from arthroplasty as opposed to the fusion surgery represents a diagnostic challenge and must be based on patient history, manual and neurological examination, radiological findings, and functional evaluation.

The cardinal MRI features of disc degeneration are loss of height, annular tears, and decreased signal intensity in T2-weighted images, indicating reduced water content, loss of internal architecture, and loss of contour. There is little correlation between imaging evidence of disc degeneration and clinical symptoms.

In 1984, Modic described magnetic resonance signal changes in the subchondral vertebral bone, the so-called Modic changes [22]. They indicate different stages of disc degeneration. Type I changes (subchondral hypointensity in T1-weighted images, hyperintensity in T2-weighted images) are related to a reactive hypertrophic trabecular structure and fibrotic granulation tissue replacing the bone marrow. Type II changes (hyperintensity in T1-weighted images, isointensity in T2-weighted images) correlate with trabecular hypertrophy and fatty degeneration of the marrow. Type III (hypointensity in both T1-weighted and T2-weighted images) represents sclerosis of the endplates and fibrosis of the bone marrow. There is some evidence to suggest that patients with LBP, disc degeneration, and Modic changes can be diagnosed as having specific LBP.

Other functional tests with additional imaging such as provocative discography with subsequent CT scan, CT-guided facet, or periradicular injections play an important role in preoperative evaluation. Their value is still under discussion [23].

## 25.5
## Fusion Surgeries

Spine fusion was initially (since the beginning of the 20th century) used to treat the instability caused by tuberculous infections [1, 17]. The procedure was later adopted in the management of scoliosis and traumatic fracture. The anterior lumbar interbody fusion technique was described by Burns in 1933 [7], and the posterior lumbar interbody fusion technique by Cloward in 1940 [9]. Recently, the transforaminal lumbar interbody fusion was described by Harms [16].

De Palma and Rothman [10] were among the first to discuss lumbar fusion for back pain. The idea was to eliminate intervertebral motion once the abnormal motion was identified as the major cause of LBP. Uninstrumented posterolateral fusion became the standard method. There was, however, a significant group of patients who experienced no relief of their LBP, despite solid bony fusion. Attention was thus directed toward the disc itself.

New knowledge of nociceptive annular microinnervation strengthened the argument in favor of the disc as the source of the pain. Thus, in the group of patients who had no relief from LBP after successful posterolateral fusion, discogenic pain was postulated as a nonmechanical explanation for their persistent symptoms. As a consequence, interbody fusions became the most popular procedure for discogenic back pain treatment.

Intervertebral fusion cages were introduced in the late 1980s by Kuslich et al. [19], Ray [24], and Brantigan et al. [6]. Posterior and anterior lumbar interbody fusions (with stand-alone cages or with an additional posterior screw) as well as transforaminal lumbar interbody fusion with posterior screw stabilization, have become the standard techniques for the surgical treatment of dysfunctional segmental motion and discogenic lumbar pain (Figs. 1 and 2). Recently, a prospective randomized trial showed significantly better clinical results following arthrodesis in comparison to nonoperative treatment [14].

Despite the progress from uninstrumented posterolateral fusion to more complex methods of instrumented 360° fusion, with complete removal of the disc and eliminated segmental motion, the clinical outcome of these procedure are quite different, leading to continuing controversy about the indications. A comprehensive literature survey reported satisfactory outcome in 65–87% of patients after an arthrodesis, with monosegmental fusions having better results than bi- or trisegmental fusions [5].

## 25.6
## Nonfusion Techniques for the Lumbar Spine

According to Bertagnoli [4], disc-related spinal problems could be treated according to the state of degenerative segmental alterations. Those at an earlier stage of disc degeneration may respond to conservative treatment or various percutaneous intradiscal procedures. More advanced disc degeneration may require open disc surgery, especially in concomitant nerve root compression. Fusion surgery is usually indicated in more advanced segmental degeneration. Since the 1990s, new concepts for the treatment of degenerative disc disease have emerged, summarized as "spine arthroplasty." Three major additional treatment choices are currently under evaluation: (1) TDR, (2) disc nucleus replacement, and (3) posterior dynamic stabilization systems.

The rationale underlying the use of an artificial disc is to replace a painful disc, to restore a reduced disc height, and to preserve segmental motion. It represents a logical alternative to fusion surgery but does not cover an identical range of indications. It is indicated in specifically

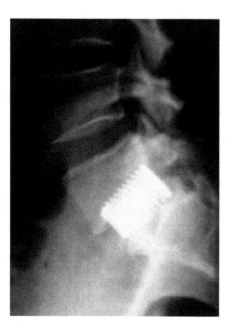

Fig. 1 Stand-alone cages L5/S1

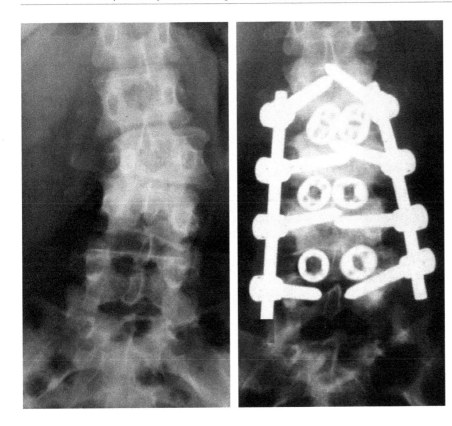

Fig. 2  Cages and posterior fixation in degenerative scoliosis L2–L5

patients with discogenic pain, provided other pain generators, such as the facet joints or canal stenosis, causing spinal claudication are excluded. The list of contraindication includes lytic or high-degree spondylolisthesis, herniation with migrated fragment causing neural compression, scoliosis, osteoporosis, central or lateral recess stenosis, and facet arthrosis. A disc prosthesis (Fig. 3) has load-bearing capacity, provides restoration of the intervertebral disc space height, may open the neuroforamina, and is, to some degree, capable to reinforce segmental stability. It is assumed that in preserving or restoring segmental mobility, adjacent levels above and below may be protected from the degenerative changes accelerated by otherwise altered load transfer.

Among the TDRs, the SB-Charité artificial disc now has a history of 24 years. In the beginning, the pioneers of disc replacement, Büttner-Janz and Schellnack, had to face difficulties with the durability of the materials [20], which have now, after three generations of development, been overcome. A variety of other artificial disc designs are currently in clinical use, mainly in Europe, but increasingly also in North America and other parts of the world. All of these devices are implanted by an anterior transperitoneal or retroperitoneal approach. The different devices may be unconstrained or own varying degrees of constraint. The increased constraint is intended to prevent hypermobility and unphysiological loading of the facets, which could cause pain and accelerated degeneration. Some devices incorporate metal on polyethylene, others metal-on-metal articulations in order to reduce wear and the risk of long-term osteolysis. Different implant geometries try to imitate natural motion patterns with the aim of overcoming some of the long-term complications, including facet degeneration and material wear, which have been identified during earlier evaluations. Thus far, there is no evidence-based knowledge supporting the superiority of this new concept. On the other hand, with the more widespread use of TDRs, there are an increasing number of reports of insufficient pain relief and challenging revision surgeries.

Rather than replacing the entire disc, several devices have been designed to replace only the nucleus pulposus (Fig. 4). These devices could be effective in patients at an early stage of disc degeneration, before the annulus has suffered significant degeneration. The goal is to repressurize the nucleus and to restore adequate tension to the annulus fibrosus, thereby eliminating the mechanical consequences that may be responsible for further degeneration. In 1995, Ray developed a hydrogel nucleus replacement covered with a polyethylene fiber jacket, called

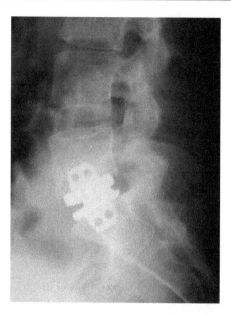

Fig. 3 Total disc replacement L5/S1

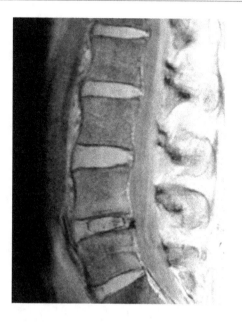

Fig. 4 Magnetic resonance imaging of disc nucleus replacement L4/L5

a prosthetic disc nucleus [25]. This prosthesis could be implanted in a dehydrated state via a posterior or lateral transpsoatic approach. After hydration, the volume of the prosthesis increases, at the same time increasing disc height and annulus tension. The primary source of complication with this device has been device migration and endplate subsidence [25]. Other nucleus replacements, such as injectable protein polymers, are under early investigation.

Posterior dynamic stabilizing implants are intended to realign and stabilize one or more linked vertebral segments without complete immobilization of the segments (Fig. 5). Surgery aims to achieve a position as close as possible to normal anatomy with realignment and some distraction of the facets. One of the devices consists of a titanium pedicle screw placed laterally to the facet joints. They are connected longitudinally with flexible polyurethane spacers that are held in place by a central polyethylene cord fixed in the screw heads under tension. The length of the spacers defines the degree of segmental distraction and unloading of the facets and – to some extent – also the disc. The system increases segmental stiffness, counteracting minor degrees of instability. Motion – albeit reduced – is preserved, thus, it is thought, protecting adjacent levels against increased stress. There are also reports of recovery of the disc signal T2-weighted MRI 6 months after implantation.

The indication for this procedure is for the treatment of chronic LBP caused by segmental hypermobility that is evident during flexion-extension movements. Contra-

indications are advanced structural damage of the facets or anterior elements as well higher degrees of instability (spondylolisthesis more than grade I). Two other devices, one allowing motion between the head of the screw and the longitudinal rod, and another with some motion within the plate, are commercially available.

## 25.7
## Conclusion

Over the past 20 years, spinal surgery has changed dramatically. The technical improvements in achieving fusion with the help of new implants and less invasive surgical techniques, together with the concept of nonfusion devices have significantly widened our range of individually tailored surgical options for the treatment of chronic LBP. These developments have also brought about noticeable improvements in patient evaluation and patient selection. Patient history and manual and neurological examination are as necessary for adequate patient selection as adequate imaging functional examinations (provocative discography, probatory facet or periradicular injections, functional myelography, or dynamic MRI). We still are lacking in evidence-based results, which are extremely important in order to support our concepts and indications. Randomized studies evaluating the different devices and techniques are also lacking. Unfortunately, more and more devices are emerging before proper long-term evaluations of their predecessors have been done.

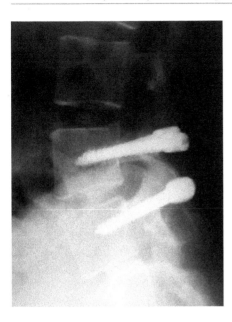

Fig. 5  Dynamic stabilization L4/L5

We bear the responsibility not only for the welfare of our patients, but also for economical stewardship of the resources of our healthcare system.

## References

1. Albee FH (1911) Transplantation of a portion of the tibia into the spine for Pott's disease. JAMA 57:885–886
2. Anderson SR, Flanaga B (2000) Discography. Curr Rev Pain 4:345–352
3. Benzel EC (1995) Biomechanics of Spine Stabilization. Principles and Clinical Practice. McGraw-Hill, New York
4. Bertagnoli R (2002) Review of modern treatment options for degenerative disc disease. In: Kaech DL, Jinkins JR (eds) Spinal Restabilization Procedures. Elsevier Science, Amsterdam, pp 365–375
5. Boos N, Webb JK (1997) Pedicle screw fixation in spinal disorders: a European view. Eur Spine J 6:2–18
6. Brantigan J, Steffe A, Lewis M, et al (2000) Lumbar interbody fusion using Brantigan I/F cage for posterior lumbar interbody fusion and variable pedicle screw placement system. Spine 25:1437–1446
7. Burns BH (1933) An operation for spondylolisthesis. Lancet 1:1233
8. Buttner-Janz K, Schellnack K, Zippel H (1987) Eine alternative Behandlungsstrategie beim lumbalen Bandscheibenschaden mit der Bandscheibenendoprothese Modulartyo SB Charite. Z Orthop Ihre Grenzgeb 125:1–6
9. Cloward RB (1940) The treatment of ruptured intervertebral disc by vertebral body fusion. Ann Surg 136:987–992
10. DePalma AF, Rothman RH (1969) Surgery of the lumbar spine. Clin Orthop 63:162–170
11. Eck JC, Humphreys SC, Hodges SD (1999) Adjacent-segment degeneration after lumbar fusion: a review of clinical, biomechanical, and radiologic studies. Am J Orthop 28:336–340
12. Enker P, Steffe A, Mcmillin C, et al (1993) Artificial disc replacement. Preliminary report with a 3-year minimum follow-up. Spine 18:1061–1070
13. Fernström U (1966) Arthroplasty with intercorporal endoprosthesis in herniated disc and in painful disc. Acta Chir Scand 357:154–159
14. Fritzell P, Hagg O, Wessberg P, Nordwall A (2001) Volvo Award Winner in Clinical Studies. Lumbar fusion versus nonsurgical treatment for chronic lox back pain: a multicenter randomized controlled trial from the Swedish Lumbar Spine Study Group. Spine 26:2521–2532
15. Guyer RD, Ohmeiss DD (1995) Lumbar discography. Position statement from the North American Spine Society Diagnostic and Therapeutic Committee. Spine 20:2049–2059
16. Harms J, Roliger H (1982) A one-stage procedure in operative treatment of spondylolisthesis: dorsal traction-reposition and anterior fusion. Z Orthop Grenzgeb 120:343–347
17. Hibbs RA (1911) An operation for progressive spinal deformities. N Y Med J 93:1013–1016
18. Kirkaldy-Willis WH, Farfan HF(1982) Instability of the lumbar spine. Clin Orthop Relat Res 165:110–123
19. Kuslich SD, Ulstrom CL, Griffith SL, et al (1998) The Babgy and Kuslich method of lumbar interbody fusion. History, techniques, and 2-year follow-up results of a United States prospective, multicenter trial. Spine 23:1267–1279
20. Kurtz S (2006) Total disc arthroplasty. In: Kurtz SM, Edidin AA (eds) Spine Technology Handbook. Elsevier Academic, New York, pp 303–370
21. Lee CK, Vessa P, Lee JK (1995) Chronic disabling low back pain syndrome caused by internal disc derangements. The results of disc excision and posterior lumbar fusion. Spine 20:356–361
22. Modic MT, Steinberg PM, Ross JS, et al (1999) Degenerative disk disease: assessment of changes in vertebral body marrow with MR imaging. Radiology 166:193–199
23. Nachemson A (1989) Lumbar discography: where are we today? Spine 14:555–557
24. Ray CD (1997) Threaded titanium cages for lumbar interbody fusion. Spine 22:667–680
25. Ray CD (2002) Prosthetic disc nucleus: 300 case update. Proceedings of the International Intradiscal Therapy, 14th Annual Meeting, May 24–26, Phoenix, Arizona
26. Waddell G (2004) The epidemiology of back pain. In: Waddell G (ed) The Back Pain Revolution. Churchill Livingstone, Edinburgh, pp 71–89
27. Waddell G (2004) Diagnostic triage. In: Waddell G (ed) The Back Pain Revolution. Churchill Livingstone, Edinburgh, pp 9–26
28. Walsh TR, Weinsteis JN, Spratt KF, et al (1990) Lumbar discography in normal subjects. J Bone Joint Surg Am 72:1081–1088

# Managing the Degenerative Cervical Spine: The Role of Interbody Fusion and Motion-Preserving Techniques

**26**

Fernando Schmidt and Robert Schönmayr

## Contents

## 26.1
## Introduction

The degenerative spine diseases are the leading causes of pain that induce the patient to consult a doctor as well as being responsible for temporary and permanent disability, mainly at an age when the human being is at its most productive (from 20 to 50 years old). Therefore, the treatment demands attention from the doctors, as well from the community and government to achieve a better quality of life for the population.

The cervical spine consists of seven vertebrae (from C1 to C7), five intervertebral discs, and many ligaments and muscles in the anterior and posterior part. The cervical spine, due to its great mobility, is a locus of painful syndromes caused mainly by degenerative disc disease.

The upper cervical spine consists of two atypical vertebrae, which together form the atlantoaxial segment and have their own anatomy, function, and biomechanical qualities, and the middle and lower cervical spine, known as the subaxial portion, consists of the other five vertebrae (C3–C7). The intervertebral disc in the anterior portion of the cervical spine forms a cushion that minimizes the forces applied to the posterior facet joints. The cervical spine, in comparison with the other segments (dorsal and lumbar), is characterized by a major mobility in flexion/extension/rotation and lateral flexion.

The degenerative changes of the cervical spine begin with the disc degeneration that affects spinal dynamics and starts a series of alterations known as disc arthrosis and cervical spondylosis, which can eventually cause the radicular and/or spinal cord compression responsible for neurological syndromes that need treatment. For these degenerative conditions, the conservative treatment is, in the majority of the patients, sufficient and efficient. However, when this treatment fails to alleviate symptoms, we may indicate the surgical treatment. The surgical indications are based on compressive radicular/spinal-cord neurological syndromes, deformities, and/or instabilities that do not respond to conservative treatment.

In the latter 20 years of the last century, the objective of surgical treatment was only to decompress the neurological structures or decompress and fusion. In the beginning of this new millennium, the introduction of new procedures with motion preservation has brought about some new paradigms of surgical treatment for degenerative cervical spine diseases.

In this chapter we will provide a brief revision of the anatomy, biomechanics, and physiopathology of neurological compressive degenerative cervical spine disease (disc herniations and spondylitic myelopathy), which may be treated surgically via anterior discectomy and fusion, and the evolution of all of theses fusion techniques from the last 25 years until the development of the new nonfusion techniques, which in the cervical spine are represented by the artificial discs.

## 26.2
## Functional Anatomy of the Cervical Spine

The cervical spine under normal conditions has a lordotic curve and consists of seven vertebrae (C1–C7) [15]. The two first vertebrae, the atlas and axis, have a unique anatomic arrangement. They do not have intervertebral discs and the movements of flexion, extension, and axial rotation are performed in the facet joints, which are localized laterally. The transverse ligament, part of the cruciform ligament, has a key function in the stability of the C1–C2 complex [1]. Due to the lack of an intervertebral disc, this area is seldom involved in the usual degenerative process; however, they are more affected by chronic inflammatory processes like rheumatoid arthritis, and there are no indications for either anterior cervical discectomy and fusion (ACDF) or artificial disc prosthesis in this region.

The inferior vertebrae (C3–C7) comprise a body, superior and inferior articular processes, lamina, bifurcated spinous processes, transverse processes, and uncinate processes, which form the uncovertebral joints. These uncovertebral joints limit the lateral translation and contribute to the coupled movements of lateral flexion and cervical rotation. The intervertebral disc of this region has an average height of 4 mm close to the anterior edge and an average height of 2.5–3 mm close to the posterior edge [15]. The superior and inferior endplates are the cranial and caudal limits of the intervertebral disc; they are essential for maintaining disc function and are typically less than 1 mm thick. They are formed by hyaline cartilage and are thicker in this periphery.

The cervical joints of C2–C3 to C6–C7 are synovial, articulous joints and have an orientation of approximately 45° [1] relative to the horizontal plane and are orientated such that its facets lie in the coronal plane. This orientation does not limit excessive movements in any plane except for extension. In these cervical regions, the primary movements are dependent on the integrity of the intervertebral disc. Flexion–extension movements are distributed along the whole cervical spine in a range of 65–75°. The limit of translation is 2–3 mm.

The nuchal ligament is located in the posterior portion, in the midline, and starts in the external occipital protuberance and ends in the spinous processes of C7; it has the important function of limiting excessive flexion of the cervical spine.

The intervertebral foramen is the place where the nerve roots emerge, and is limited anteriorly part by the lateral portion of the intervertebral disc and the uncovertebral joints, superiorly and inferiorly by the pedicles, and posteriorly by the lateral masses. The root corresponds to the inferior vertebrae, which means that the C6 root emerges from the C5/C6 intervertebral foramen.

## 26.3
## Pathophysiology

The intervertebral disc begins to degenerate early in its biochemical and mechanical structure, which alters its ability to resist compression, or act as a cushion. The amount of proteoglycan in the disc nucleus pulposus be-

gins to change and the ratio of keratin sulfate to chondroitin sulfate tends to increase, progressively desiccating the disc. The degeneration of an intervertebral disc promotes loss of its height. The approximation of the vertebral bodies alters the biomechanical forces present in the uncovertebral and zygapophyseal joints. As the disc bulges or herniates, the osteophytes may impose on the adjacent nerve root and dorsal root ganglion and excite nociceptors, causing radicular pain. In the same way, reactive osseous reactions can form in the posterior part of the vertebral body. Nerve root impingement can also be caused by soft disc bulging contained in the posterior longitudinal ligament, or a free disc fragment in the spine canal.

A transverse spondylitic spur can form in the posterior part of the vertebral body with dorsal annular bulging, followed by more osteophyte formation and hypertrophy of the soft-tissue and ligaments. Additional collapse of the intervertebral space causes deformation of the yellow ligament in the spine canal, mainly during extension. This combination of events can produce a spondylitic compromise of the anterior/posterior diameter of the cervical spinal canal and cause a clinical picture of spondylitic myelopathy. The diagnosis is confirmed by a physical examination in combination with neuroradiological tests, mainly magnetic resonance imaging, MRI, and, eventually, electrophysiological tests such as electromyography.

Pathologic degenerative processes in the cervical spine can manifest as mainly three different clinical syndromes: (1) patients with only chronic, axial, neck pain and eventually referred pain in the shoulder or interscapular area; (2) patients with radicular pain; (3) patients with the clinical picture of spondylitic myelopathy [7].

## 26.4
## Surgical Treatment

Surgery is the preferred option for advanced disc disease in the cervical spine where there is no pain relief with conservative therapy. The main indications for surgery in patients with degenerative disc disease are neck pain with radiculopathy and/or neurological deficit because of the spondylitic myelopathy. The decision to advocate surgical treatment for patients with only cervical pain must be made with caution, and we must be aware of the possibility of other diseases like myofascial syndromes and depression. Eventually, discography can be used as a method to confirm that the intervertebral disc is the origin of a putative discogenic pain.

The classic indications for surgical intervention for compressive radiculopathy include: failure of over 3–6 months of conservative treatment modalities and/or progressive neurological deficit. The clinical symptoms must be correlated with the diagnostic imaging (MRI or computed tomography).

The indications for the surgical treatment of cervical myelopathy are not well defined. A patient with mild, nonprogressive, sign of myelopathy, can be treated conservatively. The surgical intervention is indicated in a progressive myelopathy from moderate to serious, stable but with short evolution (up to 1 year).

In the cervical spine, the roots as much as the spinal cord can be decompressed either via a ventral approach or a dorsal approach. In the anterior approach, decompression is performed with a discectomy or a corpectomy. In the posterior approach, foraminotomy and laminectomies/laminotomies are used to decompress the neurological structures.

The ventral cervical discectomy and fusion have been the surgical intervention of choice for the majority of patients with degenerative cervical spine disease with discogenic pain, compressive radicular symptoms, or myelopathy. Although only decompression can alleviate radicular pain or cervical myelopathy signs [6], the consensus of opinion is that it is better to put in place some material to maintain or restore the disc height at the time of discectomy, since many patients experience persistent cervical pain and a kyphotic deformity in the postsurgical period. The gold standard is the autograft bone, but cages with osteoinductive and/or osteoconductive material can also be used.

## 26.5
## Anterior Cervical Discectomy and Fusion

Due to the anterior location of most compressive agents in degenerative cervical diseases, the anterior approach seems to be the most elegant way of decompression [9]. Cervical discectomy via the ventral approach, known as anterior cervical discectomy or ACDF, is one of the most common procedures performed by spine surgeons [10].

Ventral discectomy in the cervical spine for the treatment of degenerative cervical spine diseases was introduced by Robinson and Smith in 1955, and by Cloward in 1958 [5, 16]. The main difference in the techniques is the shape of the autograft bone. In the Smith and Robinson procedure, a horseshoe tricortical iliac crest autograft is used, and in the Cloward procedure, an autogenous dowel iliac crest graft with only cortical bone in its anterior portion is used. By the end of the 20th century, these procedures became the most commonly performed operation in the surgical treatment of degenerative cervical spine diseases. The surgeon must consider the possibility of graft complications in using these techniques. The main complications are: graft displacement, graft fracture, pseudoarthrosis, subsidence, and donor site morbidity.

In the 1980s, Caspar developed a new anterior cervical spine system with plates and bicortical screw to be used in conjunction with the bone graft, as well as a unique system of instruments like retractors and a new vertebral body distractor for the ventral intervertebral approach

[4, 12]. In the beginning, these instruments were used in cases of major instability like cervical trauma and tumors, but then became routinely used for the treatment of degenerative diseases. The classical Caspar implants are a trapezoidal, titanium plate and screws that are not locked to the plate. This is an unconstrained system. With cervical plates, we reduce the complications of graft migration and collapse and obviate the need for external bracing. The screw is not-self-tapping and must be placed into the posterior cortex of the vertebral body to avoid pullout. The plate function raises the stiffness of the segment by limiting the movements of extension and rotation, therefore reducing the percentage of pseudoarthrosis and graft displacement. Otherwise, the plate does not reduce the donor site morbidity, and, in case of graft resorption or collapse, we can have pullout or fracture of the screws, because there is more axial load to the plate.

The design of new plates (constrained) changes to a monocortical screw that is fixed to the plates by a screw-plate locking mechanism to prevent pullout, such as the Morche cervical spine locking plate system [12]. Actually, there is a tendency to use a new kind of plate, known as dynamic plates, which have evolved to address the issues of minimizing graft dislodgement and reducing the stress shielding of the graft [3].

In Europe in the 1980s, polymethylmethacrylate (PMMA, bone cement) was introduced as an isolated spacer in the intervertebral space after discectomy to minimize the donor site morbidity in the iliac crest [14]. The technique consists of injection of liquid PMMA bone cement after the complete discectomy, preparation of a small burr hole in the superior and inferior platos, and protection of the dura with Gelfoam. After 5–10 minutes, the polymer is generously irrigated with saline solution to prevent termic lesion of the spinal cord; the polymer is thus firmly attached to the disc space. This technique was very cheap and simple. However, subsidence of the material and consequent lost of the disc space height occurred in the postoperative period because the PMMA has a higher elastic modulus than the vertebral bone. In addition, PMMA has neither osteoinductive nor osteoconductive properties. Therefore, this material was gradually replaced by different spacer models of different sizes, and using different materials like titanium, polyether-etherketone (PEEK) or carbon fiber, filled with autologous bone material or other bone substitutes with osteoconductive or osteoinductive properties, like hydroxyapatite and tricalcium phosphate. These cages are designed to make possible restoration of the physiological disc height and allow contact of the autograft or other material inside the cages with both vertebral bodies to promote intersomatic arthrhodesis.

The geometric configuration of the cage is the main factor in the prevention of instability, displacement, and disc height failure because of subsidence. Considering these aspects and with the purpose to have maximal security of the construction and with minimal morbidity, since 2000 we have routinely been using an integrated cage with plate made of titanium or PEEK with osteoconductive (hydroxyapatite and tricalcium phosphate) material inside it (Fig. 1).

New artificial ceramics have been introduced as osteoconductive graft material, which can provide a scaffold into which newly forming bone can grow. There are many kinds of materials of naturally occurring, animal tissue or pure synthetics such as hydroxyapatite and tricalcium phosphate. These bioceramics are chemically inert and have a porous structure similar to the trabecular cancellous bone, creating an environment that permits the implantation of osteoprogenitor cells and bone growth.

These materials can be used in the form of particles to fill the cage or spacer themselves, directly into the intervertebral space. In the first case it is used as bone void filler and in the second as a graft substitute, obviating the need and complications associated with autogenous bone harvesting, although its osteoconductive potential is lower than that of autologous bone, increasing the likelihood of pseudoarthrosis.

The original plate-cage implant, which was designed by Professor Bezenech in France, provides immediate anterior stability of a plate combined with cage technology to obtain solid fusion [2]. Titanium cages, because of their radiopaque nature, hamper evaluation of bony fusion, and their rigidity cause stress shielding.

PEEK-OPTIMA, for medical use, is a nondegradable polymer with an elastic modulus of 3.6 Gpa, which is very close to that of cortical bone, and is radiolucent, thus permitting the evaluation of bone fusion. Because its elastic modulus is close to that of bone, it optimizes the load transfer between the cage and the adjacent vertebral bodies and reduces the stress shielding on the graft material. The plate-cage implant is available in five sizes, varying in heights between 5 and 7 mm, is wedged, with a pos-

terior height greater than the anterior, and has a convex roof and horizontal base, which is in accordance with the normal disc space anatomy in the cervical spine. The graft material is compressed inside the cage with parallel pliers before the cage is introduced into the disc space. The superior part of the plate has a posterior inclination of 12°, and the inferior part of the plate has no inclination with regard to the vertical plane. The plates have an oblique orientation in the sagittal plane, permitting the fixation of two plates on the same vertebra, and facilitating use in many adjacent spaces. Two monocortical screws are used. The rigidity of the cage meets biomechanical imperatives. Its radiolucency permits the course of consolidation to be monitored, unlike the metal cages (Fig. 2).

To date, it remains debatable whether cages in the cervical spine should be filled with any kind of bone or bone substitute.

In the field of spine implant technology and with the knowledge of biomechanics and bioengineering, the ideal implant for intervertebral arthrodesis is about to be developed. We believe that the polymer-based bioresorbable materials, especially the polylactides [17], probably integrated with osteoconductive and osteoinductive material like human bone morphogenetic protein-2, will be the most appropriate intersomatic device, once they have achieved a stiffness comparable with that of bone. They are radiolucent and resorb with time, transferring the axial load to the graft and enhancing the fusion rate.

## 26.6
## Nonfusion Techniques for the Cervical Spine

Over the last 30 years in the orthopedic field, despite the fact that arthrodesis of a joint was not considered a good solution and the development of arthroplasties with prosthesis has improved the clinical result and thus gained

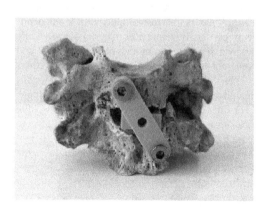

Fig. 1   Integrated cage with plate in a cadaver spine

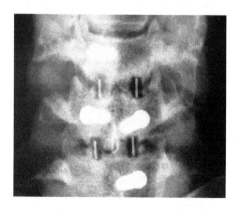

Fig. 2   Intersomatic arthrodesis with a polyetheretherketone (PEEK) cage

wide acceptance [8], nowadays cervical discectomy in combination with intersomatic arthrodesis remains the gold standard in the surgical treatment of degenerative cervical spine diseases. However, in a great number of patients, the clinical recovery doesn't reach the expected level, and the more arthrodeses are performed, the greater the incidence of advanced degenerative changes at the adjacent levels. The intervertebral arthrodesis of a motor segment can put in risk the adjacent level due to overload.

The mainstay of the surgical treatment in degenerative disc disease must be not only to re-establish the disc height and the spinal alignment, but also to recompose the hydraulics of the disc and maintain the biomechanical quality of the motor segment. The latter two objectives can not be achieved with intervertebral fusion.

Recently, many kinds of cervical disc prosthesis are available in the spinal implant market; even though the clinical studies are preliminary, they seem to have clinical results that are comparable to those achieved with intervertebral fusion. We are likely to see a reduction in the incidence of degenerative changes at the adjacent spinal levels with this nonfusion technology. The long-term success and stability of the disc prosthesis depends on the technology used. It may provide immediate stability among the vertebral bodies and allow osteointegration over time.

Some prostheses applied in great articulation have been problematic with regard to the articulating surfaces, either metal-to-metal or metal-to-polyethylene, the particulate wear debris inducing osteolysis. The first attempt to implant a prosthesis in the disc space was done by Fernström in 1962, who produced a stainless steel ball for lumbar use. This was also used in some cervical degenerative disc diseases cases [8, 11]. Because of the hypermobility, migration, and subsidence of the balls in the vertebral bodies, the technique became useless.

Historically, the first disc prosthesis was introduced into clinical practice in the 1980s and was improved in the 1990s for use in the lumbar spine. The SB-Charité artificial disc was the first to gain wide acceptance and was invented by Kurt Shellnack and Karin Buettner-Janz in Germany. It consists basically of two metallic endplates fixed to the adjacent vertebral bodies, and it articulates against a central core of polyethylene. Nowadays, this artificial disc is in its third generation.

In 1991, a cervical prosthesis named the Bristol disc was developed. It was made of stainless steel in the ball-and-socket system, for use in the cervical spine. Many implant-related complications were noted with the use of this prosthesis. Since 1997, the next successful artificial disc to be developed was the Bryan disc, which has remained essentially unchanged since then. This is the most widely used cervical disc replacement in clinical use today. It comprises two titanium endplates and a polymer core.

In many ways, nonfusion technology is more attractive to the cervical spine than to the lumbar spine. The cervical spine must support only the weight of the head. The indication for cervical arthroplasty is the same as for anterior cervical fusion, that is spondylitic radiculopathy and myelopathy, and the surgical access to the anterior cervical spine is more familiar to the spine surgeon than the anterior lumbar access, and carries with it fewer complications, even for revisions [11].

White and Panjabi described the normal movements of the subaxial cervical spine, restoration of which is the objective of spine arthroplasty. Coupling movements are very important in the motion of the cervical spine. For example, when one laterally flexes the cervical spine, there is a simultaneous movement of rotation of the spinous process to the convex side of the cervical curve. Because of its own biomechanical characteristics, coupled movements and some translation movements in the articulate facets make the cervical spine different from the lumbar spine, and therefore the technique for motion preservation appeared later in this region, probably 10 years later.

The actual main concern with this new technology is to test all of these new devices to ensure its durability; once implanted, these artificial discs must work for the rest of the patient's life without failure. Although the best clinical experience thus far is with four artificial cervical discs, the long-term clinical results are not yet known. These artificial discs include: Bryan, Prestige, Prodisc-C, and Porous Coated Motion (PCM). The first three are semiconstrained implants and the last is an unconstrained implant.

Different design models and biomaterials are used. Theoretically, an artificial disc that uses metal-to-polyethylene may produce more wear debris than the one made by metal-to-metal. Among the different devices, we have experience with the PCM (Fig. 3). This is unconstrained (or minimally constrained), with a convex polyethylene

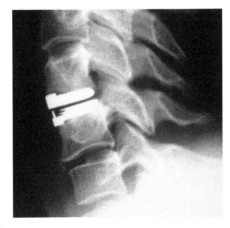

Fig. 3 Porous Coated Motion (PCM) artificial disc

core fixed to the cobalt chrome alloy caudal endplate that moves against the concave cephalad endplate. The endplate surfaces are also coated with titanium and calcium phosphate to allow for osteointegration and enhance the stability. My colleague, the neurosurgeon Pimenta, conducted a prospective pilot study that began in December 2002 and included 52 patients [11, 13]. There were only two complications, a migration and a case of heterotopic bone formation. The preliminary clinical results were good to excellent in 97% of the cases.

The surgical access for the PCM is the same as for ACDF. A transverse incision, the division of the platysma and blunt dissection until the anterior part of the cervical spine are executed. After the initial excision of the disc material, we put a screw in each vertebral body parallel to the endplates for distraction of the intervertebral space. The use of illumination with a headlight, or magnification with the microscope might be useful during this stage. Complete removal of the disc, herniated disc fragments, and osteophytes is carried out, ensuring that the uncovertebral joints are clearly visible. Preparation of the endplates with the implant forceps, followed by insertion of the prosthesis into the intervertebral space is then completed.

The success of disc replacement has to be compared with spine arthrodesis, the current gold-standard in the treatment of cervical spondylosis. The future will show us if the nonfusion technology will produce similar or better results than fusion and whether the incidence of degenerative changes of adjacent segments can be avoid by this new technique.

## References

1. An HS (1998) Anatomy of the spine. In: An HS (ed) Principles and Techniques of Spine Surgery. Williams and Wilkins, Baltimore, pp 1–30
2. Benezech J (2001) Cervical fusion with monocomponent PCB plate. In: Szpalski M, Gunzburg R (eds) The Degenerative Cervical Spine. Lippincott Williams and Wilkins, Philadelphia, pp 265–273
3. Benzel EC (1995) Biomechanics of Spine Stabilization. Principles and Clinical Practice. McGraw-Hill, New York
4. Caspar W (1982) Advances in cervical spine surgery. First experiences with the trapezial osteosynthetic plate and a new surgical instrumentation for anterior interbody stabilization. Orthop News 4:6
5. Cloward R (1958) The anterior approach for removal of ruptured cervical discs. J Neurosurg 15:602–614
6. Dunsker SB (1977) Anterior cervical discectomy with or without fusion. Clin Neurosurg 25:516–521
7. Emery SE (1998) Cervical disc disease and cervical spondylosis. In: An HS (ed) Principles and Techniques of Spine Surgery. Williams and Wilkins, Baltimore, pp 401–412
8. Golfin J (2005) Artificial disc prosthesis for the cervical spine. In: Benzel EC (ed) Spine Surgery. Techniques, Complication Avoidance, and Management. Elsevier, Amsterdam, pp 1627–1638
9. Grob D (2003) Surgery of the degenerative cervical spine. Coluna 2:75–82
10. Heary RF, Benzel EC, Vaicys C (2005) Single and multiple single interbody fusion techniques. In: Benzel EC (ed) Spine Surgery. Techniques, Complication Avoidance, and Management. Elsevier Academic, New York, pp 351–362
11. Kurtz S (2006) Total disc arthroplasty. In: Kurtz SM, Edidin AA (eds) Spine Technology Handbook. Elsevier Academic, New York, pp 303–370
12. Papavero L (2000) Microsurgery of the cervical spine. In: Mayer HM (ed) Minimally Invasive Spine Surgery. Springer, Berlin, pp 17–42
13. Pimenta L, McAfee PC, et al (2004) Clinical experience with the new artificial cervical PCM (Cervitech) Disc. Spine J 4:315S–321S
14. Roosen K (1982) Bone cement as replacement material for cervical discs. Fortschr Med 100:2120–2126
15. Roy PV, Barbaix E, Clarijs JP (2001) Functional anatomy of the cervical spine. In: Szpalski M, Gunzburg R (2001) The Degenerative Cervical Spine. Lippincott Williams, and Wilkins, Philadelphia, pp 3–27
16. Smith G, Robinson R (1958) The treatment of cervical spine disorders by anterior removal of intervertebral disc and interbody fusion. J Bone Joint Surg 40:607–624
17. Wuisman PIJM, Smit TH (2006) Bioresorbable polymers: heading for a new generation of spinal cages. Eur Spine J 15:133–148

# Surgical Reconstruction of Musculocutaneous Nerves in Traumatic Brachial Plexus Injuries

## 27

Gustavo Adolpho de Carvalho

Contents

### 27.1
## Introduction

In traumatic lesions of the brachial plexus, which are caused mainly by car and motorcycle accidents, discontinuation of the neural structures may occur at the level of the roots (intra- or extraspinal), trunks, cords, peripheral nerves or in various combinations [2, 3, 5, 6]. This usually results in severely disabling symptoms, especially when the dominant arm is affected, in these often very young patients [1, 41, 42]. Therefore, considerations about the surgical management to improve the restoration of the functional integrity of at least part of the injured brachial plexus seems to be highly warranted. Possible strategies to reconstruct the brachial plexus include nerve grafting using one of the cervical roots (e.g. C5 or C6) or when all the cervical roots are avulsed, neurotisation (nerve transfer) using the intercostal nerves, the accessory nerve, or in some special cases the phrenic nerve [4, 9, 21, 29, 35, 36]. However, surgical outcome and functional restoration of the affected arm is still very limited [7, 8, 11, 13,

17, 18, 30]. A complete restoration of the arm function after a severe traction injury of the brachial plexus is almost impossible in the majority of the cases. Avulsion of all the cervical roots is often present after such traumatic lesions, and surgical reconstruction is therefore restricted and should focus on the main functions of the arm that could be successfully surgically repaired [31, 39]. Nerve grafting or transfer to the musculocutaneous nerve is undoubtedly one of the main goals of the surgical management [33, 41, 47]. Many important preoperative and intraoperative parameters, like the accurate neuroradiological diagnosis of root avulsion, the time interval between injury to surgery, the extent of the lesion, choice of the donor nerve for transplantation and surgical technique may play an important role in the final outcome.

### 27.2
## Preoperative Neuroradiological Diagnosis of Root Avulsion

In traction injuries, lesion of the brachial plexus may occur very often at the intraspinal level (root avulsion) or at the supra- and/or infraclavicular regions [5, 32]. Therefore, the exact preoperative diagnosis of cervical root avulsion in traumatic lesions of the brachial plexus is fundamental for the surgical planning and reconstruction of the brachial plexus [5]. Extradural inspection of the cervical roots via the usual supraclavicular approach may be misleading. Surgical experience on brachial plexus surgery has shown cases in which the extradural roots are still anatomically intact despite their disruption intradurally [5].

Computed tomography (CT) myelography from the C4 to the T1 level with 3-mm axial slices and/or magnetic resonance imaging (MRI), also with 3-mm axial slices, can be performed to diagnose cervical root avulsion. In the late 1900s, we performed a prospective study with total of 75 cervical roots that were radiologically analysed by two different observers regarding the presence of root avulsion. In order to confirm the integrity or avulsion of the cervical roots and further evaluate the accuracy of the radiological findings, an intradural surgical exploration of these cervical roots was performed via a hemilaminectomy from levels C5 and C7 on the affected side (Figs. 1 and 2). Our results showed that in around 85% of cases, CT-myelography and MRI correlated with the intraoperative root inspections and therefore displayed exactly the presence of cervical root avulsion. In recent years, new sequences of MRI with an excellent myelographic effect can certainly improve these results (Figs. 3 and 4).

## 27.3
## Intraoperative Electrophysiological Diagnosis of Root Avulsion

Concerning the intraoperative electrophysiological studies; unfortunately, nerve action potentials (NAPs) and somatosensory evoked potentials (SEPs) of the cervical roots during the peripheral exposure of the brachial plexus do not answer completely the question of continuity of the motor axons within the spinal cord. Root SEPs allow only the determination of the continuity of some vital axons within the spinal cord, but do not distinguish between motor and sensory fibres. On the other hand, intraoperative NAP recording with a stimulating electrode placed as proximal as possible and a recording electrode distal to the expected level of the lesion will adequately reveal or exclude regenerating motor axons at the periphery, but still not exclude the possibility of root avulsion. Stimulation of the nerve at a distal level and recording NAPs at the root level is also possible. In cases of preganglionic injury, NAPs are positive due to the preservation of the dorsal root ganglion and post-ganglionic sensory fibres. Conversely, in post-ganglionic injuries, distal sensory conduction is lost due the degeneration of the post-ganglionic sensory fibres. Thus, NAP recordings are negative and the integrity of the cervical root could be suspect [21]. However, electrophysiological intraoperative monitoring is based on sensory conduction, and intraspinal cervical root inspection displayed some cases in which the ventral (motor) root is avulsed with preserved continuity of the dorsal root at the same level, and vice versa. In such cases of partial root avulsion, electrophysiological methods, mainly based on sensory fibres, do not reliably determine the integrity of the intraspinal course of the motor rootlets.

## 27.4
## Time Interval Between Trauma and Surgery

The time interval between the lesion (trauma/injury) and the surgery is one of the most important factors for the final surgical result [10, 22, 34, 45]. Many authors advocate, in cases of no spontaneous recovery, that surgery should be done between 4 and 6 months after the accident. Surgical results for both grafting and neurotisation (nerve transfers) of the brachial plexus decline substantially if the surgery is performed 8–12 months after injury [28–30]. One of the main factors responsible for these poor results is the progressive degeneration of the muscle fibres, formation of fibrosis, and scar tissue within the muscle [27, 33]. Histopathogical studies demonstrate this degeneration as soon as 3–4 weeks after the injury, and the complete replacement of the muscle fibres into scar tissue after 2–3 years in cases of no spontaneous muscle reinnervation [20, 21, 25]. Surgical findings in such cases usually display an atrophic muscle with some ischemic signs [31, 33]. Besides that, the lack of movement in the affected arm may commonly lead to arthrosis of the elbow, hand and finger joints, which will handicap the final surgical result, even in cases of good post-operative muscle reinnervation.

## 27.5
## Length of the Nerve Grafts

Experimental works in the 1970s have shown no correlation between the length of the nerve graft and the final surgical results of reconstruction of the brachial plexus [37, 38, 44]. Graft vascularisation, for example, occurs not from the proximal nerve donor, but from the surrounding tissue in which the nerve graft is lying [12, 14, 43, 44]. Thus, compared with short grafts, longer grafts will not suffer from more ischemic events.

On the other hand, nerve grafts with a larger diameter will have a tendency to establish an insufficient vascularisation compared with grafts of small diameter. An analysis of the length of the grafts used in our series to reconstruct the musculocutaneous nerve displayed a better result in patients with grafts shorter than 12 cm. One underlying reason may be that the extent of the brachial plexus lesion was smaller in these cases than in those where longer grafts were necessary. Therefore, the length of the graft may be taken as an indicator of the extent of the injury, which also determines the chances of a functional recovery.

## 27.6
## Nerve Grafting Using C5 or C6 Cervical Roots

Radiological and surgical findings demonstrate the avulsion of C7 and C8 cervical roots in about 50–75% of the traction injuries of the brachial plexus [7, 9]. Therefore, common nerve donors to reconstruct the brachial plexus are the C5 and/or C6 cervical roots [5, 21]. There has been some discussion in the literature concerning a better surgical outcome using C5 roots for reconstruction the musculocutaneous nerve (elbow flexion) in traumatic

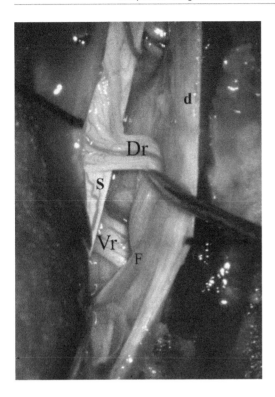

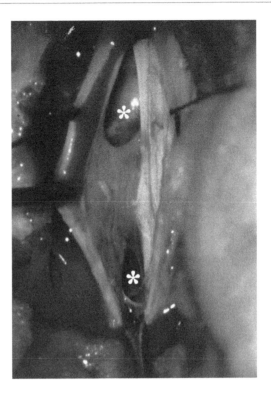

Fig. 1 Intraspinal surgical findings after a hemilaminectomy. Intact ventral and dorsal rootlets (*Vr* and *Dr*, respectively) from the cervical spinal cord (*S*) entering the intervertebral foramen (*F*). *d* Dura

Fig. 2 Intraspinal surgical findings after a hemilaminectomy. Complete root avulsion. Note the empty intervertebral foramen (*)

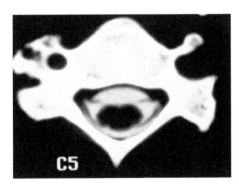

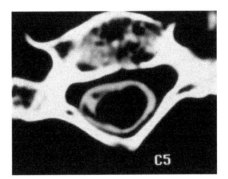

Fig. 3 Myelo computed tomography (CT) scan performed for the preoperative evaluation of cervical root avulsion after traumatic brachial plexus (BP) lesion. Note on both sides intact ventral and dorsal rootlets and absence of post-traumatic pseudomeningocele

Fig. 4 Myelo CT scan performed for the preoperative evaluation of cervical root avulsion after traumatic BP lesion. Note complete root avulsion of the ventral and dorsal roots at this level, despite the absence of a traumatic meningocele. Note the intact ventral and dorsal rootlets on the other side

brachial plexus lesion [15, 16, 27]. However, most series compared heterogeneous groups of patients with different preoperative time intervals. The analysis of our cases for the reconstruction of the musculocutaneous nerve with a similar preoperative time interval between injury and surgery failed to show a significant difference outcome of using the C5 rather than C6 nerve roots. Indeed, based on the fact that both of these cervical roots (C5 and C6) have almost the same number of motor fibres (around 25,000), and that just one-quarter of a cervical root may be actually enough for the reinnervation of the musculocutaneous nerve (around 6000 motor fibres), it is unlikely that the final surgical result would differ between roots [27, 29].

Thus, it seems that the main limiting factor is not which root is used for the transplantation or nerve grafting, but rather the "quality" of the root. Retrograde degeneration of a cervical root after trauma, which may occur in about 15–80% of the nerve fibres, and the presence of scar tissue within and around the nerve structure are the main drawbacks that may influence negatively the final surgical outcome [28–30].

Our results on nerve grafting of cervical roots C5 or C6 with the musculocutaneous nerve to restore elbow flexion in traumatic brachial plexus lesions shows an overall reinnervation rate of 62%. There is a significantly impaired functional outcome in patients operated 12 months after the original injury compared with cases that underwent surgery earlier (1 month; Fig. 5). However, by correlating the final results between patients operated between 7 and 12 months after the injury with patients treated 13 months after, no significant ($p < 0.05$) difference could be found. Other authors have also stressed the importance of early exploration of the brachial plexus in cases with no signs of regeneration, and divided this time interval into an early phase (3–6 months) and late phase of direct repair (6–12 months) [19, 23–26]. We also observed some isolated cases with proximal muscle reinnervation in patients who underwent surgery 12–18 months after the injury. However, reinnervation was only minor to moderate with no useful function reinnervation of the muscles (biceps muscle strength grade M1–M3 out of M5; Fig. 6). Finally, in our experience, in early operated cases (1–6 months after injury), surgical outcome can be improved by up 72% of reinnervation of the biceps muscles in cases of grafting C5 or C6 roots with the musculocutaneous nerve (Figs. 7 and 8).

## 27.7
## Neurotisation of the Musculocutaneous Nerve to Restore Elbow Flexion

In patients with complete avulsion of the cervical roots from the brachial plexus, different types of nerve transfers (neurotisations) can be done in order to regain important basic functions like elbow flexion and upper arm abduction. In 1963, Seddon was the first pioneer to perform a nerve transfer for restoration of elbow flexion, using one intercostal nerve to the musculocutaneous nerve [41]. The principle of this technique opened a whole new avenue for reconstructive surgery in patients with root avulsions following traumatic brachial plexus injuries [25–29].

Elbow flexion in patients with complete brachial plexus lesions has usually first priority for reconstruction by nerve transfer, and can be accomplished by using the following nerves as axon donors: accessory nerve, motor branches of the cervical plexus, intercostal nerves,

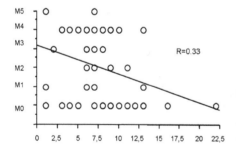

Fig. 5 Linear regression showing the relationship between the preoperative time interval from trauma to surgery, and the post-operative surgical result (grade of strength from the biceps muscle). The best final results were obtained by patients who underwent surgery between 2 and 6 months after the original trauma

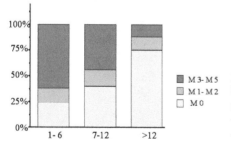

Fig. 6 Comparison of the functional and non-functional restoration of the biceps strength as a function of the different preoperative time intervals (1–6 months, 7–12 months, and over 12 months). A better functional recovery of the patients who underwent surgery between 1 and 6 months after the injury was achieved, compared to those operated later

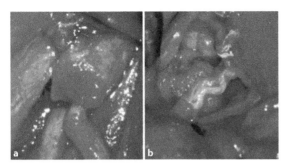

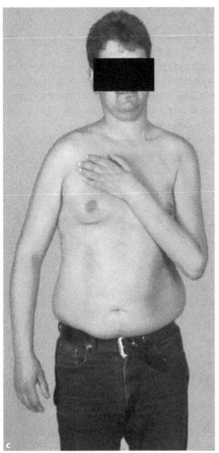

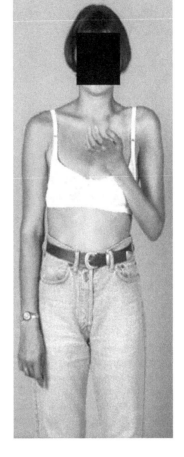

Fig. 7 **a** Intraoperative findings: the stump of the root at C5 cut just after the foramen after a supraclavicular approach do the BP. The root of C5 will be connected with two sural grafts. **b** The two sural grafts are then connected to the musculocutaneus nerve in the infraclavicular region. **c** Patient 2 years after the anastomosis of C5 to the musculocutaneus nerve via two sural grafts, showing a good recovery of elbow flexion

Fig. 8 Patient operated after a complete traumatic BP injury with no spontaneous recovery. An anastomosis of the root of C6 to the musculocutaneus nerve was performed via two sural grafts. After 2.5 years the patient show an excellent recovery of the biceps muscle (M4)

phrenic nerve, hypoglossus nerve and even the C7 root of the contralateral side [32, 35, 41].

In our experience, a branch of the accessory nerve can be often used as a donor to the musculocutaneous nerve to regain elbow flexion following brachial plexus injuries

with root avulsions. Despite the preoperative time interval and length of the sural grafts, overall reinnervation (M1–M5) of the biceps muscle can be reached in about 72% of the patients with a post-operative follow-up mean of 36±13 months (range: 1.9–7.25 years). In patients who

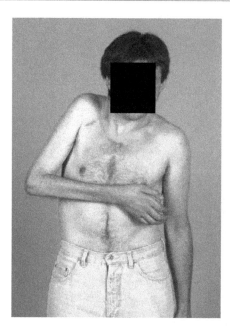

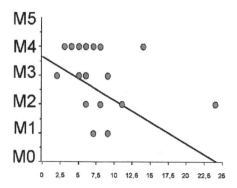

Fig. 10 Linear regression showing the relationship between the preoperative time interval from trauma to surgery, and the postoperative surgical result (grade of strength from the biceps muscle) after nerve transfer from the accessory nerve (branch) to the musculocutaneus nerve. Note that the outcome decreases in patients operated at longer time intervals after the initial injury. There was a significantly better result in the group of patients who underwent early surgery (1–6 months following injury)

Fig. 9 Patient operated after a complete traumatic BP injury with no spontaneous recovery and complete avulsion of the cervical roots from the BP. In this case an anastomosis of a branch of the accessory nerve with the musculocutaneus nerve was done with a single sural graft. After 1.5 years, the patient achieved a good recovery of elbow flexion (M4)

have been operated from 1 to 6 months after the injury, overall reinnervation improves to 86% of the cases; and functional reinnervation (M3–M5) can be reached in 71% of all patients who received early surgery (Fig. 9).

On the other hand, functional reinnervation (M3–M5) was reached in only 43% of all patients who received surgery 7–12 months after injury. In our analysis, a significantly better outcome for elbow flexion after nerve transfer with the accessory nerve was seen in patients treated during the first 6 months (Fig. 10). Similar results can also be achieved by transferring the phrenic nerve to the musculocutaneous nerve via a sural graft. Several other retrospective clinical studies have also shown an overall functional recovery of elbow flexion in approximately 64–84% of cases following nerve transfers with different donor nerves (accessory, phrenic and intercostal) [35, 41, 46].

1. In cases of no spontaneous reinnervation, surgery should be performed within 3–6 months of the injury.
2. Preoperative radiological diagnosis with CT myelography and/or MRI should be performed to evaluate cervical root avulsions.
3. Surgical results do not differ or depend on the donor nerve C5 or C6, but on the intraoperative characteristic of the roots (presence of scar tissue or degeneration).
4. The length of the grafts used for the transplantation will indirectly influence the final result, as it represent the extent of the brachial plexus injury.
5. In cases of root avulsion, a branch of the accessory nerve or the phrenic nerve can be used with a good surgical outcome.
6. One of the major points is the surgical technique on both nerve grafting and nerve transfer; perfect coaptation with no tension on the anastomosis site should always be attempted. A bad coaptation and further tension on the site of the anastomosis will stimulate the proliferation of scar tissue and formation of fibrosis and granulomas, which can impair the regeneration of growing axons [40].

## 27.8
## Summary

Different parameters that play an important role in the reconstruction of the musculocutaneous nerve after the traumatic injury of the brachial plexus:

### References

1. Allieu Y (1977) Exploration and direct treatment of neural lesions in traumatic paralysis caused by stretching of the brachial plexus in the adult. Rev Chir Orthop Reparatrice Appar Mot 63:107–122

2. Alnot JY, Daunois O, Oberlin C, et al (1992) Total paralysis of the brachial plexus caused by supra-clavicular lesions. Rev Chir Orthop Reparatrice Appar Mot 78:495–504

3. Alnot JY, Jolly A, Frot B (1981) Direct treatment of nerve lesions in brachial plexus injuries in adults – a series of 100 operated cases. Int Orthop 5:151–168

4. Berger A, Becker MH (1994) Brachial plexus surgery: our concept of the last twelve years. Microsurgery 15:760–767

5. Carvalho GA, Nikkhah G, Matthies C, et al (1997) Diagnosis of root avulsions in traumatic brachial plexus injuries. The value of myelo computed tomography and magnetic resonance imaging. J Neurosurg 86:69–76

6. Clarke D, Richardson P (1994) Peripheral nerve injury. Curr Opin Neurol 7:415–421

7. Comtet JJ, Sedel L, Fredenucci JF, et al (1988) Duchenne-Erb palsy. Experience with direct surgery. Clin Orthop 17–23

8. Davis P (1994) Managing brachial plexus injuries. Nurs Stand 8:31–34

9. Dolenc V (1986) Contemporary treatment of peripheral nerve and brachial plexus lesions. Neurosurg Rev 9:149–156

10. Dubuisson A, Kline DG (1992) Indications for peripheral nerve and brachial plexus surgery. Neurol Clin 10:935–951

11. Ferraresi S, Garozzo D, Griffini C, et al (1994) Brachial plexus injuries. Guidelines for management: our experience. Ital J Neurol Sci 15:273–284

12. Fesser Z, Radek A, Sokolowski Z (1991) Comparative evaluation of using autologous cable transplants and the classical microsurgical method of nerve anastomosis. Neurol Neurochir Pol 25:208–213

13. Fisher TR (1990) Nerve injury. Injury 21:302–304

14. Freilinger G, Gruger H, Holle J, et al (1975) Zur Methodik der sensomotorisch differenzierten Faszikelnaht peripherer Nerven. Handchirurgie 7:133

15. Glasby MA, Hems TE (1995) Repairing spinal roots after brachial plexus injuries. Paraplegia 33:359–361

16. Harat M, Radek A (1993) Management tactics in brachial plexus injuries. Neurol Neurochir Pol 27:829–837

17. Henke R (1985) Microsurgical reconstruction of the brachial plexus. Zentralbl Chir 110:749–757

18. Hentz VR, Narakas A (1988) The results of microneurosurgical reconstruction in complete brachial plexus palsy. Assessing outcome and predicting results. Orthop Clin North Am 19:107–114

19. Jamieson A, Hughes S (1980) The role of surgery in the management of closed injuries to the brachial plexus. Clin Orthop Relat Res 147:210–215

20. Kline DG (1979) Macroscopic and microscopic concomitants of nerve repair. Clin Neurosurg 26:582–606

21. Kline DG (1983) Operative management of selected brachial plexus lesions. Neurosurg 58:631–649

22. Mehta VS, Banerji AK, Tripathi RP (1993) Surgical treatment of brachial plexus injuries. Br J Neurosurg 7:491–500

23. Millesi H (1969) Reconstruction of transsected peripheral nerves and nerve transplantation. Munch Med Wochenschr 111:2669–2674

24. Millesi H (1977) Interfascicular grafts for repair of peripheral nerves of the upper extremity. Orthop Clin North Am 8:387–404

25. Millesi H (1987) Surgical treatment of traumatic brachial plexus lesions. Orthopade 16:434–440

26. Millesi H (1988) Brachial plexus injuries. Nerve grafting. Clin Orthop 36–42

27. Narakas A (1977) Indications and results of direct surgical treatment in lesions caused by stretching of the brachial plexus. Indications for direct surgical treatment. Rev Chir Orthop Reparatrice Appar Mot 63:88–106

28. Narakas A (1980) The surgical treatment of traumatic brachial plexus lesions. Int Surg 65:521–527

29. Narakas A (1982) Neurotization or nerve transfer for the brachial plexus. Ann Chir Main 1:101–108

30. Narakas A (1985) The treatment of brachial plexus injuries. Int Orthop 9:29–36

31. Oberlin C, Beal D, Leechavengvongs S, et al (1994) Nerve transfer to biceps muscle using a part of ulnar nerve for C5–C6 avulsion of the brachial plexus: anatomical study and report of four cases. J Hand Surg Am 19:232–237

32. Pazolt HJ (1986) Microsurgical treatment of brachial plexus injuries. Zentralbl Chir 111:589–596

33. Penkert G (1991) Beurteilung und Behandlung peripherer Nervenverletzung. Neurologie 7:57–64

34. Penkert G (1993) Periphere Nervenvertzung–Aktueller Behandlunsstandard. Zentralbl Neurochir 54:47–51

35. Penkert G, Carvalho GA, Nikkhah G, et al (1996) Nerven – Reinnervation bei Wurzelausrissen des Plexus brachialis mittels des N. accessorius als Spendernerv. In: Berghaus A (ed) Plastische und Wiederherstellungschirurgie. Einhorn, Reinbeck, pp 468–470

36. Samardzic M, Sekulovic N, Grujicic D (1991) Microsurgical reconstruction of peripheral nerve injuries. Srp Arh Celok Lek 119:14–17

37. Samii M (1972) Interfaszikuläre autologe Nerventransplantationen. Indikation, Technik und Ergebnisse. Dtsch Ärztebl 70:1257–1262

38. Samii M (1975) Use of the microtechniques in peripheral nerve surgery – experience with over 300 cases. In: Handa H (ed) Microneurosurgery. Igoku Shoin, Tokyo, pp 85–92

39. Samii M, Kahl RI (1972) Klinische Resultate der Autologen Nerventransplantationen. Med Mitt 42:189

40. Samii M, Wallenborn R (1972): Tierexperimentelle Untersuchungen über den Einfluss der Spannung auf den Regenerationserfolg nach Nervennaht. Acta Neurochir 27:87

41. Samii M, Carvalho GA, Nikkhah G, et al (1996) Nerven – Neurotization des Plexus brachialis: Interkostalennerven mit dem N. musculocutaneus. In: Berghaus A (ed) Plastische und Wiederherstellungschirurgie. Einhorn, Reinbeck, pp 471–472

42. Samii M, Carvalho GA, Nikkhah G, et al (1996) Nerven – Zur funktionellen Rekonstruktion des N. axillaris bei traumatischen Armplexus Läsionen: In: Berghaus A (ed) Plastische und Wiederherstellungschirurgie. Einhorn, Reinbeck, pp 466–467

43. Samii M, Schürmann K, Scheinpflug W, et al (1971) Experimental studies comparing grafting with autogenous and irradiated freeze dried homologous nerves. Mod Asp Neurosurg 3:263–266

44. Seddon HJ (1975) Surgical Disorders of the Peripheral Nerves. Churchill Livingstone, London

45. Sedel L (1982) The results of surgical repair of brachial plexus injuries. J Bone Joint Surg Br 64:54–66

46. Sedel L (1988) Repair of severe traction lesions of the brachial plexus. Clin Orthop Relat Res 237:62–66

47. Thomeer RT (1991) Recovery of brachial plexus injuries. Clin Neurol Neurosurg 93:3–11

# Peripheral Nerve Entrapment Syndromes of the Lower Extremity

## 28

Eduardo Fernandez, Francesco Doglietto, Liverana Lauretti, Alessandro Ciampini, and Luca Denaro

Contents

## 28.1

## General Concepts on Peripheral Nerve Entrapment Syndromes

Patients affected by peripheral nerve entrapment syndromes generally complain of paresthesias, pain, and/or motor weakness in the territory supplied by the involved nerve. Clinical manifestations can be divided into three stages [8]:

1. Stage I: Rest pain and intermittent paresthesias that are worse at night.
2. Stage II: Constant paresthesias and numbness that can occasionally be associated with muscle weakness.
3. Stage III: Constant pain, muscle atrophy, and permanent sensory loss.

Symptoms depend on the internal anatomy of the affected nerve. Compression, stretching, and friction are the mechanisms that cause peripheral nerve entrapment syndromes. On physical examination, changes in temperature or pain sensation and motor atrophy or weakness in the area of the involved nerve may be observed. Symptoms may be provoked or exacerbated by direct compression of the nerve or by changes in the position of the extremity. Tinel's sign is often present, being evoked by percussion over the nerve, which causes an electrical-like sensation that radiates along the nerve and over its innervated territory. A suspected entrapment syndrome is generally confirmed by conventional nerve conduction studies and electromyography, which allows the differentiation between nerve entrapments and several other pathologies like ischemic mononeuropathies, generalized peripheral neuropathies, radiculopathies, or plexopathies [12]. Surgical treatment of nerve entrapment syndromes with purely sensitive symptoms should be reserved only for cases where symptoms persist despite medical and physical therapy. Conversely, surgical treatment should be performed promptly when motor deficits and positive electrophysiology exist. In fact, functional recovery depends strongly on the duration of symptoms. Surgery serves to free the nerve from the mechanisms of entrapment (i.e., compression, stretching, or friction). By eliminating any compressive factor, mobilization of the nerve is obtained.

This chapter is dedicated to entrapment syndromes involving nerves of the inferior extremity.

## 28.1.1

## Entrapment of the Sciatic Nerve: the Piriformis Syndrome

The sciatic nerve originates from nerve roots L4–S2, arising from the lumbosacral plexus and leaving the pelvis through the greater sciatic foramen. It passes over the obturator internus muscle and beneath the gluteal and

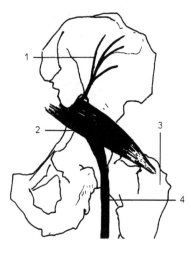

Fig. 1 Schematic drawing of the posterior aspect of the hip and femur illustrating the site of entrapment of the sciatic nerve. *1* Superior gluteal nerve, *2* piriformis muscle, *3* femur greater trochanter, *4* sciatic nerve

the piriformis muscles (Fig. 1). The nerve courses posterior and medial to the hip joint and then deep in the thigh and posterior to the femur: its two distinct trunks separate generally at the distal portion of the thigh to form the common peroneal and tibial nerves. Branches coming off the tibial division in the proximal thigh innervate all except one of the hamstring muscles (the short head of the biceps femoris); all muscles below the knee receive innervation from the sciatic nerve and, except the saphenous nerve, all sensory nerves derive from the sciatic nerve [20].

The most common entrapment syndrome of the sciatic nerve is the piriformis syndrome, representing the cause of nondiscal sciatica in almost 70% of 239 patients in a recent report by Filler et al. [4]. The most prominent symptom is pain in the buttock radiating down into the posterior thigh; weakness, numbness, and paresthesias are generally mild if present [4, 20]. Stretching of the piriformis muscle against the sciatica nerve by passive internal rotation and adduction of the thigh (Freiberg sign) or active contraction of the piriformis muscle by active external rotation and abduction of the thigh against resistance (Pace sign) have been proposed as diagnostic signs. Magnetic resonance imaing (MRI) neurography of the lumbosacral plexus and sciatic nerve might allow a more accurate diagnosis in suspected cases and can exclude other possible causes of sciatic nerve lesion [4, 11]: unilateral hyperintensity of the sciatic nerve at the sciatic notch appears to be a relatively specific sign of piriformis syndrome [4].

Computed tomography (CT)- or MRI-guided injection of a local anaesthetic (Marcaine) is a procedure with diagnostic and sometimes therapeutic value: Filler et al [4] reported permanent relief in 37 patients (23% of all patients) after one or two injection, possibly due to relief from muscle spasm. Excellent or good outcome was reported in 82% of surgically treated patients: the surgical procedure consists of a transgluteal approach to the piriformis muscle, with resection of the muscle and neuroplasty of the sciatic nerve.

A myofascial band is a rare cause of sciatic nerve entrapment in the thigh [3, 17, 20].

### 28.1.2
### Entrapment of the Lateral Femoral Cutaneous Nerve

The lateral femoral cutaneous nerve (LFCN) is primarily a sensory nerve that innervates the anterolateral aspect of the thigh. The origin of this nerve is generally from the ventral branch of the second lumbar nerve. It then passes behind the posterior aspect of the psoas muscle, runs in the iliac fossa beneath the fascia of the iliac muscle, and reaches a fibro-osseous tunnel delimited by the anterior superior iliac spine, the anterior inferior iliac spine, and the inguinal ligament (Fig. 2). The nerve exits the pelvis, crossing a narrow tunnel between two slips of the attachment of the inguinal ligament, then pierces the fascia lata, becoming superficial. After running for 2–3 cm in the fascia lata, lateral to the sartorious muscle, it provides the terminal gluteal and femoral branches, which have a highly variable location and course [2].

Meralgia paresthetica (MP) is an entrapment of the LFCN at the level of the inguinal ligament with an incidence rate of about 4.3/10,000 persons/year, being more prevalent among males and those aged between 41 and 60 years. It is often associated with carpal tunnel syndrome, pregnancy, and obesity [6, 18]. It is mostly unilateral, but 8–12% of patients experience bilateral symptoms [9]. Clinically, MP is characterized by dysesthesia or anesthesia, intermittent or persistent burning, coldness, lightning pain, tingling, and hair loss in the anterolateral aspect of the thigh. Patients usually complain of a characteristic increased sensitivity to clothing.

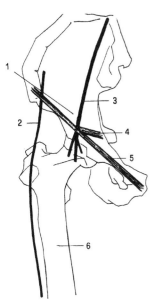

Fig. 2 Schematic drawing of the anterior aspect of the hip and femur illustrating the sites of entrapment of the femoral and lateral femoral cutaneous nerves. *1* Lacuna musculorum, *2* lateral femoral cutaneous nerve, *3* femoral nerve, *4* ileo-pectineal ligament, *5* inguinal ligament, *6* femur

The LFCN can also be irritated by the wearing of tight clothes or belts, by prolonged standing or walking, by an abdominal mass [6], and by iatrogenic causes like surgical scars, iliac crest bone graft removal, laparoscopic hernia repair, and prolonged wrong position during a surgical operation. The nerve can also be the site of a metabolic neuropathy correlated with diabetes mellitus, alcoholism, or lead poisoning [19].

The diagnosis of MP is primarily clinical, the neurological dysfunction being only sensory. It is necessary to exclude any other cause of compression along the course of the nerve. Lumbar and pelvis CT or MRI scanning should exclude L2–L3 pathology and pelvic masses. Electrophysiology, such as conduction studies and somatosensory evoked potentials, can confirm the diagnosis of an LFCN lesion and, above all, exclude other causes of thigh pain and numbness.

The initial treatment of MP is nonsurgical. Nonsteroidal anti-inflammatory drugs, local injection of steroids and anesthetics, weight loss, and avoidance of local physical constricting factors can be recommended [16]. Conservative treatment reduces symptoms to an acceptable level, and long-lasting relief is achieved in 60–90% of cases. Surgical therapy is necessary when the complaints are intractable and disabling. One method advocates transection of the LFCN under the inguinal ligament. Another method, which we prefer, consists of microsurgical decompression and neurolysis, eliminating any compressive factor under the inguinal ligament. Very recently, Siu and Chandran [16] reported their experience on the surgical treatment of 42 patients: decompression was achieved by freeing the nerve at three levels: (1) the tendinous arch from the iliac fascia, (2) the inguinal ligament anteriorly and a sling of fascia posteriorly, and (3) the deep fascia

of the thigh along each division. Six weeks after surgery, 43% experienced complete relief, 40% partial relief, and 17% of no relief; at a median follow-up of 4 years, complete relief was obtained in 73% of patients, and partial and no relief in 20% and 7%, respectively [16].

### 28.1.3
## Entrapment of the Common Peroneal Nerve

In the upper popliteal fossa, the sciatic nerve divides into two terminal branches, the peroneal and the tibial nerve. From its origin, the peroneal nerve diverges from the tibial nerve going downward and externally along the medial margin of the long head of the biceps femoris muscle and its tendon. It then passes laterally around the fibular head (the floor of the "fibular tunnel") under the soleus and peroneus longus muscles (the roof of the "fibular tunnel"), entering the anterolateral aspect of the leg and dividing into two terminal branches, the deep and the superficial peroneal nerves (Fig. 3).

Common peroneal mononeuropathy occurs more frequently in men than women and is idiopathic in 16% of cases, iatrogenic in 21.7%, correlated to posture or weight loss in 23.2% and 14.5%, respectively, due to external compression in 5.8%, to artrogenic cyst at the fibula in 1.4%, and is post-traumatic in 10% of cases [1]. It is also reported in 7.3% of bedridden patients [1]. The common peroneal nerve may be compressed in the popliteal fossa by abnormal deposition of fatty tissue or by a Baker's cyst. At the fibular head, superficiality and fixation to the bone by dense connective tissue renders the nerve particularly vulnerable to pressure and traction. The most common cause of compression is cross-leg palsy. A sudden and en-

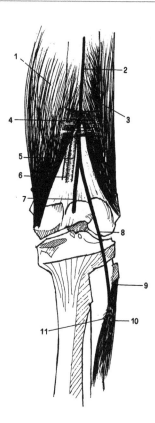

Fig. 3 Schematic drawing of the posterior aspect of the thigh illustrating the sites of entrapment of the sciatic and peroneal nerves. *1* Great adductor muscle, *2* sciatic nerve, *3* biceps femoris, *4* fibrous band, *5-6* politeal artery and vein, *7* tibial nerve, *8* peroneal nerve, *9* long peroneal muscle insertion, *10* superficial peroneal nerve, *11* deep peroneal nerve

ergic flexion and inversion of the foot is one of the most common mechanisms of injury. Deficit of the common peroneal nerve is expressed by:

1. Weakness/atrophy of the muscles located in the anterior compartment of the leg resulting in impaired foot flexion, with consequent foot drop or equine foot, and foot eversion.
2. Sensory impairment over the anterolateral aspect of the foreleg and the dorsum of the foot; pain is variable and less common.

Clinical examination and electrophysiological and radiological studies of the popliteal fossa and the lumbar spine serve to recognize this syndrome. In cases in which an external compressive factor is clearly recognized, a good recovery occurs spontaneously; in other instances, operative exploration should be proposed.

A skin incision is performed on the popliteal area and superior third of the anterolateral aspect of the leg. After opening the fascia, the nerve is isolated and gradually released along its course up to its terminal branches, elimi-

nating any compression exerted by scar tissue, fibrous bands, and ganglia. Microsurgical external and internal neurolysis can complete the procedure. Functional recovery is related to the duration and severity of symptoms.

## 28.1.4
### Entrapment of the Deep Peroneal Nerve: Anterior Tarsal Tunnel Syndrome

From its origin, the deep peroneal nerve goes downward and anteriorly in front of the interosseous membrane of the leg and reaches the anterior tarsal tunnel over the dorsal aspect of the ankle, lateral to the tibialis anterior muscle. At the ankle, the nerve and the anterior tibial vessels pass under the inferior extensor retinaculum or cruciate ligament of the ankle and over the extensor hallucis longus muscle and tendon (Fig. 4). Close to this ligament, the deep peroneal nerve divides into a lateral branch, innervating the extensor digitorum brevis muscle, and a medial branch, innervating the skin of the dorsal aspect of the foot between the first and second toes. Here, at the anterior tarsal tunnel, the deep peroneal nerve can be entrapped. Symptoms are aching or tightness at the ankle and dorsum of the foot, and numbness and paresthesias in the first dorsal web space. Clinical examination may reveal plantar and medial deviation of the foot, as an antalgic attempt, weakness-atrophy of the extensor digitorum brevis muscle, and hypoesthesia in the first dorsal web. Electrophysiological studies, as well as lumbar CT or MRI scanning and radiological studies of the ankle can easily detect the cause of the deep peroneal nerve neuropathy [14]. Like other entrapment syndromes, operative release of the entrapped nerve is indicated only when nonsurgical treatments fail. The skin incision is made on the dorsum of the foot centered on the painful area. Then, the cruciate ligament of the ankle, which is often thickened, is skeletonized and sectioned, and the deep peroneal nerve and its branches are released from the adhesions to the surrounding tissues, including the cruciate ligament itself. Results are very satisfactory.

## 28.1.5
### Entrapment of the Superficial Peroneal Nerve

The superficial peroneal nerve lies between the extensor digitorum lungus and peroneal muscles. It innervates the peroneus longus and brevis muscles. About 10 cm proximally to the ankle, on the anterolateral aspect of the leg, the nerve pierces the fascia, becoming a cutaneous nerve, and gives rise to its sensitive terminal braches. The point where the nerve exits the fascia may be a site of nerve entrapment. Symptoms are purely sensitive, characterized by pain and paresthesias in the anterolateral aspect of the leg, ankle and foot. Compression and percussion at the fascia exit of the superficial peroneal nerve elicit regional

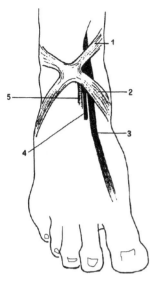

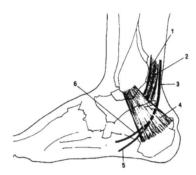

Fig. 4  Schematic drawing showing the dorsal aspect of the right ankle and foot illustrating the site of entrapment of the deep peroneal nerve. *1* Cruciate ligament, *2* medial inferior branch of the cruciate ligament, *3* tendon of the extensor hallucis longus muscle, *4* deep peroneal nerve, *5* dorsal artery of the foot

Fig. 5  Schematic drawing of the medial aspect of the right ankle and foot illustrating the site of entrapment of the tibial nerve. *1* Tendon of the posterior tibial muscle, *2* tendon of the flexor digitorum longus muscle, *3* tibial nerve, *4* flexor retinaculum, *5* medial plantar nerve, *6* lateral plantar nerve

pain and paresthesias. After a longitudinal skin incision, centered on the positive point of Tinel's sign, the superficial peroneal nerve is recognized at its fascia exit. The fascia is then incised to release the nerve. Results are good.

### 28.1.6
### Entrapment of the Tibial Nerve: Posterior Tarsal Tunnel Syndrome

From its origin, the tibial nerve goes downward through the popliteal fossa and reaches the leg deep to the gastrocnemius muscle. In the distal third of the leg, the nerve becomes more superficial, passes medial to the Achilles tendon, reaches the ankle and the sole, passing posterior to the medial malleolus, under the flexor or medial retinaculum, in the tarsal tunnel (Fig. 5). It then divides in its terminal branches: the medial and lateral plantar nerves. The term tarsal tunnel syndrome (also called "posterior" or medial tarsal tunnel syndrome) indicates entrapment of the tibial nerve at the ankle, in the tarsal tunnel. Post-traumatic fibrosis due to fracture, tenosynovitis, ganglia jogging, and misdirected movements of the foot are favoring factors. The main symptoms are plantar burning pain and/or paresthesias, which can be exacerbated by prolonged standing and walking. A positive Tinel's sign is evoked with percussion or pressure over the flexor retinaculum. Electrophisiological examination is essential to confirm the diagnosis. In addition, MRI may be useful to delineate the tarsal tunnel more accurately or if a local lesion or tumor is suspected [15]. More commonly, tarsal

tunnel syndrome must be differentiated with Achilles tendonitis and plantar fasciitis. Surgical treatment consists of a skin incision between the medial malleulus and the Achilles tendon extended distally toward the medial margin of the foot. Then, the flexor retinaculum is skeletonized and sectioned after locating the tibial nerve proximal to the retinaculum. Neurolysis of the tibial nerve and its terminal branches is then carried out and the nerve is completely released. This procedure is generally followed by complete relief of the entrapment syndrome. An endoscopic technique has been described, reporting good results [10].

### 28.2
### Morton's Metatarsalgia

The common plantar digital nerves are the terminal branches of the medial and lateral plantar nerves that originate from the tibial nerve. Morton's metatarsalgia is a paroxysmal neuralgia that is associated with a spindle-shaped swelling or neuroma of a common plantar digital nerve, just before its bifurcation into the proper plantar digital nerves, at the level of the metatarsal heads (Fig. 6). Most frequently, the common plantar digital nerve of the third intermetatarsal space is involved, and about 80% of the patients are women. Chronic trauma, ischemia, bursitis, and entrapment neuropathy have been proposed as possible etiologic factors [7]. The symptom is a burning pain in the sole of the foot, between the head of the third and fourth metatarsal bones and the corresponding two

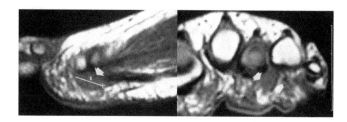

Fig. 6 Magnetic resonance images of a Morton's neuroma (*arrows*) in lateral (*left*) and coronal (*right*) views

toes. Pain can be elicited by walking or can be continuous, radiating proximally. Pressure on the sole or moving the heads of metatarsals III and IV or IV and V against each other will trigger intense pain. A dorsal injection of a local anesthetic into the third intermetatarsal space blocks the common plantar digital nerve at its bifurcation site, eliminating pain and confirming the diagnosis. Morton's metatarsalgia can be also confirmed electrophysiologically. Ultrasonography and especially MRI are useful in demonstrating the neuroma. Some patients obtain significant improvement with conservative measures such as shoe modifications. Interdigital injection of local anesthetic, steroid combinations, and phenol have been reported to provide long-term relief [5, 13]. If incapacitating pain persists, surgical treatment is required. The interdigital neuroma is excised under local anesthesia. The common plantar digital nerve of the third intermetatarsal space can be reached either by a plantar or a dorsal approach. The dorsal approach requires more preparation and is generally presented as having the advantage that the patient can bear weight on the sole earlier than the patient treated with a plantar approach. Either neurectomy or neurolysis can be performed. To reach nerves that are plantar, we prefer a plantar approach. Furthermore, we prefer neurolysis, instead of neurectomy, using microsurgical techniques to eliminate any external compression such as local fibrous bands. Compared with neurectomy, neurolysis permits both preservation of nerve function and relief from pain. Microsurgery minimizes the surgical trauma and permits a better understanding of the local anatomy and better view of compressive factors.

## References

1. Aprile I, Caliandro P, Giannini F, et al (2005) Italian multicentre study of peroneal mononeuropathy at the fibular head – study design and preliminary results. Acta Neurochir Suppl 92:63–68

2. Aszmann OC, Dellon ES, Dellon AL (1997) Anatomical course of the lateral femoral cutaneous nerve and its susceptibility to compression and injury. Plast Reconstr Surg 100:600–604

3. Banerjee T, Hall CD (1976) Sciatic entrapment neuropathy. Case report. J Neurosurg 45:216–217

4. Filler AG, Haynes J, Jordan SE, et al (2005) Sciatica of non-disc origin and piriformis syndrome: diagnosis by magnetic resonance neurography and interventional magnetic resonance imaging with outcome study of resulting treatment. J Neurosurg Spine 2:99–115

5. Greenfield J, Rea J Jr, Ilfeld FW (1984) Morton's interdigital neuroma: indications for treatment by local injections versus surgery. Clin Orthop 185:142–144

6. Gregory K (2000) Meralgia paresthetica, the elusive diagnosis. Ann Surg 232:281–286

7. Hassouna H, Singh D (2005) Morton's metatarsalgia: pathogenesis, aetiology and current management. Acta Orthop Belg 71:646–655

8. Hirose CB, McGarvey WC (2004) Peripheral nerve entrapments. Foot Ankle Clin 9:255–269

9. Kitchen C, Simpson J (1972) Meralgia paresthetica. A review of 67 patients. Acta Neurol Scand 48:547–555

10. Krishnan KG, Pinzer T, Schackert G (2006) A novel endoscopic technique in treating single nerve entrapment syndromes with special attention to ulnar nerve transposition and tarsal tunnel release: clinical application. Neurosurgery 59:89–100

11. Lewis AM, Layzer R, Engstrom JW, et al (2006) Magnetic resonance neurography in extraspinal sciatica. Arch Neurol 63:1469–1472

12. Mabin D (1997) Distal nerve comprssion of the leg. Clinical and electrophysiologic study. Neurophysiol Clin 27:9–24

13. Magnan B, Marangon A, Frigo A, Bartolozzi P (2005) Local phenol injection in the treatment of interdigital neuritis of the foot (Morton's neuroma). Chir Organi Mov 90:371–377

14. Masciocchi C, Catalucci A, Barile A (1998) Ankle impingement syndromes. Eur J Radiol 27:70–73

15. McCrory P, Bell S, Bradshaw C (2002) Nerve entrapment of the lower leg, ankle and foot in sport. Sport Med 32:371–391

16. Siu TLT, Chandran KN (2005) Neurolysis for meralgia paresthetica – an operative series of 45 cases. Surg Neurol 63:19–23

17. Sogaard I (1983) Sciatic nerve entrapment. Case report. J Neurosurg 58:275–276

18. Van Slobbe AM, Bohnen AM, Bersan RMD, et al (2004) Incidence rates and determinants in maralgia paresthetica in general practice. J Neurol 251:294–297

19. Williams PH, Trzil KP (1991) Managment of meralgia paresthetica. J Neurosurg 74:76–80

20. Yuen EC, So YT (1999) Sciatic neuropathy. Neurol Clin 17:617–631

# Hypoglossal–Facial Nerve Anastomosis

# 29

Eduardo Fernandez, Francesco Doglietto, Liverana Lauretti, Alessandro Ciampini, and Luca Denaro

## Contents

## 29.1
## Introduction

Facial nerve (FN) palsy is one of the most devastating nerve injuries with important functional and psychological impact on the patient's life [40]. Among the various aetiologies, the neurosurgeon is most likely to deal with the traumatic [32] and neoplastic ones. FN palsy indeed remains one of the major complications of vestibular schwannoma surgery, and though its incidence has significantly diminished in recent decades thanks to microsurgery and neuromonitoring, it is reported at between 3% and 19% of major modern series [23, 29, 41].

A multitude of reconstructive techniques using muscle transfers, free muscle grafts, shortening or plication of weakened muscles, dermal transplants, fascial transplants, and the removal of redundant skin, have been described for reanimation of the paralysed face [37]. When the proximal FN stump is not available, in the presence of viable facial muscles, the use of an intact donor nerve to neurotise the distal FN is the ideal choice. The most commonly used donor nerve is the hypoglossus, which is connected to the FN at the level of the stylomastoid foramen (SMF).

Here, we present the anatomical and physiological bases of the hypoglossal–FN anastomosis (HFA) as well as the indications, timing and surgical techniques of this operation. Animal experimental data are also presented.

## 29.2
## Brief History

Detailed historical overviews of HFA have been recently provided by Hammerschlag [18] and by Streppel et al [44].

At the end of the 19th century, initial attempts at FN reinnervation used the spinal accessory nerve as a donor nerve [18, 44]. Charles Ballance was probably among the first to accomplish an accessory–FN anastomosis in 1895 in London [5, 44] and the technique was also later used by other surgeons. Due to its disappointing results, Ballance speculated on the use of other cranial nerves for facial reanimation: "we considered whether it might not be practicable to select for anastomosis with the distal segment of the paralysed facial some other healthy nerve supplying muscles whose cortical centre is nearer to the face centre than in the case of the shoulder" [3, 44].

Körte [25] was the first to perform a HFA in 1901 for a facial paralysis due to temporal bone resection following infection; he used a so-called "end-to-side" nerve anastomosis [30, 44]. Since the very beginning of HFA, attempts to avoid the resulting hemitongue atrophy were made, but after extensive experience with the "end-to-side" HFA, Ballance's opinion was that the curing of facial palsy justified the sacrifice of movements of half the tongue as the end-to-side anastomosis may militate against a better restoration of the facial movement [4, 18]. In 1932, Ballance and Duel were actually the first to propagate a complete transection of the hypoglossal nerve (HN) to perform an end-to-end HFA [4, 30].

As reported by Hammerschlag [18], Körte also contemplated the possibility of central nervous system plasticity: "it is a most remarkable physiologic fact that ganglion cells of the hypoglossal or the accessory nerve-nucleus can acquire under voluntary influence the ability to induce contractions of muscles originally innervated from other nerve centres. We cannot yet decide whether there are connections between the two areas of nerve ganglia or whether by willpower, the nerve centre can adopt or become accustomed to stimulating a newly acquired muscle system" (translated by Stennert) [18, 43]. The theoretical speculations on the functional recovery after HFA remain indeed up-to-date [44].

Over the following several decades, many authors observed that HFA proved to be a reliable method of achieving reinnervation of the facial musculature. Most authors observed that loss of hypoglossal function following HFA has minimal disabling sequelae unless there are concomitant ipsilateral lower cranial nerve deficits [18].

With the subsequent advent of the microscope, different variations of the classic end-to-end HFA have been suggested, with the aim of achieving a good facial function restoration without impairing tongue function (Table 1).

## 29.3
## Indications

Neurotisation techniques (i.e. the use of a donor nerve to reinnervate the FN), are indicated when a direct nerve repair is not possible and the facial muscles are viable. More precisely, a neurotisation technique is indicated in the following three situations [40]: (1) loss of the proximal part of the FN at the brainstem in the cerebellopontine angle (CPA); (2) destruction of the facial motor nucleus, as in pontine haemorrhages due to pontine cavernomas; (3) internal axonotmesis, as can be presumed in cases in which, during a CPA operation, the nerve appeared to be anatomically in continuity, but functional recovery does not occur after 12 months. Possible donor nerves used for reanimation procedures are the phrenic, spinal accessory, hypoglossal and contralateral FNs [40].

While the spinal accessory–FN anastomosis achieves evident reinnervation of the facial muscles, the functional and cosmetic results are poor. In fact, the innervation is only sufficiently present on movement of the shoulder. The gross shoulder movements are not apt to equal the fine and differentiated pattern of facial innervation [40].

Facio-facial ("cross face") anastomosis [40, 41] can yield good results and may be used in patients in whom

no other cranial nerve can be sacrificed. This procedure entails the use of up to one-half of the plexiform FN branches on the healthy side of the face, which remains without a discernible deficit. These contralateral branches can be connected, using sural nerve grafts, to the corresponding branches of the paralysed side. Since the consequent reinnervation is fairly weak, most authors recommend additional muscle transfers [6, 18, 40, 41].

HFA yields the chance of strong reliable reinnervation and is the most popular operation for facial reanimation (Table 1) [40]. When the hypoglossus cannot be sacrificed, either the less powerful facio-facial anastomosis or the alternative types of HFA techniques, aiming to preserve tongue function, can be used.

## 29.4
## Timing

On one hand, facial movement after spontaneous recovery of the FN is generally better than after HFA. On the other hand, several degenerative phenomena occur after FN injury, such as muscular atrophy, nerve fibrosis, pontine nucleus degeneration, and degeneration and loss of plasticity and information in the facial area of the motor cortex [40, 41]. The closer the interruption is located to the proximal nuclei (i.e. at the FN origin at the brainstem), the faster these degenerative processes will occur. Timing is therefore a fundamental issue in HFA, especially after FN injury in CPA, as in vestibular schwannoma surgery. To achieve an optimal result, the reanimation procedure should be performed before the degenerative mechanisms can negatively influence its final result.

Although some investigators initially reported that the onset of FN remission can occur as late as 2 years after tumour resection [34], others reported that this is quite rare [26–28]. Kunihiro et al [27, 28] noted that two-thirds of their patients recovered spontaneously from complete facial paralysis; signs of recovery appeared most frequently between 3 and 4 months after surgery, and never after 12 months.

Although initial reports did not document any difference between early and late repair of the FN [34], it is now generally recommended that the nerve reanimation procedure should be performed within 6 months and, in any case, never scheduled later than 1 year after the onset of the paralysis [28, 31, 41]. Good results are obtained more frequently when patients are operated before 1 year of persistent paralysis, rather than later [26, 40]. Experimental research in guinea pigs has revealed that nerve regeneration and rearrangement in the central nucleus were better in early HFA [8]. However, if a patient is treated as late as 2 years after onset of paralysis, HFA offers some opportunity of facial muscle reinnervation, but a very satisfying result is less probable [41].

Table 1 Review of some of the major series of hypoglossal–facial nerve anastomosis and its suggested variations. *HHFA* HFA with longitudinal splitting of the hypoglossal nerve, *JIG* Jump interpositional nerve graft, *HN* hypoglossal nerve, *FN* transposition: rerouting of the intratemporal facial nerve and/or parotid release manoeuvre, *H-B* House-Brackmann scale

| Technique | Author (year) | No. of patients | Facial restoration (%) (H-B scale) | | | | | Hemitongue atrophy (%)/swallowing, chewing and speech disturbances (%) |
|---|---|---|---|---|---|---|---|---|
| | | | II | III | IV | V | VI | |
| HFA | Conley and Baker (1979) [9] | 137 | | 65 | 18 | 17 | | 100/45 |
| | Pensak et al. (1986) [33] | 61 | | 42 | 48 | 10 | | 100/74 |
| | Samii and Matthies (1997) [41] | 29 | | 96 | 4 | | | 100/7 |
| HHFA with longitudinal split of the HN (without JIG) | Cusimano and Sekhar (1994) [10] | 1 | | 100 | | | | 100/100 |
| | Arai et al. (1995) [1][b] | 8 | | 100 | | | | 100/13 |
| HHFA[a] with JIG | May et al. (1991) [31] | 20 | | 80 | 15 | 5 | | 10/3 |
| | Hammerschlag (1999) [18] | 17 | 22 | 61 | 11 | | | 0 |
| | Manni et al. (2001) [30] | 29 | 21 | 45 | 24 | 7 | 3 | 3/0 |
| HHFA with FN transposition | Atlas and Lowinger (1997) [3][a] | 3 | | 100 | | | | 0 |
| | Sawamura and Abe (1997) [42] | 4 | | 75 | | 25 | | 0 |
| | Darrouzet et al. (1999) [11] | 6 | | 83 | 17 | | | 33/33 |
| | Donzelli et al. (2003) [13] | 3 | | 33 | 67 | | | 100/0 |
| | Rebol et al. (2006) [35] | 5 | | 40 | 20 | 20 | 20 | 0 |
| | Roland et al. (2006) [36][b] | 10 | | 100 | | | | 0 |
| End-to-side HFA | Ferraresi et al. (2006) [16][c] | 2 | | 100 | | | | 0 |
| | Koh et al. (2002) [24][b] | 4 | | 50 | 50 | | | 0 |

[a] Frequently or [b]sometimes combined with regional reanimation techniques (mostly eyelid weight implantation, but also spring implantation, temporalis muscle transposition)
[c]With an HN endoneurial window

## 29.5
## Surgical Anatomy

The surgical anatomies of the hypoglossus and FNs for HFA have recently been extensively studied by Asaoka et al. [2] and Salame et al. [38, 39].

### 29.5.1
### Cervical Segment of the HN

The HN exits the skull through the hypoglossal canal, which is anterior-inferior to the jugular foramen in the posterior cranial base. It continues medial to the internal jugular vein, internal carotid artery and cranial nerves IX, X and XI, descending in a plane between the styloid process anteriorly and the transverse process of the atlas posteriorly [20, 38]. Below the level of the mandibular angle, the HN passes medial to the posterior belly of the digastric muscle, which is a reliable guide to identify the nerve. The HN is crossed superficially by the occipital artery. Assuming a horizontal course, the nerve continues forward, inferomedially to the digastric posterior belly to enter the submandibular triangle. This triangle is bounded superiorly by the mandible, anteriorly by the anterior belly of the digastric muscle, and posteriorly by the posterior belly of the same muscle. Whereas the nerve can be either superior or inferior to the digastric tendon [38], it is always superior to the body of the hyoid bone.

The descending ramus (ramus descendens; descendens hypoglossi), long and slender, quits the hypoglossal where it turns around the occipital artery and descends in front of or in the sheath of the carotid vessels [20]. It gives a branch to the superior belly of the omohyoideus and then joins the communicantes cervicales from the second and third cervical nerves, just below the middle of the neck, to form a loop, the ansa hypoglossi.

The shortest distance between the HN and the bifurcation of the FN trunk (pes anserinus) is approximately 16–17 mm [1, 38]. Asaoka et al. [1] reported that the length of the FN from the external genu to the pes anserinus was 30.5±4.4 mm. Salame et al. [39] found that the length of the FN trunk from the SMF to the bifurcation was 16.44 mm. The minimal distance between the HN immediately before entering the submandibular triangle and the SMF was 33.54±12.71 mm [38].

According to Salame et al. [38, 39], in formaldehyde-fixed cadavers, the diameter of the HN just before its entrance into the submandibular triangle was 2.69±0.36 mm and its cross-sectional area was 6.88 mm². The diameter of the ansa hypoglossi, 10 mm after its separation from the HN, was 1.62±0.36 mm.

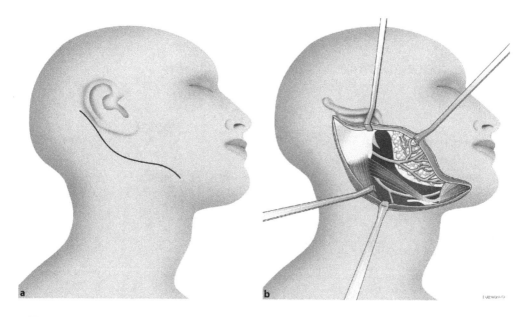

Fig. 1a,b Schematic rendering of the skin incision (**a**) and basic anatomy (**b**) pertinent to hypoglossal-facial nerve anastomosis (HFA): the sternocleidomastoid muscle is displaced and the digastric muscle is visible. The hypoglossal and facial nerves are coloured in *yellow* and *blue*, respectively

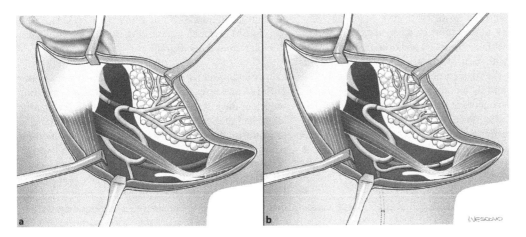

Fig. 2a,b  Schematic rendering of surgical techniques for HFA. **a** Classic HFA. **b** HFA + anastomosis of the descending branch of the hypoglossal nerve (HN) to the distal cut HN

## 29.5.2
## FN Trunk

The FN exits from the skull through the SMF, bound medially by the styloid process and laterally by the mastoid tip. The distance between the mastoid tip and the SMF was 17.22±3.18 mm. The FN is relatively superficial and Kempe [21] has pointed out the common error of looking for the nerve too deeply. In fact, the FN runs under the deep cervical fascia, the mean minimal distance from the skin surface being 22.4±3.8 mm [39].

The FN trunk runs anteriorly in an oblique caudal–external direction with a slight upward concavity. It traverses the styloid process, the posterior belly of the digastric muscle, the external carotid artery, the posterior division of the retromandibular vein and the ramus of the mandible. The number of branches arising from the FN between the SMF and the parotid gland varies from two to four. The posterior auricular nerve and the branch to the digastric muscle are the most commonly found and they originate approximately 3 and 3.6 mm, respectively, from the SMF [39]. The stylomastoid artery usually supplies the FN trunk and enters the skull through the SMF.

As reported by Salame et al. [39], in 45 out of 46 dissections, the FN terminated in a bifurcation within the parotid gland. The length of the FN trunk from the SMF to its bifurcation was 16.44±3.20 mm (range: 12.20–18.68 mm). The distance between the bifurcation and the mastoid tip was 16.11±3.92 mm (range: 12.10–25.10 mm). The distance between the bifurcation and the mandibular angle was 33.35±4.41 mm (range: 26.46–54.88 mm) [39].

According to Asaoka et al. [1], the mean number of myelinated axons in the FN is approximately 75% of that in the HN; the myelinated axons in the FN have a smaller calibre than those in the HN. The cross-sectional area of the FN is then usually smaller than that of the HN, and the difference can significantly increase when the FN has been severed and has undergone degeneration [1].

## 29.6
## Surgical Technique

### 29.6.1
### Hypoglossal–Facial Nerve Anastomosis

Access to the anterior neck muscles is gained by a skin incision following the submandibular chin line (Fig. 1a). Anterior to the sternocleidomastoid muscle and to its origin at the mastoid process, the FN is to be identified where it leaves the skull at the SMF (Fig. 1b). It is possible to expose and mobilise the nerve trunk either with or without mastoidectomy. The styloid process is a reliable landmark for exposure of the FN trunk, either by identifying the nerve lateral to this bony spicule or by leading the surgeon to the SMF, where the nerve can be identified [1, 38–40]. The stylohyoid muscle and the digastric muscle, which originate at the stylomastoid process, need to be followed distally to find the HN crossing under the occipital artery. The FN is sectioned as proximal as possible at the SMF, whereas the HN is sectioned immediately before it passes in the submandibular triangle. After section, the proximal stump of the HN is mobilised so that it can be connected to the distal stump of the FN (Fig. 2a). With the aid of an operating microscope, nerve coaptation is performed and stabilised by two 10/0 monofilament sutures or using fibrin glue.

The main principles of nerve suturing should be followed [40]. First, the nerve stumps must be inspected and prepared to be vital with healthy nerve axons, all at the same length and not distorted against each other. Second, the nerve stumps must be adapted exactly against one another, without distortion and overlapping, without any tension, with nerve diameters of similar sizes. Third, sutures to fix the adapted nerve stumps should not lead to distortion and should not be led through the nerve fibres. Fourth, handling of the nerve stumps has to be performed with utmost care to prevent secondary scarring. Therefore, the nerves must not be torn, rotated, or treated with more than two sutures; the application of fibrin glue might simplify the procedure, leading to the same results [40].

## 29.6.2
## Hemitongue Atrophy and Variations of HFA

Hemitongue atrophy is a consequence of total section of the HN. Its functional consequences have been stressed by some authors. Conley and Baker reported that 10–12% of patients complained of post-operative difficulty in swallowing that was attributed to tongue dysfunction [9]. Pensak et al. [33] reported in 74% of patients some functional difficulties with eating, of which 21% were debilitating; few patients had problems with swallowing. Hammerschlag [18] observed both speech and swallowing problems in 45% of his patients.

Recently, several surgical techniques aiming to preserve the glossal function have been reported.

Variations of the classic HFA include:

1. Anastomosis of a descending branch of the HN to the FN [9].
2. After a classic HFA, an anastomosis of a descending branch of the HN to the distal stump of the same HN (Fig. 2b) [7, 22, 34].

3. Hemihypoglossal–FN anastomosis (HHFA), with (Fig. 3b) [31] and without (Fig. 3a, Fig. 4a) [9, 12, 22] an interposed nerve graft.

Conley and Baker reported their experience with 12 cases of HHFA and three cases of anastomosis of a descending branch of the HN to the FN [9]. They concluded that the use of half of the HN or a descending branch of the HN, to neurotise the FN was not advisable because of disappointing results in expected facial reanimation and improvement in dexterity of the tongue. Other authors [7, 22, 34] used a descending branch of the HN after a classic HFA to neurotise the distal stump of the same HN, but they failed to achieve improvement in tongue dexterity.

HHFA has been advocated by some authors, with the aim of preventing post-surgical hemiparalysis and hemiatrophy of the tongue muscles [10]. This procedure has been justified by the minor diameter of the FN trunk in comparison with the diameter of the HN [1, 38, 39, 45]. May et al. [31] and Dellon [12] reported good results in facial reanimation and facility of the tongue after HHFA, which was performed with and without a nerve graft, respectively. Frequently though, the neurotisation procedure was combined with other reanimation techniques (e.g. eyelid weight implantation), depending on the specific areas of weakness [18]: May et al. [31] indeed emphasised that ancillary reanimation techniques significantly contributed to the excellent results.

Atlas and Lowinger [3] introduced a technique of hypoglossal–facial crossover involving a smaller, bevelled, partial incision of the HN and mobilisation of the intratemporal FN, following the Hitselberger technique [19] of mobilisation of the intratemporal FN with a mastoidectomy (Fig. 4a).

Other authors have also suggested the use of a "pure" end-to-side technique, with an epineurial window in the

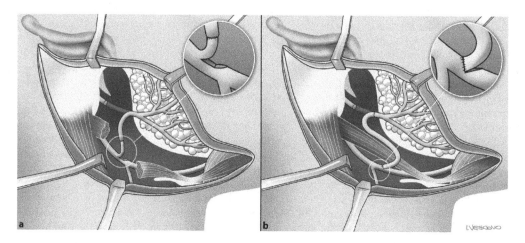

Fig. 3a,b Schematic rendering of surgical techniques for HFA. **a** HFA with longitudinal splitting of the HN (HHFA). **b** HHFA + jump interpositional graft (*green*)

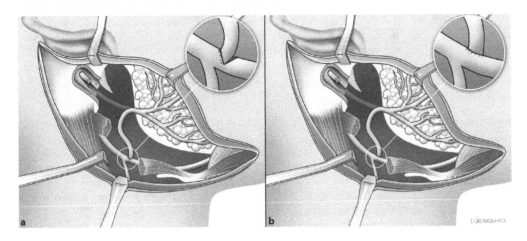

Fig. 4a,b Schematic rendering of surgical techniques for HFA. **a** HHFA + facial nerve transposition. **b** End-to-side HFA + facial nerve transposition

donor HN (Fig. 4b) [16, 24]. The effectiveness of these operations needs to be demonstrated in larger series of patients than those published to present these questionable end-to-side techniques.

## 29.7
## Post-surgical Care

Improved facial tone and symmetry usually precede initial facial movements. The average time to initial facial movements seems to be proportional to the time of FN palsy prior to the reanimation technique [26–28]. Older people seem to have a lesser ability to recover [17].

Post-operative-specific physiotherapy is indispensable. Samii et al. [40, 41] provided a succinct but detailed description of specific exercises that the physiotherapist dealing with these patients should be familiar with.

## 29.8
## Discussion

When reviewing the literature on HFA, it is clear that different series are not always comparable, as very frequently different facial reanimation techniques are used together and significant variations in the classification of results are present.

One of the major concerns in the literature is hemitongue atrophy, but, as it is recognised by many authors, complaints regarding mastication and speech differ greatly among patients with even marked or severe hemiglossal atrophy, and some patients complain of difficulty whereas others do not. Moreover, even after alternative HFA techniques, patients with a moderate tongue atrophy can complain of prolonged difficulty in mastication and speech [1].

While the results and limitations of the classic HFA have been widely reported and investigated, those concerning variations of HFA techniques are more limited (Table 1). However, we believe that the best operative option among such variations is that in which the classic HFA is combined with an anastomosis of the descending branch of the HN to the distal stump of the same HN. In fact, with such an operation, the reanimation of facial muscle function is indeed privileged over the hemiglossal muscle function, but an attempt to preserve the function of the tongue is made [15].

We believe that animal experiments in HFA might be useful to investigate the mechanisms of facial reinnervation, which will help us to better treat patients and will answer the questions that were posed by the pioneers of this surgery.

In a recent article [14] we investigated the difference between the HFA and HHFA in a rat model: we found that, in a comparison with intact rats, facial muscles were innervated by a lower number of motoneurons after either HFA (–48%) or HHFA (–75%). Therefore, both HFA and HHFA performed immediately after section of the FN in rats did not result in a phenomenon of motor hyperinnervation. In fact, if we consider the ideal possible HN nucleus motoneurons/FN axon ratio to be 0.8, after HFA and HHFA, this ratio was only 0.5 motoneuron/axon and 0.2 motoneuron/axon, respectively. We therefore documented what might appear intuitive; that is, the HHFA gives half the innervation provided by HFA, which should correspond to near 25% of normal innervation. Therefore, with HHFA the risk of obtaining a percentage of innervation of facial muscles insufficient for good functional results is increased compared to HFA. Unexpectedly, after both HFA and HHFA, facial motoneurons also reinnervated the facial muscles, as demonstrated by the study with the retrograde axonal tracer horseradish peroxidase, even after the extensive exclusion of possible contamination. Such a phenomenon should be the expression of axonal projections from facial motoneurons to the regenerating HN into the FN, and so of neural plasticity, of which we still know so little.

## 29.9
## Conclusions

The connection of the HN end-to-end directly to the FN is a popular technique with consistent and satisfying results [41]. Reinnervation occurs over a period of between 4 and 12 months. About 70% of patients obtain good results. Hypertonia and spastic contractions only occasionally give clinical problems. The frontal muscle regains poor function in most patients. In about 25% of patients, emotional mimic expression can be observed. Most patients can be classified as "good" or as House-Brackmann grade III [3, 41]. Tolerance of speech difficulty varies from patient to patient, also depending on their occupation. Currently, HHFA should be taken in consideration when speech is crucial to the patient's occupation, and especially when facial palsy is associated with other cranial nerves deficits.

As well as clinical investigations, experimental studies are needed to further develop the field of neurotisation techniques.

## References

1. Arai H, Sato K, Yanai A (1995) Hemihypoglossal–facial nerve anastomosis in treating unilateral facial palsy after acoustic neurinoma resection. J Neurosurg 82:51–54
2. Asaoka K, Sawamura Y, Nagashima M, Fukushima T (1999) Surgical anatomy for direct hypoglossal–facial nerve side-to-end "anastomosis". J Neurosurg 91:268–275
3. Atlas MD, Lowinger DS (1997) A new technique for hypoglossal-facial nerve repair. Laryngoscope 107:984–991
4. Ballance C, Duel AB (1932) The operative treatment of facial palsy by introduction of nerve grafts into fallopian canal and by other intra-temporal methods. Arch Otol 15:1–70
5. Ballance C, Ballance H, Stewart P (1903) Remarks on the operative treatment of chronic facial palsy of peripheral origin. BMJ 1:1009–1013
6. Braam M J, Nicolai JP (1993) Axonal regeneration rate through cross-face nerve grafts. Microsurgery 14:589–591
7. Chang CGS, Shen AL (1984) Hypoglossofacial anastomosis for facial palsy after resection of acoustic neurinoma. Surg Neurol 21:282–286
8. Chen YS, Hsu CJ, Liu TC, et al (2000) Histological rearrangement in the facial nerve and central nuclei following immediate and delayed hypoglossal–facial nerve anastomosis. Acta Otolaryngol 120:551–556
9. Conley J, Baker D (1979) Hypoglossal–facial nerve anastomosis for reinnervation of the paralysed face. Plast Reconstr Surg 63:3–72
10. Cusimano MD, Sekhar L (1994) Partial hypoglossal to facial nerve anastomosis for reinnervation of the paralyzed face in patients with lower cranial nerve palsies: technical note. Neurosurgery 35:532–533
11. Darrouzet V, Guerin J, Bebear JP (1999) New technique of side-to-end hypoglossal–facial nerve attachment with translocation of the infratemporal facial nerve. J Neurosurg 90:27–34
12. Dellon AL (1992) Restoration of facial nerve function: An approach for the twenty-first century. Neurosurg Q 2:199–222
13. Donzelli R, Motta G, Cavallo LM, et al (2003) One stage removal of residual intracanalicular acoustic neuroma and hemihypoglossal intratemporal facial nerve anastomosis: technical note. Neurosurgery 53:1444–1447
14. Fernandez E, Lauretti L, Denaro L, et al (2004) Motoneurons innervating facial muscles after hypoglossal and hemihypoglossal–facial nerve anastomosis in rats. Neurol Res 26:395–400
15. Fernandez E, Pallini R, Palma P, et al (1997) Hypoglossal–facial nerve anastomosis. J Neurosurg 87:649–650
16. Ferraresi S, Garozzo D, Migliorini V, et al (2006) End-to-side intrapetrous hypoglossal–facial anastomosis for reanimation of the face. Technical note. J Neurosurg 104:457–460
17. Guntinas-Lichius O, Streppel M, Stennert E (2006) Postoperative functional evaluation of different reanimation techniques for facial nerve repair. Am J Surg 191:61–67
18. Hammerschlag PE (1999) Facial reanimation with jump interpositional graft hypoglossal facial anastomosis and hypoglossal facial anastomosis: evolution in management of facial paralysis. Laryngoscope 109:1–23
19. Hitselberger WE (1979) Hypoglossal–facial anastomosis. In: House WF, Luetje CM (eds) Acoustic Tumors. University Park Press, Baltimore, pp 97–103
20. Jones N (1995) The hypoglossal nerve. In: Williams PL (ed) Gray's Anatomy, 38th edn. Churchill Livingstone, New York, pp 1256–1258
21. Kempe LG (2004) Hypoglossal–Facial Anastomosis. In: Salcman M, Heros RC, Laws ER, Sonntag VHS eds (2004) Kempe's Operative Neurosurgery. Springer, Berlin, Heidelberg, New York, pp 219–223
22. Kessler LA, Moldaver J, Pool JL (1959) Hypoglossal–facial anastomosis for treatment of facial paralysis. Neurology 9:118–125
23. Koerbel A, Gharabaghi A, Safavi-Abbasi S, et al (2005) Evolution of vestibular schwannoma surgery: the long journey to current success. Neurosurg Focus 18:e10
24. Koh KS, Kim JK, Kim CJ, et al (2002) Hypoglossal–facial crossover in facial-nerve palsy: pure end-to-side anastomosis technique. Br J Plast Surg 55:25–31

25. Körte W (1903) Ein Fall von Nervenpropfung: des Nervus facialis auf den Nervus hypoglossus. Deutsche med Wihnschr 17:293–295

26. Kunihiro T, Kanzaki J, O-Uchi T (1991) Hypoglossal–facial nerve anastomosis. Clinical observation. Acta Otolaryngol Suppl [Stockh] 487:80–84

27. Kunihiro T, Kanzaki J, Shiobara R, et al (1999) Long-term prognosis of profound facial nerve paralysis secondary to acoustic neuroma resection. ORL J Otorhinolaryngol Relat Spec 61:98–102

28. Kunihiro T, Kanzaki J, Yoshihara S, Satoh Y (1994) Analysis of the prognosis and the recovery process of profound facial nerve paralysis secondary to acoustic neuroma resection. ORL J Otorhinolaryngol Relat Spec 56:331–333

29. Lanman TH, Brackmann DE, Hitselberger WE, et al (1999) Report of 190 consecutive cases of large acoustic tumors (vestibular schwannoma) removed via the translabyrinthine approach. J Neurosurg 90:617–623

30. Manni JJ, Beurskens CH, van de Velde C, et al (2001) Reanimation of the paralyzed face by indirect hypoglossal–facial nerve anastomosis. Am J Surg 182:268–273

31. May M, Sobel SM, Mester SJ (1991) Hypoglossal–facial nerve interpositional jump graft for facial reanimation without tongue atrophy. Otolaryngol Head Neck Surg 204:818–826

32. Odebode TO, Ologe FE (2006) Facial nerve palsy after head injury: case incidence, causes, clinical profile and outcome. J Trauma 61:388–391

33. Pensak ML, Jackson CG, Glasscock ME 3rd, et al (1986) Facial reanimation with the VII–XII anastomosis: analysis of the functional and psychologic results. Otolaryngol Head Neck Surg 94:305–310

34. Pitty LF, Tator CH (1992) Hypoglossal–facial nerve anastomosis for facial nerve palsy following surgery for cerebellopontine angle tumors. J Neurosurg 77:724–731

35. Rebol J, Milojkovic V, Didanovic V (2006) Side-to-end hypoglossal–facial anastomosis via transposition of the intratemporal facial nerve. Acta Neurochir 148:653–657

36. Roland JT Jr, Lin K, Klausner LM, et al (2006) Direct facial-to-hypoglossal neurorrhaphy with parotid release. Skull Base 16:101–108

37. Rosenwasser RH, Liebman E, Jimenez DF, et al (1991) Facial reanimation after facial nerve injury. Neurosurgery 29:568–574

38. Salame K, Masharawi Y, Rochkind S, et al (2006) Surgical anatomy of the cervical segment of the hypoglossal nerve. Clin Anat 19:37–43

39. Salame K, Ouaknine GE, Arensburg B, et al (2002) Microsurgical anatomy of the facial nerve trunk. Clin Anat 15:93–99

40. Samii M, Matthies C (1994) Indication, technique and results of facial nerve reconstruction. Acta Neurochir 130:125–139

41. Samii M, Matthies C (1997) Management of 1000 vestibular schwannomas (acoustic neuromas): the facial nerve-preservation and restitution of function. Neurosurgery 40:684–694

42. Sawamura Y, Abe H (1997) Hypoglossal–facial nerve side-to-end anastomosis for preservation of hypoglossal function: results of delayed treatment with a new technique. J Neurosurg 86:203–206

43. Stennert E (1979) Hypoglossal facial anastomosis: its significance for modern facial surgery. Clin Plast Surg 6:471–485

44. Streppel M, Heiser T, Stennert E (2000) Historical development of facial nerve surgery with special reference to hypoglossal–facial nerve anastomosis (in German). HNO 48:801–808

45. Vacher C, Dauge MC (2004) Morphometric study of the cervical course of the hypoglossal nerve and its application to hypoglossal facial anastomosis. Surg Radiol Anat 26:86–90

# Facial Pain – Diagnosis and Therapy

**30**

Hans-Werner Bothe

## Contents

## 30.1
## Introduction

Correct diagnosis facilitates treatment; it may therefore be helpful to classify facial pain. According to Hapak et al. [6] facial pain can be classified as musculoligamentous, dentoalveolar and neurological categories of pain origin.

Temporomandibular joint disorders, facial arthromyalgia, salivary gland disease and rhinosinus-related headache are assigned to the musculoligamentous group and are mostly treated by maxillary surgeons. Bruxism, increased or reduced saliva production, local swelling, fever, pain aggravated by eye movements and other clinical signs can help to make a probable diagnosis in the field of musculoligamentous disorders.

Concerning the dentoalveolar group, which is extremely common, we have to consider dentinal, periodontal, pulpal, thermal sensitivity and other causes of pain. Patients suffering from dentoalveolar disorders are best referred to dentists. Pain character and duration include the whole range of possibilities and can show some degree of diagnostic overlap with trigeminal neuralgia (TN).

The last, but for neurosurgeons not the least, group of facial pain is the neurological one. This includes pain caused by nerve compression (e.g. neurinoma of the fifth nerve), cranial arteritis (temporal arteritis), Tolosa-Hunt syndrome (unspecific inflammation of the cavernous sinus and adjacent neural structures of the orbit) and vari-

ous neuralgias, among which the most important is TN. A sudden, intense, sharp, lancinating pain lasting from a few seconds to less than 2 min and recurring within short periods of time is characteristic for neuralgias. Given that the majority of neurosurgeons treat only TN, this chapter will deal mainly with this condition (tic douloureux): epidemiology, natural course, diagnosis, treatment, and prognosis.

## 30.2
## Epidemiology

TN is the most frequently occurring facial neuralgia, with a prevalence of 107.5/100,000 (0.1%) [12]. In Germany, there are about 80,000 people with TN and about 8000 new cases every year. Incidence increases with age: 4–5/100,000/year for patients younger than 60 years, 20/100,000/year for patients older than 60 years, and 25/100,000/year in those older than 70 years. Therefore, about 70% are older than 60 years at onset [14]. The female-to-male ratio is about 3:2. TN is commoner in the lower areas of the face than in the upper areas. Several case studies show that pain is more right sided, but this finding is not backed up statistically.

TN is associated with certain disorders. The risk for TN in arterial hypertension is doubled (odds ratio 1.96, 95% confidence interval 1.2–3.1) [9]. There is a report of 15 cases of Charcot-Marie-Tooth neuropathy (hereditary chronic motor and sensory polyneuropathy) combined with TN [15]. The association between multiple sclerosis and TN was estimated at between 1.9% and 4% (relative risk 20%, 95% confidence interval 4.1–58.6) [7]. Furthermore, co-morbidity exists between glossopharyngeal neuralgia and TN. In 217 patients suffering from glossopharyngeal neuralgia, Rushton [13] found as many as 25 also suffering from TN. In nine cases of that series, those two forms of neuralgia occurred simultaneously. Elderly and immunosuppressed patients are at risk of developing acute *Herpes zoster*. Watson [18] found that in about 25% of all *Herpes zoster* cases, the trigeminal nerve is involved. Therefore, it can be assumed by extrapolation of this data that the incidence of post-herpetic TN is 3.3/100,000/year and 20/100,000/year before and after age 60 years, respectively.

## 30.3
## Natural Course of Typical Trigeminal Neuralgia

It is generally accepted that focal demyelination in the root of the trigeminal nerve is one of other reasons of TN [3]. The frequent impingement of the nerve by arterial and venous vessels in the posterior fossa with often observable indentation of the root [5] was another rationale why vascular compression together with demyelination was thought to be involved in the pathogenesis of TN. To generation of "neuralgic pain", the compression and demyelination should occur at the Obersteiner-Redlich line (the level of the central and peripheral myelin junction). The mechanism involves ectopic excitation and ephaptic connections at that junction line. This may be the explanation as to why innocuous stimulation of trigger zones within the distribution of the same trigeminal branch causes an attack of pain.

The natural progression of TN shows an increase in the frequency and strength of attacks and shortening, or sometimes disappearance of remission periods. The response to conservative treatment usually wanes. Patients were presented frequently to dentists, and tooth extractions are common therapeutic approaches. Strength of pain increases progressively. Scoring using the visual analogue scale (VAS) occasionally reaches 10 on a scale of 10 points. Therefore, it is not unusual that patients attempt suicide to escape from that state of unbearable pain.

Untreated TN also shows worsening of nerve function and presents occasionally "negative" phenomena (in contrast to "positive" symptoms) like sensory dysfunction [4]. The character of the pain also changes in advanced disease: Dull pain sensation overlaps regions of previous lancinating pain allotted to the same trigeminal branch. The response to carbamazepine decreases over time. The characteristic of pain changes from triggered, sharp, shooting, lancinating, electric-shock-like, lasting several seconds, with pain-free intervals that are described by adjectives like constant, dull, boring, gnawing, and lasting permanently. Therefore, during progression of TN, there may develop different entities of pain syndromes: "typical" trigeminal neuralgia is followed by the so-called "atypical" trigeminal neuralgia.

Eventually, the symptomatology of "atypical" TN may be caused by various other than vascular lesions of the trigeminal nerve. In this group of disorders sensation in the trigeminal distribution is usually altered. In addition to pain hypaesthesia, hyperalgesia or allodynia are possible findings. The underlying pathology can be localised to any level of the trigeminal pathway (nerve, ganglion, roots, nuclei and tracts) and comprises infections (herpes), demyelination (multiple sclerosis), trauma (tooth extraction), destructive operations for typical TN (anaesthesia dolorosa after percutaneous radiofrequency trigeminal rhizotomy) and tumours (e.g. neurinoma of the trigeminal nerve).

A comparison (prospective cohort study, evidence level: 2b) of pharmacological and surgical treatment of typical TN (caused by vascular compression) reveals that after a 16-year observation period, 75% of all patients needed surgery [19]. Outcome after any type of surgery was better than that following pharmacological treatment, and 66% of the patients who underwent surgery felt that they should have done so earlier.

## 30.4
## Diagnosis

Careful history and examination is the basis for diagnosis. One has to determine both the pain disease (typical or atypical TN) and the pain illness (suffering). History is facilitated if patients are given questionnaires to complete before the consultation. For chronic pain diseases, there are several questionnaires used as standard [17]: the Brief Pain Inventory uses a VAS (0: no pain – 10: maximum conceivable pain) to determine severity of pain and the impact on quality of life, considering mood, relationship and work. Another routinely applicable questionnaire is Beck's Depression Index. Using the McGill Pain Questionnaire, we gauge both the sensory component of pain and the affective and evaluative aspects. Of cause for every chronic pain it is important to ascertain whether patients have other pain complaints and symptoms that might suggest a need to undertake further evaluations of their mental state.

The International Headache Society defines five criteria of typical TN (Table 1) [8]. Pain must have an electrical quality that gives the patient the sensation that an exposed nerve is being manipulated, such as might be experienced when a dentist drills into the pulp of unanaesthetised tooth. Ordinarily, no neurological deficits are present unless the pain results from multiple sclerosis, a tumour, or other morphologic abnormality along the course of the trigeminal nerve, such as dolichoectasia of the vertebrobasilar arterial system or an arteriovenous malformation.

An imaging study of the brain should be performed early in the course of management. Not only the aforementioned causes of TN, but particularly compression of the trigeminal nerve by blood vessels can be demonstrated by magnetic resonance imaging (MRI; Fig. 1). The high sensitivity of MRI for the detection of vascular compression is 88.5% and the low specificity is 50% [2] elucidates the fact that typical TN is correlated in most cases with vascular compression. In contrast to that fact, neuralgia does not necessary follow from a contact of a vessel to the trigeminal nerve root. There are clearly other causes (for example demyelination) underlying the development of neuralgia. In conclusion, decision making to operate upon a patient with typical TN relates to criteria that are summarised in Table 2.

Table 1 Five diagnostic criteria for typical trigeminal neuralgia (International Headache Society) [14]

1. Typical history and examination according to International Headache Society criteria

2. Pain has at least four of the following characteristics:
   2a. Distribution along one or more divisions of the trigeminal nerve
   2b. Sudden, intense, sharp, superficial, stabbing in quality
   2c. Intensity severe
   2d. Precipitation from trigger areas
   2e. Between paroxysms history and examination

3. No neurological deficit

4. Attacks are stereotyped in the individual patient

5. Exclusion of other causes of facial pain by history, examination or special investigations

Table 2 Indications for neurovascular decompression surgery in patients suffering from trigeminal neuralgia.

1. Attacks of facial pain that last a few seconds to less than 2 min

2. No other pain complaint as a sign of somatisation of chronic pain disease

3. Exclusion of morphological abnormalities along the course of the trigeminal nerve by MRI

4. Vascular compression of the trigeminal nerve (facultative criterion)

5. Exclusion criterion is not age, but bad ASA classification

*MRI* magnetic resonance imaging, *ASA* American Society of Anesthesiologists

## 30.5
## Treatment

The operation is performed with the patient supine and the head turned to the contralateral side (if preoperative evaluation of the cervical spine by x-ray reveals degenerative lesions or preoperative probe positioning provokes neurological deficits, we select the semi-sitting position for the procedure). The head is held by a Mayfield three-point head holder. The chin is flexed somewhat forward and the vertex is tilted toward the floor to maximise the working space between the retromastoid space and the shoulder, which is drawn towards the foot and to the floor by tape (care must be taken not to stretch the brachial plexus!). Electrodes necessary for the intraoperative monitoring of auditory evoked potentials and facial stimulation are attached to the patient. Hair is shaved only ipsilaterally in the retromastoid region.

After preparing and draping of the operative area, a skin incision is made behind the hairline along the mastoid crease. Michel clips are applied to the skin edges and the underlying fascial and muscular layers are dissected along the same line. The soft tissue is stripped from the bone and held aside with retractors. The craniectomy is placed high and lateral in the posterior fossa. The superior and lateral edges of the bony opening expose the inferior margin of the transverse sinus and the medial margin of the upper sigmoid sinus. The craniectomy measures 3 cm in craniocaudal and mediolateral length. Mastoid cells that have been opened are sealed with muscle pieces bonded by tissue glue at the end of the operation. Before the dura mater is opened, the patient is given mannitol intravenously.

After the microscope is brought into field, a dura incision is made along the margin of the transverse and sigmoid sinus. If the edge of sinus is incised, a piece of Gelfoam will staunch the bleeding without interfering with venous flow in the sinus. A cottonoid is placed superficially supralaterally over the cerebellum. A first look should now be made in the posterolateral direction as there can be bridging veins in this area, and these are dif-

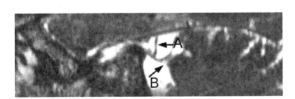

Fig. 1a,b A 44-year-old woman suffering from trigeminal neuralgia (TN) of the right third branch for 7 years. Parasagittal magnetic resonance imaging (MRI) along the course of the trigeminal nerve, constructive interference in steady-state (T2 subgroup) protocol with high resolution (0.7 mm). It can be seen an aberrant loop of the superior cerebellar artery (**a**) is compressing the trigeminal nerve (**b**) from above (that means that the nerve fibres of the third branch are affected!) within a few millimetres of the entry into the pons (MRI protocol developed and performed by Dr. Papke, Department of Neuroradiology, University of Münster, Germany)

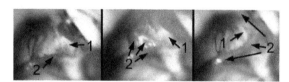

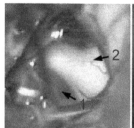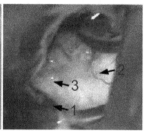

Fig. 2a–c Intraoperative microphotographs showing right trigeminal nerve (*1*) which is compressed by superior cerebellar artery (*2*). **a** The caudal loop of the superior cerebellar artery is behind the trigeminal nerve on its anteromedial edge. **b** The main trunk has been brought up from behind the nerve to its cranial border. **c** The artery is mobilised from the nerve and located on its lateral aspect

Fig. 3a,b Intraoperative microphotographs showing the right trigeminal nerve (*2*), which is compressed by superior cerebellar artery (*1*). **a** The caudal loop of the superior cerebellar artery is at the superior aspect of the trigeminal nerve. **b** A piece of muscle (*3*) has been inserted between the artery (*1*) and the nerve (*2*)

ficult to treat if they are torn. If the cerebellum is "full", rather than approaching rostrally one should lift the cerebellum off the occipital plate and the subarachnoid cistern around the nerves IX and X to allow cerebrospinal fluid to escape. As a consequence, the cerebellum will lower by gravity. Now the self-retaining retractor can be slid over the cottonoid towards the petrous bone.

The superior petrosal vein is encountered at or near the anteromedial end of the line of attachment of the tentorium to the petrous ridge. This vein must usually be coagulated to permit adequate visualisation of the trigeminal nerve. Sometimes, just one branch must be taken. The eighth nerve is identified, and the fifth nerve appears deeply anterior and rostral to it.

Now the surgeon looks for vascular compression. The general rule is that rostral compression of the nerve causes lower facial TN; caudal compression causes neuralgia of the first branch, and lateral or medial compression causes second branch neuralgia. Frequently, the superior cerebellar artery loops down anteromedial to the nerve (Fig. 2a). The main trunk can be brought up and mobilised away from the nerve (Fig. 2b and 2c). A piece of muscle is inserted between the nerve and the artery, and bonded in place with tissue glue (Fig. 3). If there is a compression by a small vein, it can be coagulated and divided. Simple coagulation should be avoided because of the danger of recanalisation. Larger veins should be decompressed by means of muscle implants. Sometimes the artery is adherent to the nerve; sharp dissection may then be necessary. Before closure, multiple Valsalva manoeuvres are performed after the retractor has been removed for detecting and servicing lesioned and bleeding veins.

The cerebellopontine angle is filled with a warm-water irrigation solution. Afterwards, the dura is closed in a watertight fashion with the aid of an operating microscope, which is subsequently removed. Open mastoid cells are closed with muscle pieces bonded by tissue glue. To fill

the bony defect, the epidural space is filled with absorbable gelatine sponge. Muscles, fascia and subcutaneous tissue are closed in layers with interrupted sutures. The skin is closed with single stitches according to Donati, using 3-0 nylon sutures.

Post-operatively, the patient is monitored overnight in an intermediate care unit. Preoperatively, given medication should be slowly reduced rather then stopped suddenly, to avoid withdrawal syndrome. Suture removal is done on the 7th day after operation, discharge from hospital after 10 days, and return to work 1 month later.

If the clinical character of the pain is atypical and its cause is a lesion along the course of a peripheral trigeminal branch or of the central pathway, and if there is no response to pharmacological treatment and no way for a classical surgical approach, then we recommend stimulation of the motor cortex (MC) [10].

We perform a MRI under stereotactic conditions with the patient under general anaesthesia, to localise the central sulcus (CS) and the MC. The CS can be seen optimally in its full length not on the surface of the brain, but 1 cm underneath on a plane perpendicular to the surface (Fig. 4b). The target for facial pain is located at the junction of the caudal part of the MC and the elongation of the inferior frontal sulcus, immediately anterior to the CS (Fig. 4a).

After positioning, preparation, and draping of the patient we make a linear oblique skin incision parallel to the estimated position of the MC. A small craniotomy, 5 cm in diameter, is performed around the CS. The centre of the craniotomy should correspond to the target as determined by imaging and stereotactic frame. Now an electrode array with four plate electrodes (diameter 5 mm, separation 10 mm) is placed on the dura. The location of the precentral and post-central gyrus is confirmed from the phase reversal of the $N_{20}$ wave of the somatosensory evoked potential. Subsequently, we seek the final target

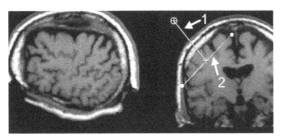 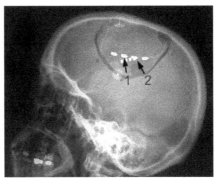

Fig. 4a,b MRI under stereotactic conditions for navigation of motor cortex stimulation. **a** One can see the trajectory, plane 1, perpendicular to the surface of the cortex. **b** Plane 2 is 1 cm underneath the cortex surface. The target for facial pain is at the bottom of the motor cortex (*2* in **a**) at the junction of the central sulcus (*1* in **a**) and the elongation of the inferior frontal sulcus, immediately anterior to central sulcus

Fig. 5 A 39-year-old woman suffering from atypical left facial pain (third branch of the trigeminal nerve) after a tooth extraction. The epidural electrode is orientated perpendicularly to the right central sulcus. The second contact (*1*) of the electrode is negative and placed over the right caudal motor cortex. The third contact (*2*) is positive and placed over the sensory cortex

point by stimulating epidurally the MC until we get a muscle contraction within the painful facial area. For intraoperative motor stimulation, we use electrodes with an interpolar distance of 20 mm, monophasic pulses with a relatively long duration of minimally 500 ms to 1 s and a low frequency of 1–5 Hz (higher frequencies are susceptible to habituation and tend to cause seizures). The intensity of current is adjusted between 5 and 15 mA. For permanent placement, we position the electrode (Resume, model 3587A, Medtronic, Minneapolis, US; length 44 mm, width 8 mm, four contacts, separation 10 mm) perpendicular to the CS on the evaluated region of the caudal MC with the contact "1" (second contact from the end of the electrode), which is negative over the target and contact "2" (third contact from the end of the electrode), which is positive over the sensory cortex dorsal to the CS (Fig. 5).

The electrode is fixed to the dura with two stitches and the bone is replaced and fixed. If the patient complains after the operation of a painful sensation at the stimulation site, we isolate the dura around the electrode by incision and resuturing. Before permanent implantation of the stimulator (Itrel II, Medtronic), we perform a test stimulation for a period of 5 days. In general, the parameters for chronic stimulation are as follows: frequency 20–60 Hz, pulse width 60–200 m, amplitude 1–4 V, bipolar stimulation with the negative pole over the MC and the positive pole over the sensory cortex. We adjust the stimulator such that it is switched on for 2 h and switched off for 3 h. Pain relief is reported to occur not until several minutes after starting the stimulation, and is long lasting after stopping stimulation, amounting to several hours. If test stimulation shows successful results, a permanent stimulator is implanted after 1 week. Suture

removal takes place 7 days later, discharge from hospital after 10 days and control visits to check the system every 3 months.

Destructive procedures for facial pain (especially percutaneous radiofrequency electrocoagulation) usually result in a worsening of the pain level after a time period of precious few months. However, if a patient suffering from TN presents in a generally bad condition with an American Society of Anaesthesiologists classification of 3 (severe systemic disease, but not incapacitating) or 4 (severe systemic disease that is a constant threat to life) that argues against general anaesthesia and operability, then we choose a method for treatment of TN that represents an advancement of the classical percutaneous electrocoagulation of the ganglion Gasseri: percutaneous electrical stimulation of the ganglion Gasseri.

The procedure is done under local anaesthesia. A standard needle with an inner diameter of 1.4 mm that allows the introduction of a deep-brain stimulation electrode (model number 3389, Medtronic) is inserted freehand under fluoroscopic monitoring. The patient is placed in the supine position on the fluoroscopic table with their head rotated about 15° contralateral to the side of pain. The foramen ovale is identified by angling the fluoroscopic beam approximately 40° from the vertical in the caudocranial direction. If the central ray passes a point 2.5 cm lateral to the angle of the mouth on the side of the pain, one can visualise the foramen between the ramus of the mandible laterally and the maxilla medially. It sits as a so-called "setting sun" on the shadow of the petrous ridge. Along that fluoroscopically evaluated pathway, the needle is inserted with a gloved finger inside the month to avoid penetration of the oral mucosa. It is guided towards the foramen ovale under intermittent fluoroscopic

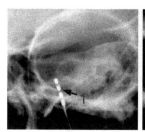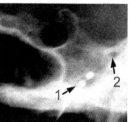

Fig. 6a,b A 71-year-old man with left-sided atypical trigeminal pain of the third branch, which has persisted despite five destructive procedures in his history. This patient also suffers from severe heart failure (American Society of Anesthesiologists classification 3). **a** Anteroposterior view of the deep-brain stimulation electrode (*1*) in situ with projection to the left orbit. **b** Lateral view with the electrode (*1*) 5 mm apart from the clivus (*2*)

control. The optimal point for penetration is the centre of the medial half of the foramen. Lateral puncture of the foramen places the needle beneath or in the temporal lobe (complications: haematoma, abscess and seizures!). As soon as the needle penetrates the foramen (resistance dissipates), the patient's head is rotated into the neutral position and the fluoroscopic unit is turned to the lateral view to assess the depth of the tip of the needle. For pain in the mandibular division, the needle is placed about 5 mm anterior to the clivus, as viewed on the lateral fluoroscopy. For pain in the second division, the needle is advanced to a distance of 1 mm to the clivus, and for the first division the needle is inserted 1 mm posterior to the clivus. If the needle has reached its target, the electrode is introduced (Fig. 6) and test stimulation is performed. The electrode is moved along the trajectory until the patient reports paraesthesia in the region of facial pain. Thereafter, the needle is withdrawn and the electrode was sutured to the skin. Test stimulation is done for 5 days.

## 30.6
## Prognosis

For typical TN, the immediate relief from pain after operation is complete in 82% of patients [1]. One year after decompression, 75% of patients don't have pain; 10 years after surgery, 70% present excellent results, which means that they are free of pain without medication. The four predictors of recurrences are female sex, symptoms lasting more than 8 years, venous compression and the lack of immediate cessation of TN. Most recurrences of TN occur within the first 2 years after surgery.

Concerning the safety of microvascular decompression, it has been reported [20] that atypical facial pain traditionally associated with nerve injury occurred in 37% of cases after radiofrequency rhizotomy, in comparison to 13% following microvascular decompression. An unsuccessful radiofrequency-lesion procedure before microvascular decompression was a significant risk factor for post-operative burning and aching pain. Rare major complications are death (0.2%), brainstem infarction (0.1%), and hearing loss (1.0%).

Definite pain relief in patients suffering from atypical TN is achieved by MC stimulation in 75% [11] over a

time period of 3 years. Progressive loss of effect can be observed in about 20% of patients during the first 3 months. In 80% of those cases, electrodes are not correctly placed in relation to the somatotopy of the MC. In atypical TN treated by MC stimulation, VAS scores improve from 85 out of 100 (maximum of pain) to 24 out of 100.

Complications of epidural MC stimulation are observed in less than 1% of cases. Among those complications are subcutaneous infection, dehiscence of the stimulator pocket, and local pain at the stimulation site treated by isolation of the dura around the electrode.

Peripheral stimulation of the ganglion Gasseri leads to a substantial pain reduction of between 100 and 75% [16]. No serious complications occur. One common problem with that therapy is electrode dislocation, alterations at the site of the pulse generator and infection.

## References

1. Barker FG, Jannetta PJ, Bissonette DJ, (1996) The long-term outcome of microvascular decompression for trigeminal neuralgia. N Engl J Med 334:1077–1083
2. Boecher-Schwarz HG, Bruehl K, Kessel G, et al (1998) Sensitivity and specificity of MRI in the diagnosis of neurovascular compression in patients with trigeminal neuralgia: a correlation of MRI and surgical findings. Neuroradiology 40:88–95
3. Burchiel KJ (1980) Abnormal impulse generation in focally demyelinated trigeminal roots. J Neurosurg 53:674–683
4. Burchiel KJ, Slavin KV (2000) On the natural history of trigeminal neuralgia. Neurosurgery 46:152–155
5. Hamlin PJ, King TT (1992) Neurovascular compression in trigeminal neuralgia, a clinical and anatomical study. J Neurosurg 76:948–954
6. Hapak L, Gordon A, Locker D, et al (1994) Differentiation between musculoligamentous, dentoalveolar, and neurologically based craniofacial pain with a diagnostic questionnaire. J Orofac Pain 8:357–368
7. Hooge JP, Redekop WK (1995) Trigeminal neuralgia in multiple sclerosis. Neurology 45:1294–1296
8. International Headache Society (1988) Classification and diagnostic criteria for headache disorders, cranial neuralgias and facial pain. Headache classification committee of the international headache society. Cephalgia 8:S1–S96

9.  Katusec S, Beard M, Bergstralh E, et al (1990) Incidence and clinical features of trigeminal neuralgia. Ann Neurol 27:89–95

10. Meyerson BA, Lindblom U, Linderoth B (1993) Motor cortex stimulation as treatment of trigeminal neuropathic pain. Acta Neurochir Suppl 58:150–153

11. Nguyen JP, Lefaucheur JP, Decq P, et al (1999) Chronic motor stimulation in the treatment of central and neuropathic pain. Correlations between clinical, electrophysiological and anatomical data. Pain 82:245–251

12. Penman J (1968) Trigeminal neuralgia. In: Vinken PJ, Bruyn GW (eds) Handbook of Clinical Neurology. North Holland, Amsterdam, pp 296–322

13. Rushton JG, Stevens C, Miller RH (1981) Glossopharyngeal neuralgia. Arch Neurol 38:201–205

14. Siccoli MM, Bassetti CL, Sandor PS (2006) Facial pain, clinical differential diagnosis. Lancet 5:257–267

15. Smyth P, Greenough G, Stommel E (2003) Familial trigeminal neuralgia, case reports and review of the literature. Headache 43:910–915

16. Steude U (1998) Chronic trigeminal nerve stimulation for the relief of persistent pain. In: Gidenberg PL, Tasker RR (eds) Textbook of Stereotactic and Functional Neurosurgery. McGraw-Hill, New York, pp 1557–1564

17. Wall P, Melzack R (1999) Textbook of Pain. Churchill Livingstone, London

18. Watson CP (2004) Management issues of neuropathic trigeminal pain from a medical perspective. J Orofac Pain 18:366–373

19. Zakrzewska JM, Patsalos PN (2002) Long-term cohort study comparing medical (oxcarbazepine) and surgical management of intractable trigeminal neuralgia. Pain 95:259–266

20. Zakrzewska JM, Thomas DGT (1993) Patient's assessment of outcome after three surgical procedures for the management of trigeminal neuralgia. Acta Neurochir 122:225–230

Eduardo Vellutini, Eliana Garzon,
Luciana Midori Inuzuka, Roger Schimdt
Brock, and Jose Erasmo Dal 'Col Lucio

## Contents

## 31.1
## Introduction

Almost 50,000,000 people in the world are estimated to have epilepsy, with a prevalence of 1–2 cases per 1000 persons in developed countries [20], and 18 per 1000 persons in developing ones [4]. While most epileptic patients can achieve seizure control with the use of antiepileptic drugs (AEDs), about 25–45% of them continue to have refractory seizures despite an appropriate clinical treatment [20, 26]. Medical refractoriness should be suspected when two appropriately chosen, well-tolerated, first-line AEDs or one monotherapy and one combination regimen have failed to achieve acceptable seizure control [5, 23].

Surgical treatment may be an important alternative for those patients whose quality of life is significantly impaired by the seizures or by the adverse effects of medication. Surgical candidates must be evaluated by a specialized multidisciplinary team after an extensive presurgical study based on video-electrographic monitoring, neuroimaging, and neuropsychological study. Surgery is best indicated for those whose seizures start in a noneloquent brain area, which can be removed without causing a severe neurological deficit. In some cases, palliative procedures are performed in order to reduce the frequency and severity of the seizures, even when the expectation of a cure is low.

A wide variety of surgical options are available today. The most frequent is temporal lobectomy with amygdalo-hippocampectomy. Other procedures are lesionectomies, neocortical resections, multiple subpial transections (MSTs), hemispherectomy, and corpus callosotomy.

Surgery for the treatment of epilepsy in children and adolescents has been indicated in earlier ages. Factors like neuronal plasticity and the effect of epilepsy on early brain development reinforces this indication [11].

## 31.2
## Presurgical Evaluation

The main goal of presurgical evaluation in patients with intractable epilepsy has been the identification of the epileptogenic zone. This includes not only the actual area that is generating the patient's habitual seizures, but also those regions with potential epileptogenicity [7].

Five zones should de identified in the evaluation: (1) the symptomatogenic zone: (cortical area that, when activated by the epileptic discharge, reproduces the patient's typical ictal symptoms), (2) the epileptogenic zone (cortical area capable of generating seizures, and whose removal or disconnection will result in seizure freedom), (3) the irritative zone (cortical area capable of generating interictal spikes on the electroencephalogram, EEG), (4) the ictal onset zone (cortical region from which we can objectively demonstrate that seizures are arising), and (5) the functional deficit zone (area that shows abnormal functioning in the interictal period) [46]. These results can be achieved with careful analysis of seizure semiology and electrophysiological studies (video-EEG, VEEG) associated with dates from anatomical and functional neuroimaging. Neuroimaging is particularly important for the evaluation of patients and the identification of focal lesions such as tumors, cortical dysplasia, areas of gliosis, neuronal loss with atrophy, and other developmental abnormalities

Functional imaging studies using radiotracers, such as positron emission tomography (PET) and single-photon-emission computed tomography (SPECT), are performed to identify or confirm the ictal focus in preparation for surgery). In some cases it is necessary to perform the Wada test, when the language and memory function on the same side are tested after sodium amytal infusion into the homolateral carotid artery.

Magnetoencephalography (MEG) is a recent method that is not available at all centers. MEG is a method used to localize epileptic activity and consists of the evaluation of the magnetic fields produced by electrical activity in the brain.

The gold standard for surgical localization in intractable epilepsy is the ictal EEG pattern identified by long-term scalp-recorded VEEG monitoring [8]. The rationale underlying ictal recordings includes confirmation of seizure type, evaluation of ictal semiology, and surgical localization. Trained personnel perform peri-ictal speech and memory testing and ensure the patient's safety. Ictal scalp recordings alone may suffice if results are concordant with those of other neurodiagnostic studies [8]. This method has some limitations for identification of ictal EEG changes in patients with simple or frontal lobe partial seizures. Myogenic and electrode artifacts during seizures may obscure an ictal electrographic seizure pattern, and patients may not have a typical, habitual seizure during prolonged EEG recordings despite the withdrawal of AEDs [8, 32].

Invasive procedures become necessary when noninvasive means of preoperative investigation cannot determine in a reliable manner the epileptogenic zone for surgery, or due to its close proximity to the eloquent cortex. They should be indicated only if the noninvasive evaluation results in at least a reasonable hypothesis regarding the possible localization of the epileptogenic zone.

## 31.3
## Temporal Lobe Epilepsy

Temporal lobe epilepsy is the most frequent form of adult refractory epilepsy and also presents the best prognosis after surgical treatment. These refractory forms can be classified as neocortical or mesial temporal epilepsies. While the neocortical forms are similar to extratemporal neocortical epilepsies in terms of evaluation and surgical treatment, most patients with mesial temporal epilepsy present clinical, electrophysiological, and imaging signs and symptoms suggestive of mesial temporal sclerosis (MTS) with hippocampal sclerosis.

MTS typically causes complex partial seizures in young adult patients with a history of prolonged febrile seizures during childhood [2, 19]. Despite intensive investigation, it has not been determined whether MTS is the cause (disorders of neuronal migration in the hippocampus) [15] or the consequence (hippocampus vulnerable to the tissue damage induced by prolonged seizures) of the febrile episodes.

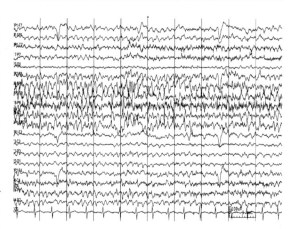

Fig. 1 Video electroencephalogram (EEG): ictal EEG showing rhythmical theta activity in electrodes in the right mesial temporal lobe

The difficulty in controlling seizures increases progressively over the years, with the disorder becoming refractory to medicamentous treatment within a period of 1–15 years [31]. The seizures usually arise with epigastric or psychic auras followed by behavioral arrest and oroalimentary or hand automatisms. The latter are usually homolateral to the temporal lobe involved, while the contralateral limb presents dystonic postures [21]. The difficulty in speaking during the seizure and during the postictal period may suggest lateralization to the dominant temporal lobe [16].

Electrophysiological investigations demonstrate the presence of rhythmic activities in the mesial electrodes of the interictal EEG. Ictal investigation by VEEG, in addition to correlating the clinical seizure with the electrographic seizure (lateralized rhythmic theta activity is usually observed; Fig. 1), permits radioisotope study (SPECT), which identifies local metabolic changes, facilitating the location of the epileptogenic area.

Over recent years, improvements in imaging techniques such as magnetic resonance imaging (MRI) have represented a major advance, permitting a precise evaluation of the changes mainly located in the hippocampus. MTS is characterized by atrophy of this structure in the T1-weighted sequence or in the volumetric reconstructions and by an increase of the signal in T2-weighted and the fluid-attenuated inversion recovery sequence (Fig. 2) [9].

In patients with MTS, the congruence of these data (clinical, interictal EEG, VEEG, SPECT, and MRI) suggests a better prognosis for surgical treatment. When doubts exist, especially regarding the lateralization of the seizures, invasive evaluation can be used by bilateral implantation of deep electrodes into the hippocampus.

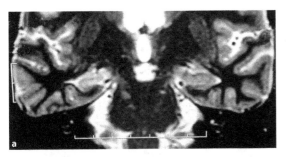

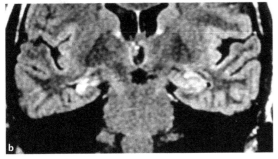

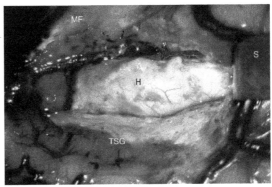

Fig. 3 Surgical exposure of right hippocampus (*H*). *TSG* Temporal superior gyrus, *MF* medial fossa, *S* spatula

Fig. 2a,b Right mesial temporal sclerosis. **a** Hippocampal atrophy on T1-weighted imaging. **b** Signal increase in fluid-attenuated inversion recovery sequence

Surgery is the recommended treatment. Randomized studies have demonstrated that after 1 year, seizure control is at least twice as efficient in patients who submit to surgical treatment as in patients receiving medicamentous treatment [59].

Surgical treatment of MTS is based on two interventions: anterior temporal lobectomy and selective amygdalohippocampectomy sparing resection of the temporal neocortex. No statistical difference has been demonstrated between these two methods regarding the efficiency of seizure control or the prevention of cognitive disorders [31].

Anterior temporal lobectomy starts with resection of the temporal neocortex including the middle and inferior temporal gyri, permitting a better view of the mesial structures. The posterior extension differs according to the side: about 5–6 cm in the nondominant hemisphere and 3–4 cm in the dominant hemisphere [51]. Using a subpial technique, the entire lateral temporal parenchyma and uncus are removed up to the limit consisting of the medial margin of the tent. This permits the exposure laterally through the pia mater, of cranial nerve III and the posterior cerebral artery, and of the internal carotid, posterior communicating, and choroidal arteries medially. This resection in a posterior direction creates a space that permits the lateral retraction of the hippocampus, facilitating the coagulation of its hilus. The next

step is the opening of the ventricular cavity in order to expose the amygdala and the hippocampus. To facilitate the location of these structures, a corticectomy is performed from the superior temporal sulcus, 3 cm posterior to the tip of the temporal lobe, in the direction of the free margin of the previously exposed tent. The amygdala is the first structure to be removed using, as a reference, the upper limit of the line formed between the emergence of the choroidal artery into the internal carotid artery and its entry into the choroidal fissure of the temporal horn (choroidal point). This limit is important in order to prevent damage to the optic tract [58]. Resection of the hippocampus starts from the anterior portion (head) and extends posteriorly through its medial surface, with coagulation of the hilus and of the branches originating from the posterior cerebral artery. The hippocampus is removed in a block of 2.5–3 cm up to the posterior portion of the cauda, permitting the complementary removal of the parahippocampal gyrus in its more medial portion (Figs. 3 and 4).

Regarding the results of anterior temporal lobectomy, 65–80% of patients have been reported to remain seizure free. This difference is due to different criteria for the evaluation of the results and to refractoriness for surgical indication. In our series of 60 patients with temporal lobe epilepsy followed up for at least 2 years, 69% showed results compatible with Engell Ia or Ib [12]. However,

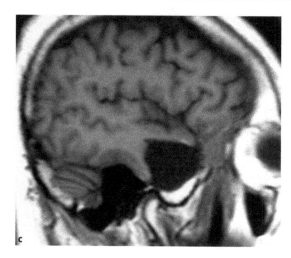
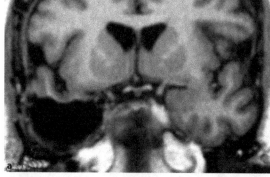
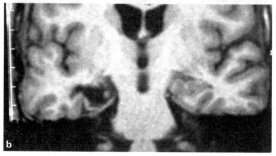

Fig. 4a–c Postoperative magnetic resonance imaging (MRI) showing resection of the right neocortex (**c**), amygdala (**a**) and hippocampus (**b**)

if we consider only patients with MTS, this rate reaches 80% (Fig. 5).

Several complications have been reported regarding this procedure: superior quadrantopsy, hemianopsia, hemiplegia due to lesion of the choroidal artery, and memory and speech disorders. In our series we observed a patient with late osteomyelitis, a patient with temporary dysfunction of cranial nerve III, and two asymptomatic patients with a chronic subdural hematoma revealed by postoperative MRI.

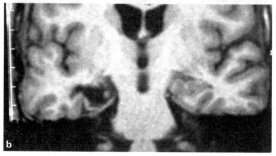

Fig. 5 Results in temporal lobe surgery. Percentage of patients with Engell Ia–Ib results. *MTS* Mesial temporal sclerosis, *Dual* MST and lesional

## 31.4
## Extratemporal Epilepsies

While about 80% of patients with temporal epilepsy present with an anatomical substrate (hippocampal sclerosis), the extratemporal epilepsies are heterogeneous in terms of their etiology. Recent advances in imaging examinations have led to a rapid increase in the number of identifiable lesions, especially cortical dysplasias, which play an important role in the genesis of extratemporal epilepsies. However, approximately 50% of refractory extratemporal epilepsies are not definitely identified by neuroimaging studies [52].

Historically, the first surgeries for extratemporal epilepsies date back to the work of Rasmussen and Penfield at the Neurological Institute of Montreal [44, 45, 47]. These investigators classified the pre- and postcentral gyri as a specific region, denoted the central area. On this basis, surgical epilepsies were identified as being 56% temporal, 18% frontal, 7% in the central region, 6% in the parietal lobe, and 1% in the frontal lobe [45]. Mutilobar resections or hemispherectomy was used to treat 11% the patients. Other series focusing on surgical treatment of extratemporal epilepsies identified 45–64% of the surgeries as being performed after seizures starting in the frontal lobe, 7–13% starting in the parietal lobes, 2–23% as being occipital, and 23–44% as multilobar foci [25]. In the surgical series published by Eriksson et al. [13], while 75% of adult surgeries involved the temporal lobe, only 25% of children's surgeries involved this lobe.

The semiology of extratemporal syndrome is varied and is not well characterized, even when limited to a single lobe. Extratemporal epilepsies also tend to spread rapidly, impairing their location on the basis of clinical characteristics. In some cases, especially those involving the frontal lobe, the seizures rapidly cross to the contralateral side, also impairing their lateralization [38].

The presence of a focal finding in MRI is probably the most important factor in the approach to extratemporal epilepsies, since a focal lesion classifies the epilepsy as lesional, with a better surgical prognosis. Other imaging studies such as ictal or interictal SPECT, PET, and spectroscopy can be of help for the focal diagnosis when MRI is normal [35].

Most patients with extratemporal epilepsies refractory to medicamentous treatment present extensive irritative multilobar surface areas in their EEG monitoring [35, 38]. In a series of 30 patients with localized forms of cortical dysplasia, more than half of the subjects presented a greater distribution of interictal findings than the structural lesion, with two-thirds of them being multilobar [36]. The identification of lobar distribution, in turn, is insufficient for a precise topographic definition. In addition, extensive neocortical areas located in the interhemispheric and basal regions, and therefore "far" from the surface electrodes, may be initial firing foci. These factors, together with the property of extratemporal foci, especially of the frontal lobe, to rapidly propagate also to the contralateral hemisphere, lead to an inconclusive, or even "false-positive," location of the epileptogenic foci [24]. Thus, it is necessary, especially when the structural lesion cannot be located, to use invasive monitoring (i.e., the placement of electrodes in the cerebral parenchyma (deep electrodes) or on the cortical surface (subdural electrodes) [36].

Deep electrodes are fine cables with cylindrical contacts along their terminal extremity, which are placed inside the encephalic parenchyma. They are used when there is a suspicion of epileptogenic areas deeply located or, more commonly, in patients with temporal epilepsy who cannot be correctly lateralized due to the rapid propagation of the impulse to the contralateral temporal lobe. They are commonly implanted stereotaxically by trephining along the direction of the hippocampus (entering through the occipital lobe) or orthogonal to the axis of the hippocampus (entering through the temporal lobe; Fig. 6).

The need for implantation involves a 1–4% risk of infection and a risk of cerebral hemorrhage of 3% in parasagittal placement and of 1% in lateral placement [42]. The placement of bilateral intrahippocampal electrodes may be associated with a postoperative decline of verbal memory [41].

Subdural electrodes are used to map the surface of the encephalon and to delimit the region of seizure onset in the neocortex. The electrodes are fine platinum or stain-

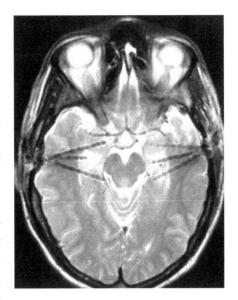

Fig. 6 Deep bilateral temporal electrodes

less steel discs attached to a fine plastic surface arranged in the configuration of striae or plates. They are placed in intimate contact with the cerebral parenchyma by craniotomy, and they can be placed in mesial structures. Subdural electrodes are used not only for ictal recording and for the determination of the zone of seizure onset, but also for cortical stimulation and mapping of cortical function on this area [52]. Six cases of infection (two cases of meningitis, one abscess, and three infections of the surgical wound) were reported in a series of 350 patients. In another series of 131 patients, 2.5% of them presented small hematomas that did not require surgical drainage [41]. Analyses of a limited amount of cortical surface and enhancement or reduction of the epileptiform activity over the underlying cortex are disadvantages of this method (Figs. 7–11) [7].

Eloquent areas such as the motor cortex, sensitive cortex, language areas (Broca's area, Wernicke's area, supplementary motor area, basal temporal area), and visual areas can be identified by cortical stimulation either in the operating theater (motor and language) or during the period of invasive VEEG evaluation when subdural electrodes are implanted.

The interictal epileptiform activity can be recorded directly form the cerebral cortex during surgery (eletrocorticography), and is considered to be an indispensable technique for defining the irritative zone in the intraoperative evaluation. During the subdural grid implantation it is useful for better defining the areas of the cerebral cortex to be evaluated. After electrode removal and cortex resection, it is a tool for determining any residual epileptiform activity.

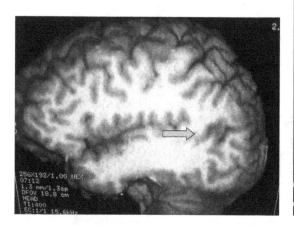

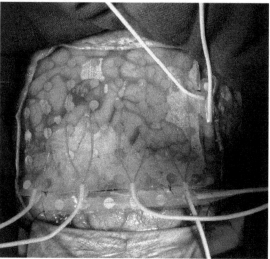

Fig. 7 Gliotic area near the left angular gyrus (*arrow*) in a 40-year old man with partial seizures

Fig. 8 Subdural electrodes in the same patient as shown in Fig. 7

Patients with extratemporal epilepsy who submit to surgical treatment are divided into two major groups: patients with lesional epilepsies and patients with cryptogenic epilepsies whose imaging exams do not identify lesions. Patients with lesional epilepsies have a better prognosis regarding seizure control. In a representative study of 60 patients with extratemporal epilepsy, 61% of the patients with identified structural lesions were seizure free over a period of 5 years, as opposed to 20% of nonlesional patients [60]. In a review of frontal epilepsies from 1987 to 1994, 72% of the lesional patients had adequate seizure control (Engel I or II), after 5 years, as compared to 40% of nonlesional patients [29].

## 31.4.1
### Lesional Epilepsies

Of patients with refractory extratemporal epilepsies, 50% present identifiable structural lesions, representing up to 80% of patients in the surgical series [35]. Focal abnormalities such as tumors, vascular lesions, and cortical abnormalities show different degrees of differentiation from the parenchyma, a fact that influences the surgical programming [25].

Neoplasias such as low-grade astrocytomas, oligodendrogliomas, dysembryoplastic neuroepithelial tumors, and others may often be the origin of epileptic foci (Figs. 12–14). Epileptogenic tumors usually grow slowly, occur in young individuals, and involve the gray matter. Epileptogenic control is better when resection of the entire lesion and the marginal area (extended lesionec-

tomy) is possible, with a rate of seizure control of about 80% [25].

Cavernomas and arteriovenous malformations are vascular lesions commonly associated with epileptic seizures [25]. Lesionectomy with the removal of marginal areas by impregnation with hemosiderin leads to seizure control in 73% of patients [22].

As diagnostic imaging methods evolve with increasing sensitivity, anomalies of cortical development are becoming increasingly more frequent as the cause of focal epilepsy. The most common developmental anomaly is cortical dysplasia, followed by malformations of the cortical gyri such as polymicrogyria. Developmental lesions are observed more frequently in children, often involving large extensions of the cortex [13]. Cortical dysplasias are associated with a particular pattern of epileptogenicity, with some authors believing that intraoperative electrocorticography is a necessary tool [37]. In large series, 49% of the patients with dysplasia became seizure free, with 58% have been submitted to complete resection and 27% to incomplete resection. Cortical dysplasia with Taylor's balloon cells was completely removed with a 100% success rate in a series of 16 patients [41].

## 31.4.2
### Nonlesional Epilepsies

Patients with nonlesional epilepsy represent the greatest challenge for the surgical treatment of epilepsies, with a lower success rate ranging from 20 to 55% of the patients. The use of invasive preoperative electrocorticography ap-

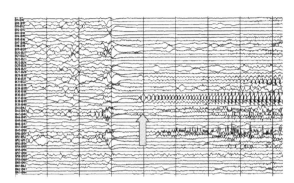

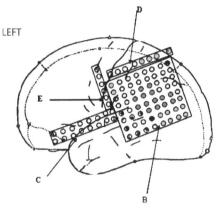

Fig. 9 Ictal EEG recording during a partial seizure from the patient of Fig. 7. Repetitive spikes in contacts B38, 42, 51 corresponding to the area surrounding the language area. The *arrow* marks the electrographic seizure onset

Fig. 10 Results of electrical stimulation of the cortex from the patient in Fig. 7 with subdural electrodes in the left hemisphere. Key: *red* ictal zone, *green* visual area, *blue* sensitive area, *black and white* language area

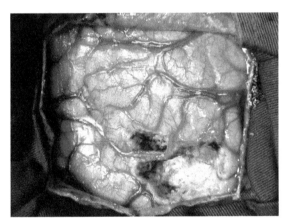

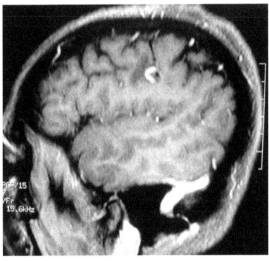

Fig. 11 Postresection with preservation of the arterial supply for the adjacent cortex from the patient in Fig. 7

Fig. 12 A 35-year-old woman with left frontal granuloma

pears to play a fundamental role in this type of patient. A study conducted on 24 patients with epilepsy and normal MRI did not reveal a significant difference in seizure-free evolution in patients submitted to invasive monitoring. However, the use of invasive monitoring was of fundamental importance for the surgical strategy by establishing a clear definition between the epileptogenic zone and the motor and language areas [10].

In a study conducted by Chapman et al. [10], 78% of patients with frontal epilepsy and a normal MRI received

a diagnosis of dysplasia after a postoperative anatomopathological exam.

Among the surgical possibilities for nonlesional patients are neocortical resection and disconnection procedures such as MST and callosotomy. Resection of the cerebral cortex is denoted topectomy, corticectomy, or neocortical resection. The margins of this resection are determined by invasive subdural recordings and by the mapping of eloquent areas. Mapping can be performed by a preoperative methodology with functional MRI and

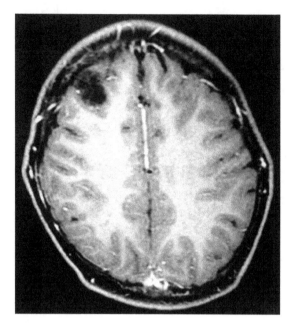

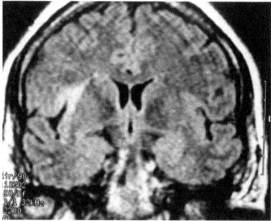

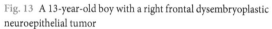

Fig. 13 A 13-year-old boy with a right frontal dysembryoplastic neuroepithelial tumor

Fig. 14 A 51-year-old woman with a right insular dysplasia

magnetoencephalography in addition to cortical stimulation and somatosensory evoked potential recording using subdural electrodes.

## 31.5
## Disconnective Surgery

The objective of disconnective surgery for the treatment of intractable epilepsies is to isolate or disconnect the epileptogenic area of the ipsilateral hemisphere or to prevent the propagation of the seizure to the contralateral hemisphere. The main types of disconnective surgery used are multiple subspinal transection (MST), corpus callosotomy, and hemispherectomy,

### 31.5.1
### Multiple Subpial Transection

MST was developed by Morrel [28, 49] for the treatment of epilepsies originating from a cortex that cannot be resected, such as the motor cortex. The technique is based on the principle of the columnar organization of the cerebral cortex, whereby the fibers belonging to the long descending tracts would not be affected by the section of horizontal segments. The theory that the generation of electroencephalographic and clinical seizures depends on the horizontal propagation of the epileptiform discharge in the cortex, while functional activity such as motor and speech control depends on an intact vertical column of the cortex, is the physiological basis of this technique. MST consists of lesion of the horizontal connections that run between the cortex, which are crucial for the synchronization of neural activity (a key point of the seizures), without involving the fibers of ascending and descending projections responsible for cortical functioning. A small hook-shaped blade is used to cut through the gray matter, while leaving the pia and vessels intact. The transections should be performed at right angles along the axis of the gyri at 5-mm intervals. Invasive recording and electrocorticography can be used to determine the area to be submitted to the procedure, with an intraoperative seizure-free recording being the determinant of the functional final point of the procedure. Most patients present temporary deficits during the postoperative period, with improvement within 2–4 weeks and a return to the previous functional status. The incidence of permanent deficits is about 5% [27].

MSTs can be used for the treatment of continuous partial epilepsy; focal seizures of the sensory, somatosensory, or visual cortex; resection with evidence of epileptiform activity in the adjacent eloquent areas; Landau-Kleffner syndrome and Rasmussen encephalitis. The procedure is also used when the extension of resection increases the surgical risk [6].

A meta-analysis of international experience with 53 patients submitted to MST and 158 submitted to cortical resection plus MST reported a successful reduction of seizures in 95% of the patients who submitted to resection and in 68% of the patients submitted to MST alone [25]. Another study, however, demonstrated a late increase in the incidence of seizures in up to 19% of the patients [34].

The efficacy of treatment of patients with Landau-Kleffner syndrome has been promising, with favorable results in 62% of patients with isolated MST [48].

## 31.5.2
## Corpus Callosotomy

Median section of the corpus callosum is a palliative form of treatment for patients with generalized tonic-clonic, tonic or myoclonic seizures, or seizures with drop attacks refractory to medicamentous treatment. Some authors perform corpus callosotomy in patients with primarily generalized epileptiform discharges or in patients who show secondary bilateral generalization [18]. First introduced by Van Wagenen and Herren in 1939 [53], section of the corpus callosum is performed in order to prevent the bilateral synchrony of a cortical epileptiform activity that may result in seizures with bilateral motor manifestations.

The corpus callosum performs interhemispheric connection, unifying motor function and sensory, visual, and somatosensory perception. The axons that connect the frontal lobes occupy the more rostral portions, whereas the connections of the parietal, temporal, and occipital cortex occupy the more caudal portion. In a feline model of generalized epilepsy, Musgrave and Gloor [30] demonstrated that total section of the corpus callosum and of the anterior commissure leads to the disappearance of the bilateral synchrony of epileptiform discharges of the slow-wave-spike type.

Direct right frontal craniotomy is performed, with the anterior limit located 2 cm from the coronary suture and the medial limit located in the superior sagittal suture, exposing the superior sagittal sinus. An opening of the dura mater is performed toward the superior sagittal sinus until the interhemispheric portion is exposed. The interhemispheric fissure is dissected following the ascending branch of the pericallosal artery, with identification of the cingulate gyrus and of the corpus callosum. The anterior two-thirds or three-quarters of the corpus callosum are then opened longitudinally, while the splenium is left intact because it contains fibers connecting the supplementary motor areas. Complete section of the corpus callosum is reserved for patients whose response to anterior section is unsatisfactory [50]. Phillips and Sakas [40] reported that surgical section of the corpus callosum reduced the frequency of seizures by 70% in 16 of 20 patients (80%). Gates and dePaola [17] reported a reduction of generalized tonic-clonic seizures in 50–80% of their patients.

Feichtinger et al. [14] evaluated the efficacy of anterior callosotomy by radiosurgery in a group of eight patients with intractable drop attacks. One of these patients required radiosurgical callosotomy of the middle third after 17 months and two patients were submitted to partial hemispherotomy. This was an effective and safe noninvasive method for the treatment of these patients.

In addition to the complications inherent to the surgical act, the typical complications of corpus callosotomy are mainly neuropsychological [3]. Varied degrees of disconnection syndrome characterized by lethargy, apathy, mutism, incontinence, apraxia, and a bilateral Babinski sign may be present during the first postoperative week. There is a direct relationship between symptoms and the extension of section. The more posterior the disconnection, the greater the possibility of neuropsychological alterations.

Total callosotomy should be performed as the initial procedure only in patients whose initial cognitive deficit is so severe that no functional impairment will derive from the institution of disconnection syndrome [25].

## 31.5.3
## Hemispherectomy

The first description of hemispherectomy was reported in 1928 by Walter Dandy [1] for the treatment of a patient with glioblastoma multiforme. Ten years later, Mackenzie described the use of this technique for a patient with epilepsy. In 1950, Krynauw reported the use of hemispherectomy in a patient with hemiplegia since childhood, intractable epilepsy, and behavioral alteration [55].

In 1966, Oppenheimer and Griffith [33] reported a late complication of hemispherectomy consisting of small and repeated bleedings in the subdural space causing obstructive hydrocephalus and superficial hemosiderosis of the central nervous system. In the 1970's, numerous modifications were introduced in the anatomical technique of hemispherectomy in order to prevent late complications. In 1982 Rasmussen [43] introduced the surgical technique of functional hemispherectomy, anatomically incomplete but functionally complete, leaving more brain tissue and considerably reducing late complications. More recently, the hemispherotomy technique of Delalande and the peri-insular hemispherotomy technique of Villemure [57] represent an attempt to obtain complete functional disconnection with a smaller cerebral resection.

This technique is indicated for patients who present severe motor seizures associated with other types of seizures that originate from the same brain hemisphere and who present contralateral hemiparesis, with a nonfunctioning hand and homonymous hemianopsia. Patients with Rasmussen and Sturge-Weber syndrome, and hemimegaloencephaly are frequent candidates for this type of treatment. Other malformation disorders and cerebral

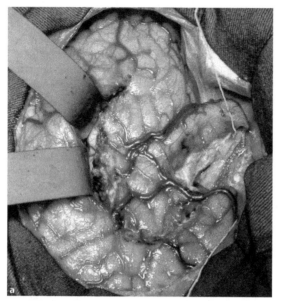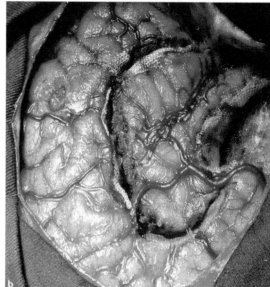

Fig. 15a,b Operative view of a right hemispherotomy. **a** Temporal lobe resection and intraventricular exposure. **b** Final view, with a small amount of tissue removed

ischemias leading to unilateral cortical atrophy or porencephaly also benefit from this surgery.

Anatomical hemispherectomy was the original technique [54]. Lobar or en bloc resection of the brain hemisphere is performed, with preservation of the base nuclei. Peacock et al. [39] recommend anatomical hemispherectomy for patients with a small lateral ventricle and with dysplastic syndromes, because of the risk of hemorrhage and because of the consistency of brain tissue.

The technique of functional hemispherectomy proposed by Rasmussen [43] consists of temporal lobectomy with amygdalohippocampectomy followed by suprasylvian central corticectomy extending to the fornix. The initial disconnection is performed and then extended by callosotomy and by disconnection of the temporal and parieto-occipital lobes. The frontal lobe is disconnected through a plane corresponding to the wing of the sphenoid bone.

Hemispherotomy, proposed by Delalande in 1992, consists of a disconnection technique above the resection. The lateral ventricle is accessed and callosotomy is performed, followed by transection of the ganglia from the base to the inferomesial frontal region. In 1995, Villemure [57] described peri-insular hemispherotomy. The frontal, parietal, and temporal opercles are resected by means of suprainsular and infrainsular corticectomies, and callosotomy is performed through the lateral ventricle. Disconnection of the frontal lobe on the coronal plane follows the level of the greater wing of the sphenoid bone. After callosotomy, the procedure is continued with

subpial aspiration through the fimbria-fornix. Amygdalohippocampectomy is then performed (Figs. 15 and 16).

The complication of hemispherectomy [56], especially in patients with incomplete motor deficit, is flaccid hemiplegia, which usually improves over a period of months. Preservation of arteries and veins in functional hemispherectomy is important for the prevention of cerebral infarctions and edema during the immediate postoperative period, as well as late progressive brain atrophy. Hydrocephalus can be an acute complication requiring a temporary or definitive external shunt. Many patients develop aseptic meningitis, which is characterized by low fever, headache, irritability, and lethargy. Infections and hemorrhages are late complications. Hemispherectomy, when properly indicated, provides an excellent result in terms of the control of epileptic seizures, leading to intellectual and behavioral improvement of the patient.

## References

1.  Andermann F, Freeman JM, Vigevano F, et al (1993) Surgical remediable diffuse hemispheric syndromes. In: Engel J Jr (ed) Surgical Treatment of Epilepsies, 2nd edn. Raven, New York, pp 87–101

2.  Annegers JF, Hauser WA, Shirts SB, et al (1987) Factors prognostic of unprovoked seizures after febrile convulsions. N Engl J Med 316:493–498

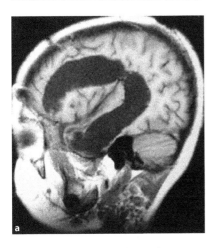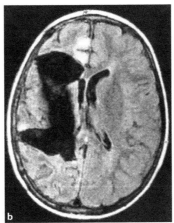

Fig. 16 Postoperative, posthemispherectomy MRI

3. Black PM, Holmes G, Lombroso CT (1992) Corpus callosum section for intractable epilepsy in children. Pediatr
Neurosurg 18:298–304

4. Borges MA, Min LL, Guerreiro CA, et al (2004) Urban
prevalence of epilepsy: populational study in Sao Jose do
Rio Preto, a medium-sized city in Brazil. Arq Neuropsiquiatr 62:199–204

5. Bourgeois BF (2001) General concepts of medical intractability. In: Lüders HO, Comair YG (eds) Epilepsy Surgery,
2nd edn. Lippincott Williams Wilkins, Philadelphia, pp
63–68

6. Byrne RW, Whisler WW (2004) Multiple subpial transection. In: Winn HR (ed) Youmans Neurological Surgery, 5th
edn. Saunders, Philadelphia, pp 2635–2642

7. Carreño MAR, Lüders HO (2001) General principles of
presurgical evaluation. In: Lüders HO, Comair YG (eds)
Epilepsy Surgery, 2nd edn. Lippincott Williams Wilkins,
Philadelphia, pp 185–200

8. Cascino GD (2006) Recognition of potential surgical candidates and video-electroencephalographic evaluation. In:
Wyllie E (ed) The Treatment of Epilepsy: Principles and
Practice, 4th edn. Lippincott Williams Wilkins, Philadelphia, pp 993–1008

9. Cendes F, Andermann F, Gloor P, et al (1993) MRI volumetric measurement of amygdala and hippocampus in
temporal lobe epilepsy. Neurology 43:719–725

10. Chapman K, Wyllie E, Najm I, et al (2005) Seizure outcome
after epilepsy surgery in patients with normal preoperative
MRI. J Neurol Neurosurg Psychiatry 76:710–713

11. Cross JH, Jayakar P, Nordli D, et al (2006) Proposed criteria
for referral and evaluation of children for epilepsy surgery:
recommendations of the subcommission for pediatric epilepsy surgery. Epilepsia 47:952–959

12. Engel J Jr, Van Ness PC, Rasmussen TB, et al (1993), Outcome with respect to epileptic seizures. In: Engel J Jr (ed)
Surgical Treatment of the Epilepsies. Raven, New York,
pp 609–621

13. Eriksson S, Malmgren K, Rydenhag B, et al (1999) Surgical
treatment of epilepsy – clinical, radiological and histopathological findings in 139 children and adults. Acta Neurol
Scand 99:8–15

14. Feichtinger M, Schrottner O, Eder H, et al (2006) Efficacy
and safety of radiosurgical callosotomy: a retrospective
analysis. Epilepsia 47:1184–1191

15. Fernandez G, Effenberger O, Vinz B, et al (1998) Hippocampal malformation as a cause of familial febrile convulsions and subsequent hippocampal sclerosis. Neurology
50:909–917

16. Gabr M, Luders H, Dinner D, et al (1989) Speech manifestations in lateralization of temporal lobe seizures. Ann
Neurol 25:82–87

17. Gates JR, dePaola L (1996) Corpus callosum section. In:
Sliovon S, Dreifuss F, Fisher D, et al (eds) The Treatment of
Epilepsy. Blackwell Scientific, London, pp 722–738

18. Gates JR, Courtney W, Ritter FJ, et al (1993) Reevaluation
of corpus callosotomy. In: Engel J (ed) Surgical Treatment
of the Epilepsies. Raven, New York, pp 637–648

19. Harvey AS, Grattan-Smith JD, Desmond PM, et al (1995)
Febrile seizures and hippocampal sclerosis: frequent and
related findings in intractable temporal lobe epilepsy of
childhood. Pediatr Neurol 12:201–206

20. Hauser WA, Hesdorffer DC (2001) Epidemiology of intractable epilepsy. In: Lüders HO, Comair YG (eds) Epilepsy
Surgery, 2nd edn. Lippincott Williams Wilkins, Philadelphia, pp 55–61

21. Kotagal P, Luders H, Morris HH, et al (1989) Dystonic pos-
turing in complex partial seizures of temporal lobe onset: a
new lateralizing sign. Neurology 39:196–201

22. Kraemer DL, Griebel ML, Lee N, et al (1998) Surgical outcome in patients with epilepsy with occult vascular malformations treated with lesionectomy. Epilepsia 39:600–607

23. Kwan P, Brodie-Martin J (2006) Issues of medical intractability for surgical candidacy In: Wyllie E (ed) The Treatment of Epilepsy: Principles and Practice, 4th edn. Lippincott Williams Wilkins, Philadelphia, pp 983–991

24. Laskowitz DT, Sperling MR, French JA, et al (1995) The syndrome of frontal lobe epilepsy: characteristics and surgical management. Neurology 45:780–787

25. Leiphart JW, Fried I (2004) Surgery for extratemporal lobe epilepsy. In: Winn HR (ed) Youmans Neurological Surgery, 5th edn. Saunders, Philadelphia, pp 2587–2604

26. Mattson RH, Cramer JA, Collins JF, et al (1992) A comparison of valproate with carbamazepine for the treatment of complex partial seizures and secondarily generalized tonic-clonic seizures in adults. N Eng J Med 327:765–771

27. Morrel F, Kanner A, Whisler WW (1998) Multiple subpial transection. In: Stefan H, Andermann F (eds) Plasticity in Epilepsy. Lippincott-Raven, New York, pp 219–234

28. Morrel F, Whisler WW, Bleck T (1989) Multiple subpial transection: a new approach to the surgical treatment of focal epilepsy. J Neurosurg 70:231–239

29. Mosewich RK, So EL, O'Brien TJ, et al (2000) Factors predictive of outcome of frontal lobe epilepsy surgery. Epilepsia 41:843–849

30. Musgrave J, Gloor P (1980) The role of corpus callosum in bilateral interhemispheric synchrony of spike and wave discharge in feline generalized penicillin epilepsy. Epilepsia 21:369–378

31. Najm IM, Babb TL, Mohamed A, et al (2001) Mesial temporal lobe sclerosis. In: Lüders HO, Comair YG (eds) Epilepsy Surgery, 2nd edn. Lippincott Williams Wilkins, Philadelphia, pp 95–104

32. Nordli DR (2006) Usefulness of video-EEG monitoring. Epilepsia 47:26–30

33. Oppenheimer DR, Griffith HB (1966) Persistent intracranial bleeding as a complication of hemispherectomy. J Neurol Neurosurg Psychiatry 29:229–240

34. Orbach D, Romanelli P, Devinsky O, et al (2001) Late seizure recurrence after multiple subpial transections. Epilepsia 42:1130–1133

35. Palmini A, Costa da Costa J (1998) Cirurgia das epilepsias extratemporais: a difícil arte de definir alvos e fronteiras. In: Costa da Costa J, Palmini A, Yacubian EMT (eds) Fundamentos Neurobiológicos das Epilepsias – Aspectos Clínicos e Cirúrgicos. Lemos Editorial, São Paulo, pp 1141–1161

36. Palmini A, Andermann F, Olivier A, et al (1991) Focal neuronal migration disorders and intractable partial epilepsy: a study of 30 patients. Ann Neurol 30:741–749

37. Palmini A, Gambardella A, Anderman F, et al (1995) Intrinsic epileptogenicity of human dysplastic cortex as suggested by corticography and surgical results. Ann Neurol 37:476–487

38. Palmini A, Portal K, Costa da Costa J, et al (1992) Espectro de manifestações clônicas, eletrográficas e de neuroimagem em pacientes com provável epilepsia do lobo frontal. JLBE 5:175–183

39. Peacock WJ, Wehby-Grant MC, Shields WD, et al (1996) Hemispherectomy for intractable seizures in children: a report of 58 cases. Childs Nerv Syst 12:376–384

40. Phillips J, Sakas DE (1996) Anterior callosotomy for intractable epilepsy: outcome in a series of twenty patients. Br J Neurosurg 10:351–356

41. Pilcher WH (2003) Epilepsy surgery: outcome and complications. In: Winn HR (ed) Youmans Neurological Surgery, 5th edn. Saunders, Philadelphia pp 2565–2585

42. Pilcher WH, Ojemann GA (1993) Presurgical evaluation and epilepsy surgery. In: Apuzzo MLJ (ed) Brain Surgery: Complications, Avoidance and Management. Churchill Livingstone, New York, pp 1525–1555

43. Rasmussen T (1983) Hemispherectomy for seizures revisited. Can J Neurol Syst 10:71–78

44. Rasmussen T (1991) Tailoring of cortical excisions for frontal lobe epilepsy. Can J Neurol Sci 18:606–610

45. Rasmussen T (1991) Surgery for central, parietal and occipital epilepsy. Can J Neurol Sci 18:611–616

46. Rosenow F, Luders H (2001) Presurgical evaluation of epilepsy. Brain 124:1683–700

47. Salanova V, Andermann F, Rasmussen T, et al (1995) Parietal lobe epilepsy: clinical manifestations and outcome in 82 patients treated surgically between 1929 and 1988. Brain 118:607–627

48. Schramm J, Aliaskevich A, Grunwald T (2002) Multiple subpial transection: outcome and complications in 20 patients who did not undergo resection. J Neurosurg 97:39–47

49. Smith MC (1998) Multiple subpial transection in patients with extra-temporal epilepsy. Epilepsia 39:S81–S89

50. Spencer SS, Katz A, Ebersole J, et al (1993) Ictal EEG changes with corpus callosum section. Epilepsia 34:568–573

51. Spencer DD, Spencer SS, Masttson RH, et al (1984) Access to the posterior medial temporal lobe structures in the surgical treatment of temporal lobe epilepsy. Neurosurgery 15:667–671

52. Swartz BE, Halgren E, Delgado-Escueta AV (1989) Neuroimaging in patients with seizures of problable frontal origin. Epilepsia 30:547–558

53. Van Wagenen WP, Herren RY (1940) Surgical division of commissural pathways in the corpus callosum: relation to spread of an epileptic attack. Arch Neurol Psychiatry 44:740–759

54. Villemure, JG (1991) Hemispherectomy techniques. In: Lüders H (ed) Epilepsy Surgery. Raven, New York, pp 569–578

55. Villemure JG (1992) Anatomical to functional hemispherectomy from Krynauw to Rasmussen. Epilepsy Res 5:209–215

56. Villemure JG (2004) Hemispherectomy: techniques and complications. In: Wyllie E (ed) The Treatment of Epilepsy: Principles and Practice, 2nd edn. Williams Wilkins, Baltimore, pp 1081–1086

57. Villemure JG, Macott CR (1995) Peri-insular hemispherectomy: surgical principles and anatomy. Neurosurgery 37:975–981

58. Wen HT, Rhoton AL Jr, de Oliveira E, et al (1999) Microsurgical anatomy of the temporal lobe. Part 1: mesial temporal lobe anatomy and its vascular relationships as applied to amygdalohippocampectomy. Neurosurgery 45:549–591; discussion 591–592

59. Wiebe S, Blume WT, Girvin JP, et al (2001) A randomized, controlled trial of surgery for temporal-lobe epilepsy. N Engl J Med 345:311–318

60. Zentner J, Hufnagel A, Ostertun B, et al (1996) Surgical treatment of extratemporal epilepsy: clinical, radiologic, and histopathologic findings in 60 patients. Epilepsia 37:1072–1080

# Bypass and Vascular Reconstruction for Anterior Circulation Aneurysms

Laligam N. Sekhar,
Sabareesh K. Natarajan, Gavin W. Britz,
and Basavaraj Ghodke

## Contents

## 32.1
## Introduction

Complex aneurysms are defined as those with a dome to neck ratio of 1.5:1, those larger than 2 cm without a defined neck, those that have a major artery originating from the neck or sac, those that have considerable atherosclerotic changes in the neck, those with a significant thrombus in the lumen, fusiform aneurysms, and blister aneurysms (Table 1). Such aneurysms cannot be occluded by simple microsurgical clipping or standard endovascular coiling techniques without occluding the parent vessel or its major branches. Available strategies for preserving or reconstructing the parent vessel or major branches are: microsurgical (clip reconstruction or bypass) or endovascular (balloon-assisted coiling or stent-assisted coiling, endovascular parent vessel occlusion). The strategy of choice for a particular case has to be individualized and depends on multiple patient and aneurysm characteristics. A simplified protocol we use in making treatment decision is shown in Fig. 1.

Table 1 Complex aneurysms

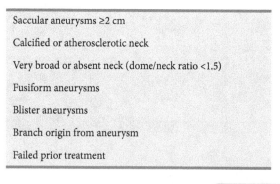

Saccular aneurysms ≥2 cm

Calcified or atherosclerotic neck

Very broad or absent neck (dome/neck ratio <1.5)

Fusiform aneurysms

Blister aneurysms

Branch origin from aneurysm

Failed prior treatment

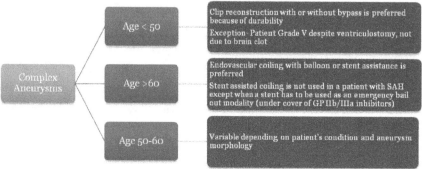

Fig. 1 Protocol for managing complex aneurysms. Note that age is given in years. *SAH* Subarachnoid hemorrhage, *GP* glycoprotein

## 32.2
## Parent Vessel Occlusion

When the intracranial internal carotid artery (ICA) is occluded, whether or not a bypass is needed in all patients is controversial. A selective approach bases this decision on a balloon occlusion test, with monitoring of cerebral blood flow by single photon emission computed tomography (SPECT), transcranial Doppler ultrasound (TCD), or xenon blood flow studies. A universal approach recommends a bypass in all patients. The senior author followed a selective approach in his earlier patients. However, based on a review of his patients who were not revascularized and suffered strokes, and the reports of other surgeons with a similar experience [4, 6, 8, 14], a universal approach is presently followed if the ICA has to be occluded surgically. A selective approach is used in patients who can have a vascular occlusion via an endovascular technique. However, even in such patients we have observed the occurrence of delayed ischemia, necessitating a protracted, hypertensive management in the intensive care unit, or the need for bypass in a delayed fashion in some patients.

The potential long-term consequences of large-vessel occlusion – increased incidence of flow aneurysms,

enlargement of existing aneurysms, and increased incidence of hypertension – have to be kept in mind. Therefore, an endovascular occlusion of the parent vessel harboring an aneurysm is performed presently in patients older than 60 years of age if there is a good collateral circulation demonstrated by anatomic and physiological tests. In case of the carotid artery, a balloon occlusion test is performed for 15 min under normotensive conditions. Simultaneously, TCD monitoring is performed, making sure that the middle cerebral artery (MCA) velocity does not fall below 30% of the baseline. Xenon blood flow or SPECT scanning may also be performed when possible to assess the cerebral perfusion. It is important to note the sources of collateral circulation and to ensure that they will not be occluded by the treatment. If all criteria are fulfilled, then the ICA may be occluded with coils.

In all other patients wherein the ICA is significantly involved by the aneurysm, a cross-compression angiogram (with compression of the cervical common carotid artery) is performed, to determine the adequacy of the collateral circulation during temporary occlusion at surgery. This enables surgical decision-making regarding the risk of temporary occlusion, and selection of the proximal donor vessel for the bypass (e.g., the ICA or external carotid artery, ECA).

## 32.3
## Endovascular Options for Preserving or Reconstructing the Parent Vessel

Balloon-assisted coiling is used for wide-necked aneurysms with a dome to neck ratio between 1.5 and 2. However, there are no long-term studies (>2 years follow up) demonstrating the durability of aneurysms coiled with balloon assistance. The recurrence rate of wide-necked aneurysms due to coil compaction at short-term follow up has been 35–60% [5].

Stent-assisted coiling is an option for more complex aneurysms. It is preferred for older patients because of questions about the durability and long-term safety of endovascular stents. Recurrence rates after stent-assisted coiling have been reported to be around 23% [1] at a mean follow up of 4.6 months. When the vessel wall is totally diseased (e.g., dissection, fusiform aneurysms) or when branches are arising from the wall, stent-assisted coiling may not be an option. Stent-assisted coiling is also not preferred in a patient with subarachnoid hemorrhage (SAH), since the patient has to be loaded and maintained on antiplatelet therapy with aspirin and clopidogrel. For the same reasons, stent-assisted coiling may be contraindicated even in patients with unruptured aneurysms with associated gastric or duodenal ulceration, other intestinal pathology, or intolerance to antiplatelet therapy.

## 32.4
## Microsurgical Options for Reconstructing the Parent Vessel

Clip reconstruction is possible for aneurysms provided that a distinct portion of the artery wall (at least 270° of circumference) is healthy, and not aneurysmal. Potential problems include the need for 15–30 min of temporary occlusion of the artery, multiple trials of clipping, the need for intraoperative angiography, and the occurrence of neck remnant or occlusion of the artery by the clipping process. Frequently, such aneurysms have an atherosclerotic wall or extensive thrombus inside, which complicates the operation.

Surgical reconstruction options for complex aneurysms include local techniques such as resuture, interposition graft, and side-to-side anastomosis, as well as extra- to intracranial bypass techniques using the superficial temporal artery (STA), saphenous vein, or the radial artery. In addition, in some patients, a temporary bypass using the radial artery may be required to provide adequate collateral circulation to the brain during protracted temporary clipping and occlusion of an intracranial aneurysm [11, 12].

## 32.5
## Preoperative Preparation, Anesthesia, and Monitoring

If a bypass procedure is planned to treat an aneurysm, the patient is placed on aspirin, 325 mg by mouth preoperatively for 1 week before the surgery, or at least for 2 days prior to the surgery. A prophylactic antibiotic, usually ceftriaxone 1 g, is administered intravenously 1 h prior to the incision and continued for 48 h postoperatively. The patient should have central-venous- and arterial-line monitoring. In case of radial artery grafts (RAGs), the graft extraction site is marked before the operation to avoid the placement of the radial artery line in that arm. When an RAG or saphenous vein graft is planned, the vessel is imaged preoperatively by duplex ultrasound in order to evaluate the vessel size, and in the case of the saphenous vein, to mark its course on the skin. A lumbar drain or a ventriculostomy is inserted prior to surgery in order to achieve adequate brain relaxation, in addition to the administration of intravenous mannitol upon skin incision.

A balanced neuroanesthetic technique is employed. Intraoperative neurophysiological monitoring is performed with the monitoring of somatosensory evoked potentials, electroencephalogram, and motor evoked potentials. When prolonged temporary occlusion of the intracranial vessels is anticipated during the aneurysm treatment (>30 min), or during the bypass procedure itself, 5000 units of heparin are given intravenously; the activated clotting time is monitored to maintain it above 250 s until flow is resumed in the occluded vessels and the bypass. Patients are placed in burst suppression using propofol in order to protect the brain during temporary arterial occlusion for bypass [7], but care must be taken to avoid hypotension during such burst suppression. Normal blood pressure and volume are maintained during burst suppression in cases of ruptured aneurysms, and in case of unruptured aneurysm the blood pressure is elevated 20% above the patient's normal value. Autoregulation of cerebral blood flow may be impaired or absent in aneurysm patients with high-flow bypasses used for revascularization. Hence, systemic hypertension (more than 20 mmHg above the baseline) must be avoided after the operation, for 48 h. Intraoperative angiography is often (but not always) performed during the management of complex aneurysms [11].

## 32.6
## Choice of Graft

The choice of graft depends upon four factors: (1) the size of the recipient vessel, which is the major determinant, (2) the availability of a donor vessel, (3) the availability of graft material, and (4) the extent of blood flow augmentation required. A low-flow vessel (<50 ml/min) such as the STA is generally inadequate if a large parent artery such as the ICA has to be sacrificed during the bypass operation, unless another collateral source exists (such as a good anterior communicating, ACOM, artery). If the STA is large in caliber, it may be anastomosed to an $M_3$ branch of the MCA, and this may provide adequate flow when the volume demand for replacement is low.

High-flow grafts (>100 ml/min) such as the RAG or the saphenous vein graft are more reliable when the occlusion of the ICA is planned. The radial artery provides a flow rate of between 100 and 300 ml/min acutely and the flow can increase significantly over the ensuing days, as measured by TCD [11]. The radial artery is easier to harvest. However, one major problem with its use is the occurrence of vasospasm, which can be prevented by the use of the pressure distension technique [11, 13].

A saphenous vein graft is used when the radial artery is not available as a suitable vessel. It is better to extract the saphenous vein from the upper leg and the lower thigh, where it has a fairly uniform caliber. The saphenous vein has a much thicker wall than the intracranial vessels and because of the high flow through it, it is more prone to kinking the distal anastomotic site and is technically more difficult to perform than the RAG. Graft flow in the saphenous vein has been measured at 100–350 ml/min. In children below the age of 12 years, where the RAG is small in diameter, the saphenous vein graft is the only alternative. Because of the high flow through the saphenous vein graft, there may be a flow mismatch when it is anastomosed into the MCA; this could lead to turbulence and graft flow problems.

Long-term results for saphenous vein grafts and RAGs in the intracranial circulation are not available at present. A study from the Mayo Clinic about the long-term patency of saphenous vein grafts indicates that these grafts have an average failure rate of 1–1.5% per year after the 1st year after surgery [9]. However, this study only measured the patency of grafts by palpation behind the ear. In the cardiac literature, however, RAGs appear to have a better patency rate than saphenous vein grafts, and internal mammary artery grafts exhibited an even better long-term patency [2].

## 32.7
## Exposure of the STA

The STA is traced out using a Doppler probe, and marked on the skin surface with a marking pen. After draping, an incision is made over the outline of the STA through the epidermis using a Colorado microneedle-tip monopolar cautery (Stryker Leibinger, Kalamazoo, Michigan, USA) at a low setting of 8, with the aid of a surgical microscope. The incision is carefully deepened through the dermis until loose areolar tissue is reached. Using a fine

scissors, the soft tissue is dissected, exposing the surface of the artery, which overlies the temporalis fascia or periosteum. The artery is exposed from its origin anterior to the tragus of the ear. A 0.5-cm pedicle, lateral to the artery on each side, is isolated by cutting the galea down to the temporalis fascia or periosteum. The artery becomes more superficial (runs in the dermal layer) more distally, and care should be taken not to damage it. Side branches are coagulated at a safe distance from the artery. The periadventitial tissues are cleared from the artery distally, near the site of the anastomosis. The vessel is left in situ until the bypass procedure.

A T-incision is created from the incision made to expose the artery to facilitate the muscle dissection and performance of the craniotomy. When the vessel is extracted prior to the surgery, a temporary clip is placed proximally; the vessel is ligated distally, and divided. A small blunt-tipped needle is inserted into the vessel at the distal end, and the vessel is irrigated with heparinized saline with the temporary opening of the temporary clip in order to clear the blood from the arterial segment beyond the clip.

## 32.8
## Radial Artery Exposure

The presence of adequate perfusion to the hand must be confirmed by the Allen test preoperatively, prior to the extraction of the radial artery [3]. During the procedure, a pulse oximeter is placed on the index or middle finger to further test the adequacy of the collateral circulation. The radial artery pulse is palpated just above the wrist and a vertical incision is made through the skin and subcutaneous tissue and deep fascia. This is extended as a gently curved, longitudinal incision on the ventral aspect of the forearm following the course of the artery. The artery is identified distally on the volar aspect of the forearm between the tendons of the flexor carpi radialis and brachioradialis muscles (Fig. 2). It is then traced proximally from this point, upward to just below the bend of the elbow, where it lies under the brachioradialis. Once the artery is well exposed, it should be gently occluded between the fingers of the surgeon to verify that there are no changes in pulse oximetry, to confirm the patency of the ulnar artery and the palmar arch. Small arteries and veins emerging from the neurovascular bundle are occluded with tiny titanium clips and further cauterized with bipolar cautery beyond the clip, and then divided. The venae commitantes are left attached to the artery except near the ends. The artery is left in situ and harvested just prior to the anastomosis.

At extraction, the artery is ligated proximally and distally, sectioned sharply, and removed. It is first cleared of intraluminal blood with heparinized saline using a small blunt needle. Following this, the pressure distension technique (Fig. 3) is used to expand the vessel. This is done by

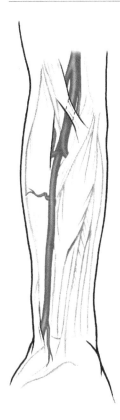

Fig. 2  Course of the radial artery in the forearm. Courtesy of Laligam N. Sekhar

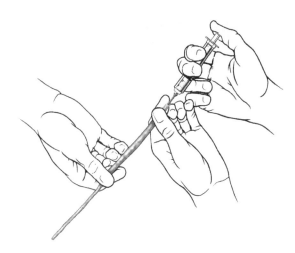

Fig. 3  Pressure distention technique. Courtesy of Laligam N. Sekhar

compressing the graft around the needle and then pinching the graft sequentially in segments and distending the graft with heparin saline to expand it. After removing the RAG, the adventitia is removed from the artery at either end of the graft, for about 1 cm.

## 32.9
## Saphenous Vein Exposure

The best way to find the vein is by preoperative duplex ultrasound imaging and mapping. The ideal location for vein harvest is the upper leg and the lower thigh, where the vein is of uniform caliber. During surgery, the leg is positioned with the thigh rotated outward (Fig. 4). The vein exposure is started at the lower end and traced up at least 20 cm superiorly; branches are ligated or occluded with titanium hemoclips, and divided. The vein is left in situ until extraction. At extraction, both the ends beyond the graft segment are ligated, and the vein is sectioned and removed. After extraction, it is flushed through with heparinized saline and distended at a slight pressure to release the spasm of the vessel. The adventitia of either end of the vein must be trimmed adequately before implantation. The vein should be transferred cranially without reversal, to avoid valve-related blood flow obstruction. The flow direction in the vein is confirmed before

anastomosis by flushing the graft with heparinized saline and confirming free flow of fluid from the other end. The vein is marked longitudinally with methylene blue to detect torsion.

## 32.10
## Choice of Recipient Vessel

In order to perform the bypass, the appropriate vessel must be selected beforehand. In the anterior circulation, this is generally an $M_2$ branch of the MCA. The $M_1$ segment is unsuitable for bypass due to the presence of lenticulostriate perforators, and temporary ischemia is poorly tolerated in this vascular territory. The vessel chosen as the recipient should be at least 2 mm in diameter. Saphenous vein grafts require a larger vessel for implantation and it is often best to implant the vein into the bifurcation of the MCA or into a vessel at least 2.5 mm in diameter. In some patients, the MCA branches very proximally with a short $M_1$ segment and the perforators will be arising from the various branches. This may make the MCA unsuitable as a recipient vessel for a high-flow bypass. In such cases and if the aneurysm is infraclinoid, then the supraclinoid ICA may be chosen to serve as the recipient vessel for the bypass. When the ICA is used in this fashion, the patient must have some collateral circulation from the

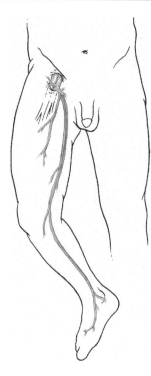

Fig. 4 Course of great saphenous vein until its drainage into the femoral vein. Courtesy of Laligam N. Sekhar

contralateral anterior cerebral artery, since it may be necessary to temporarily occlude the posterior communicating artery during the bypass. RAGs can be implanted into arteries 1.5–2.5 mm in diameter.

## 32.11
## Intracranial Anastomosis

We prefer the addition of a skull-base approach to the standard craniotomy to enhance the exposure and to reduce brain retraction in the case of large or giant aneu-

rysms of the ICA. Such an approach may not be necessary for distal MCA aneurysms. Prior to dural opening, epidural hemostasis must be carefully secured. This is very important in cases where a bypass is performed because heparin is administered intravenously during the procedure. The dura mater is opened with the aid of a surgical microscope. The early steps of the operation are to expose the aneurysm with minimal trauma to the brain and to occlude very few veins. In cases of paraclinoid and ophthalmic aneurysms, an intradural optic nerve decompression and clinoidectomy are performed.

The intracranial anastomosis is performed first to allow the graft vessel to be flipped easily after the first side has been sutured. Generally, the anastomotic time should be less than 45 min, and preferably less than 30 min. After the patient has been placed in burst suppression, with the systemic blood pressure being maintained at normal or elevated levels, temporary clips are placed on the recipient artery. An oval-shaped arteriotomy is then created into the recipient artery (Fig. 5). In the case of RAGs, this arteriotomy should be about 3–4 mm in length; in the case of saphenous vein grafts it should be 4–5 mm in length. The distal end of the graft is then anastomosed to the side of the recipient vessel by anchoring sutures on either end of the anastomosis. Following this, the suturing is started on the more difficult side, near the heel of the graft, because this is where leaks are more likely, and a continuous suture is performed. Once the suturing has been performed on one side, the graft is flipped over and the lumen of the vessel is carefully inspected to make sure that there has been no suturing of the opposite wall. Another suture is then started near the heel-end of the graft vessel and the suture can either be run to the apical region, or two sutures, one from the heel and one from the apex, may be run to the middle of the anastomotic line where they are be tied. Prior to completing the last sutures, the graft is flushed with heparinized saline and a temporary clip is placed on the graft, usually about 2 cm proximal to the distal anastomosis in case of the radial

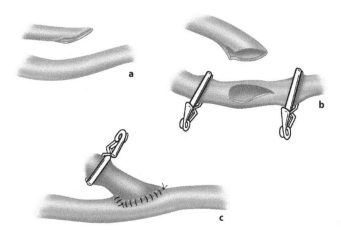

Fig. 5a–c Radial artery graft distal anastomosis. **a** A fish-mouthed graft. **b** Tear-drop shaped arteriotomy in the recipient vessel. **c** The completed anastomosis. Courtesy of Laligam N. Sekhar

artery and about 1 cm proximal to the anastomosis in case of the saphenous vein (distal to any valves that may exist). The graft is then carried to the donor vessel in the neck area. Wherever possible, because of the potential for constriction of the graft vessels in the tunnel, we prefer to use an incision that connects both the cranial and cervical incisions with dissection of soft tissue, which avoids all tunnel-related issues. The graft is placed in the subcutaneous space under direct vision.

In the case of the STA-to-MCA anastomosis, the STA is connected to the largest branch of the MCA possible, usually an M₃ branch, using 10/0 nylon sutures. A continuous suturing technique is frequently employed.

## 32.12
## Extracranial Anastomosis

We generally perform a high carotid exposure (Fig. 6) in order to reduce the length of the graft. If the anastomosis is planned to the ICA (Fig. 7), the ICA must be traced above the level of the digastric muscle, which is divided in order to facilitate the exposure. If grafting is into the ECA (Fig. 8), it should be exposed for at least 2 cm distal to the carotid bifurcation, until its major branching into the superficial temporal and internal maxillary arteries. The proximal anastomosis is performed either in an end-to-end, or an end-to-side fashion. End-to-end anastomosis

can always be performed to the ECA. End-to-end anastomosis also can be performed to the ICA if the patient has some collateral circulation. End-to-side anastomosis to the ICA can be done with temporary occlusion of the ICA proximal and distal to the anastomosis. In such a case, the graft flow is checked with Doppler measurements and intraoperative angiography after temporary ICA occlusion, and the ICA is permanently occluded if the graft flow is good and fast.

Before tying the last suture of the proximal anastomosis, the graft and the recipient vessels are bled by releasing the temporary clips transiently, to clear air bubbles in the case of an RAG; in the case of a vein graft, it is not possible to back bleed the graft after removing the proximal clips. However, if any air bubbles are observed, these can be extracted using a fine needle placed into the vein just prior to the distal clip on the graft or by opening a side branch to allow blood to wash the air bubbles through. The distal clip on the graft is then removed and the graft is carefully observed and palpated. A micro-Doppler probe is then used to check the graft flow. If a nonquantitative Doppler flow probe (Mizuho micro Doppler, Mizuho America, Beverly, MA, USA) is used, then both systolic and diastolic flow must be present. If a quantitative Doppler flow is employed (Transonic Doppler Flow Probe, Transonic Systems, Ithaca, NY, USA) then one should observe at least 35 cm³ of graft flow. The quantitative Doppler flow probe does not give a very accurate measurements of flow

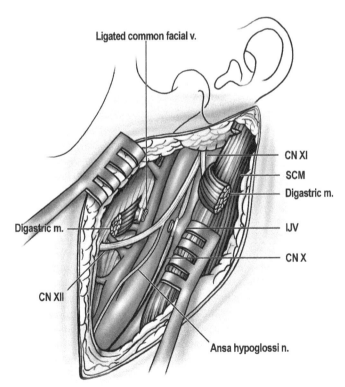

Ligated common facial v.

CN XI
SCM
Digastric m.

Digastric m.

IJV

CN X

CN XII

Ansa hypoglossi n.

Fig. 6 High cervical exposure of carotid arteries for proximal anastomosis. Courtesy of Laligam N. Sekhar

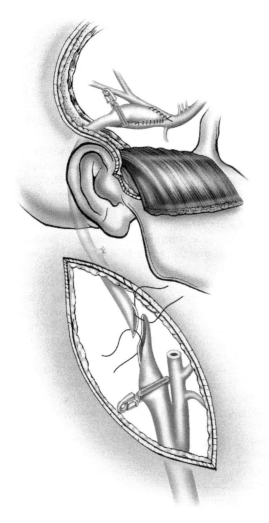

Fig. 7 Cervical internal carotid artery (ICA)-to-middle cerebral artery (MCA) saphenous vein bypass. Courtesy of Laligam N. Sekhar

velocity in our experience; however, it does give a very clear idea about whether or not flow is present.

## 32.13
## Management of Aneurysms

In aneurysms that are extradural (infraclinoid aneurysms), proximal occlusion is adequate. In case of intradural aneurysms, it is better to trap the aneurysm. Alternatively, the aneurysm may be clipped with the preservation of perforator vessels, such as the anterior choroidal artery, even though the parent vessel may be occluded in the process. Once the graft has been completed, is patent, and is flowing, then one can expect an

increase in the intra-aneurysmal pressure, and therefore, the treatment of the aneurysm must be performed fairly quickly. After the bypass grafting, heparin is not reversed. The dura mater is closely loosely with sutures, and may be supplemented with Duragen® (Integra Life Sciences, Plainsboro, NJ, USA), and Durasil® (Confluent Surgical, Waltham, MA, USA). The graft is checked again with TCD after the affixation of the bone flap. A sizeable segment is cut into the bone flap to allow the passage of the graft intracranially. An intraoperative angiogram is usually done after dural closure and bone reimplantation.

## 32.14
## Reconstruction Options for Complex ACOM Aneurysms

During the management of complex ACOM artery aneurysms it may be necessary to occlude one or both A2 vessels, most commonly one. This may also happen as a complication during the endovascular management of small ACOM aneurysms. Some patients have good collateral circulation to the A2 vessels, and may be able to tolerate permanent occlusion. However, the experience of the senior author has shown that this is difficult to predict, and a stroke in the ACOM artery and Heubner's territory may occur in a delayed fashion, due to vasospasm or unanticipated hypotension. Because of this, a revascularization procedure is recommended in every case wherein the A2s are occluded or severely stenosed by the clipping procedure. When one A2 is occluded, an A3–A3 side-to-side bypass is performed using the callosomarginal or pericallosal arteries (Fig. 9).

In the case of unruptured large or giant aneurysms, both A2s may have to be occluded as a part of the aneurysm treatment. In such cases, both A2s have to be revascularized using an RAG (or a saphenous vein if radial artery is not available). To keep the length of the graft short, one of the MCA–M₂ branches or the STA near the zygomatic arch is chosen as the donor vessel. The bypass is then performed to one A2 or A3 vessel, with an additional A3–A3 side-to-side bypass. Alternatively, a Y graft may be anastomosed to both vessels (Figs. 10 and 11) [10].

## 32.15
## Postoperative Care

Postoperative monitoring of graft patency usually consists of palpation of the graft and Doppler evaluation. A computed tomography angiogram (CTA) is usually done to evaluate the graft at 12 h postoperatively. If there is any doubt regarding the functioning of the graft, intra-arterial angiography is performed. If the radial artery has been used, vascular checks of the hand are performed

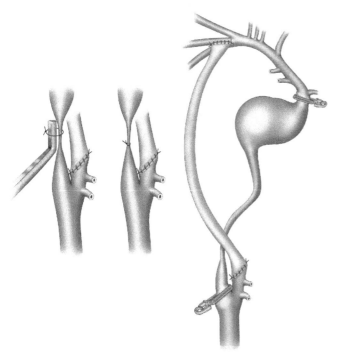

Fig. 8 Cervical external carotid artery (ECA)-to-MCA bypass. Courtesy of Laligam N. Sekhar

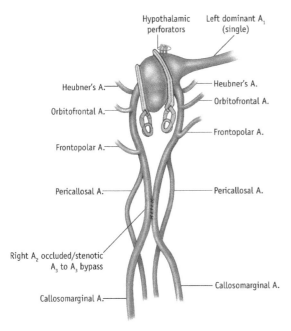

Fig. 9 Revascularization option when one A2 is occluded: A3–A3 side-to-side bypass is performed using the callosomarginal arteries. Courtesy of Laligam N. Sekhar

for the first 24 h. Patients are maintained on subcutaneous heparin, 5000 U, every 12 h, and started on aspirin, 81 mg once daily. Duplex Doppler studies are performed to follow the volume flow through the graft.

## 32.16
## Follow Up

Following discharge (7–10 days), the patients are kept on aspirin, 81 mg per os, once daily for life in case of the vein grafts and at least for 1 year in case of RAGs. The graft is followed by three-dimensional (3D)CTA or magnetic resonance angiography at 3 months postoperatively, and if possible, also by using graft flow measurements by Doppler imaging. Subsequently, a 3DCTA is performed annually. The frequency of the radiographic follow up may be reduced after 5 years.

## 32.17
## Troubleshooting of a Bypass

Two types of graft occlusion problems may occur with a bypass. There may be no flow inside the graft initially. Flow may be present in the beginning, but diminish or stop after a few minutes. In both cases, investigation must be performed as to the cause of the problem. If the patient had not been adequately heparinized during the by-

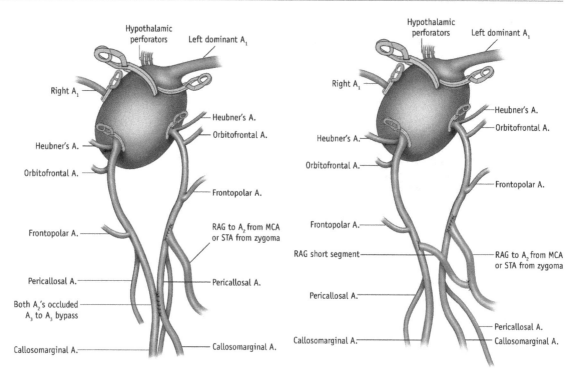

**Fig. 10** Revascularization option when both A2s are occluded: radial artery graft from the MCA or superficial temporal artery (STA) to A3 vessel followed by A3–A3 side-to-side bypass. Courtesy of Laligam N. Sekhar

**Fig. 11** A second revascularization option when both A2s are occluded: "Y" radial artery graft from MCA or STA to both A3 vessels. Courtesy of Laligam N. Sekhar

pass, then the patient must be reheparinized during any exploration of the graft, and the activated clotting time is checked. We have observed a hypercoaguable state in some patients, which leads to the occlusion of the graft. Temporary clips are replaced on the recipient artery, proximal and distal to the anastomotic site (Fig. 12a). A temporary clip is placed on the donor vessel and then a small arteriotomy is performed in the graft about 1 cm proximal to the anastomosis. The graft is irrigated out with heparinized saline. The temporary clips are then removed from the distal vessel to see whether or not there is backflow. If there is no back bleeding, this indicates that the problem is in the distal anastomotic site. If there is good backflow, then the clips are replaced on the recipient artery and the temporary clips are removed from the donor artery to see if there is antegrade flow. If there is no flow, then this indicates that the problem is at the proximal anastomosis or in the tunnel (if a tunneler was used to get the graft from the proximal to the distal side). If, on the other hand, there is good backflow and good antegrade flow, this means that the graft kinks the recipient vessel when there is full force of flow. This has been observed only with saphenous vein grafts due to the

very high flow through the graft, and this can be solved by placing a traction suture from the graft to the dura mater to relieve the kink (Fig. 12b,c). Sometimes there is a kink in the proximal anastomosis site that may require some type of a "pexy" in order to relieve it. Such a pexy may be performed by suturing the site of the graft to the proximal vessel (Fig. 12d). If the graft clots in the first 24 h (this is rare if flow was good), then endovascular thrombolysis may be tried. If this is not feasible, it will be necessary to do another anastomosis with a fresh graft using the saphenous vein or the radial artery. It is not possible to surgically reopen the same graft if it is clotted (Fig. 13).

## 32.18
## Illustrative Cases

### 32.18.1
### Giant Cavernous Aneurysm with Another Aneurysm on the Other Side

A 65-year-old woman presented with a 1-month history of complete right VIth-nerve palsy, which led to the dis-

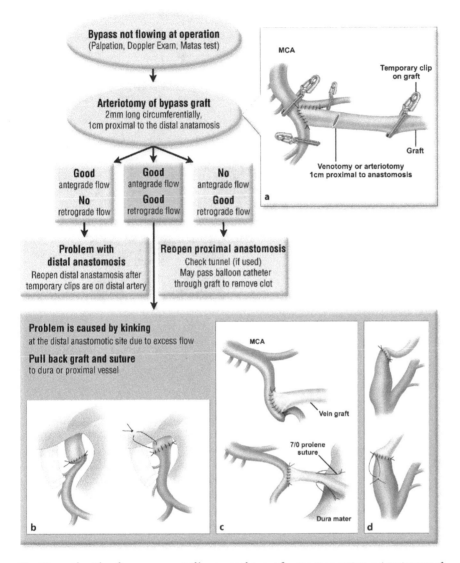

Fig. 12a–c Algorithm for management if bypass graft is not flowing at operation. **a** Arteriotomy of the graft to check the direction of flow. **b** Pexy of graft to dura to avoid kinking. **c** Pexy of graft to adventitia of proximal vessel to avoid kinking. Courtesy of Laligam N. Sekhar

covery of a giant intracavernous and a superior hypophyseal aneurysm. The intracavernous aneurysm ended at the edge of the ophthalmic artery and considerably eroded the petrous bone laterally, up to the geniculate ganglion (Fig. 14). Due to an equivocal Allen's test, a brachial artery angiogram was performed, which revealed only a single communicating branch between the ulnar and the radial arteries in the hand instead of the usual superficial and deep palmar arches (Fig. 15). Because of this, a saphenous vein graft was planned instead of an RAG. The patient underwent a right frontotemporal craniotomy with an orbital osteotomy. This was followed by a cervical ICA-to-M$_2$ bypass using a saphenous vein graft. The cavernous an-

eurysm was then trapped after clip ligation of the cervical ICA by placing a clip on the supraclinoid ICA proximal to the origin of the posterior communicating artery (Fig. 16). We also clipped the superior hypophyseal aneurysm, which was heavily calcified. Postoperatively, the cavernous aneurysm continued to thrombose, causing delayed facial nerve palsy after 3 days. This patient also had a left paraclinoid ICA aneurysm, which was managed by balloon-assisted coiling 1 year after the previous surgery. (Fig. 17). At recent follow up, the patient has completely recovered from her facial nerve palsy. An angiogram at this time revealed a widely patent graft, complete thrombosis, and involution of the cavernous aneurysm (Fig. 18).

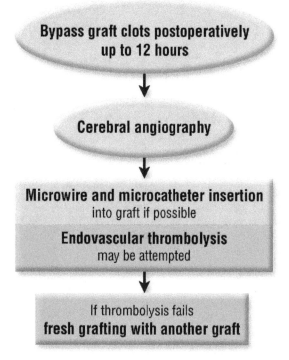

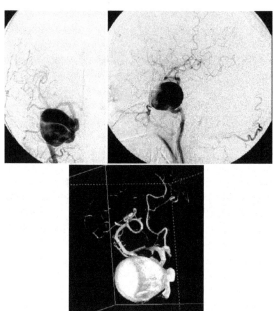

Fig. 13 Algorithm for management if bypass graft clots up to 12 h postoperatively. Courtesy of Laligam N. Sekhar

Fig. 14a–c Anteroposterior, lateral view and three-dimensional reconstruction of a right carotid angiogram showing a right giant cavernous ICA aneurysm and right posterior paraclinoid aneurysm. Courtesy of Laligam N. Sekhar

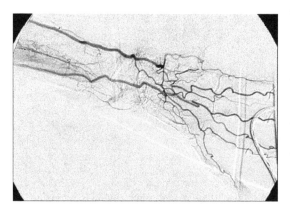

Fig. 15 Brachial angiogram showing only single communicating artery between the radial and ulnar arteries. Courtesy of Laligam N. Sekhar

### 32.18.2
### Giant Supraclinoid Aneurysm

A 45-year-old doctor presented with severe headache and visual problems. On examination it was found he had a left hemianopsia. An angiogram showed a giant fusiform supraclinoid aneurysm (Fig. 19) and poor crossflow to the MCA through the ACOM artery. The anterior choroidal artery was arising from the aneurysm. The aneurysm was trapped with preservation of the anterior choroidal artery after an ECA-to-MCA M$_2$ bypass (Fig. 20). He had a caudate stroke after the surgery, but was free of neurological deficits. The postoperative angiogram showed obliteration of the aneurysm, bypass filling the MCA, and a patent anterior choroidal artery (Fig. 21).

### 32.18.3
### Acoustic Neuroma and Large ICA Aneurysm (Stent-Assisted Coiling)

A 71-year-old female with 5 years of decreasing hearing was diagnosed with a left acoustic neuroma and a broad-based aneurysm of the left ICA in the region of the posterior communicating artery, measuring 10.5×6.5 mm, with

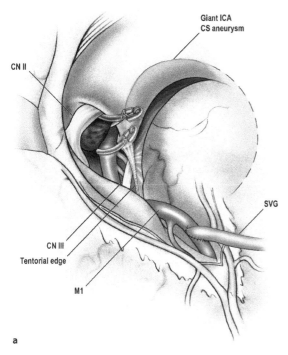

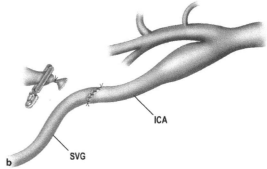

Fig. 16 **a** Transylvian approach showing a giant cavernous ICA aneurysm, occlusion of the supraclinoid ICA distal to the cavernous ICA aneurysm, clipping of paraclinoid ICA aneurysm and saphenous vein to MCA–M₂ anastomosis. **b** Trapping of the ICA aneurysm by proximal clipping of the cervical ICA, and end-to-end cervical ICA-to-saphenous vein anastomosis. Courtesy of Laligam N. Sekhar

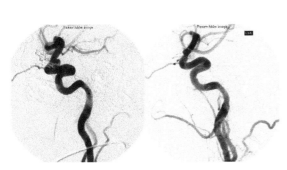

Fig. 17 Left ICA-paraclinoid aneurysm, which was coiled. Courtesy of Laligam N. Sekhar

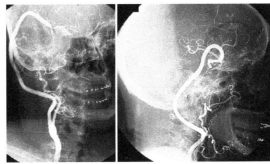

Fig. 18a,b Postoperative right carotid angiogram: **a,b** Showing the clips on the cervical ICA and supraclinoid ICA, trapping of the cavernous ICA aneurysm and ICA to MCA–M₂ bypass. Courtesy of Laligam N. Sekhar

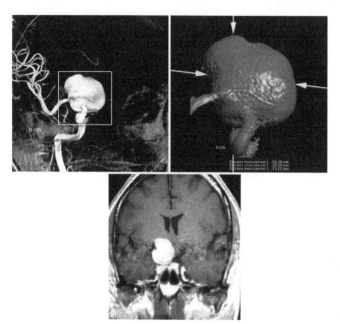

Fig. 19 Giant supraclinoid ICA aneurysm. Courtesy of Laligam N. Sekhar

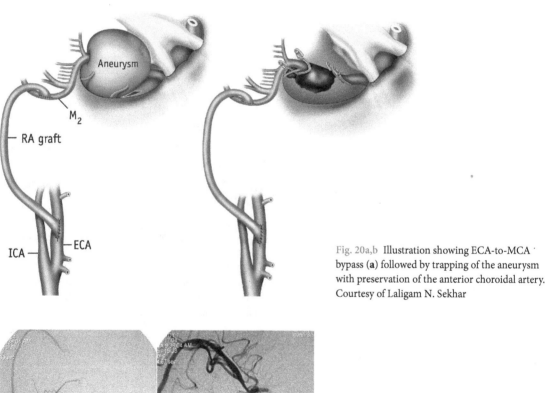

Fig. 20a,b Illustration showing ECA-to-MCA bypass (**a**) followed by trapping of the aneurysm with preservation of the anterior choroidal artery. Courtesy of Laligam N. Sekhar

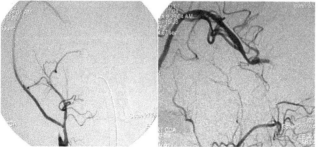

Fig. 21 Postoperative angiogram showing complete obliteration of the aneurysm and filling of the anterior choroidal artery. Courtesy of Laligam N. Sekhar

a neck dimension of 6.5 mm (Fig. 22). She underwent stent-assisted coiling of the aneurysm. After deployment of two coils, the procedure was terminated as the microcatheter kicked out and the stent was moving (Fig. 23). The aneurysm was coiled subtotally with eight additional coils after 2 weeks (Fig. 24). After 3 months, clopidogrel was stopped and she underwent surgical removal of the acoustic neuroma (Fig. 25). Her hearing and facial nerve function were preserved after surgery.

### 32.18.4
### MCA Aneurysm, RAG into the Upper Branch, and Clipping

A 59-year-old woman was being investigated for back pain and numbness involving the left and then the right lower extremity. This lead to the diagnosis of a left MCA aneurysm, which measured 1×1.3 cm. This was a very broad-necked aneurysm with two branches coming right out of the neck of the aneurysm (Figs. 26 and 27A). She was scheduled for angiography and possible endovascular coiling, but the endovascular coiling procedure was abandoned, since the aneurysm could not be coiled completely. She was explored by another surgeon with the understanding that if it was possible, the aneurysm would be clipped. However, the neck of the aneurysm was extremely atherosclerotic, and the upper $M_2$ branches arising from the neck of the aneurysm, and its origin was sclerotic. Because of this, the operation was aborted and the patient was referred to our center for the performance of a radial artery bypass graft to the two vessels, followed by a trapping procedure of the aneurysm.

As a consequence, this patient underwent a left frontotemporal craniotomy and orbital osteotomy, RAG bypass into the superior branch of the MCA, and clipping of aneurysm with the preservation of the inferior branch (Fig. 27b). A postoperative angiogram was obtained and showed good flow into the superior branch through the graft, and into the inferior branch from the parent MCA itself (Fig. 28). Hemostasis was achieved. After 7 months, MRA revealed that the RAG was widely patent. The inferior branch of the MCA, which was preserved during surgery, was also patent.

### 32.18.5
### MCA Aneurysm, Reimplantation of the Branch Vessel, and Clipping

This 70-year-old man presented with an unruptured left MCA aneurysm, 5 mm in diameter with a 4-mm neck, which was complex due to the origin of the anterior temporal branch of the MCA directly from the neck of the aneurysm (Fig. 29). This was not suitable for endovascular coiling, nor was it suitable for direct clipping without occlusion of the branch. Therefore, the aneurysm was

clipped and the anterior temporal branch was reimplanted into the $M_2$ segment of the MCA (Fig. 30). The postoperative angiogram showed obliteration of the aneurysm and filling of the anterior temporal branch (Fig. 31).

### 32.18.6
### Bilateral Mycotic MCA Aneurysms: STA–MCA on One Side and RAG Interposition on the Other

This 47-year-old man had an infected pancreatic pseudocyst complicated by enterococcal sepsis, endocarditis, and mycotic aneurysm of the left MCA $M_2$ segment, and was managed conservatively with intravenous antibiotics. He presented with a rapidly enlarging right-sided mycotic aneurysm when he has receiving home antibiotic therapy (Fig. 32). The right-sided aneurysm was resected emergently with a right-sided STA–MCA bypass (Fig. 33). The aneurysm on the left side was larger than that on the right, and was in the $M_2$ segment of the left MCA (Fig. 34). Two weeks after the first surgery, the aneurysm was excised and a radial artery interposition graft was used to establish flow in the parent vessel (Fig. 35).

### 32.18.7
### Recurrent ACOM Aneurysm with SAH A3-to-A3 Bypass and Clipping, with Occlusion of A2

This patient had a ruptured ACOM artery aneurysm (Fig. 36–39), which was managed by clipping. She had a dominant right A1 and an aplastic left A1. Postoperative angiography demonstrated complete aneurysm obliteration. The patient presented 1 month after clipping with a recurrent SAH. Angiography revealed growth of an aneurysm remnant posterior to the left A2 that had not been obliterated by the previous clipping (Figs. 40 and 41). The aneurysm was approached by a subfrontal and interhemispheric approach. The remnant was more posterior to the tip of the clip, and the left A2. The aneurysm could only be obliterated by clipping the neck of the aneurysm and the ACOM artery (Fig. 42). An A3–A3 bypass (Fig. 43) was performed to restore blood flow in the left A2. Postoperative angiography (Fig. 44) revealed complete obliteration of the aneurysm and good flow in both A2 segments from the right A1. She was independent for all daily activities after 3 months of follow up.

### 32.19
### Results

Table 2 shows a summary of patients who underwent revascularization for anterior circulation aneurysms, the types of bypass, graft patency, outcome of patients (in-

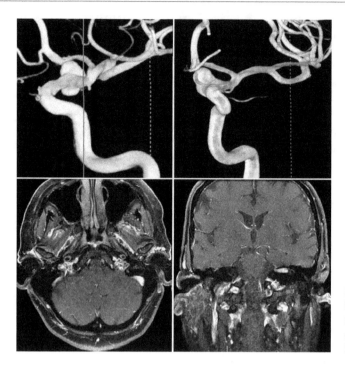

Fig. 22a–d Angiogram showing a broad-based ICA-posterior communicating artery aneurysm (**a,b**) and magnetic resonance imaging (MRI) scan showing a left acoustic neuroma (**c,d**). Courtesy of Laligam N. Sekhar

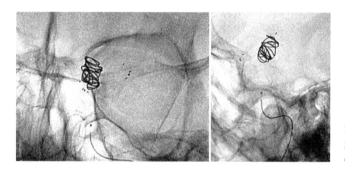

Fig. 23 Stent assisted coiling stopped after deploying two coils as the stent was moving. Courtesy of Laligam N. Sekhar

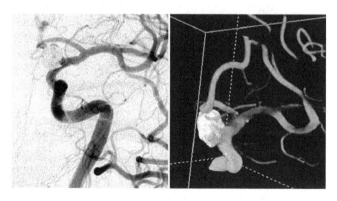

Fig. 24 Complete obliteration by additional coiling after 2 weeks. Courtesy of Laligam N. Sekhar

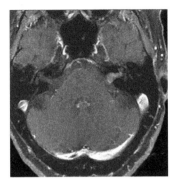

Fig. 25 Postoperative MRI showing complete removal of the acoustic neuroma after 3 months. Courtesy of Laligam N. Sekhar

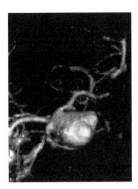

Fig. 26 Three-dimensional reconstruction of a computed tomography angiogram showing a large left MCA bifurcation aneurysm. Courtesy of Laligam N. Sekhar

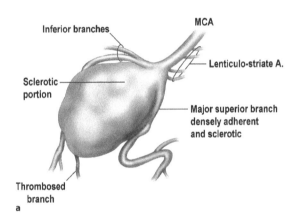

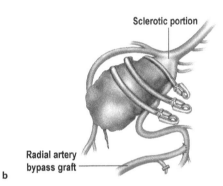

Fig. 27 **a** Large MCA bifurcation aneurysm with adherent superior branch and inferior branch arising from the aneurysm. **b** Clipping of the MCA aneurysm with the superior branch, excluding the inferior branch, and radial artery grafting to the superior branch of MCA. Courtesy of Laligam N. Sekhar

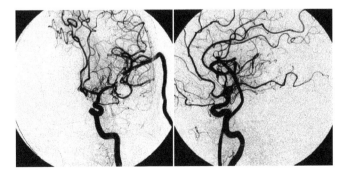

Fig. 28a,b Anteroposterior and lateral view of left carotid angiogram showing the graft filling the superior branch of MCA, and filling of the inferior branch of MCA from MCA proper. Courtesy of Laligam N. Sekhar

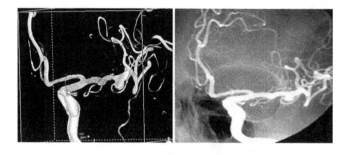

Fig. 29 Angiogram showing an MCA aneurysm with the anterior temporal branch of the MCA directly from the neck of the aneurysm. Courtesy of Laligam N. Sekhar

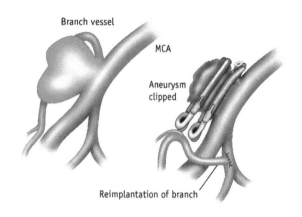

Fig. 30 Illustration showing clipping of the and implantation of anterior temporal branch into the M₂ segment of the MCA. Courtesy of Laligam N. Sekhar

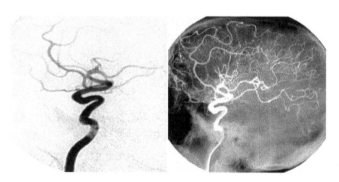

Fig. 31 Angiogram showing complete obliteration of the aneurysm and filling of the anterior temporal branch. Courtesy of Laligam N. Sekhar

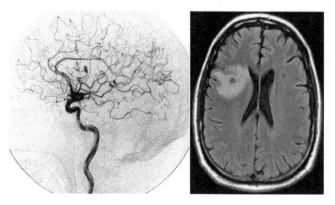

Fig. 32a,b Angiogram showing a right MCA mycotic aneurysm (**a**), and MRI showing edema around the aneurysm (**b**). Courtesy of Laligam N. Sekhar

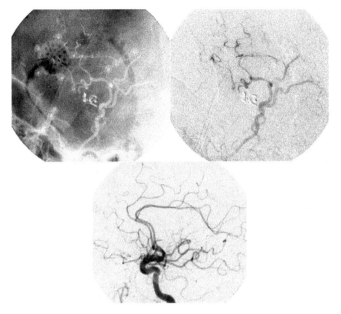

Fig. 33 Angiogram showing filling of the MCA from the STA and obliteration of the right-sided aneurysm. Courtesy of Laligam N. Sekhar

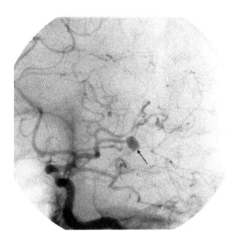

Fig. 34 Angiogram showing a left MCA mycotic aneurysm. Courtesy of Laligam N. Sekhar

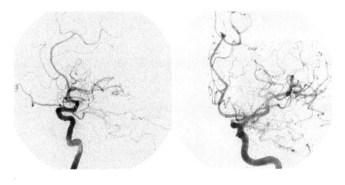

Fig. 35 Angiogram after complete excision of a left MCA aneurysm and radial artery interposition grafting. Courtesy of Laligam N. Sekhar

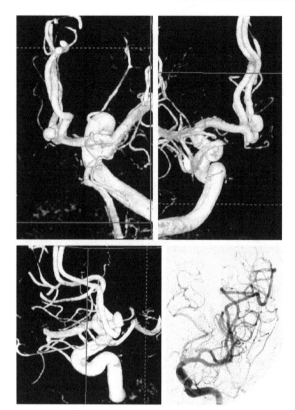

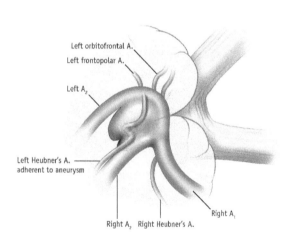

Fig. 36 Preoperative angiography showing an anterior communicating artery aneurysm arising from a totally dominant right anterior cerebral artery. Courtesy of Laligam N. Sekhar

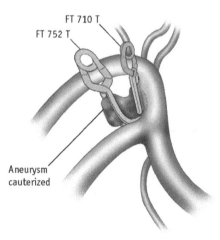

Fig. 37 Illustration showing the anatomy of the anterior communicating artery complex, the aneurysm, and their relationships. Courtesy of Laligam N. Sekhar

Fig. 38 Illustration showing the technique of clipping of the aneurysm. Courtesy of Laligam N. Sekhar

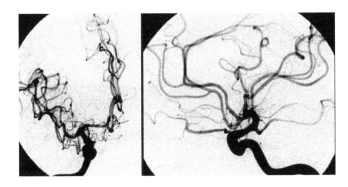

Fig. 39 Postoperative angiography showing complete obliteration of the aneurysm. Courtesy of Laligam N. Sekhar

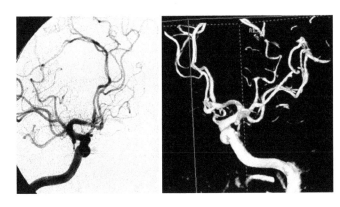

Fig. 40 Angiogram taken 1 month after the previous clipping showing an aneurysm remnant posterior to the left A2. Courtesy of Laligam N. Sekhar

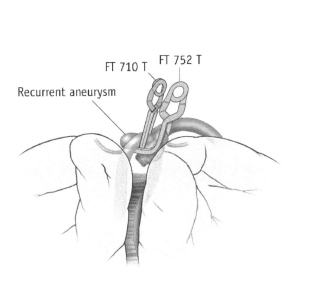

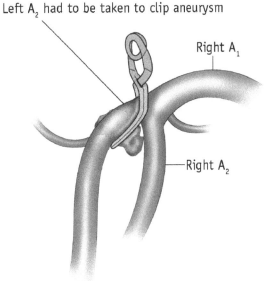

Fig. 41 Illustration showing the relationship between the recurrent aneurysm and the anterior communicating artery complex. Courtesy of Laligam N. Sekhar

Fig. 42 Illustration showing the technique of clipping of the recurrent aneurysm with the anterior communicating artery. Courtesy of Laligam N. Sekhar

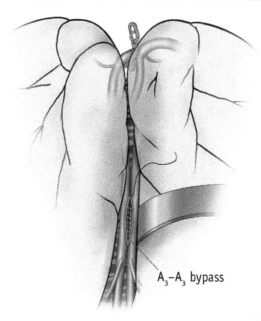

Fig. 43 Illustration showing the technique of A3–A3 side-to-side anastomoses. Courtesy of Laligam N. Sekhar

Table 2 Revascularization for anterior circulation aneurysms 1988–2006. *RAG* Radial artery graft, *SVG* saphenous vein graft, *RA* radial artery, *STA* superficial temporal artery, *GOS* Glasgow Outcome Scale

| Patients | Grafts | | |
|---|---|---|---|
| 90 | 91 | | |
| High-flow bypass | | | |
| **RAG** | **SVG** | | |
| 37+4 Temporary | 38 | | |
| Low-flow bypass | | | |
| Reimplantation | 4 | | |
| Primary repair | 1 | | |
| RA patch | 1 | | |
| A3 to A3 | 2 | | |
| Superior thyroid artery | 1 | | |
| STA bypass | 3 | | |
| Graft patency | | | |
| **Immediate** | **After salvage** | | |
| 88/91 (97.4%) | 89/91 (98.7%) | | |
| Outcome | | | |
| GOS score | **5** | **4** | **0** |
| | 69 (78%) | 15 (16%) | 6 (6%) |
| Complication/complete recovery | | | |
| Major stroke | 1/0 | | |
| Minor stroke | 5/3 | | |
| Brain swelling | 2/2 | | |
| Emergency bypass-grafts performed after major stroke had occurred | | | |
| **Number** | **Outcome** | | |
| 2 | Died | | |

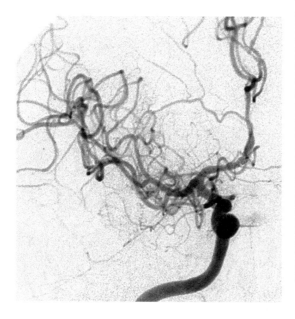

Fig. 44 Postoperative angiography showing complete obliteration of the aneurysm. Courtesy of Laligam N. Sekhar

cluding management, morbidity of SAH, and vasospasm), and major complication related to grafts and recovery. Included in these patients are two in whom bypass was carried out as a desperate measure after a major stroke had occurred before or during surgery.

## 32.20
## Conclusion

Cerebral revascularization may be necessary when surgical treatment of complex aneurysms requires sacrifice of the ICA or other major vessels. With a variety of techniques available to treat complex intracranial aneurysms, it is important to tailor the management of each patient. Not all aneurysms can be coiled, even with advent of stent/coil strategies. Therefore, the technique of arterial bypass grafting can greatly add to the vascular neurosurgeon's armamentarium.

## References

1.  Fiorella D, Albuquerque FC, Deshmukh VR, McDougall CG (2005) Usefulness of the Neuroform stent for the treatment of cerebral aneurysms: results at initial (3–6-mo) follow-up. Neurosurgery 56:1191–1201; discussion 1201–1192

2.  Fisk RL, Brooks CH, Callaghan JC, Dvorkin J (1976) Experience with the radial artery graft for coronary artery bypass. Ann Thorac Surg 21:513–518

3.  Jarvis MA, Jarvis CL, Jones PR, Spyt TJ (2000) Reliability of Allen's test in selection of patients for radial artery harvest. Ann Thorac Surg 70:1362–1365

4.  Larson JJ, Tew JM Jr, Tomsick TA, van Loveren HR (1995) Treatment of aneurysms of the internal carotid artery by intravascular balloon occlusion: long-term follow-up of 58 patients. Neurosurgery 36:26–30; discussion 30

5.  Lylyk P, Ferrario A, Pasbon B, Miranda C, Doroszuk G (2005) Buenos Aires experience with the Neuroform self-expanding stent for the treatment of intracranial aneurysms. J Neurosurg 102:235–241

6.  McIvor NP, Willinsky RA, TerBrugge KG, Rutka JA, Freeman JL (1994) Validity of test occlusion studies prior to internal carotid artery sacrifice. Head Neck 16:11–16

7.  Ogilvy CS, Chu D, Kaplan S (1996) Mild hypothermia, hypertension, and mannitol are protective against infarction during experimental intracranial temporary vessel occlusion. Neurosurgery 38:1202–1209; discussion 1209–1210

8.  Origitano TC, Al-Mefty O, Leonetti JP, DeMonte F, Reichman OH (1994) Vascular considerations and complications in cranial base surgery. Neurosurgery 35:351–362; discussion 362–353

9.  Regli L, Piepgras DG, Hansen KK (1995) Late patency of long saphenous vein bypass grafts to the anterior and posterior cerebral circulation. J Neurosurg 83:806–811

10.  Sekhar LN, Natarajan SK, Britz GW, Ghodke B (2007) Microsurgical management of ACOM aneurysms: operative nuances. Neurosurgery (in press)

11.  Sekhar LN, Bucur SD, Bank WO, Wright DC (1999) Venous and arterial bypass grafts for difficult tumors, aneurysms, and occlusive vascular lesions: evolution of surgical treatment and improved graft results. Neurosurgery 44:1207–1223; discussion 1223–1204

12.  Sekhar LN, Duff JM, Kalavakonda C, Olding M (2001) Cerebral revascularization using radial artery grafts for the treatment of complex intracranial aneurysms: techniques and outcomes for 17 patients. Neurosurgery 49:646–658; discussion 658–649

13.  Sekhar LN, Kalavakonda C (2002) Cerebral revascularization for aneurysms and tumors. Neurosurgery 50:321–331

14.  Sekhar LN, Patel SJ (1993) Permanent occlusion of the internal carotid artery during skull-base and vascular surgery: is it really safe? Am J Otol 14:421–422

# Cerebral Bypass and Vascular Reconstructions for Posterior Circulation Aneurysms

**33**

Laligam N. Sekhar,
Sabareesh K. Natarajan, Gavin W Britz,
and Basavaraj Ghodke

## Contents

## 33.1
## Introduction

Posterior circulation aneurysms are among the most challenging problems facing the cerebrovascular neurosurgeon. Aneurysms of the vertebrobasilar system may be broad-necked or fusiform, and may involve critical branches, such as the cerebellar vessels, brainstem perforators, or the posterior cerebral arteries (PCAs). Furthermore, optimal exposure of these lesions often requires specialized expertise in cranial-base anatomy and microvascular surgery. Parent vessel or perforator occlusion may result in a devastating stroke or death. Direct surgical repair, Hunterian ligation or trapping, and endovascular stenting or coiling are treatment options that may not always be feasible [1]. These challenges and the poor natural history of symptomatic posterior fossa aneurysms have fueled interest in continuing the development of techniques of posterior circulation revascularization to improve the management of these difficult cases.

## 33.2
## Indication for Bypasses and Vascular Reconstruction

Due to the advances in endovascular techniques, bypasses and vascular reconstruction are likely to be used in the following situations (Fig. 1): fusiform aneurysms that cannot be adequately treated by stent-assisted coiling, origin of large branches from an aneurysm that will have to be sacrificed during endovascular coiling or microsurgical clipping, dissecting and blister aneurysms that require parent vessel occlusion, those without adequate collaterals, and patients with failed endovascular stent-assisted coiling.

## 33.3
## Collateral Circulation and Parent-Vessel Sacrifice

The effect of occlusion of the posterior circulation arteries depends upon the collateral circulation. Such collaterals may exist through the circle of Willis (posterior communicating arteries), pial collateral circulation around the

cerebellum or brainstem, and deep collaterals through the cerebellum and brainstem. The presence of pial collaterals and perforating collaterals may or may not be observed angiographically, and are more likely to be present in young patients without vascular risk factors such as hypertension, and absent in older patients with multiple risk factors.

When parent-vessel occlusion is done, it is best done using an endovascular technique. Major vessel sacrifice may be preceded by a balloon occlusion test for 15 min under normotensive conditions. The actual occlusion is done under general anesthesia, and the patient must be heparinized for at least 24 h perioperatively.

The nondominant vertebral artery cab be occluded safely provided the posterior inferior cerebellar artery (PICA) is preserved. The dominant vertebral artery (VA) can be occluded if there is one other (small) VA and at least one large posterior communicating artery.

With regard to the mid- and lower basilar artery (BA; including vertebrobasilar aneurysms), some type of bypass procedure is necessary unless both posterior communicating arteries are of large caliber. The origin of the anterior inferior cerebellar artery (AICA) is an important consideration. In two patients, we performed only a distal

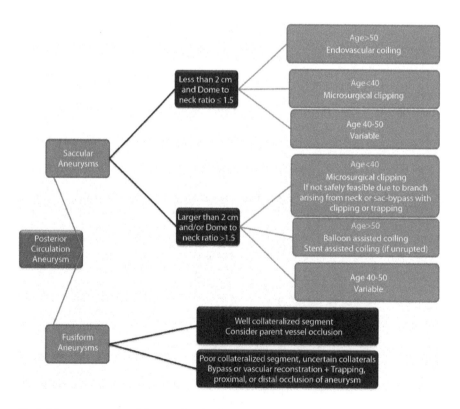

Fig. 1 Management protocol for posterior circulation aneurysms. Note that age is given in years

occlusion procedure, which successfully preserved the AICA. This is feasible only when the aneurysm is unruptured. In the case of ruptured aneurysms, the aneurysm and the BA can be occluded in a way that preserves the AICA and any major perforators. There is concern about the perforating vessels arising from the mid- and lower basilar segments; in patients with a partially thrombosed aneurysm, these vessels may already be thrombosed, and collaterals are likely to have developed through the brainstem. The length of the artery involved by the aneurysm is important, since the number of perforators in the segment increase with the length of the artery involved. However, the maximum length that can be safely occluded is not known.

For complex and giant aneurysms of the upper BA, we have relied on the experience of Drake and Peerless [2] that BA occlusion is safe when both posterior communicating arteries are more than 1 mm in diameter. Many giant aneurysms in this area are very complex and may involve the origin of both PCAs or one PCA. A bypass into the PCA can augment flow and make it safe to occlude the upper BA when the posterior communicating arteries are small in size; the use of the deep hypothermic circulatory arrest technique for clipping of the aneurysm (with neck remnant), the Neuroform stent with endovascular coiling, and bypass into one PCA with aneurysm clipping, or coiling, are treatment options [1, 4, 5, 9, 12].

With respect to second-order arteries such as the PCA (beyond the posterior communicating artery), the superior cerebellar artery (SCA), the AICA, or the PICA, occlusion testing is not possible. In most patients, perforators to the brainstem arise close to their origin from the parent artery, and therefore, occlusion of the proximal segment should be avoided. Effects of occluding the more distal segments are variable and depend on the size of the artery and the collateral circulation available. Occlusion of the P3 segment in the treatment of aneurysms or other lesions is sometimes but not always followed by hemianopsia. Occlusion of the SCA near or beyond the trigeminal root is often followed by infarction, but of a variable size. Occlusion of the AICA proximal to the internal auditory artery is invariably followed by hearing loss, but beyond cranial nerve VIII, the effects are variable. Occlusion of the PICA close to its origin is usually followed by brainstem infarction, but the effects of occlusion further distally are dependent on the size of the PICA (which often has a seesaw relationship with the size of the AICA) and the pial collateral circulation available through the ipsilateral AICA and the contralateral PICA. The safest solution for most patients who require the occlusion of a vessel of this size is revascularization, although this may mean unnecessary revascularizations in some patients.

The effects of occlusion of brainstem perforator vessels are also uncertain. Although once thought to be "end arteries," it is clear that collateral circulation exists [2]. Although it would never be the interest of the surgeon to occlude perforating vessels intentionally, thrombosis of some perforators will frequently occur during the treatment of large, giant, or fusiform aneurysms. In most patients, such presumed thrombosis in the vertebrobasilar segments does not seem to result in stroke, but it can result in stroke and death.

## 33.4
## Learning Curve

The technical difficulties associated with posterior circulation revascularization procedures should not be underestimated. Equally important is the judgment regarding what procedure has the best chance of success and the lowest risk for the patient; the choice for an individual patient may include not doing anything, performing various types of surgical revascularization with aneurysm occlusion, an endovascular procedure, or referral to another center (this may not be possible because of logistical and financial reasons). The availability of a good endovascular colleague within the institution, with whom discussion can be held about the pros and cons of surgical, endovascular, or combined procedures, is of great benefit. Neurosurgeons should generally not attempt posterior circulation revascularization procedures before becoming adept with anterior circulation procedures.

## 33.5
## Preoperative Preparation, Anesthesia, and Monitoring

Before performing arterial grafts, we administer aspirin (325 mg orally or 650 mg rectally). During the performance of radial artery or saphenous vein grafting (RAG and SVG, respectively), 4000 U of heparin is administered intravenously. During temporary arterial occlusion, the blood pressure is increased by 20% to improve collateral flow in case of unruptured aneurysms and kept at normal levels in ruptured aneurysms. Metabolic brain suppression is induced with propofol to achieve electroencephalographic burst-suppression and achieve cessation of synaptic transmission.

## 33.6
## Neuromonitoring

Monitoring of motor evoked potentials, somatosensory evoked potentials, brainstem evoked potentials, and sometimes cranial nerves VII–XII is performed during surgery for complex posterior circulation aneurysms.

### 33.7
## Cranial-Base Approaches Used to Facilitate Posterior Circulation Revascularization

Upper basilar aneurysms located at or above the level of the dorsum sellae and those involving the PCA or SCA are managed with the frontotemporal/orbitozygomatic [13, 15] or subtemporal/transzygomatic, transpetrous apex approach [3], depending on the location of the aneurysm in relation to the dorsum sellae. The transpetrosal approach, or one of its variants, is used for aneurysms requiring exposure of the midbasilar region: transpetrosal-retrolabyrinthine or transpetrosal-partial labyrinthectomy petrous apicectomy (PLPA) with hearing preservation [14], depending on the extent of presigmoid and precerebellar exposure required. A combined presigmoid and retrosigmoid or the trans-sigmoid approach may be used with the transpetrosal approach to expose aneurysms and/or arteries that lie in the junctional region between the presigmoid-transpetrosal and retrosigmoid-far lateral approaches. A total petrosectomy is used for midbasilar fusiform or giant aneurysms that cannot be adequately exposed by the PLPA approach [8]. The far-lateral retrosigmoid and extreme lateral partial transcondylar or transjugular tubercle approaches may be used for approaching many VA, PICA, and AICA aneurysms requiring carotid–VA bypass, extradural-intradural VA bypass, occipital artery (OA)-to-AICA or PICA bypass, and

PICA–AICA anastomosis or reimplantation [7]. When an aneurysm is located directly anterior to the lower brainstem, the extreme lateral approach is expanded by removal of the occipital condyle or jugular tubercle [7]. A midline suboccipital approach may be used for performing a PICA–PICA side-to-side anastomosis [5].

### 33.8
## Vascular Reconstructions

### 33.8.1
## Direct Reconstruction

Direct reconstruction (Fig. 2) of cerebral arteries is usually performed after the excision of an aneurysm involving a short segment of a parent vessel. When the artery cannot be mobilized and sutured without tension, then a short interposition graft (Fig. 3) can be used.

### 33.8.2
## Side-to-Side Anastomosis

Side-to-side anastomosis (Fig. 4) of two adjacent arteries, such as AICA-PICA or PICA-PICA, or reimplantation of an artery (e.g., PICA reimplantation into AICA) may be performed if no adequate donor vessel is available for

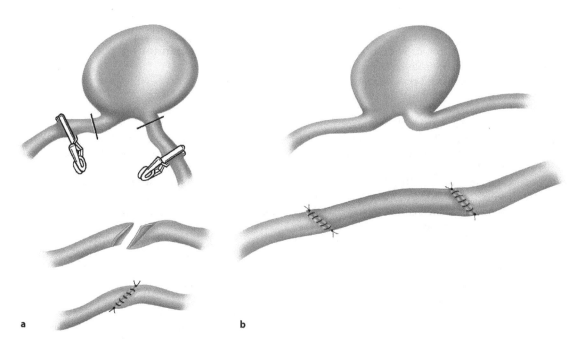

a                                    b

Fig. 2a,b After excision of the aneurysmal sac, either arterial end is sharply sectioned obliquely (a), slightly fish-mouthed, and sutured (b). Courtesy of Laligam N. Sekhar

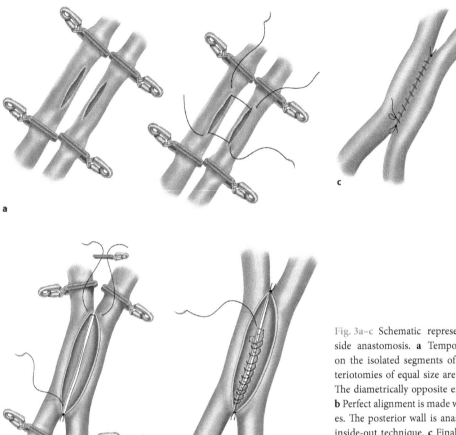

Fig. 3a–c Schematic representation of a side-to-side anastomosis. **a** Temporary clips are placed on the isolated segments of both arteries and arteriotomies of equal size are made in both vessels. The diametrically opposite ends are anchored first. **b** Perfect alignment is made with the first two stitches. The posterior wall is anastomosed first with an inside-out technique. **c** Finally, the anterior wall is sutured and the anastomosis completed. Courtesy of Laligam N. Sekhar

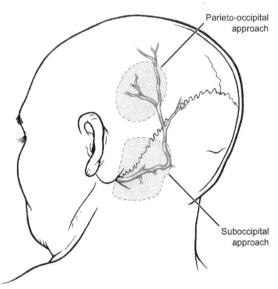

Parieto-occipital approach

Suboccipital approach

Fig. 4 The course of the occipital artery, which is usually more tortuous in the elderly. The sites of parieto-occipital and sub-occipital craniotomies are indicated (*grey patches*). Courtesy of Laligam N. Sekhar

a bypass graft. The vessels must be naturally close to each other or able to be mobilized to lie close to each other, without any tension.

## 33.8.3
### Choice of Revascularization Conduits

There are four types of vessel that can be used for surgical revascularization: (1) distant vessels such as the saphenous vein, (2) the radial artery, (3) the OA or STA, and (4) regional vessels such as the AICA, SCA, or PICA (Table 1) [6, 9, 10, 12]. The choice of grafting procedure depends on the extent of flow required, the complexity of the operation, and the surgeon's experience.

The VA and (in the very rare case) the BA are good recipient vessels for SVG, but the PCA is less reliable. The transition from a high-flow vessel (SVG) into a low-flow vessel, such as the PCA, results in marked turbulence and may lead to graft occlusion. The senior author has found the RAG to be a good solution for revascularization after VA or BA occlusion because of the better size match to the PCA and the moderate flow rate provided [6, 9, 10, 12]. The major problem in the past was one of postoperative spasm, which has been mostly solved by the pressure distention technique [6]. Smaller arteries, such as the STA, the OA, and regional blood vessels, are very reliable when the vessel being replaced is small, but less so when the BA or VA has to be occluded [6, 9, 12]. The OA and STA are used if they exhibit adequate flow and caliber on angiography and if the recipient vessel is small (2 mm or less) and supplies a territory that is appropriate for the low blood flow rate (20–40 ml/min) typically provided by these donor arteries.

## 33.8.4
### Choice of Recipient Vessel

In cases of posterior circulation aneurysm, if the PCA is chosen for the bypass, then the $P_2$ segment of the PCA is selected. It is generally devoid of major perforators. Even if perforators are present, they are not as critical as perforators arising from the $P_1$ segment, and temporary occlusion of this vessel and perforators is remarkably well tolerated. If large perforators arise from $P_2$, we occlude them temporarily with microclips during the bypass. The $P_2$ segment is exposed lateral to the midbrain. We use a transpetrosal approach with the division of tentorium, or a frontotemporal orbitozygomatic approach with tentorial division rather than a subtemporal approach for $P_2$ exposure, since this provides more space to perform the anastomosis. In some patients the $P_2$ may be very high in location, making dissection more difficult. It may also be atherosclerotic. In such a case, a nonsclerotic segment should be selected for bypass. In such cases, the SCA may also be used if it is adequate in caliber.

For aneurysms of the VA, the distal VA may be used for bypass when a segment is available for anastomosis. But a bypass to the PCA may be necessary when this vessel is not easily exposed or available. For vertebral- PICA aneurysms, the OA is used as a donor vessel. The radial artery is used as a graft when the OA is diseased. In cases of midbasilar aneurysms, we usually use the PCA as the recipient. However, in one patient, the senior author has used the BA distal to the aneurysm as the recipient vessel in a 15-year-old girl, under deep hypothermic circulatory arrest after performing a petrosectomy to expose the aneurysm on the previous day. This can only be done in young patients who have good brain plasticity. The

Table 1  Surgical revascularization options for posterior circulation aneurysms. *PICA* Posterior inferior cerebellar artery, *AICA* anterior inferior cerebellar artery, *VA* vertebral artery, *SVG* saphenous vein graft, *ECA* external carotid artery, *MCA* middle cerebral artery, *STA* superficial temporal artery, *PCA* posterior cerebral artery, *SCA* superior cerebellar artery, *BA* basilar artery

| | |
|---|---|
| PICA fusiform aneurysms | Direct suture, interposition grafting, occipital-PICA bypass; PICA–PICA reanastomosis |
| AICA fusiform aneurysms | Direct suture, interposition grafting, AICA–PICA bypass |
| VA fusiform aneurysms | Direct suture, interposition grafting, VA–VA SVG graft |
| Low-basilar/vertebrobasilar aneurysms | ECA/VA/MCA-to-PCA |
| Midbasilar aneurysms | ECA/VA/MCA-to-PCA/BA; STA–SCA bypass |
| Upper basilar aneurysms | ECA/VA/MCA-to-PCA bypass |

SCA may be used as a recipient when the terminal BA is atretic, with two fetal types of PCA.

## 33.9
## OA Exposure

Dissection of the OA is more difficult than the STA because of its deep course (Fig. 5). The OA runs horizontally deep to the mastoid tip and digastric muscle, medial to the splenius capitis muscle, medial or lateral to the longissimus capitis muscle, and lateral to the semispinalis capitis muscle. It then perforates the muscular fascia to enter the subcutaneous tissue approximately 2 cm lateral to the midline and turns to run vertically at the level of the superior nuchal line. It has a very tortuous course and gives off multiple muscular branches.

An inverted U-shaped incision is made and the skin and subcutaneous flap are reflected. The course of the OA is marked with a Doppler sonogram. The artery is dissected with the aid of an operating microscope, and bleeding may occur from accompanying veins or muscular arterial branches (Fig. 6). Tortuosity makes the dissection difficult. Smaller branches are coagulated away from the main artery and the larger ones ligated. A cuff of periadventitial tissue is left around the artery. For posterior fossa anastomoses, it is adequate to dissect the OA until it penetrates the muscular fascia and turns vertically upward.

## 33.10
## Extracranial Anastomosis

The proximal anastomosis is performed either in an end-to-end, or an end-to-side fashion. An end-to-end anastomosis can always be performed to the external carotid artery (ECA). An end-to-side anastomosis to

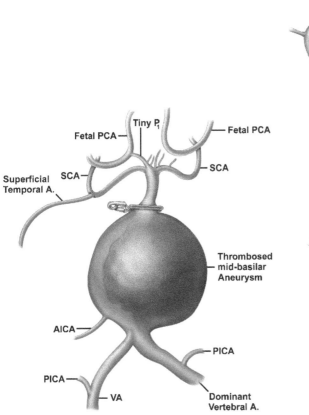

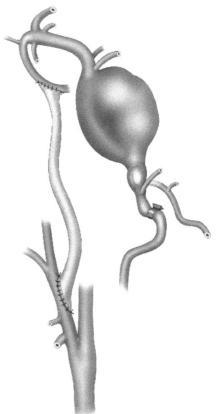

Fig. 5 A superficial temporal artery (*Superficial Temporal A.*)-to-superior cerebellar artery (*SCA*) bypass can be done when there is a fetal posterior cerebral artery (*PCA*). Courtesy of Laligam N. Sekhar. *PICA* posterior inferior cerebellar artery, *AICA* anterior inferior cerebellar artery, *VA* vertebral artery

Fig. 6 An external carotid artery to P₂ segment of the posterior cerebral artery anastomosis using the radial artery or a saphenous vein graft is used to manage a giant midbasilar aneurysm. Courtesy of Laligam N. Sekhar

the internal carotid artery (ICA) can be done with temporary occlusion of the ICA proximal and distal to the anastomosis, if the ECA is not available and the ICA has some intracranial collateral circulation. In cases of the VA, an end-to-side anastomosis is always performed in order to preserve the perfusion of branches proximal to the aneurysm.

## 33.11
## STA–SCA Bypass

This is a rare procedure used for upper basilar aneurysms when there is a fetal PCA or a hypoplastic $P_1$ (Fig. 6). A relatively large and long STA is needed. It is dissected as far distally as possible. Lumbar spinal drainage is instituted, and the SCA is approached subtemporally with division of the tentorium just posterior to the entrance of cranial nerve IV. A transpetrosal approach may also be utilized. The superior side of the anastomosis is performed first, then the STA is placed gently under the retractor and the inferior side of the anastomosis is completed. Alternatively, the inferior side can be sutured first by an inside-out suturing technique.

## 33.12
## ECA, Middle Cerebral Artery, or VA-to-PCA Anastomosis

This type of anastomosis is performed for midbasilar aneurysms (Fig. 7). A temporal craniotomy with an or-

bitozygomatic osteotomy or a petrosal approach is used for the exposure of the PCA. If a temporal craniotomy is used, a spinal drain is needed to relax the brain. The $P_2$ segment of the PCA is isolated for about 1.5 cm, and a rubber dam is placed under it. An arteriotomy to match the size of the graft is performed. The ends of the graft are anchored with 8-0 nylon. The superior edge is anastomosed first, then the graft is placed under the retractor and the inferior side of the anastomosis is completed. This is a difficult anastomosis due to the depth and usually takes about 50–60 min, but the temporary occlusion is usually well tolerated. The graft is tunneled to the ECA, middle cerebral artery (MCA), or VA proximally and anastomosed.

## 33.13
## VA-to-VA Grafting

This type of anastomosis is performed for giant aneurysms of the VA when collateral flow is poor (Fig. 8). If the anastomosis is planned as a prelude to aneurysm excision, an extreme lateral retrocondylar or partial transcondylar approach is used. Resection of the jugular tubercle may be needed to expose the aneurysm. An end-to-end anastomosis is performed into the distal VA and an end-to-side anastomosis is performed to the proximal VA at C1. The permanent clip is placed just proximal to the aneurysm intracranially, allowing preservation of the PICA and other perforating vessels originating proximal to the aneurysm. The location of the distal anastomosis, whether proximal or distal to the PICA, is dependent on

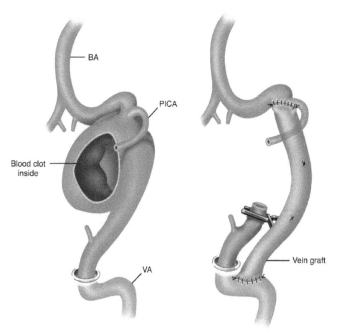

Fig. 7 A vein graft from the proximal to the distal vertebral artery. *BA* Basilar artery. Courtesy of Laligam N. Sekhar

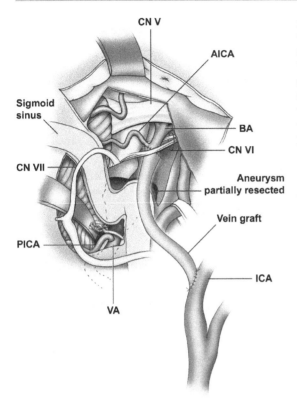

Fig. 8 The saphenous vein graft from the cervical internal carotid artery to the BA. *CN* Cranial nerve. Courtesy of Laligam N. Sekhar

the aneurysm anatomy. Proximal anastomosis to the VA is done at the level of C1–C2.

## 33.14
## VA- or ECA-to-BA Grafting

VA- or ECA-to-BA grafting is used for a very special situation in the presence of a giant midbasilar aneurysm (Fig. 9). The distal anastomosis is performed under deep hypothermic circulatory arrest. This is a technically very difficult and demanding procedure [11].

## 33.15
## Illustrative Cases

### 33.15.1
### Case 1: Recurrent Basilar Tip Aneurysm with PCA Arising from the Neck

A 72-year-old woman presented with a history of subarachnoid hemorrhage from a ruptured basilar tip aneu-

rysm 4 years ago. At that time she had undergone endovascular coiling for treatment of the aneurysm. She had suffered right third-nerve palsy as well as multiple deep brain infarcts. She had significantly recovered from her stroke but her third-nerve palsy remained unimproved and her gait was ataxic. Since then the patient had multiple recurrences of her basilar tip aneurysm on follow-up angiography, had undergone four more endovascular procedures for recoiling (Figs. 10 and 11), and had an episode of treatment for loss of consciousness. A four-vessel cerebral angiogram at this presentation revealed filling of a broad-necked basilar tip aneurysm, both in the sac and the neck due to coil compaction (Fig. 12). Stent-assisted coiling as well as a bypass procedure was considered by our team. However, due to the large amount of coils already within the aneurysm sac and the anatomy of the aneurysm neck, it was felt the best option for obliteration of the aneurysm would be a bypass procedure with distal basilar occlusion, or aneurysm clipping.

The patient underwent a right MCA-to-$P_2$ branch of the PCA bypass using an RAG. After subsequent exploration of the neck of the aneurysm, we were able to place a large straight clip across its neck, although the clip significantly narrowed the right $P_1$ due to a "funnel effect" (Fig. 13). Postoperatively, the patient had some difficulty with swallowing and mild left-sided weakness. An angiogram revealed good flow through her bypass graft and no residual filling of her aneurysm (Fig. 14). After 2 months of convalescence, her swallowing recovered and her mild left-sided weakness resolved. She was able to be discharged home for self care. Delayed angiography 3 months later revealed the bypass to be filling slowly but with re-opening of the right PCA from the BA injection, and obliteration of the aneurysm. Balloon angioplasty of the graft was done using a Hyperglide microballoon catheter (ev3 Corporate, Plymouth, MN, USA; 4×15 mm) and the graft opened up, filling the PCA.

### 33.15.2
### Case 2: Giant Mid-BA Aneurysm

A 42-year-old man was admitted after an automobile accident. The patient had been having problems with memory and had intermittent episodes of loss of consciousness for the last 2 years. Computed tomography of his head revealed a large (27×13 mm) aneurysm of the mid-BA with significant brainstem compression. Cerebral angiography showed that this aneurysm started below the origin of the anterior inferior cerebellar arteries and ended 1 cm inferior to the origin of the SCAs (Fig. 15c). An intraluminal stent placement followed by endovascular coil obliteration of the aneurysm was considered but, even with two stents, the anatomy of the aneurysm was not favorable for endovascular coiling. The collateral circulation to the BA distal to the aneurysm was poor, with a totally fetal PCA on the

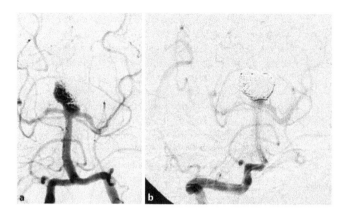

Fig. 9a,b Vertebral angiogram showing recurrence of aneurysm after coiling 3 years before surgery. Courtesy of Laligam N. Sekhar

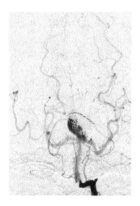

Fig. 10 Vertebral angiogram showing recurrence of aneurysm after coiling 2 years before surgery. Courtesy of Laligam N. Sekhar

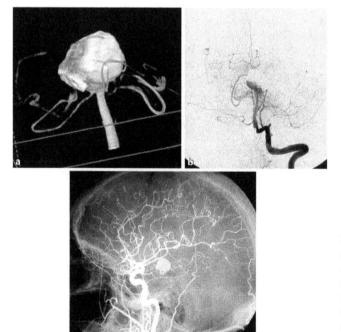

Fig. 11a–c Preoperative cerebral angiography. a Three-dimensional reconstruction of a vertebral angiogram showing of the bilateral PCA near the neck of the aneurysm. b Anteroposterior (AP) view of the vertebral angiogram showing the aneurysm filled with coils and filling of the sac and the neck of the aneurysm. c Lateral view of right carotid angiogram showing a small right posterior communicating artery (PCOM). Courtesy of Laligam N. Sekhar

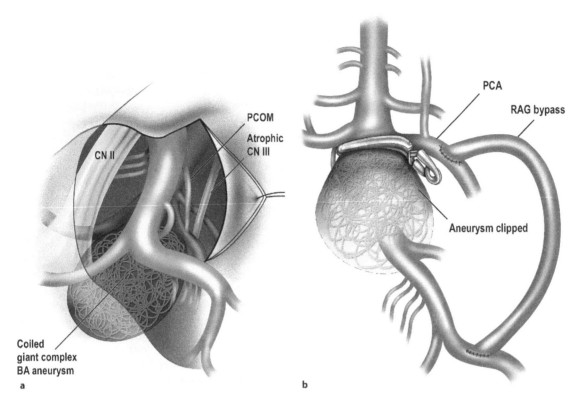

Fig. 12 **a** Giant basilar tip aneurysm with coils in situ with an atrophic CN III. **b** Clipping of the aneurysm, narrowing of the right $P_2$, and right middle cerebral artery (MCA)-to-$P_2$ bypass. Courtesy of Laligam N. Sekhar

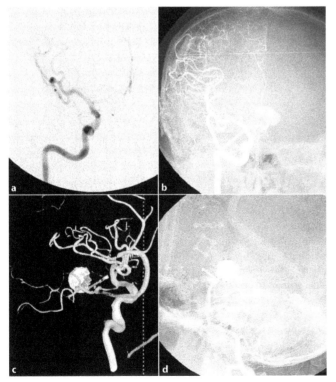

Fig. 13a–d Postoperative right carotid angiogram. **a,d** AP and lateral views, respectively, showing no residual filling of the aneurysm. **b,c** AP view and three-dimensional reconstruction, respectively, showing an MCA-to-$P_2$ graft and clipping of the aneurysm. Courtesy of Laligam N. Sekhar

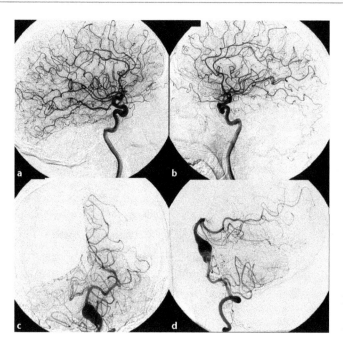

Fig. 14a–d Preoperative cerebral angiography. **a** Lateral view of the right carotid angiogram showing a fetal right PCA. **b** Lateral view of the left carotid angiogram showing a small left PCOM. **c,d** AP and lateral view, respectively, of the vertebral angiogram showing a midbasilar aneurysm below the origin of the AICA. Courtesy of Laligam N. Sekhar

right side and a small posterior communicating artery on the left side (Fig. 15a, b). We performed a left-sided ECA-to-PCA bypass graft with the radial artery (RAG) followed by distal occlusion of the aneurysm. Distal occlusion was performed in order to preserve the flow through the AICAs. The surgery was performed via a left transpetrosal approach and exposure of the ECA in the neck (Fig. 15a). An RAG bypass was performed to the left $P_2$ segment of the PCA from the ECA. Following the demonstration of flow through the graft, the BA was occluded at the upper end of the aneurysm inferior to a large perforating vessel (Fig. 16b, c). Immediate angiography demonstrated partial thrombosis of the aneurysm (Fig. 17b), which progressed to complete occlusion over the course of the next several days (Fig. 13). The graft was flowing well and flow to the AICAs was preserved (Fig. 17a, c). The patient had a transient episode of dysarthria and confusion, which gradually resolved. A cerebral angiogram 4 months after the surgery revealed that the aneurysm had completely thrombosed (Fig. 18). However, the graft had also occluded spontaneously at this time, but with the concurrent and significant enlargement of the left PCA. The occlusion of the graft was related to the spontaneous enlargement of the posterior communicating artery with the graft preserving flow in the interim period (Fig. 19). Delayed occlusion of bypasses as in this case has been observed in some patients due to spontaneous enlargement of natural collateral circulation in the patient. The patient returned to his job in an aircraft manufacturing company.

### 33.15.3
### Case 3: Giant Mid- and Lower-BA Aneurysm

This ten-year-old boy had presented with a progressively enlarging giant aneurysm of the basilar trunk (Fig. 20). The patient had previously undergone endovascular coil obliteration of the aneurysm, but it was incomplete and the aneurysm continued to grow. The patient suffered from very severe and episodic headaches and hypertension. Preoperative angiography revealed that the aneurysm was filling through both VAs, the right one being the dominant one. There was a fenestration of the BA just proximal to the aneurysm. The PICA was dominant, arising from the right, and a large anterior spinal artery was also seen to be arising from the right VA. Preoperatively, stent-assisted coiling of the aneurysm was considered, but because of the peculiar anatomy of the aneurysm and the patient's young age, the patient was not considered an optimal candidate for this. The patient underwent a right transpetrosal and extreme lateral approach, SVG from the $V_2$ segment of the VA to the right PCA, followed by proximal occlusion of the aneurysm using aneurysm clips on the right VA and the left VA. The intraoperative angiogram showed complete occlusion of both VAs proximal to the aneurysm. However, delayed cerebral angiography (Fig. 21) revealed that the left VA was stenotic at the site of the previously placed aneurysm clip, but the aneurysm was still filling. The SVG was filling from the right VA to the right PCA and the upper BA through this. The left

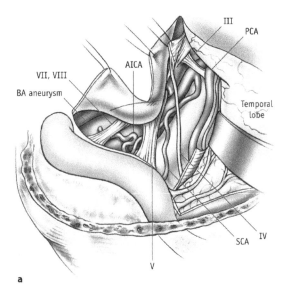

a

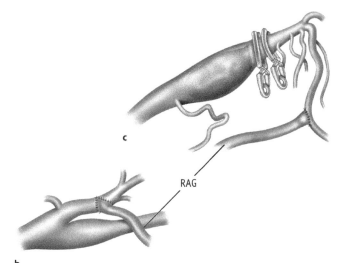

c

RAG

b

Fig. 15 **a** Left transpetrosal approach to a midbasilar aneurysm. **b,c** Radial artery grafting from the external carotid artery (ECA) to the P₂ segment of the PCA and distal occlusion of the BA. Courtesy of Laligam N. Sekhar. *III, IV, V, VII, VIII* Cranial nerves III, IV, V, VII and VIII, respectively

posterior communicating artery was also patent. Because of this, we performed endovascular coiling of the proximal sac of the aneurysm and the neck of the aneurysm extending into the VA using multiple Guglielmi detachable coils. The aneurysm was obliterated completely. A repeat angiogram that was performed the next day (Fig. 22) showed that the aneurysm was completely thrombosed with the exception of a small portion leading into the AICAs at the apex. The SVG was filling the PCA on the right side very nicely and there was retrograde flow back into both AICAs and the distal portion of the aneurysm. The patient has had a complete neurological recovery and cessation of his headaches.

### 33.15.4
### Case 4: Giant Mid- and Lower-BA Aneurysm; Hypothermic Circulatory Arrest Used for Bypass

A 15-year-old girl presented with a giant fusiform lower and midbasilar aneurysm (Fig. 23) and progressive quadriparesis and stupor. The aneurysm was approached by a total
 approach. Using hypothermic circulatory arrest a saphenous vein bypass (SVG) was done from the cervical ICA to the BA (Fig. 24). The aneurysm was trapped, and emptied. Magnetic resonance angiography at 9 years follow

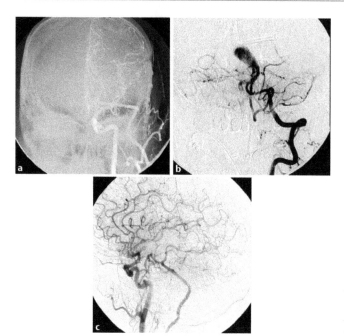

Fig. 16a–c Postoperative cerebral angiography. **a,c** AP and lateral views of the left carotid angiogram showing an ECA-to-P$_2$ bypass. **b** Vertebral angiogram showing clips on the distal BA and sluggish filling of the aneurysm. Courtesy of Laligam N. Sekhar

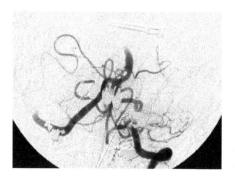

Fig. 17 Vertebral angiogram 3 days after surgery showing no filling of the aneurysm. Courtesy of Laligam N. Sekhar

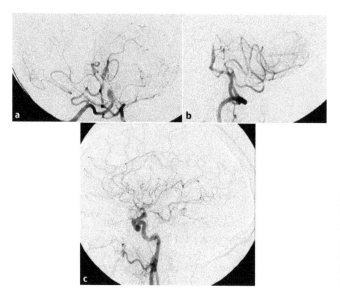

Fig. 18a–c Four months after surgery. **a,b** AP and lateral views of vertebral angiogram at showing no filling of the aneurysm and occlusion of the graft. **c** Lateral view of the left carotid angiogram showing left PCA filling through opened left PCOM from the internal carotid artery (ICA). Courtesy of Laligam N. Sekhar

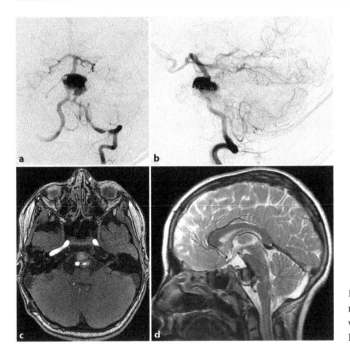

Fig. 19a–d Angiogram (**a,b**) and magnetic resonance imaging (MRI) scan (**c,d**) showing a giant vertebrobasilar junction aneurysm. Courtesy of Laligam N. Sekhar

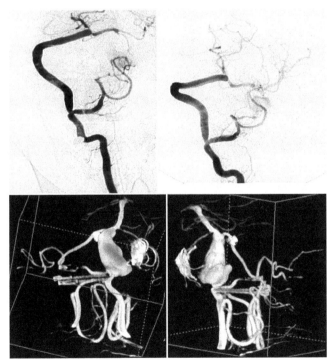

Fig. 20 The saphenous vein graft is filling from the right vertebral artery to the right PCA and the upper BA. The left VA is stenosed by the clip, but not completely occluded, and the aneurysm is filling. Courtesy of Laligam N. Sekhar

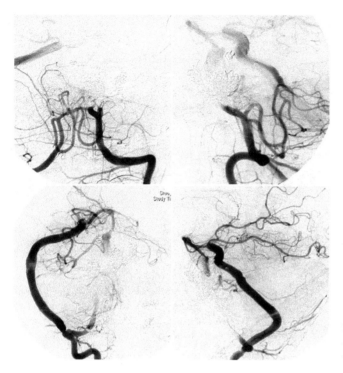

Fig. 21 Angiogram showing complete obliteration of the aneurysm after endovascular coiling. Courtesy of Laligam N. Sekhar

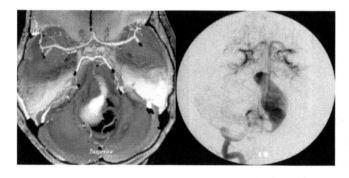

Fig. 22 Preoperative angiograms showing a giant lower- and mid-BA fusiform aneurysm. Courtesy of Laligam N. Sekhar

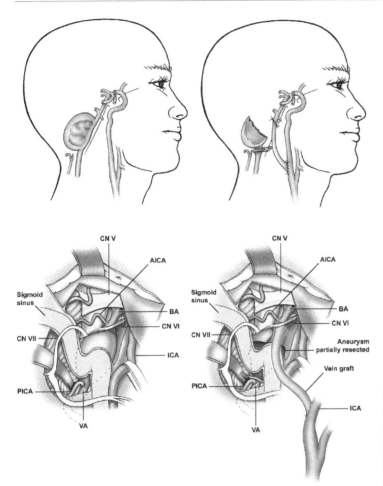

Fig. 23 Drawing illustrating a lateral view of the aneurysm preoperatively, and postoperative drawing illustrating a lateral view of the proximal clipping and partial decompression of the aneurysm and the right ICA-to-BA bypass using a saphenous vein graft (SVG). Courtesy of Laligam N. Sekhar

up (Fig. 25) shows a widely patent graft and filling of the posterior circulation. At last follow-up, this patient has a Brackmann-House grade II facial paresis and right-sided hearing loss.

### 33.15.5
### Case 5: Giant Vertebrobasilar Aneurysm Involving Both VAs

A 57-year-old man presented with recent subarachnoid hemorrhage. The patient was found to have a giant, fusiform aneurysm involving both VAs and the lower BA (Fig. 26). The right VA ended in the aneurysm just distal to the PICA, but the left VA entered the aneurysm and the left PICA arise from the aneurysm. With the idea that the left PICA would occlude when the aneurysm thrombosed, a PICA-to-PICA anastomosis was planned but could not be performed because the vessels were too far apart in the midline. A combined extreme-lateral, transpetrosal approach was used to place a radial artery bypass (RAG) from the left VA to the left PCA (Fig. 27). The left VA was occluded proximal to the aneurysm and PICA, and the right VA was occluded distal to the PICA. Initially, the patient did well postoperatively, but as the aneurysm thrombosed, the patient developed a cerebellar infarct that required reoperation for decompression and partial resection of the cerebellum (Fig. 28). The patient improved, but as the aneurysm thrombosed progressively in the subsequent days, the patient sustained a progressive neurological decline, presumably related to thrombosis of the basilar perforators. The patient recovered partially but remained ventilator-dependent and eventually died. Possibly a better option for the patient might have been the occlusion of only one VA after the bypass, with delayed endovascular occlusion, if possible, of the other VA. Alter-

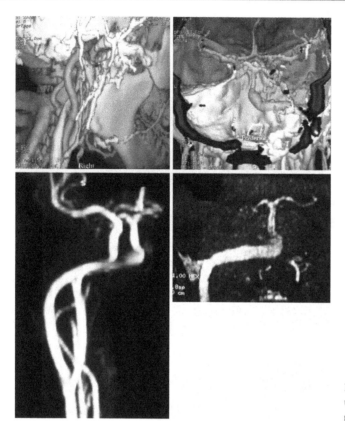

Fig. 24 Magnetic resonance angiogram at follow-up, showing a patent bypass graft. Courtesy of Laligam N. Sekhar

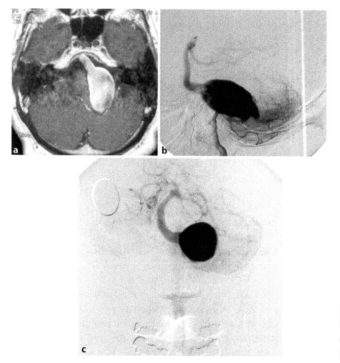

Fig. 25 **a** Preoperative axial T1-weighted, contrast MRI scan. **b** Preoperative lateral left VA angiogram. **c** Preoperative AP vertebral angiogram. Courtesy of Laligam N. Sekhar

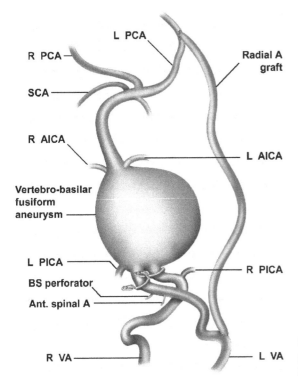

Fig. 26 Diagram of the left cervical VA-to-PCA radial artery graft (RAG) and bilateral VA proximal occlusion. Courtesy of Laligam N. Sekhar. *R* Right, *L* left, *Ant.* Anterior, *BS* brainstem

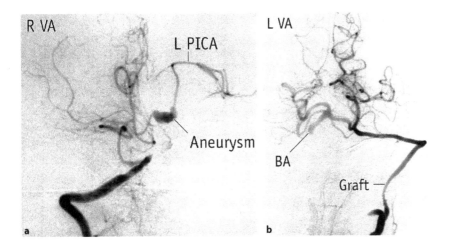

Fig. 27 **a** Right vertebral angiogram showing filling up to the level of the PICA and obliteration of the aneurysm. **b** Left VA angiogram showing filling of the RAG and obliteration of the aneurysm. Courtesy of Laligam N. Sekhar

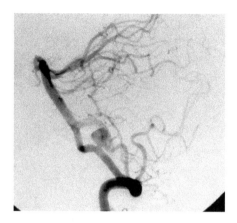

Fig. 28 Preoperative lateral right VA angiogram. Courtesy of Laligam N. Sekhar

natively, some other type of revascularization procedure of the PICA (such as reimplantation) or occipital PICA bypass could have preserved the collateral circulation.

### 33.15.6
### Case 6: Vertebral PICA Aneurysm (OA-to-PICA Bypass)

This patient presented with a ruptured 2.0- to 1.5-cm fusiform aneurysm located at the origin of the PICA from the VA (Fig. 29). After exposure of the aneurysm by a far-lateral approach, a right sided OA-to-PICA bypass was performed with clipping of the aneurysm (Fig. 30). At follow-up, the patient was doing very well and was neurologically intact, and a transient difficulty with cranial nerve X resolved completely.

### 33.16
### Results

Table 2 shows a summary of patients who underwent revascularization for anterior circulation aneurysms, the types of bypasses performed, graft patency, outcome of patients (including management morbidity of subarachnoid hemorrhage and vasospasm), and major complications related to grafts and recovery. Included is one patient in whom bypass was performed as a desperate measure after a major stroke had occurred before or during surgery.

Table 2 Revascularization for posterior circulation aneurysms 1988–2006. *GOS* Glasgow Outcome Scale

| Patients | Grafts | |
|---|---|---|
| 25 | 28 | |
| Location of aneurysms | | |
| Upper BA | 4 | |
| Mid BA | 6 | |
| Vertebral-BA | 2 | |
| AICA fusiform | 1 | |
| VA fusiform | 5 | |
| VA dissecting | 2 | |
| VA–PICA | 4 | |
| PICA fusiform | 1 | |
| Graft patency | | |
| **Immediate** | **After salvage** | |
| 25/28 (89.3%) | 26/28 (92.9%) | |
| Outcome | | |
| GOS score | **5** | **4** | **0** |
| | 16 (64%) | 6 (24%) | 3 (12%) |
| Complication/complete recovery | | |
| Major stroke | 1/0 | |
| Minor stroke | 2/2 | |
| Brain swelling | 1/1 | |
| Emergency bypass-graft performed after major stroke had occurred | | |
| **Number** | **Outcome** | |
| 1 | Died | |

### 33.17
### Conclusions

Revascularization can be effective in treating complex posterior circulation aneurysms. Despite the risk of serious neurologic complications, when one considers the natural history of untreated patients, revascularization remains an acceptable option.

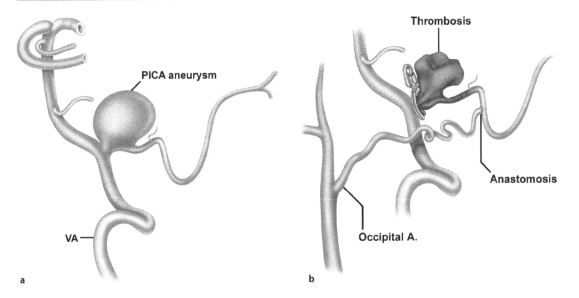

Fig. 29  **a** Diagram of the preoperative vascular anatomy. **b** Diagram of the right occipital artery (OA)-to-PICA bypass and clipped aneurysm. Courtesy of Laligam N. Sekhar

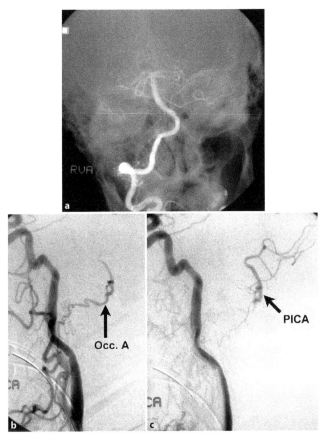

Fig. 30  **a** Postoperative AP right VA angiogram showing obliteration of the aneurysm and the PICA. **b,c** Sequential frames of a right common carotid artery angiogram showing filling of the PICA via the OA. Courtesy of Laligam N. Sekhar

## References

1. Ali MJ, Bendok BR, Tella MN, Chandler JP, Getch CC, Batjer HH (2003) Arterial reconstruction by direct surgical clipping of a basilar artery dissecting aneurysm after failed vertebral artery occlusion: technical case report and literature review. Neurosurgery 52:1475–1480; discussion 1480–1471

2. Drake CG, Peerless SJ (1997) Giant fusiform intracranial aneurysms: review of 120 patients treated surgically from 1965 to 1992. J Neurosurg 87:141–162

3. Harsh GRT, Sekhar LN (1992) The subtemporal, transcavernous, anterior transpetrosal approach to the upper brain stem and clivus. J Neurosurg 77:709–717

4. Javedan SP, Deshmukh VR, Spetzler RF, Zabramski JM (2001) The role of cerebral revascularization in patients with intracranial aneurysms. Neurosurg Clin N Am 12:541–555

5. Lawton MT, Daspit CP, Spetzler RF (1997) Technical aspects and recent trends in the management of large and giant midbasilar artery aneurysms. Neurosurgery 41:513–520; discussion 520–511

6. Mohit AA, Sekhar LN, Natarajan SK, Britz GW, Ghodke B (2007) High-flow bypass grafts in the management of complex intracranial aneurysms. Neurosurgery 60:ONS105–122; discussion ONS122–103

7. Salas E, Sekhar LN, Ziyal IM, Caputy AJ, Wright DC (1999) Variations of the extreme-lateral craniocervical approach: anatomical study and clinical analysis of 69 patients. J Neurosurg 90:206–219

8. Sekhar LN, Estonillo R (1986) Transtemporal approach to the skull base: an anatomical study. Neurosurgery 19:799–808

9. Sekhar LN, Kalavakonda C (2002) Cerebral revascularization for aneurysms and tumors. Neurosurgery 50:321–331

10. Sekhar LN, Bucur SD, Bank WO, Wright DC (1999) Venous and arterial bypass grafts for difficult tumors, aneurysms, and occlusive vascular lesions: evolution of surgical treatment and improved graft results. Neurosurgery 44:1207–1223; discussion 1223–1204

11. Sekhar LN, Chandler JP, Alyono D (1998) Saphenous vein graft reconstruction of an unclippable giant basilar artery aneurysm performed with the patient under deep hypothermic circulatory arrest: technical case report. Neurosurgery 42:667–672; discussion 672–663

12. Sekhar LN, Duff JM, Kalavakonda C, Olding M (2001) Cerebral revascularization using radial artery grafts for the treatment of complex intracranial aneurysms: techniques and outcomes for 17 patients. Neurosurgery 49:646–658; discussion 658–649

13. Sekhar LN, Kalia KK, Yonas H, Wright DC, Ching H (1994) Cranial base approaches to intracranial aneurysms in the subarachnoid space. Neurosurgery 35:472–481; discussion 481–473

14. Sekhar LN, Schessel DA, Bucur SD, Raso JL, Wright DC (1999) Partial labyrinthectomy petrous apicectomy approach to neoplastic and vascular lesions of the petroclival area. Neurosurgery 44:537–550; discussion 550–532

15. Taylor CL, Kopitnik TA, Jr, Samson DS, Purdy PD (2003) Treatment and outcome in 30 patients with posterior cerebral artery aneurysms. J Neurosurg 99:15–22

CPSIA information can be obtained
at www.ICGtesting.com
Printed in the USA
LVHW010100220423
745015LV00008B/595